Cardiac Radiology THE REQUISITES

SERIES EDITOR **James H. Thrall**, MD

Radiologist-in-Chief
Department of Radiology
Massachusetts General Hospital
Professor of Radiology
Harvard Medical School
Boston, Massachusetts

OTHER VOLUMES IN THE REQUISITES SERIES

Gastrointestinal Radiology

Pediatric Radiology

Neuroradiology

Nuclear Medicine

Ultrasound

Musculoskeletal Radiology

Genitourinary Radiology

Thoracic Radiology

Mammography

Cardiac
Radiology

THE REQUISITES

STEPHEN WILMOT MILLER, MD
Associate Professor of Radiology
Harvard Medical School
Massachusetts General Hospital
Boston, Massachusetts

with 820 illustrations

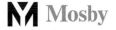 Mosby

St. Louis Baltimore Boston
Carlsbad Chicago Naples New York Philadelphia Portland
London Madrid Mexico City Singapore Sydney Tokyo Toronto Wiesbaden

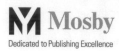
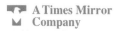

Vice President and Publisher: Anne S. Patterson
Executive Editor: Robert A. Hurley
Managing Editor: Elizabeth Corra
Associate Developmental Editor: Mia Cariño
Project Manager: Linda Clarke
Production Editor: Julie Cullen
Composition Specialist: Christine H. Poullain
Designer: Carolyn O'Brien
Manufacturing Manager: Andrew Christensen

Printed in the United States of America
Composition by Mosby Electronic Publishing, Philadelphia
Printing/binding by Maple-Vail Book Manufacturing Group

Mosby–Year Book, Inc.
11830 Westline Industrial Drive
St. Louis, MO 63146

Library of Congress Cataloging-in-Publication Data

Miller, Stephen W. (Stephen Wilmot), 1941-
    Cardiac radiology / Stephen Wilmot Miller.
        p.   cm. — (The requisites)
    Includes bibliographical references and index.
    ISBN 0-8016-6478-0
    1. Heart—Imaging. I. Title. II. Series: Requisites series.
    [DNLM: 1. Heart Diseases—diagnosis. 2. Heart Diseases—
pathology. 3. Diagnostic Imaging—methods. WG 141 M647c 1996]
RC683.I42M55   1996
616.1'20757—dc20
DNLM/DLC
for Library of Congress   95-48871
                                            CIP

96 97 98 99 00 / 9 8 7 6 5 4 3 2 1

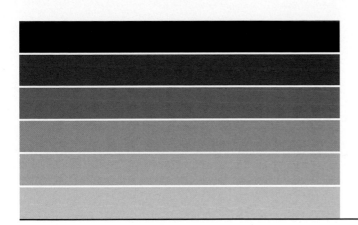

Contributors

Lawrence M. Boxt, M.D.
Professor of Clinical Radiology
Director of Cardiac Radiology
Department of Radiology
College of Physicians and Surgeons
  of Columbia University
Attending Radiologist
Columbia-Presbyterian Medical Center
New York, New York

Margaret A. Ferrell, M.D.
Clinical Assistant in Medicine
Harvard Medical School
Cardiac Unit
Massachusetts General Hospital
Boston, Massachusetts

Jose Katz, M.D., Ph.D.
Associate Professor of Medicine (Cardiology)
  and Radiology
Co-Director, Cardiovascular Nuclear Magnetic Resonance
College of Physicians and Surgeons of
  Columbia University
Co-Director, Cardiovascular Nuclear Magnetic Resonance
Staff Attending, Medicine (Cardiology) and Radiology
Columbia-Presbyterian Medical Center
New York, New York

Mary Etta E. King, M.D.
Assistant Professor of Pediatrics
Harvard Medical School
Associate Pediatrician
Children's Service
Massachusetts General Hospital
Boston, Massachusetts

Stefan Mark Nidorf, M.D., M.B.B.S.
Cardiologist
Department of Cardiovascular Medicine
Queen Elizabeth II Medical Center
Perth, Western Australia

Igor F. Palacios, M.D.
Director of Interventional Cardiology
Massachusetts General Hospital
Associate Professor in Medicine
Harvard Medical School
Boston, Massachusetts

Kathleen Reagan, M.D.
Assistant Professor
Department of Radiology
College of Physicians and Surgeons of
  Columbia University
Radiologist
Columbia-Presbyterian Medical Center
New York, New York

To **Richard Van Praagh**, *M.D., and* **Allan Goldblatt,** *M.D.*
outstanding teachers at Harvard Medical School.

S.W.M.

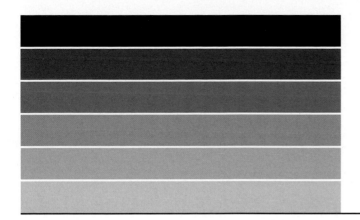

Foreword

Cardiac Radiology: The Requisites is the seventh book in a series designed to provide core material in major subspecialty areas of radiology for use by residents during their training and by practicing radiologists seeking to review or expand their knowledge.

The cardiac imaging component of radiology curriculum is difficult to develop, both because the subject matter is complex and because significant aspects of the subspecialty are not within the purview of radiology departments in many academic medical centers. The task of preparing this text was correspondingly difficult, and Dr. Stephen Miller has done an outstanding job in facing the challenge.

Dr. Miller has structured his book to provide basic information that residents should master during their training in order to correctly interpret cardiac imaging studies. He expands upon these fundamental principles by addressing questions of clinical context. For example, a correct basic interpretation of a study might result in the conclusion that aortic valvular calcification is present. Dr. Miller then raises the level of instruction by discussing the significance and meaning of such a finding within the context of clinical decisionmaking. This greater understanding is necessary for the reader to become a credible participant in such a competitive subspecialty.

Dr. Miller has also taken on the daunting task of summarizing congenital heart disease. He has masterfully presented the material in a concise and thorough fashion so that confusing details do not prevent the reader from acquiring a comprehensive understanding of the topic.

Cardiac Radiology: The Requisites embraces several imaging modalities including plain radiographs, ultrasound, magnetic resonance imaging, and computed tomography. Dr. Miller helps the reader assess the relative strengths and limitations of each modality, as well as their contemporary clinical applications. The reader should note that scintigraphy of the heart is covered in the nuclear medicine volume of the Requisites in Radiology series.

The Requisites in Radiology series includes one book specifically written for each of the major subspecialties. The length and format of each volume are dictated by the material being covered, but the principal goal is to equip the resident with a text that might reasonably be read within several days at the beginning of each subspecialty rotation and perhaps reread several times during subsequent rotations. Not intended to be exhaustive, the volumes instead provide the basic conceptual, factual, and interpretive material required for clinical practice. Each book is written by nationally recognized authorities in the respective subspecialties who, because the Requisites is a completely new series, are able to present material in the context of today's practice of radiology rather than grafting information about new imaging modalities onto a preexisting text.

Dr. Miller and his contributors have done an excellent job of sustaining the philosophy of the Requisites in Radiology series and have produced a truly contemporary text for cardiac imaging. I believe that *Cardiac Radiology: The Requisites* will serve residents in radiology as a concise and useful introduction to the subject, and as a very manageable text for review by fellows and practicing radiologists. Further, I hope that cardiologists, cardiac surgeons, and internists, as well as their resident and fellowship trainees, will consider this a user-friendly vehicle for exploring imaging of the heart.

James H. Thrall, M.D.

Radiologist-in-Chief
Massachusetts General Hospital
Juan M. Taveras Professor of Radiology
Harvard Medical School
Boston, Massachusetts

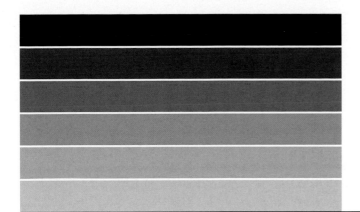

Preface

The Requisites in Radiology series was conceived by Dr. James H. Thrall as a set of books that radiology residents would find useful from the first day of their residency through 4 years of training. Based on a "spiral learning" approach, this volume seeks to present core material on the subspecialty and then enhance the information base with more complex concepts. Dr. Thrall asked me to organize a curriculum on cardiovascular imaging, defining the basic knowledge that one should have at the end of a postgraduate radiology residency. *Cardiac Radiology: The Requisites* presents this core knowledge.

The resident in radiology first needs an overview of cardiac radiology with anatomic and physiologic correlations. In that context, the first four chapters of the text feature the essentials of imaging technology for chest film, magnetic resonance imaging, echocardiography, and angiography. Subsequent chapters, organized by common cardiac diseases, build upon these essentials and correlate diagnostic possibilities with clinical context.

The radiology resident also needs to be oriented to the logic of differential diagnosis based on the analysis of the image. The process of making a diagnosis from an image is typically accomplished in two steps. First, the abnormality is detected visually and analyzed by its location, borders, calcification, and other characteristics. Because some diseases form an imaging spectrum as a gradation from normal, this first step of recognizing an abnormality may prove difficult. Shunt vascularity, for example, is a continuum ranging from normal size pulmonary arteries when the shunt is small, to large pulmonary arteries when the pulmonary flow is greater than twice the systemic flow. Further, normal structures must be distinguished from abnormal structures before a diagnosis can have any relevance, although some abnormalities are so unique—the scimitar syndrome—that

they have no differential. Second, by deductive reasoning a list matching possible diseases is constructed and then re-ordered to begin with the most likely possibility.

In this text, lists of associated conditions and differential diagnoses are highlighted in breakouts for quick reference. I have also constructed short lists of radiologic signs and split them into groups by location, physiology, or pathology for easier recall. For the difficult topic of congenital heart disease, I have developed "Aunt Marys" (Dr. Benjamin Felson's aunt was Minnie; mine is Mary) for images that should be instantly recognized. The name reflects the fact that I do not need to analyze the features of my Aunt Mary minutely to know who she is, in the same way one should instantly recognize the snowman configuration of total anomalous pulmonary venous connection.

In organizing the content of the book, I have discussed all of the common imaging modalities. I have illustrated most common cardiac diseases, as well, and have included uncommon diseases if the imaging examination is a key to the diagnosis or is so unique that it should be identified as an "Aunt Mary." Clinical and pathologic content is interwoven and correlated with the imaging so that salient points are discussed in the context of a patient's demand for a diagnosis and treatment. Finally, because I believe that good teaching results when the lecturer, seminar leader, or writer speaks directly to the students, the style of the book departs from standard medical writing in that the second person is frequently addressed.

I hope that the curriculum offered in *Cardiac Radiology: The Requisites* becomes a valuable learning tool for all its readers.

Stephen Wilmot Miller, M.D.

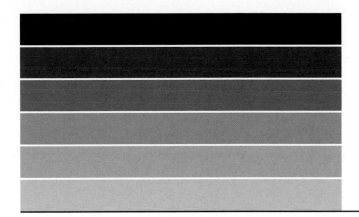

Acknowledgments

Writing a book involves the creative talents of many people besides the author. I am indebted to a number of colleagues who have contributed to the book's philosophy, organization, content, and illustrations.

Dr. James H. Thrall, Radiologist-in-Chief at the Massachusetts General Hospital, conceived the idea for this book and provided the departmental academic milieu so I could write it.

My colleagues in the Department of Radiology at the Massachusetts General Hospital have contributed ideas on the organization of the book and teaching methods for a number of the cardiovascular diseases and have provided their illustrations for some of the less common entities. I am particularly indebted to Dr. Elizabeth A. Drucker for her enthusiasm and critique. Dr. Robert E. Dinsmore has been a beacon of knowledge of cardiac radiology for staff and residents for 35 years. Drs. John A. Kaufman and S. Mitchell Rivitz were expert sources for magnetic resonance imaging and aortography. Drs. Robert Bramson, Susan Connolly, and Johan Blickman advised me on the pediatric aspects of heart disease. Dr. Godtfred Holmvang, a pioneer in magnetic resonance blood flow imaging, contributed many of the magnetic resonance images.

A book as broad as one on cardiac imaging is made immensely better by having internationally known contributors. I am privileged to work with Drs. Igor F. Palacios and Margaret A. Ferrell in the Cardiac Unit of the Department of Medicine at the Massachusetts General Hospital, who contributed the chapter on interventional cardiology. Drs. Lawrence M. Boxt, Jose Katz, and Kathleen Reagan of Columbia University contributed the chapter on magnetic resonance imaging of the heart. Drs. Mary Etta E. King and Stefan Mark Nidorf contributed the chapter on echocardiography. Dr. King founded the pediatric echocardiography section at the Massachusetts General Hospital and has been one of the pioneers in that field for over 15 years.

To paraphrase Gustave Flaubert, "God is in the details." That certainly is evident in writing a book and is a concern of many people at all stages of the publishing process. Dianne Stenwall typed the manuscript and encouraged my timely submission of chapters. Gale Abbass, a professional medical writer, edited the entire manuscript, suggested the style, developed the breakouts for lists of diagnoses, and indexed the illustrations. Nancy J. Speroni, M.Ed., illustrated the computer graphic drawings and supervised the photography. Finally I thank Mia Cariño, Julie Cullen, Anne Patterson, Susan Gay, Elizabeth Corra, Maura Leib, Linda Clarke, Christine Poullain, Andrew Christensen, Carolyn O'Brien, and Debbie Cicirello. Those talented and capable professionals at Mosby–Year Book gave me support and encouragement during the 4 years of preparing this book.

S.W.M.

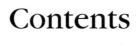

Contents

Part I   Imaging Modalities

1   The Elements of Cardiac Imaging   3

2   Echocardiography   46
       Mary Etta E. King and Stefan Mark Nidorf

3   Magnetic Resonance Imaging of the Heart   96
       Lawrence M. Boxt, Jose Katz, and Kathleen Reagan

4   Cardiac Angiography   123

Part II Specific Diseases

5   Valvular Heart Disease   149

6   Ischemic Heart Disease   199

7   Interventional Cardiology   247
       Margaret A. Ferrell and Igor F. Palacios

8   Pericardial and Myocardial Diseases   264

9   Congenital Heart Disease   298

10   Thoracic Aortic Diseases   386

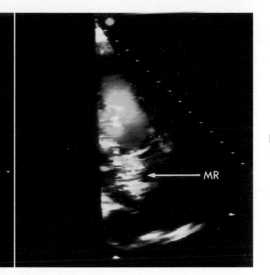

A

B

Plate 1 **A** illustrates a two-dimensional apical echocardiographic view of the mitral valve in systole. **B** shows the superimposed color Doppler flow map. A central stream of mitral regurgitation *(arrow)* is shown emerging from the leaflet coaptation point and spreading into the left atrium. The jet is blue (indicating flow away from the transducer) with yellows and greens to reflect turbulent flow. *Ao* = aorta; *LA* = left atrium; *LV* = left ventricle; *MR* = mitral regurgitation. (This figure is reproduced in black and white on page **53**.)

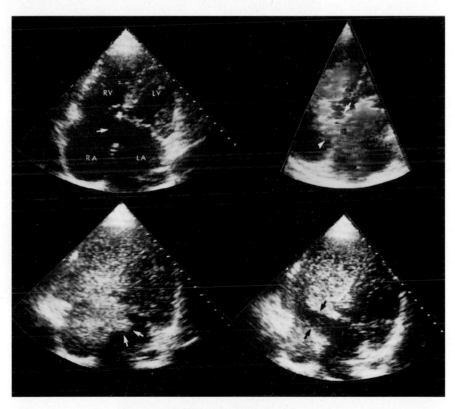

Plate 2 Series of apical four-chamber echocardiographic views in a patient with an ostium primum atrial septal defect. In the upper left panel, the dropout in the lower atrial septum *(arrow)* delineates the defect. Doppler color flow mapping *(upper right)* demonstrates a wide band of flow crossing from the left atrium to the right atrium *(arrows)*. Following intravenous injection of agitated saline, microbubbles are detected as contrast within the cardiac chambers. In the lower left panel, right-to-left shunting can be seen across the defect *(arrows)* and left-to-right negative contrast is shown in the lower right panel as unopacified blood crosses the atrial defect *(arrows)*. *LA* = left atrium; *LV* = left ventricle; *RA* = right atrium; *RV* = right ventricle. (From Levine RA et al: Echocardiography: principles and clinical applications, in Eagle KA et al (eds): The practice of cardiology, Boston, 1989, Little Brown.) (This figure is reproduced in black and white on page **83**.)

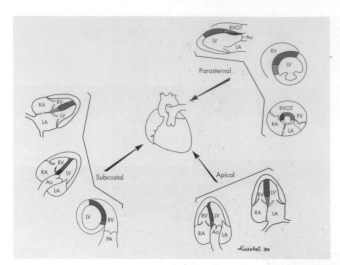

Plate 3 Diagrammatic representation of multiple echocardiographic views of the interventricular septum with color encoding of the subdivisions of the septum. The muscular septum is shown in blue, the inlet septum in green, the infundibular septum in orange, and the membranous septum in red. *Ao* = aorta; *LA* = left atrium; *LV* = left ventricle; *RA* = right atrium; *RV* = right ventricle; *RVOT* = right ventricular outflow tract; *PA* = pulmonary artery. (From Levine RA et al: Echocardiography: principles and clinical applications, in Eagle KA et al (eds): The practice of cardiology, Boston, 1989, Little Brown.) (This figure is reproduced in black and white on page **85**.)

Plate 4 Two-dimensional echocardiographic images and color flow Doppler illustration of shunt flow across small ventricular septal defects. **A,** Following repair of a malalignment VSD, a small residual defect is present at the upper edge of the patch *(arrow)*. **B,** The jet of shunt flow is seen as a mosaic-like stream emerging from the right ventricular aspect of the defect. Flow accelerates along the left ventricular septal surface *(arrows)* as it approaches the defect. **C,** Two small defects in the midmuscular septum are present *(arrows)*. Two discrete jets can be detected by color Doppler, shown in **D.** *Ao* = aorta; *LA* = left atrium; *LV* = left ventricle; *RA* = right atrium; *RV* = right ventricle. (This figure is reproduced in black and white on page **86**.)

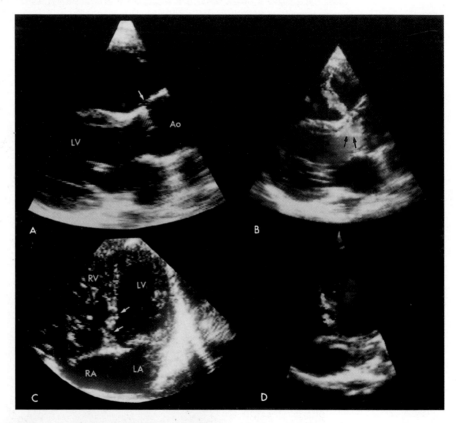

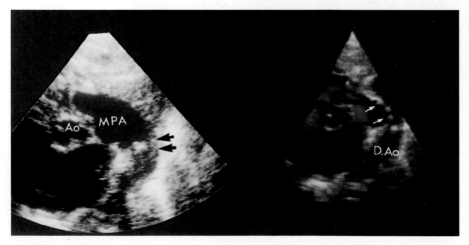

Plate 5 Parasternal short-axis images at the base of the heart depicting a patent ductus arteriosus *(black arrows)* on the left, and the color Doppler appearance of the shunt flow from the descending aorta into the pulmonary artery *(white arrows)* on the right. *Ao* = aorta; *D Ao* = descending aorta; *MPA* = main pulmonary artery. (This figure is reproduced in black and white on page **87**.)

IMAGING MODALITIES

PART

I

The Elements of Cardiac Imaging

Cardiac Shape and Size
Age and its visible effects
Evaluation of heart size
Cardiothoracic ratio
Chamber enlargement
Right atrium
Right ventricle
Left atrium
Left ventricle
Cardiac and Pericardial Calcifications
Aortic valve calcification
Distinguishing characteristics
Calcific aortic stenosis
Mitral annulus calcification
Distinguishing patterns
Clinical significance
Mitral valve calcification
Causes
Appearance
Myocardial calcification
Left Atrial calcification
Pericardial calcification
Causes
Radiologic appearance
Use of CT scan
Coronary calcification
Appearance
Association with stenosis
Pulmonary Vasculature
Determining the vascular pattern
Segmental analysis
Central pulmonary arteries
Hilar structures
Upper and lower lung zones and bronchoarterial ratios
Pattern recognition
Diminished vasculature
High-output states
Segmental analysis
Flow ratios
Contributing diseases, lesions, and defects
Pulmonary artery hypertension
Pressure measurements and patterns of pulmonary vasculature
Eisenmenger syndrome
Venous hypertension
Pulmonary venous hypertension
Fluid and water exchange
Radiologic appearance
Skeletal Abnormalities in Heart Disease
Cardiac surgery
Thoracic cage and heart disease
Congenital syndromes with heart disease
Coronary Sinus and the Left Superior Vena Cava
Coronary sinus
Anatomy and relation to the left superior vena cava
Location from catheter position
Left superior vena cava
Mediastinal position
Catheter course
Suggested Readings

The anatomic and physiologic effects of heart disease have many common imaging features. Chamber dilatation, valve calcification, and anomalous connections are morphologic signs of cardiac abnormalities. Increased or decreased blood flow and segmental wall motion disorders are physiologic signs of heart disease. The analysis for cardiovascular disease on the chest film, echocardiogram (ECG), computed tomography (CT) scan, and magnetic resonance image (MRI) begins with a search for these common elements. Then a more systematic imaging examination can be devised to address particular questions.

The chest film is often the first imaging procedure performed when heart disease is suspected, and, more commonly, it is used to assess and follow the severity of cardiac disease. Because the chest film forms images by projection, this technique detects only those cardiopulmonary abnormalities that change the shape of the heart, mediastinum, and lungs and those that alter the structure of the pulmonary vasculature. Clinically silent heart disease may also be detected on a chest film taken for other reasons. Extracardial structures, particularly in the abdomen and the thoracic cage, may produce additional clues indicating heart disease. Calcification in the aortic valve, for example, identifies the abnormal structure and directs the differential diagnosis toward a particular pathologic lesion.

To evaluate cardiac disease in the thoracic film you should interpret the following structures:

1. The shape and size of the heart and its individual chambers
2. The pulmonary vasculature, which mirrors the physiologic pressure and volume state of the cardiopulmonary system
3. The mediastinum, for the size and location of the aorta and major systemic veins
4. Extracardial anomalies that may be associated with heart disease

CARDIAC SHAPE AND SIZE

Age and Its Visible Effects

The age of the patient greatly influences what is considered the normal appearance of the heart and lungs, and there are some normal variants that may at times mimic disease. In the infant, the thymus typically obscures the upper portion of the mediastinum and may overlay the pulmonary hilum. In rare instances it extends inferiorly, causing the transverse heart size to appear falsely large. In the first day of life, the pulmonary vasculature has a fuzzy appearance. This normally represents the complex and rapidly changing pressures and flows in the lungs, but can suggest pulmonary abnormalities (such as transient tachypnea of the newborn or respiratory distress syndrome) or cardiac disease. In sick children under prolonged stress, the thymus may shrink to a small size but usually is still partially visible. The thymic shadow is invisible in transposition of the great arteries.

In the child and adolescent, the bronchopulmonary markings become more distinguishable, and the thymic

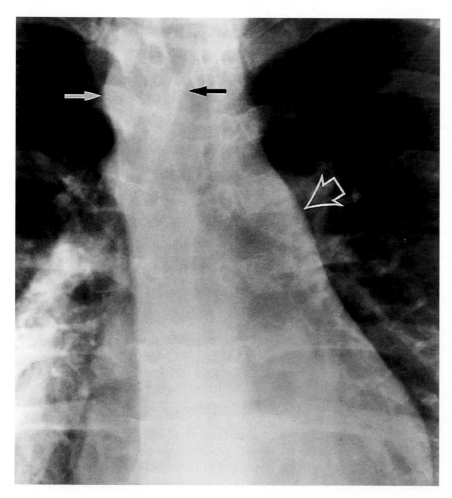

Fig. 1-1 Convex main pulmonary artery. The moderate convexity of the main pulmonary artery segment *(arrowhead)* is a normal variant in this young adult even though the aortic arch *(arrows)* is on the right side. The space usually occupied by a left aortic arch contains the aberrant left subclavian artery.

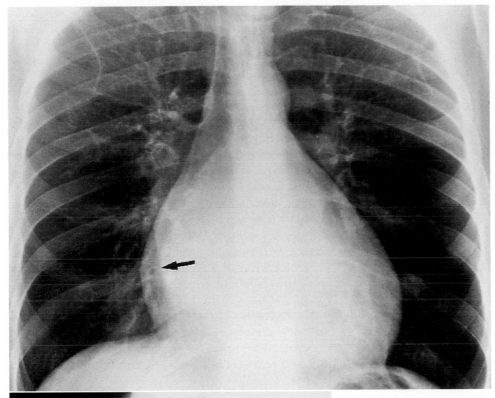

A

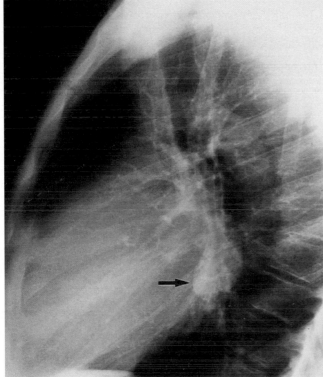

B

Fig. 1-2 Confluence of the pulmonary veins. The superior and inferior right pulmonary veins may join and connect with the left atrium as a common vein. This normal variant may look similar to an enlarged left atrium *(arrow)* on the frontal film **(A)** and a pulmonary nodule *(arrow)* on the lateral film **(B).**

shadow regresses and becomes inapparent so you can see the aortic arch and pulmonary trunk. A convex pulmonary trunk in girls in their late teens may suggest pulmonary artery enlargement, but in the absence of a heart murmur this is usually a normal variant (Fig. 1-1).

However, an ECG may be necessary to exclude entities such as pulmonary stenosis and left-to-right shunts. The "double density" of the pulmonary veins may mimic an enlarged left atrium (Fig. 1-2), but a large left atrium has a rounder curve and extends medially above the diaphragm.

In the young adult, the major changes in the cardiac silhouette are the mild prominence of the aortic arch and the vertical orientation of the heart. In the elderly, the thoracic aorta may become elongated and tortuous. The cardiac apex becomes more rounded and the overall heart size is smaller, which possibly reflects aging changes but more likely results from the loss of heart muscle because of lack of exercise.

Evaluation of Heart Size

Cardiothoracic ratio

The determination of heart size, both subjectively and quantitatively, has been assessed from the chest film for more than 70 years. Then Danzer described the cardiothoracic ratio, which is still one of the most common measurements of overall heart size. This ratio was constructed to measure left ventricular dilation. Because it measures the transverse heart diameter, the cardiothoracic ratio usually is normal when either the left atrium or the right ventricle is quite enlarged, because neither of these two chambers is reflected in the transverse dimension. Rose and colleagues noted that changes in left ventricular volume up to 66% in excess of normal are needed for the cardiothoracic ratio to reliably detect enlargement of the left ventricle (see table below).

$$\text{Cardiothoracic ratio} = \frac{\text{Widest transverse cardiac diameter}}{\text{Widest inside thoracic diameter}}$$

Patient characteristics	Normal ratio	Mean
Newborn	< 0.6	•••
> 1 month old	< 0.5	0.47

Sensitivity = 0.45 (Many patients with left ventricular dilatation are not detected.)
Specificity = 0.85 (When ratio exceeds the normal value, heart is clearly large.)
Accuracy = 0.59

Modified with permission from Rose CP, Stolberg HO: The limited utility of the plain chest film in the assessment of left ventricular structure and function, *Invest Radiol* 17:139-144, 1982.

When the heart size is subjectively evaluated based on the configuration of the heart with respect to the thorax, the sensitivity and specificity are quite similar to the measured cardiothoracic ratio. For this reason and because quantitative measurements from tomographic imaging methods are commonly available, the cardiothoracic ratio is now used mainly as an adjunct in assessing heart size on the chest film. Although the cardiothoracic ratio is moderately variable among individuals, it is a useful indicator in an individual who is being watched for potential cardiac dilatation, such as in chronic aortic regurgitation. In this instance, an abrupt change in the cardiothoracic ratio suggests the need for urgent clinical reevaluation.

Marathon runners with heart rates in the range of 30 to 40 beats/min occasionally have a cardiothoracic ratio between 0.50 and 0.55, reflecting the normal physiologic dilatation of the heart, rather than any overall hypertrophy.

Several other measurements can be made from the standard posteroanterior and lateral chest film. Examples include total heart volume, left atrial dimension on the frontal film, width of the right descending pulmonary artery, and the distance of the left ventricle behind the inferior vena cava. These, however, are rarely used now in clinical evaluation.

Most measurements made from the chest film have poor correlation with left ventricular size from quantitative angiographic measurements. Therefore, the measurements of specific chamber diameters, volumes, and wall thicknesses should be made from techniques that show the chamber cavities (for example, ECG, angiography, and MRI).

Measurements of the heart and mediastinum are dramatically affected by the height of the diaphragm and the intrathoracic pressure and less so by the body position and status of the intravascular volume (see table below).

Typical Variations of Heart and Mediastinum Measurements on the Chest Film

Circumstance	Variation
In expiration	Transverse diameter of heart and mediastinum widens. Indistinct appearance of pulmonary hilum can be identical to that seen with pulmonary edema.
In recumbent position	Heart is broader. Lung volumes are lower. Upper lobe arteries and veins appear more distended.
On posteroanterior film	Change in heart width between systole and diastole is typically less than 1 cm.
On right anterior oblique film	Heart size does not change between systole and diastole. Left ventricular apex appears akinetic.
On left anterior oblique film	Posterolateral wall motion is typically more than 1 cm.

Chamber Enlargement

Usually the abnormal enlargement of the heart is easily recognized by its displacement out of the mediastinum. It may also be recognized by contour changes, by a new or different interface with the adjacent lung, or by displacement of adjacent mediastinal structures.

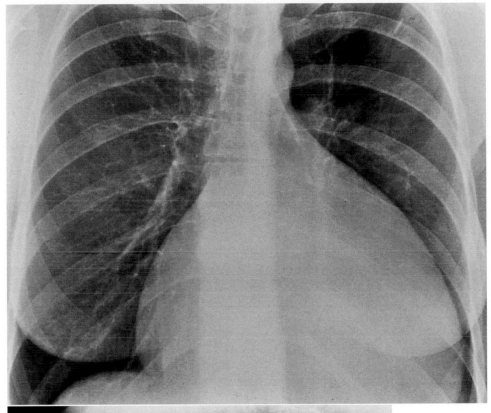

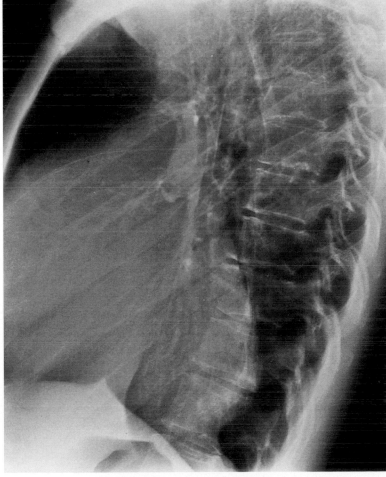

Fig. 1-3 Right heart enlargement suggesting left heart enlargement. The left ventricle is normal in this patient with Ebstein anomaly. **A,** The entire left heart border from the pulmonary artery to the diaphragm is the border of the huge right ventricle. **B,** The posterior border of the heart projected over the spine is the left ventricle, which has been pushed backward by the anterior right ventricle touching the sternum.

Each chamber basically enlarges directly outward from its normal position. Except for the right ventricle, isolated chamber enlargement does not affect the position of the heart in the mediastinum nor the identification of other chamber enlargement. When the right ventricle enlarges, it contacts the sternum and rotates the heart posteriorly and in a clockwise direction as viewed from below. Frequently in right ventricular enlargement, the normal left ventricle may falsely appear enlarged on both the frontal and lateral films because the entire heart is displaced posteriorly. If the right ventricle is dilated, the diagnosis of left ventricular enlargement may not be possible in the chest film (Dinsmore's principle). Therefore, you should assess the size of the right ventricle on the lateral film before you judge the left ventricle (Fig. 1-3).

Right Atrium

In the frontal view the right atrium is visible because of its border with the right middle lobe. Neither subtle nor moderate enlargement can be recognized accurately because there is moderate variability of its shape in normal subjects, and in expiration the right atrium becomes more round and moves to the right. The following are signs of right atrial enlargement:

1. Displacement of more than several centimeters to the right of the spine (Fig. 1-4)

2. A prominent convexity superiorly near the superior vena caval junction on the frontal film (Fig. 1-5)

3. On the lateral view, a horizontal interface with the lung above the right ventricle (the normal right atrium is not visible in the lateral view)

4. On the lateral view, displacement of the heart behind the inferior vena cava mimicking left ventricular enlargement

The right atrium, as do the other three chambers, enlarges because of increased pressure, increased blood volume, or a wall abnormality. Common causes of right atrial enlargement are tricuspid stenosis and regurgitation, atrial septal defect, atrial fibrillation, and dilated cardiomyopathy. Ebstein anomaly may have all of these features. In pulmonary atresia, the right atrium dilates in direct proportion to the amount of tricuspid regurgitation (Fig. 1-6).

All the signs of right heart enlargement that are implied on the chest film are directly visible on the CT scan. The right atrium and ventricle touch the anterior chest wall and rotate the heart posteriorly. The right coronary artery adjacent to the right atrial appendage lies to the left of the sternum (Fig. 1-7).

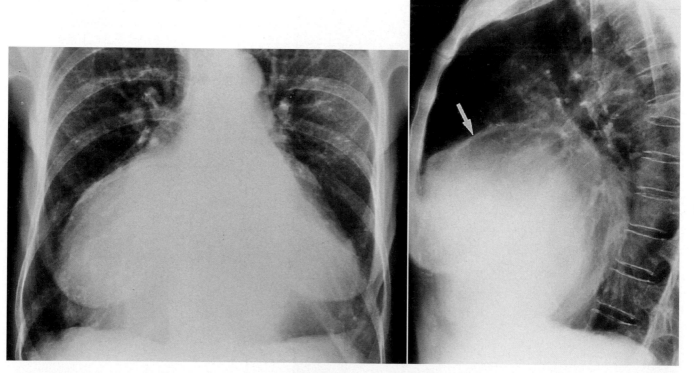

A **B**

Fig. 1-4   Right atrial enlargement in rheumatic heart disease. **A,** The unusually large right atrium compresses the right middle lobe and extends inferiorly to intersect the diaphragm. A large left atrium usually does not have a diaphragmatic interface. **B,** Enlargement of the right heart creates a sharp interface with the lung *(arrow)*. The horizontal contour suggests that this is the right atrial appendage rather than the right ventricle.

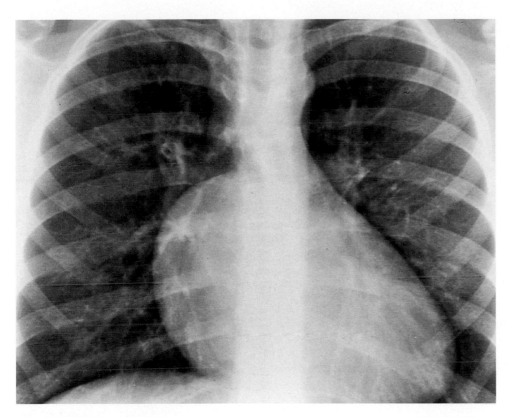

Fig. 1-5   Superior right atrial convexity. In Ebstein anomaly, the large right atrium has a characteristic round superior border.

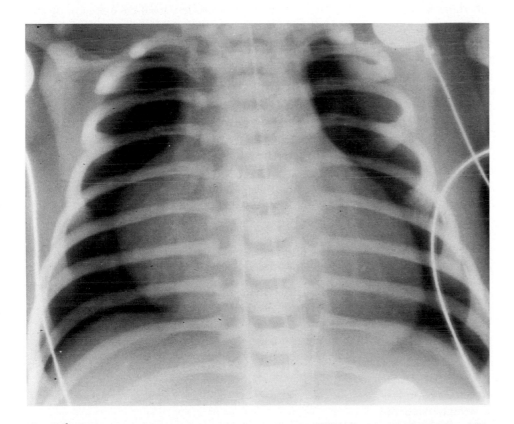

Fig. 1-6   Right atrial enlargement in pulmonary atresia with intact ventricular septum. This patient had moderate tricuspid regurgitation. Note the decreased vascularity in the lungs.

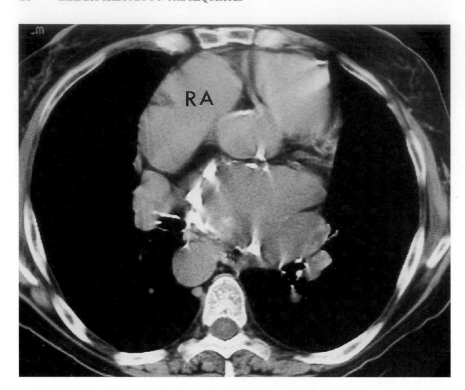

Fig. 1-7 Right atrial enlargement in rheumatic heart disease. The appendage portion of the right atrium *(RA)* touches the anterior chest wall in this patient who had a sternotomy for mitral valve replacement. The right coronary artery is visible in the fat between the right atrium and right ventricle. The left atrium is calcified and also enlarged.

Right Ventricle

On the lateral view, the normal right ventricle does not touch more than one fourth of the lower portion of the sternum as measured by the distance from the sternodiaphragmatic angle to the point at which the trachea meets the sternum. One sign of right ventricular enlargement is the filling in of more than one third of the retrosternal space. On the frontal view, the normal right ventricle is not visible, and only extreme dilatation causes recognizable signs because the heart rotates clockwise as it dilates and pushes against the sternum. In this instance, the usual contour of the left atrial appendage is rotated posteriorly and is no longer part of the left side of the mediastinum. You can recognize this sign by an unusually long convex curvature extending inferiorly from the main pulmonary artery (Fig. 1-8). In extreme instances the entire left heart border may be the right ventricle.

In tetralogy of Fallot when the fat pad is absent in the left cardiophrenic angle, the heart may have an uplifted cardiac apex (Fig. 1-9), which has been called the "boot-shaped heart," or the *coeur en sabot*. The right ventricle is not enlarged but may have hypertrophy.

Common causes of right ventricular enlargement are pulmonary valve stenosis, pulmonary artery hypertension (cor pulmonale), atrial septal defect, tricuspid regurgitation, and dilated cardiomyopathy; it can occur secondarily to left ventricular failure.

Left Atrium

There are many clues to left atrial enlargement on the frontal and lateral chest film. One of the earliest signs of slight enlargement is the appearance of the double density, which is the right side of the left atrium as it pushes into the adjacent lung. Because a prominent pulmonary vein or varix may also cause a vertical double density, for the double density to present, it should begin to curve inferiorly (Fig. 1-10). In extreme cases, the left atrium may enlarge to the right side and touch the right thoracic wall (Fig. 1-11). The etiology of this "giant left atrium" is rheumatic heart disease, mainly from mitral regurgitation.

A convex left atrial appendage on the frontal view is abnormal and usually reflects prior rheumatic heart disease. In pure mitral regurgitation, the body of the left atrium, but not the appendage, enlarges.

The following indirect signs are visible only when the left atrium is dilated at least moderately:

1. Displacement of the left main stem bronchus posteriorly on the lateral view and superiorly on the frontal view (Fig. 1-12)
2. Spreading of the carina
3. Posterior displacement of the barium filled esophagus (Fig. 1-13)
4. Double density on the left side as the left atrium extends into the left lower lobe

Common acquired causes of left atrial enlargement are mitral stenosis or regurgitation, left ventricular fail-

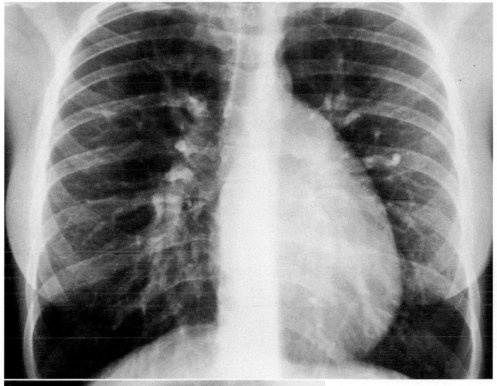

A

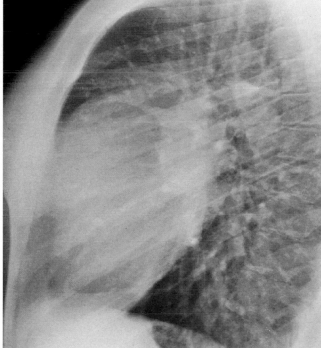

B

Fig. 1-8 Right ventricular enlargement. **A,** The broad convexity along the upper left heart border represents the dilated right ventricle. **B,** The right ventricle touches the sternum and fills one third of the retrosternal space. Shunt vascularity is also evident in this patient with atrial septal defect.

ure, and left atrial myxoma. Congenital causes include ventricular septal defects, patent ductus arteriosus, and the hypoplastic left heart complex. When atrial fibrillation occurs, the left atrial volume may increase by 20%.

Left Ventricle

Left ventricular enlargement exists if the left heart border is displaced leftward, inferiorly, or posteriorly. Inferior displacement may invert the diaphragm and cause this border to appear in the gastric air bubble. The

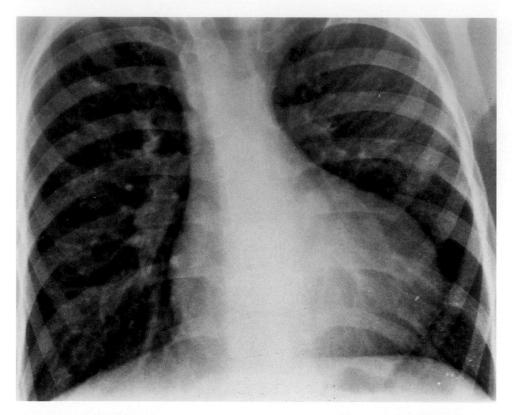

Fig. 1-9   Boot-shaped heart. In tetralogy of Fallot, the cardiac apex has an uplifted appearance. Other typical features are the concave main pulmonary artery segment and the right aortic arch.

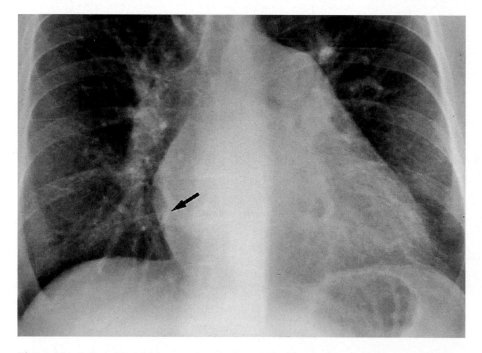

Fig. 1-10   Left atrial enlargement in mitral stenosis. The double density *(arrow)* occurs because the large left atrium pushes into the adjacent lung. The line curves inferiorly, differentiating it from a pulmonary varix. The large pulmonary artery indicates pulmonary hypertension.

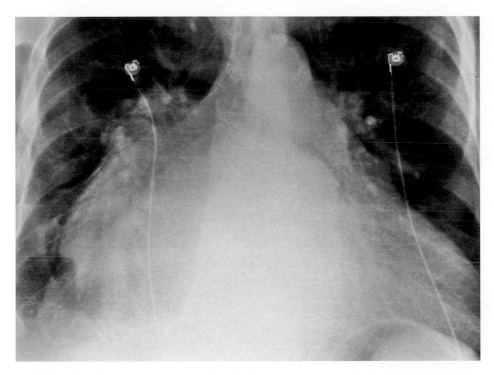

Fig. 1-11   Giant left atrium. Rheumatic mitral valve disease has caused the left atrium to enlarge so that it almost touches the right thorax wall. The carina is splayed superiorly over the atrium, and the left atrial appendage is convex.

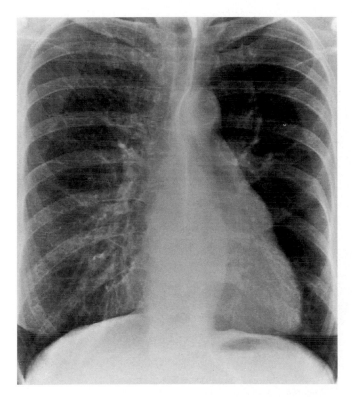

Fig. 1-12   Convex left atrial appendage. The large left atrial appendage and the redistribution of blood flow to the upper lobes indicate mitral stenosis.

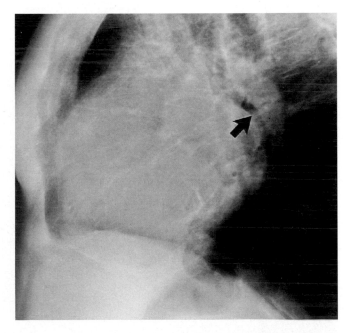

Fig. 1-13   Posterior displacement of the left main stem bronchus. The left bronchus should lie in a straight line with the trachea, but is displaced posteriorly *(arrow)* by the large left atrium. The large left pulmonary artery is seen on top of the bronchus.

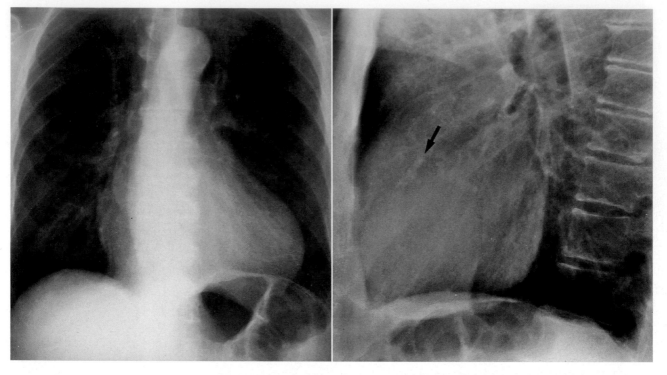

Fig. 1-14   Aortic stenosis. **A,** The left ventricle is enlarged to the left and inferiorly where it is seen through the stomach bubble. **B,** The posterior border of the left ventricle is significantly behind the inferior vena cava. Note moderate calcium in the aortic valve *(arrow).*

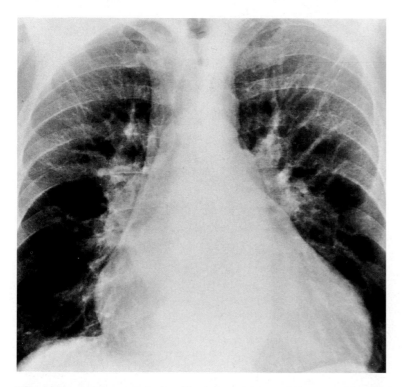

Fig. 1-15   Aortic regurgitation. The left ventricle and the aorta are both large from moderate aortic regurgitation. The indentation in the descending thoracic aorta and the absence of rib notching denote a pseudocoarctation. Because 50% of those with pseudocoarctation have a bicuspid aortic valve, this probably is the etiology of the aortic regurgitation.

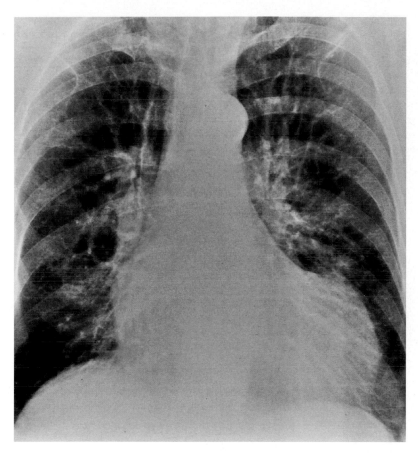

Fig. 1-16   Left ventricular aneurysm. This angular left ventricular border with the sharp superior corner is characteristic of an aneurysm. The large upper lobe vessels indicate left ventricular failure, which was caused by a rupture of the interventricular septum.

chest film cannot reliably distinguish between left ventricular dilatation and hypertrophy. With hypertrophy, the apex has a pronounced rounding and a decrease in its radius of curvature. The elderly normal heart also has this shape. When massive hypertrophy is present, the left ventricular shape is large and appears similar to one that is only dilated.

Common causes of left ventricular enlargement can be grouped into three categories: pressure overload (hypertension, aortic stenosis) (Fig. 1-14); volume overload (aortic or mitral regurgitation, ventricular septal defects) (Fig. 1-15); and wall abnormalities (left ventricular aneurysm, hypertrophic cardiomyopathy) (Fig. 1-16).

CARDIAC AND PERICARDIAL CALCIFICATIONS

Calcium in the heart is not only a marker for specific diseases, but also an aid for locating structures on the chest film. Structures that calcify usually can be located easily on routine frontal and lateral films, although in spe-

cial situations, oblique views with barium may be necessary. Most of the calcium found in the heart is dystrophic and is in tissue that has had a previous inflammatory process (for example, rheumatic mitral stenosis) or has been in a malformed structure that has degenerated (for example, bicuspid aortic valve).

Aortic Valve Calcification

Distinguishing characteristics

Calcium in the aortic valve is seen best in the lateral view, where it projects free of the spine. You can distinguish between aortic and mitral calcification by the following methods:

1. If the ascending aorta is dilated, follow its curvature back to locate the aortic valve in the middle of the cardiac silhouette.
2. On the lateral view, if you draw a line from the junction of the diaphragm and the sternum to the carina, it will pass through the aortic valve (unless the thoracic cage is quite distorted or there is

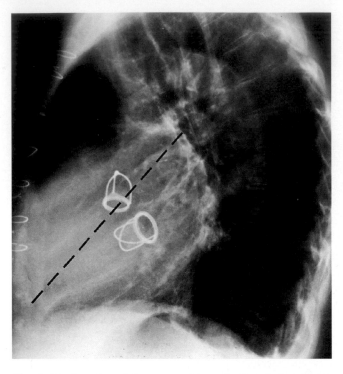

Fig. 1-17   Location of the aortic valve on the lateral chest film. A line drawn from the junction of the diaphragm and the sternum to the carina passes through the aortic valve. The mitral valve is below and posterior.

severe right heart enlargement). The mitral valve lies posterior to this line (Fig. 1-17).

3. Aortic calcification may have a specific appearance. Calcification in a bicuspid aortic valve, which never occurs before age 35, is dystrophic and involves the raphe and edges of the cusps. The calcification is linear in the raphe and may curve along the cusp edge. A nearly circular calcification with an interior linear bar in the aortic region is diagnostic of a bicuspid valve (Fig. 1-18). In older patients with bicuspid aortic stenosis, this architecture is obliterated by nodular masses of calcium; in this instance the severely calcified aortic valve looks identical to that of the three major causes of aortic stenosis: bicuspid valve, rheumatic heart disease, and elderly degeneration.

Calcific aortic stenosis

Calcium in the aortic valve may extend from the valve into the adjacent interventricular septum and cause arrhythmias. In most cases of bicuspid aortic stenosis, the mitral valve is normal and the left atrium is not enlarged. When both the aortic and mitral valves are calcified, the cause is usually rheumatic heart disease. In a patient without rheumatic heart disease or a previous episode of infected endocarditis, calcification in a tricuspid aortic

A

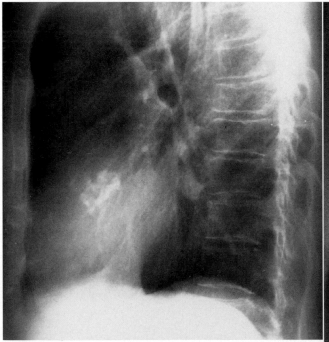

B

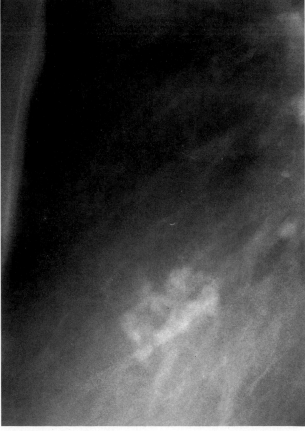

Fig. 1-18   Bicuspid aortic valve calcification. **A,** The calcification is located in the aortic valve by following the dilated ascending aorta into the heart. **B,** The distinctive bicuspid valve calcification is a ring with a linear bar through it.

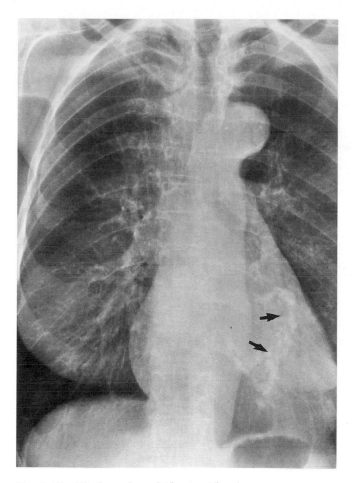

Fig. 1-19 Mitral annulus calcification. The characteristic oval calcification *(arrows)* is located below the left atrial appendage segment.

valve is rare before age 70. Patients with bicuspid aortic valves also may have had rheumatic heart disease or endocarditis and develop heavy central calcification.

The aortic valve is the only one that has a good correlation between the amount of calcium and the amount of stenosis. If the patient is over age 35, heavy calcification in the aortic valve indicates severe stenosis that probably will require a valve replacement. Conversely, if no calcium is seen by fluoroscopy in the aortic valve, it is unlikely that aortic stenosis exists.

Mitral Annulus Calcification

Distinguishing patterns

The mitral valve ring may calcify in individuals over age 60. The incidence is four times higher in women. The calcium begins to form in or below the mitral annulus at the junction between the ventricular myocardium and the posterior mitral leaflet. More severe degrees of calcification will form a pattern resembling the letter "J," the letter "O," or a reverse letter "C" (Fig. 1-19). In extreme cases, the mass of calcification can grow posteriorly into

the ventricular myocardium to produce heart block. It can also grow anteriorly into the leaflets of the mitral valve to cause mitral regurgitation and stenosis. Rarely, the calcification can erode through the endocardium and cause small systemic emboli. Mitral annulus calcification in the elderly is associated with a doubled risk of stroke, independent of the traditional risk factors.

Clinical significance

In most instances, mitral annulus calcification has little clinical significance and is a noninflammatory chronic degenerative process. Aortic stenosis and hypertension have a higher incidence of mitral annulus calcification, possibly because of increased strain exerted on the mitral valve apparatus from the left ventricular pressure overload. For the same reason, the tricuspid annulus rarely may calcify when right ventricular pressures have been chronically increased (Fig. 1-20).

Mitral Valve Calcification

Causes

Mitral leaflet calcification is almost always caused by chronic rheumatic valvular disease. Rarely the leaflets are calcified from infected endocarditis or from tumors attached to the mitral valve. There is limited correlation between the hemodynamic severity of mitral stenosis and the amount of calcium in the valve. Although a severely calcified mitral valve is usually stenotic, mitral stenosis frequently exists with no calcium in the valve.

Appearance

Radiologically, the calcium first appears as fine speckled opacities and later coalesces into larger amorphous masses (Fig. 1-21).

Mitral annulus calcification may coexist but has a different cause. As the rheumatic valvulitis progresses, causing commissural fusion, chordal shortening, and fibrosis, the leaflet calcification may extend into the chordae and to the tip of the papillary muscles. Tricuspid calcification from rheumatic valvulitis is rare, and pulmonary calcification from rheumatic heart disease does not occur.

Myocardial Calcification

A myocardial infarction can later calcify if it evolves to form either a scar or an aneurysm. You will easily recognize the thin curvilinear calcification as it projects within the left ventricular wall and inside the heart silhouette (Fig. 1-22).

Occasionally, the tip of an infarcted papillary muscle will calcify; the ensuing mitral regurgitation represents papillary muscle dysfunction. The anterolateral, apical, and septal walls of the left ventricle are the usual loca-

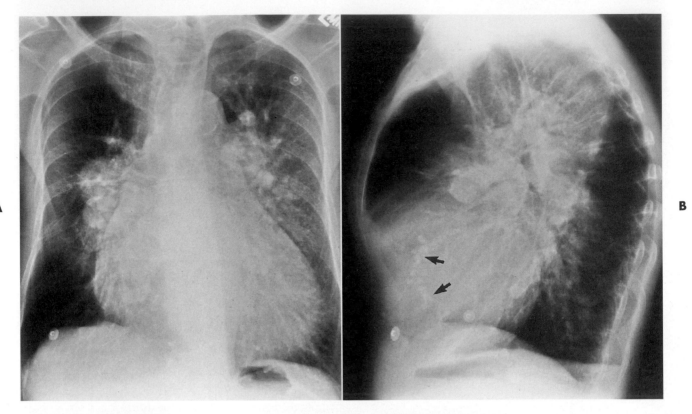

Fig. 1-20   Tricuspid annulus calcification. **A,** Adult tetralogy of Fallot with unusually large mediastinal collaterals to the pulmonary hila. **B,** The tricuspid annulus *(arrows)* calcified because of the chronic right ventricular hypertension.

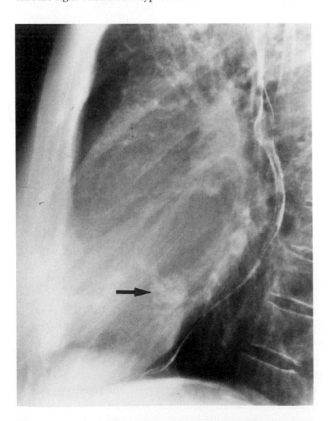

Fig. 1-21   The barium-filled esophagus is displaced posteriorly around the large left atrium. The mitral valve *(arrow)* is heavily calcified.

tions for true aneurysms, and therefore are the typical locations for myocardial calcification.

Left Atrial Calcification

Left atrial calcification is the sequela of rheumatic endocarditis. The appearance usually is curvilinear around the body of the left atrium (Fig. 1-23). The interatrial septum does not calcify, but the appendage does and has a shaggy nodular appearance. The calcium deposits may be shaggy but usually occur in an "eggshell" pattern (Fig. 1-24). Left atrial wall calcification indicates that the patient is in atrial fibrillation. Mural thrombi over the calcium are frequently present and may embolize into the systemic circuit. Tumors in the left atrium, such as myxomas, calcify with an incidence of less than 5%.

Pericardial Calcification

Causes

Calcific deposits in the pericardium represent the end stage of a nonspecific inflammatory process. Tuberculosis, viruses and many other infectious agents, rheumatic fever, uremia, and trauma all may cause local or diffuse calcification. Large localized masses of calcification suggest that the etiology was tuberculosis.

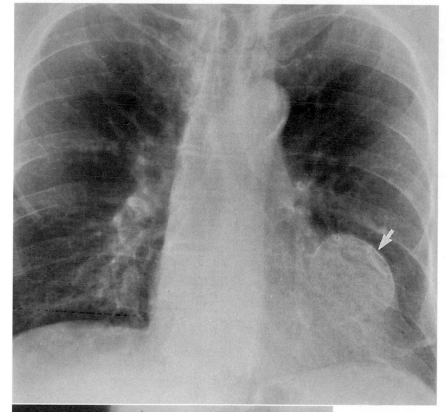

A

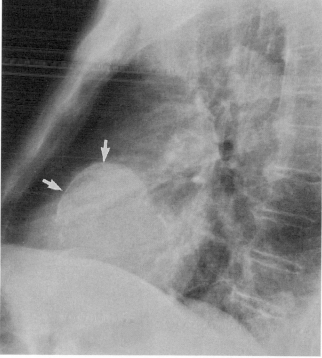

B

Fig 1-22   Calcified left ventricular aneurysm. **A** and **B**, The rim of calcium *(arrows)* outlines a saccular aneurysm in the anterolateral wall.

Radiologic appearance

The calcification radiologically appears in two forms: (1) clumpy amorphous deposits, frequently in the atrioventricular grooves; (2) diffuse eggshell calcification involving most of the cardiac silhouette, except the left atrium, which is not covered with pericardium (Fig. 1-25).

Use of CT scan

In patients with constrictive pericarditis, 50% have calcium visible on the chest film, and most have calcium on the CT scan. Because pressure tracings from the ventricles may be identical in both restrictive cardiomyopathy and constrictive pericarditis, a CT scan that shows

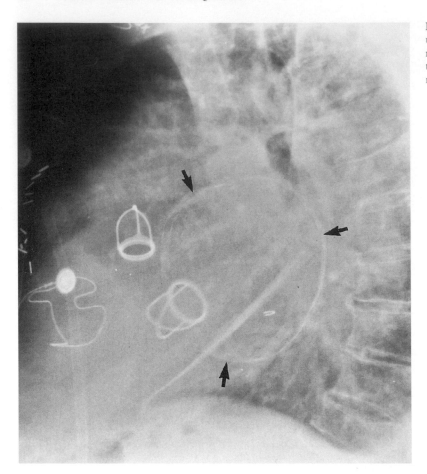

Fig. 1-23 Left atrial calcification. The large left atrium *(arrows)* has eggshell calcification extending superiorly to the left main stem bronchus and inferiorly to the mitral valve replacement. Aortic and tricuspid valve replacements are also present.

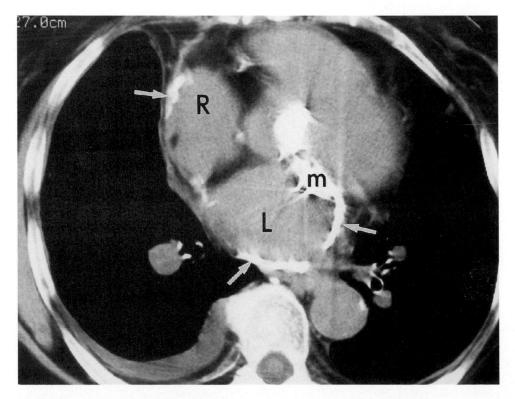

Fig. 1-24 Right and left atrial calcification. Linear nodular calcification *(arrows)* is present in the right atrium *(R)* and left atrium *(L)* in this patient who had a mitral valve replacement *(m)*.

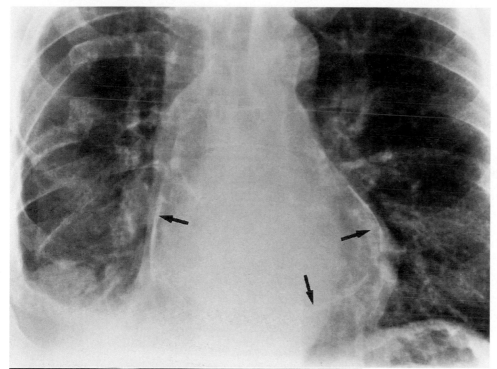

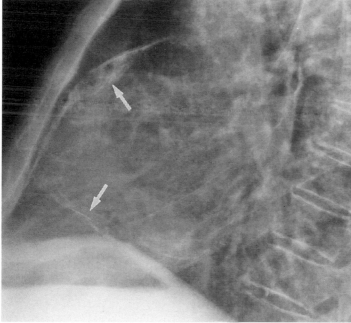

Fig. 1-25 Pericardial calcification. **A,** Eggshell calcification *(arrows)* outlines the right and left borders of the heart. **B,** Diffuse calcification projects over most of the heart and reflects circumferential deposits.

calcium in a thickened pericardium in a patient with elevated filling pressure is diagnostic of constrictive pericarditis (Fig. 1-26).

Coronary Calcification

Appearance

Coronary calcification represents atherosclerotic changes in the intima and in the internal elastic membrane of the coronary arteries. The left anterior descend-

ing artery is the most frequently calcified site, followed by the left circumflex, then the right coronary arteries (Fig. 1-27). The incidence of coronary calcification increases with age and may be part of the normal aging process. Generally, in patients under age 60, there is a strong correlation between calcification and severity of atherosclerosis; the association is less firm in older patients. Coronary calcification is influenced by risk factors such as increased cholesterol and lipids, smoking, hypertension, and a family history of coronary disease.

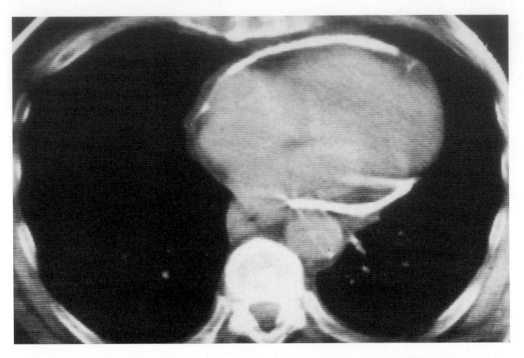

Fig. 1-26   CT scan of pericardial calcification. Calcium is seen in the anterior pericardium, in the left atrioventricular groove, and along the lateral aspect of the left atrium.

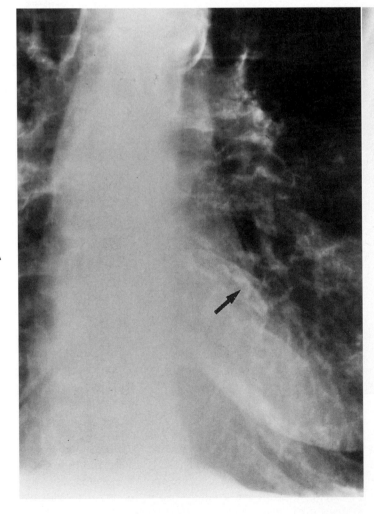

A

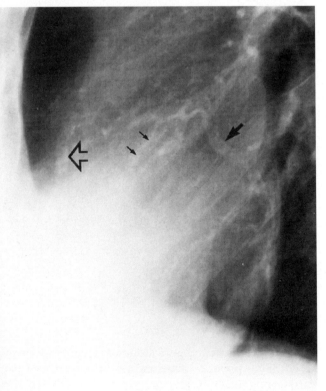

B

Fig. 1-27   Coronary artery calcification. **A,** The region just below the left atrial appendage segment is the location of the proximal left coronary artery *(arrow)*. **B,** The right coronary artery *(open arrow)* is anterior in the right atrioventricular groove. The left anterior descending artery *(small arrows)* is in the interventricular sulcus, and the left circumflex artery *(arrow)* lies in the left atrioventricular groove.

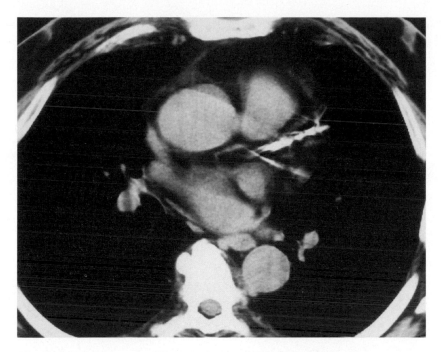

Fig. 1-28   CT scan of dense calcification in the left anterior descending and left circumflex arteries.

There is correlation between calcification and the severity of coronary stenosis; however, some severe stenoses may not be calcified, and some heavy calcifications may not denote stenotic arteries.

Association with stenosis

A number of investigators have attempted to develop a test for asymptomatic coronary artery disease by screening for coronary calcification (Moore, Fallavollita, Loecker, and Janowitz). Fluoroscopic detection should be more sensitive than the chest film because the motion of flecks of calcium in the coronary arteries should be more visible. However, Loecker and colleagues found a sensitivity and specificity of only 66% and 78%, respectively. Moore and colleagues quantitated the amount of coronary calcium with standard CT scans (Fig. 1-28) and showed similar numbers for patients with little calcification, but high specificity for stenoses that are severely calcified. Ultrafast or electron-beam CT is more sensitive (85%) but less specific (45%). Thus, these tests currently should not be used to search for subtle coronary calcification as a screening test for coronary stenosis.

PULMONARY VASCULATURE

The pulmonary vasculature is the most difficult part of the chest radiography to analyze because of the complex size and position of the bronchoarterial and pulmonary venous systems. The information gained from analyzing the pulmonary vasculature is as valuable as the shape of the heart in arriving at a cardiac diagnosis.

Determining the Vascular Pattern

Segmental analysis

Because the pulmonary arteries and veins have a complex branching pattern and are associated with many overlapping structures on the standard chest film, there is moderate variability in interpreting which pulmonary pattern is present. Segmental analysis can help to classify pulmonary vasculature patterns. In the standard upright chest film exposed at total lung capacity, the pulmonary vasculature can be divided into the following three areas:

1. The central pulmonary arteries
2. The hilar structures
3. The parenchymal arteries and veins

Central pulmonary arteries

The central pulmonary artery, below the aortopulmonary window and medial to the left hilum on the posteroanterior film, appears with a straight border or with slight curvature from early childhood to middle age; it may be more convex in the elderly. Enlargement of this segment is one of the earliest signs of pressure or volume overload in the main pulmonary artery. By Laplace's law, larger arteries dilate more than smaller arteries because of higher wall tension. An extremely dilated pulmonary artery segment on the frontal chest film will continue inferiorly as the right ventricular outflow tract. On a CT scan, the upper limit of normal for the diameter of the main pulmonary artery is 3 cm.

Hilar structures

The next components of the pulmonary arteries to enlarge are the pulmonary hilar vascular structures. The hilar enlargement on the frontal chest film can be confirmed on the lateral view by using the subjective correlation that the diameter of the normal right pulmonary artery is roughly the same size as the tracheal air column, and that the left pulmonary artery is not visible for more than a 2-cm arc. The diameter of the interlobar artery on the frontal chest film as measured from its lateral side to the wall of the intermediate bronchus should be less than 16 mm.

Upper and lower lung zones and bronchoarterial ratios

In the normal erect person, the upper lung zone vessels are smaller in width than those in the lung bases. The lung apex is barely perfused, whereas gravitational differences cause an increasing distribution of blood flow toward the lung base. This gravitational effect can be noticed on upright chest films as well as on supine or prone CT scans, where the gradient of blood vessel size then increases to the most dependent part of the lungs. In the normal subject, the pulmonary artery in the hilum is roughly the same size as its adjacent bronchus. In the upper lung zones, the pulmonary artery diameter in an erect film is 85% of the adjacent bronchial diameter. In the lower lung zones, the pulmonary arteries are one third bigger than the nearby bronchus.

Pattern recognition

The first step in analyzing the pulmonary vasculature is to classify it into one of the following five patterns:

1. Normal
2. Diminished
3. High output
4. Pulmonary arterial hypertension
5. Pulmonary venous hypertension

Diminished Vasculature

In many patients with cyanotic congenital heart disease and decreased pulmonary blood flow, the pulmonary vasculature appears normal on the chest film. In spite of this lack of sensitivity, there are several clues on the chest film that indicate abnormally diminished flow.

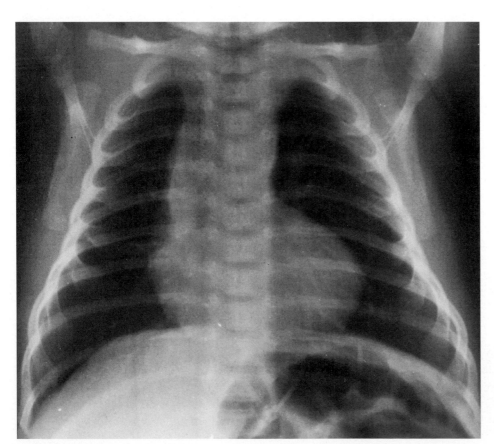

Fig. 1-29 Decreased pulmonary vasculature. The main pulmonary artery segment is concave, the hilar arteries are small, and the peripheral vessels are indistinct in this patient with tetralogy of Fallot.

Box 1-1 Examples of Decreased Pulmonary Vasculature

I. CONGENITALLY HYPOPLASTIC PULMONARY ARTERIES

A. By location

1. Diffuse hypoplasia
2. Segmental stenoses
   a. Main pulmonary artery (supravalvular pulmonary stenosis)
   b. Bifurcation of right and left pulmonary artery
   c. Branch or peripheral pulmonary arteries

B. By disease

1. Williams syndrome
2. Noonan syndrome
3. Ehlers-Danlos syndrome
4. Cutis laxa
5. Alagille syndrome (biliary hypoplasia and vertebral anomalies)

C. Complex anomalies with right-to-left shunts

1. Tetralogy of Fallot
2. Pulmonary valve atresia with or without a ventricular septal defect
3. Ebstein anomaly

II. ACQUIRED SMALL PULMONARY ARTERIES

A. Central obstruction

1. Emboli
2. Tumor

B. Hilar

1. Takayasu disease
2. Rubella
3. Emboli

C. Precapillary obstruction

1. Air trapping diseases like emphysema and Swyer-James syndrome

and destruction of a lung by previous pneumonia, abscess, or bulla all may have caused decreased pulmonary vasculature in only a single lobe. Pulmonary stenosis with any malformation that allows a right-to-left cardiac shunt can cause diminished flow to the lungs. For example, patients with tetralogy of Fallot have decreased pulmonary vasculature because of the pulmonary stenosis and right-to-left shunt across the ventricular septal defect. See Box 1-1 for examples of decreased pulmonary vasculature.

High-Output States

Segmental analysis

The size of the central, hilar, and peripheral pulmonary arteries and veins reflects in a complex way the pressure, flow, and volume in the lungs. In a high-output state, all pulmonary segments are enlarged: the central pulmonary artery segment is convex, the hilum appears engorged, and the peripheral vessels are large from apex to base.

Flow ratios

High-output states can be separated into those that have increased blood flow in both the pulmonary and the systemic circulation and those that have increased pulmonary circulation only. The chest film usually does not detect increased pulmonary flow until the flow ratio (Qp/Qs) is at least 2, that is, the pulmonary flow is twice the aorta. Increased cardiac output from both the right and left ventricles occurs in metabolic and endocrine diseases, in arteriovenous fistulas and malformations, and in aortic regurgitation.

Contributing diseases, lesions, and defects

Thyrotoxicosis (Fig. 1-30), beriberi, and pheochromocytoma are diseases that either increase the overall metabolic rate of the body or have a specific affect on the heart. They increase its rate and stroke volume. Extracardial shunts such as patent ductus arteriosus, aortopulmonary window, and arteriovenous fistulas and malformations either in the lungs or in another part of the body provide a lower-resistance parallel circuit to the systemic capillary bed for the blood to return to the heart. (The electrical analogy is a short circuit of a battery, which causes a high current to flow across its terminals.) In Paget disease there are numerous arteriolarvenous channels within the bone. In aortic regurgitation, blood flow that is regurgitated from the aorta into the left ventricle is added to the forward output to produce an augmented forward flow in the aorta. Because the lungs are in a series circuit with the aorta, the output is also increased. Intracardiac shunts have a normal aortic size and large main, hilar, and peripheral pulmonary arteries. In babies, high-output states often result in an element of pulmonary edema (Fig. 1-31). A

Using a segmental analysis approach, examine the central, hilar, and peripheral pulmonary arteries and veins. In the frontal view, a concave main pulmonary artery segment is the most reliable indicator of small main and central pulmonary arteries (Fig. 1-29). There are diminished bronchovascular markings in the hilum, and the diameters of the pulmonary arteries are smaller than their adjacent bronchus. The peripheral pulmonary arteries and veins are very small. In infants, separate arteries may be difficult to see individually, and the lung therefore appears hyperlucent.

Decreased blood flow and volume are easier to recognize when only a lobe is involved so that the adjacent lung can be used as a standard. Peripheral pulmonary emboli; congenital branch stenosis; Takayasu disease;

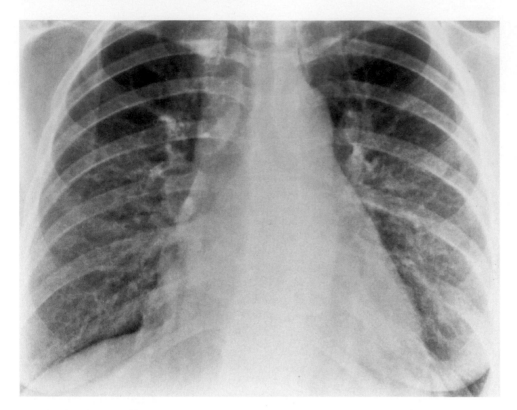

Fig. 1-30 High output state in Graves disease. The hilar pulmonary arteries are slightly large. The pulmonary arteries in the lung are larger than their adjacent bronchus in both the upper and lower lobes.

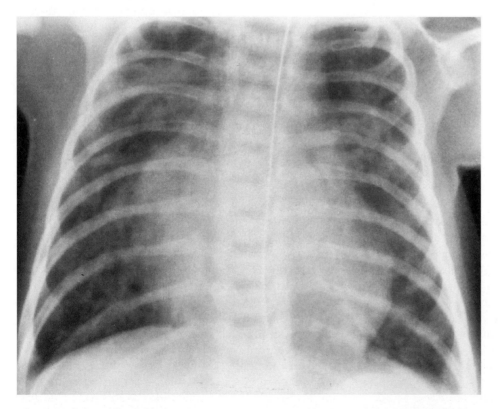

Fig. 1-31 Shunt vascularity in ventricular septal defect. The large central pulmonary arteries are indistinct because of surrounding pulmonary edema.

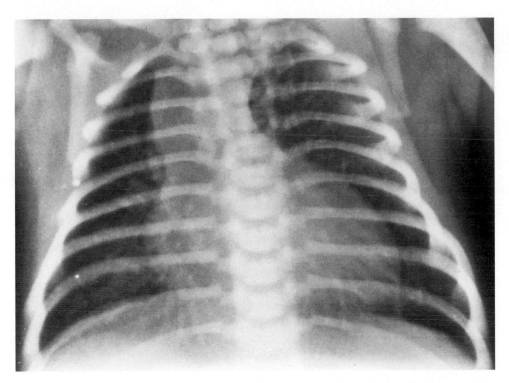

Fig. 1-32 Shunt vascularity in transposition of the great arteries with ventricular septal defect. Both upper and lower lobe pulmonary arteries and veins are large. The right-sided thymus obscures the upper lobe.

large pulmonary vasculature is also a feature of certain cyanotic congenital heart diseases (Fig. 1-32).

A convex main pulmonary artery segment suggesting a high-output state may be present in healthy individuals. Highly trained endurance athletes such as marathon runners and women in the third trimester of pregnancy and occasionally teenage girls frequently show mild enlargement of the main pulmonary artery.

Common acyanotic cardiac lesions with increased pulmonary flow include atrial septal defect, atrioventricular canal defect, and ventricular septal defect. Patients with partial anomalous pulmonary venous connection rarely have large pulmonary arteries because their Qp/Qs is usually less than 2.

Common cyanotic congenital heart defects that have increased pulmonary arterial flow are as follows:

- Transposition of the great arteries
- Truncus arteriosus (which has a ventricular septal defect)
- Total anomalous pulmonary venous connection above the diaphragm
- Tricuspid atresia with transposition of the great arteries
- Variants of these malformations (double outlet right ventricle, single ventricle)

Pulmonary Artery Hypertension

Pressure measurements and patterns of pulmonary vasculature

Pulmonary hypertension exists when the pulmonary systolic pressure is greater than 30 mm Hg and the mean pressure exceeds 20 mm Hg. Pulmonary hypertension may occur when there is increased resistance in any part of the pulmonary circulation from the pulmonary artery to the left heart. The type of pattern of the pulmonary vasculature on the chest film depends upon the location of the abnormal resistance, the chronicity, and the severity.

If the heart is structurally intact, the earliest sign of pulmonary artery hypertension is a convex main pulmonary artery segment. Severe, chronic pulmonary artery hypertension also dilates the hilar branches but, unlike a left-to-right shunt, not the peripheral arteries within the lungs (Fig. 1-33). The gradient of small vessels at the apex and large vessels at the base is preserved.

Eisenmenger syndrome

In adults with Eisenmenger syndrome the pulmonary vasculature is unusually striking because of the central arterial enlargement. The arteries dilate longitudinally forming a serpentine course (Fig. 1-34). The rapid taper

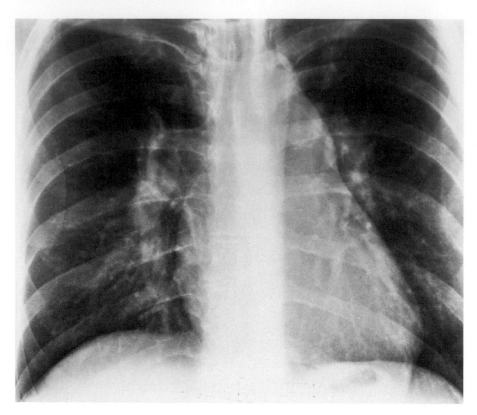

Fig. 1-33   Primary pulmonary artery hypertension. The main pulmonary artery segment is convex and the hilar arteries are large. The peripheral vessels are larger at the base, smaller at the apex, and retain their normal branching pattern.

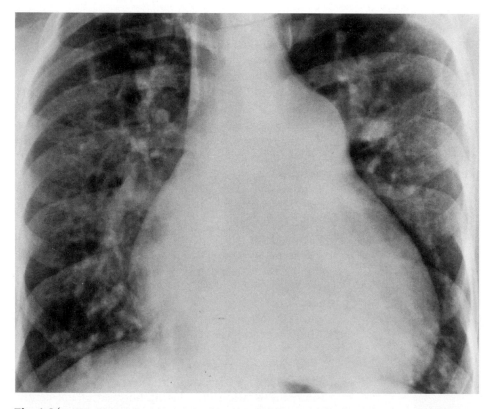

Fig. 1-34   Eisenmenger syndrome. In addition to the large main pulmonary artery segment and hilar branches, the peripheral pulmonary arteries are large and have a tortuous course.

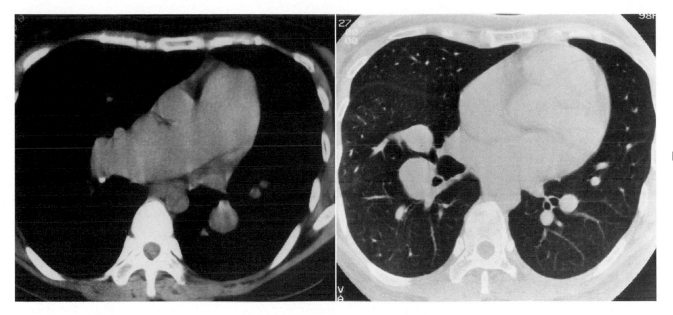

Fig. 1-35 CT scan of pulmonary artery hypertension. **A,** The diameters of the main and right pulmonary arteries are almost twice that of the adjacent aorta. **B,** The hilar pulmonary arteries are two to three times larger than their adjacent bronchus.

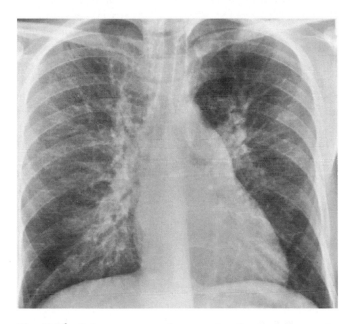

Fig. 1-36 Pulmonary artery hypertension from mitral stenosis. The central pulmonary artery is convex and the hilar arteries are large because of arterial hypertension. The large upper lobe pulmonary arteries and veins and invisible lower lobe vessels indicate pulmonary venous hypertension. Note the double density along the right side of the heart from left atrial enlargement.

Box 1-2   Common Causes of Pulmonary Artery Hypertension

I. OBSTRUCTION IN THE CENTRAL PULMONARY ARTERIES

   A. Thromboembolism or tumor
   B. Peripheral pulmonary stenosis
   C. Hypoplastic pulmonary arteries

II. INCREASED RESISTANCE IN THE CAPILLARY BED

   A. Obstructive or interstitial lung disease
   B. Widespread airspace disease such as pneumonia, tumor, atelectasis, or pneumonectomy
   C. Primary pulmonary hypertension
   D. Eisenmenger syndrome

III. OBSTRUCTION TO PULMONARY VENOUS DRAINAGE

   A. Left ventricular failure
   B. Restrictive cardiomyopathy such as amyloid
   C. Mitral stenosis (Fig. 1-36)
   D. Hypoplastic left heart syndrome
   E. Pulmonary veno-occlusive disease
   F. Fibrosing mediastinitis

of the large aneurysmal hilar pulmonary arteries to the periphery looks like a "pruned tree." This phrase is correct angiographically and pathologically; there are fewer arterial side branches than in a normal arterial tree. However, the reduced number of side branches can not be seen on a chest film. The size of the pulmonary arteries in relation to their adjacent bronchus is measurable on CT (Fig. 1-35).

Venous hypertension

The pulmonary pattern in pulmonary artery hypertension that is secondary to pulmonary venous hypertension has a different time course and appearance. After weeks to months of increased pulmonary venous pressure, the hilar and central segments of the pulmonary arteries begin to dilate. The peripheral pulmonary branches continue to suggest pulmonary venous hypertension with large vessels at the apex and small vessels at the lung base.

See Box 1-2 for common causes of pulmonary artery hypertension.

Pulmonary Venous Hypertension

Pulmonary edema—excessive fluid in the alveolar and interstitial compartments of the lung—has two clinical classifications: cardiogenic and noncardiogenic. Cardiogenic edema is caused by pulmonary venous hypertension and is most commonly the result of left ventricular failure or acute mitral regurgitation. In the infant, it may result from hypoplastic left heart syndrome or total anomalous pulmonary venous connection below the diaphragm.

Fluid and water exchange

Noncardiogenic or permeability edema is the accumulation of fluid in the lungs in the presence of normal left atrial pressures. This has many complex causes that disrupt the alveolar capillary membrane.

Pulmonary edema has many radiologic patterns, and to analyze these more exactly, it is important to have an understanding of lung architecture and physiology for gas and fluid exchange.

In the normal lung, hydrostatic and osmotic forces provide a gradient to keep fluid within the pulmonary microvasculature. Fluid exchange mainly takes place across the alveolar–capillary endothelium as well as the interstitium around the precapillary and postcapillary vessels. The alveolar septum is differentiated into one side with thin cells for gas exchange and one side with thick cells for fluid exchange. When interstitial pulmonary edema develops, the water and protein accumulate predominantly on the thick side. The lung removes excess fluid mainly by a network of pulmonary lymphatics. The mediastinal and pulmonary lymphatics serve as the major channel for fluid removal. Extensive lymphatic channels exist near the alveolar ducts and drain centrally adjacent to respiratory bronchioles, the interstitium about the minor and major bronchi, and to the major mediastinal lymph nodes. The cortex of the lung has its own lymphatic supply, which drains the peripheral portion of the lung into pleural lymphatics. This anatomic arrangement provides a pathologic correlation that explains peribronchial cuffing and hilar haze on the chest film as two signs of pulmonary edema. When there is significant accumulation of lung water, the rate of lymph

flow can increase tenfold before there is significant pulmonary edema. The excess lung fluid in the pulmonary interstitium is visible in patients with transplanted lungs because the lymphatics have been cut, thereby blocking the major pathway of fluid transport from the lung.

Radiologic appearance

The radiologic appearance of pulmonary venous hypertension with the later formation of pulmonary edema has a distinct time course and appearance that frequently separates it from other types of diffuse lung disease and noncardiogenic pulmonary edema. As the left atrial pressure rises from its normal value of less than 12 mm Hg, the size of the pulmonary veins changes and fluid begins to appear in the interstitium. The first two signs to appear on the upright chest film are that the lower lobe vessels become indistinct and the upper lobe vessels begin to dilate. In normal appearance of the lower lobe vasculature, vessel edges are sharp, multiple secondary branches are clearly visible, and the average size of vessels in the middle part of the lung between the hilum and cortex is 4 to 8 mm. At least five to eight arteries can be seen at the right base. This effect is predominantly due to gravity in the upright person, giving greater blood flow and blood volume to the lower lobes.

As left atrial pressure rises, the hilar and lower lobe vasculature becomes indistinct and the edges are less sharp. Fluid begins to accumulate in the interstitium. The number of visible side branches decreases, perhaps because of a silhouette sign as water in the interstitium partially obscures the adjacent vessel wall. In response to the higher venous pressure, the upper lobe vessels handle the blood that is meeting resistance as it enters the left atrium. You will recognize this increased blood flow to the upper lobes by the increased visibility of numerous upper lobe arteries and veins (Fig. 1-37). The width of these structures, normally 1 to 2 mm in the middle part of the lung, increases to 2 to 4 mm. The redistribution now is reflected by an increase in both the size and number of vessels in the apices. The development of pulmonary venous hypertension is a continuum in the gradient of vessel size from apex to base. The normal distribution of small apical and large basilar vessels becomes balanced with equal size in both locations; at higher pressures this reverses and the upper lobe vessels are larger. A CT scan of a supine person with pulmonary venous hypertension will show large anterior vessels and smaller posterior vessels. Roughly the same branching generation from the main pulmonary artery should be used when comparing the anterior and posterior arteries (Fig. 1-38).

There are other signs of interstitial lung water that help confirm the diagnosis of pulmonary venous hyper-

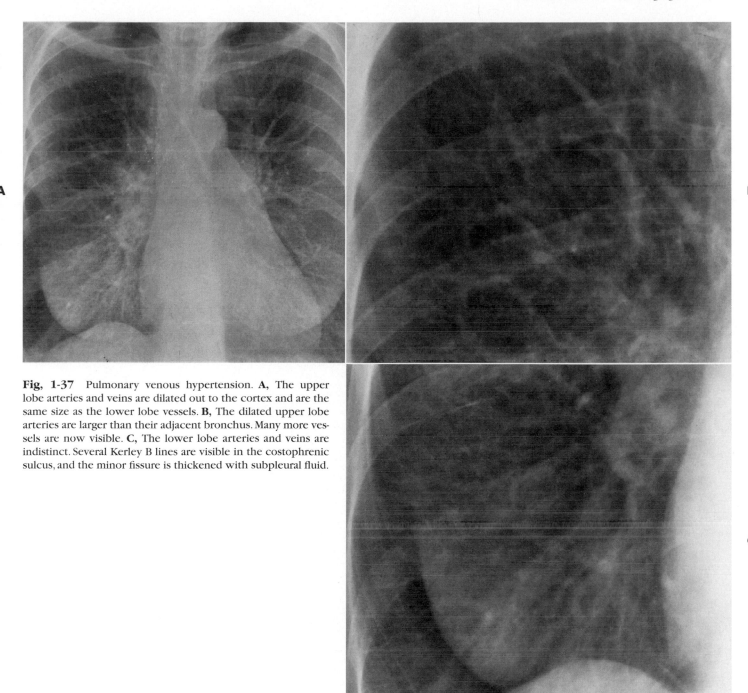

Fig, 1-37 Pulmonary venous hypertension. **A,** The upper lobe arteries and veins are dilated out to the cortex and are the same size as the lower lobe vessels. **B,** The dilated upper lobe arteries are larger than their adjacent bronchus. Many more vessels are now visible. **C,** The lower lobe arteries and veins are indistinct. Several Kerley B lines are visible in the costophrenic sulcus, and the minor fissure is thickened with subpleural fluid.

tension. In the cortex of the lung, Kerley B lines appear and represent thickening of the interlobular septum (Fig. 1-39). Kerley A lines—3- to 5-cm lines about 1 mm thick and extending from the central part of the lung—represent distended lymphatics (Fig. 1-40). The perihilar haze probably represents a combination of distended lymphatics, alveolar transudate, and interstitial thickening in lung parenchyma that lies anterior and posterior to the hilum. Thickening of the interlobular fissures

and accumulation of subpleural fluid represent excess fluid and distention of the interstitial space and lymphatics. The end-on appearance of the bronchus and its adjacent pulmonary artery also changes in pulmonary venous hypertension. The bronchial wall becomes thickened and less distinct ("cuffed") and the pulmonary artery dilates (Fig. 1-41).

As interstitial edema proceeds to alveolar edema, roseate opacities begin to appear in the perihilar

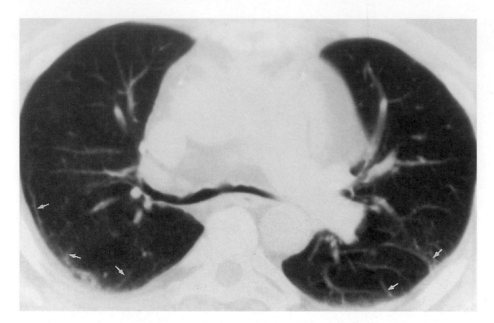

Fig. 1-38   CT scan of pulmonary venous hypertension. The anterior vessels are larger than the corresponding posterior vessels in this supine scan. Kerley B lines are adjacent to the right lung pleura posteriorly and a linear subpleural opacity in the posterior left lung *(arrows).*

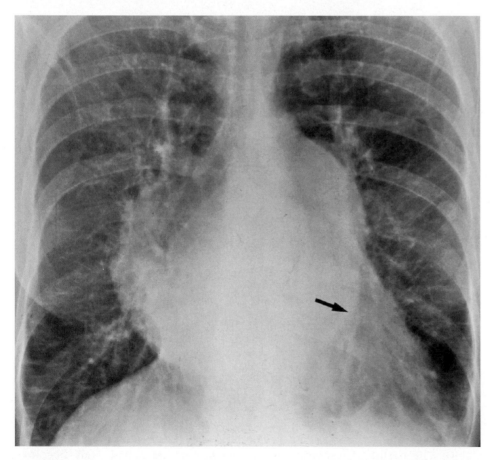

Fig. 1-39   Kerley B lines. Bilateral linear opacities in the costophrenic sulci represent distended interlobar septa. These lines may extend along the lateral wall nearly to the apex. Mitral stenosis has enlarged the left atrium and distorted the right side of the heart. A double density *(arrow)* along the left heart border is the interface of the large left atrium with the lung. The convex main pulmonary artery indicates pulmonary artery hypertension.

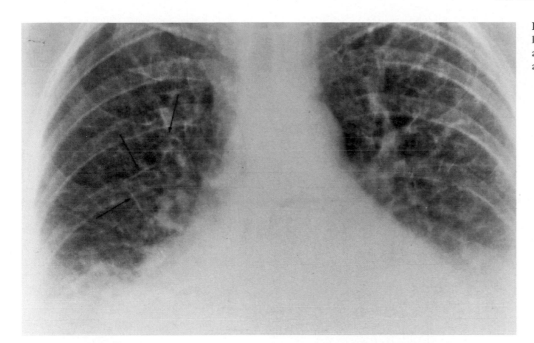

Fig. 1-40   Kerley A lines. Central linear opacities that are perihilar and do not conform with fissures are distended lymphatics.

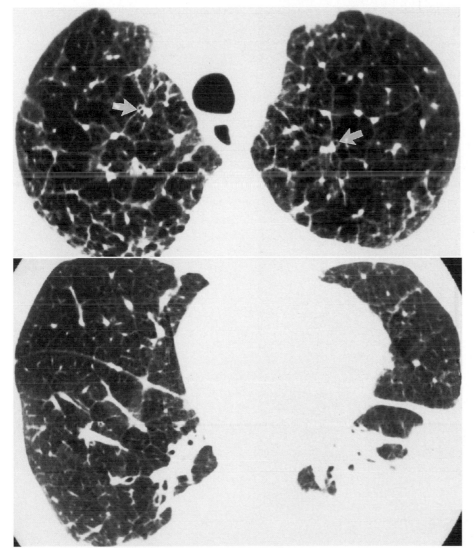

A

B

Fig. 1-41   High Resolution CT (HRCT) of cardiac interstitial edema. **A,** The secondary pulmonary lobules are outlined by the thickened interstitium in this patient with emphysema. The bronchovascular bundles *(arrows)* have a pulmonary artery larger than the adjacent bronchus. **B,** A basal section shows thickening of the major fissures with dependent posterior pleural effusions. The secondary lobules are visible because of a thickened interlobar septum. The bronchial walls are thickened, which is the plain chest film correlate of "cuffing."

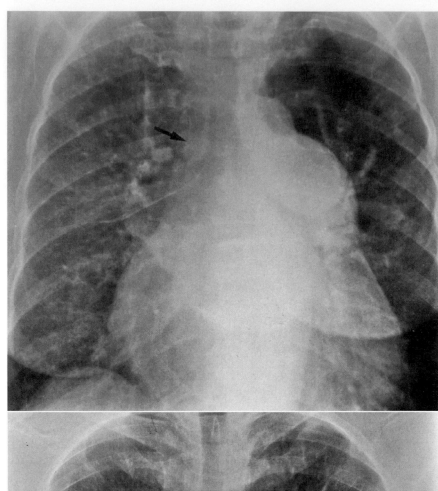

A

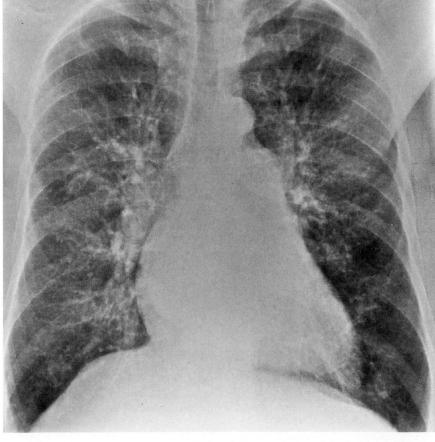

B

Fig. 1-42 Width of the vascular pedicle as an indicator of fluid status. **A,** The wide vascular pedicle measured above the aortic arch reflects a dilated superior vena cava. The azygos vein *(arrow)* is also large. **B,** This patient also has pulmonary edema, but a small vascular pedicle, probably reflecting vigorous diuretic therapy that reduced the intravascular volume. The residual pulmonary edema represents a therapeutic time lag.

region and spread peripherally to form a "butterfly pattern." This does not involve the lung cortex except in extreme cases. When the opacities involve a significant part of the lung cortex and its adjacent pleura, other disease processes, such as pneumonia and adult respiratory distress syndrome, are more likely explanations for the cortical distribution. The edema caused by a cardiac disease typically is symmetrical and perihilar and is more severe in the lung bases than in the apices. The distribution of cardiac pulmonary edema can be quite variable and asymmetric but is never completely unilateral. Asymmetric pulmonary edema is usually more severe in the right lung. These patients are often lying with their right side down so the distribution of pulmonary edema often corresponds to the gravity gradient. Patients who develop mitral regurgitation during myocardial infarction rarely may also have pulmonary edema predominantly in the right upper lobe. The jet of mitral regurgitation is directed into the right upper pulmonary vein and augments the forces in that lung that promote fluid retention.

Pleural and pericardial effusions develop in patients with left heart failure. In edema, the subpleural interstitial pressure rises sufficiently to create a net pressure into the pleural space. Generally, the pulmonary venous pressure needs to exceed 20 mm Hg to have visible pleural effusions. Isolated elevation of pulmonary arterial pressure does not produce pleural effusions.

The width of the vascular pedicle is an indirect but reliable sign of increased intravascular fluid. The width is measured just above the aortic arch from the left subclavian artery on the left side to the superior vena cava on the right side (Fig. 1-42). Dilatation of this pedicle and the adjacent azygos vein is increased in overhydration, renal failure, and chronic cardiac failure. In contrast, the vascular pedicle is usually unchanged in capillary permeability edema.

The time course of the appearance and disappearance of pulmonary edema on the chest film is variable, but in slowly progressing clinical situations, there is a rough correlation with the pulmonary capillary wedge pressure. When the wedge pressure is greater than 20 mm Hg, there are always detectable signs of pulmonary venous hypertension and pulmonary edema on the chest film.

There is only a fair correlation between redistribution of blood flow with dilatation of the upper lobe vessels and pulmonary capillary pressure between 12 and 20 mm Hg. Because the osmotic pressure of plasma protein is 25 mm Hg, it is reasonable to expect alveolar edema when the pulmonary capillary wedge pressure exceeds this number; however, alveolar opacities can be seen with pressures of only 20 mm Hg. Pulmonary edema may be visible within a few minutes after the onset of acute mitral regurgitation or left

heart failure. As the pulmonary edema resolves, there may be a therapeutic lag during which the wedge pressure returns to normal while the pulmonary edema persists. This lag may exist from several hours to several days. Although it is common to compare interpretation of the pulmonary edema on the chest film with the pulmonary capillary wedge pressure, these two observations measure different parameters and therefore are not appropriate standards of comparison. The pulmonary capillary wedge pressure

---

Box 1-3   Cardiac Causes for Pulmonary Edema

I. OBSTRUCTION

  A. At pulmonary vein level

   1. Congenital pulmonary vein atresia
   2. Pulmonary veno-occlusive disease
   3. Extrinsic pulmonary vein obstruction by tumor or fibrosing mediastinitis
   4. Total anomalous pulmonary venous connection below the diaphragm

  B. At left atrial level

   1. Cor triatriatum
   2. Left atrial myxoma or tumor
   3. Left atrial thrombus

  C. At mitral valve level

   1. Mitral stenosis or regurgitation

  D. At left ventricular level

   1. Left ventricular infarct, aneurysm, or failure
   2. Hypoplastic left heart syndrome
   3. Cardiomyopathy with stiff left ventricular walls
   4. Left coronary artery from the pulmonary artery

  E. At aortic valve level

   1. Aortic stenosis (valvular, subvalvular, or supravalvular)

  F. At aortic level

   1. Hypoplastic aorta
   2. Coarctation
   3. Takayasu aortitis

II. HIGH-OUTPUT FAILURE

   1. Systemic vasodilatation (septic shock)
   2. Mitral or aortic regurgitation
   3. Thyrotoxicosis
   4. Large ventricular septal defect
   5. Patent ductus arteriosus
   6. Peripheral arteriovenous fistula

measures the instantaneous pulmonary venous and left atrial pressures. The radiologic signs of pulmonary edema are an integrated history of the production and resorption of lung water. Particularly in the resorption phase, these signs more accurately mirror the amount of lung water present rather than the pulmonary venous pressure. A patient with an acute myocardial infarction who has a chest film showing pulmonary edema and a normal pulmonary wedge pressure has stiff and noncompliant lungs because of the unresorbed interstitial fluid.

See Box 1-3 for cardiac causes for pulmonary edema.

SKELETAL ABNORMALITIES IN HEART DISEASE

Cardiac Surgery

The appearance of the thoracic cage can indicate previous surgery and frequently suggests certain types of heart disease. Most cardiac surgery begins with a median sternotomy because it gives excellent access to the heart's anterior structures and to the ascending aorta. A sternotomy also causes less postoperative pain than a posterior thoracotomy. After many types of cardiac surgery, there may be sternal wire sutures, mediastinal clips, and epicardial pacing wires. A myriad of vascular clips following the course of the left internal mammary artery indicates a graft to the left anterior descending or diagonal arteries. Most prosthetic mitral and aortic valve replacements are easily seen, except for the St. Jude valve, whose ring is usually not visible. The leaflets of this valve appear as one or two straight lines, and are seen in about 30% of chest films when the leaflets are tangential to the x-ray beam. You can identify a posterior thoracotomy by a surgical absence of the fifth rib or by uneven spacing between the fourth, fifth, and sixth ribs. Left posterior thoracotomies are performed to repair a coarctation of the aorta, to ligate a patent ductus arteriosus, to repair a vascular ring, and to create a left Blalock-Taussig shunt between the left subclavian artery and the left pulmonary artery. Right posterior thoracotomies are performed to create a right Blalock-Taussig shunt or to approach a coarctation in the right aortic arch.

Thoracic Cage and Heart Disease

The thoracic cage also has several distinctive signs associated with heart disease. The chest film of a patient with Marfan syndrome may show a tall person with a narrow anteroposterior diameter and a pectus excavatum (Fig. 1-43). However, a normal variation is a narrow posteroanterior diameter of the thorax, which has a structurally normal heart that is rotated to the left side.

The lateral chest film then shows a straight thoracic spine lacking the normal kyphosis and diminished retrosternal and retrocardiac spaces.

Congenital Syndromes with Heart Disease

Spine abnormalities also may indicate surgery or disease. An acquired scoliosis may occur where the ribs on the side of a posterior thoracotomy have been pulled tightly together. Vertebral anomalies, such as hemivertebra and "butterfly" vertebra, are frequently associated with congenital heart disease (Fig. 1-44).

Chest radiographs of infants with trisomy 21, or Down syndrome, may be distinctive enough to diagnose not only the heart disease but also the syndrome. Of patients with trisomy 21, roughly half have atrioventricular canal defects. Conversely, of those infants who have atrioventricular canal defects, about half have trisomy 21. Other indicative chest radiographic findings include 11 pairs of ribs (Fig. 1-45) and multiple manubrial ossification centers (Fig. 1-46), both of which are more prevalent in infants with trisomy 21 than in normal newborn infants.

The bony abnormalities in neurofibromatosis mimic the rib notching seen in coarctation of the aorta. The spine and ribs reflect the mesodermal dysplasia. Scoliosis, kyphosis, and distortion of numerous ribs are common. The ribs may appear notched from neurofibroma in the neurovascular groove (Fig. 1-47). The overconstricted ribs appear like ribbons with bowing and apathologic fractures. Occasionally you may see pseudoarthrosis in the clavicle; interstitial lung disease; and aneurysms of the mediastinal arteries, veins, or lymphatic system.

Patients with the Holt-Oram syndrome (heart-hand syndrome) have abnormalities in the upper limbs with congenital heart diseases such as atrial septal defect and ventricular septal defect. The upper extremity defects are usually bilateral and affect the radial ray. The thumb is almost always affected and is either absent or part of a hand complex with three phalanges, focal phocomelia, or carpal bone fusions (Fig. 1-48).

Other bone diseases associated with heart disease can be recognized on the chest film. Osteogenesis imperfecta is a disease that causes diffuse aortic ectasia, aortic regurgitation, or coarctation. The bony abnormalities include variable bone density, multiple fractures in many bones, kyphoscoliosis, and biconcave vertebra with anterior wedge deformities. Sickle cell disease and thalassemia major, which are associated with cardiomyopathy and thoracic cage abnormalities, are representative of severe anemias. In sickle cell disease the ribs have diffuse sclerosis and a coarsened trabecular pattern; the vertebral bodies have squared-off corners. Ischemia of the central portion of the cartilaginous end plate results in a steplike depres-

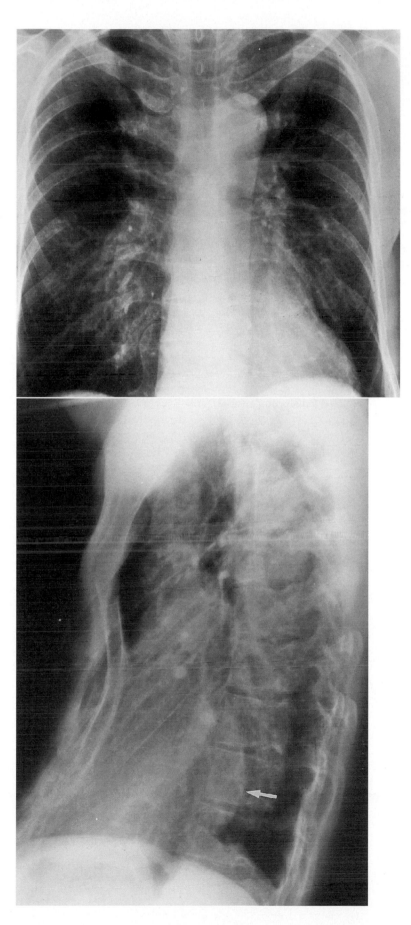

Fig 1-43   Marfan syndrome. **A,** The heart is shifted into the left hemithorax because the right atrial border is not seen. The lungs have large volume. The aorta and the main pulmonary artery are dilated. **B,** The narrow antero-posterior diameter is accentuated by the pectus excavatum. The left ventricle *(arrow)* is not enlarged, but is rotated posteriorly by the skeletal deformity.

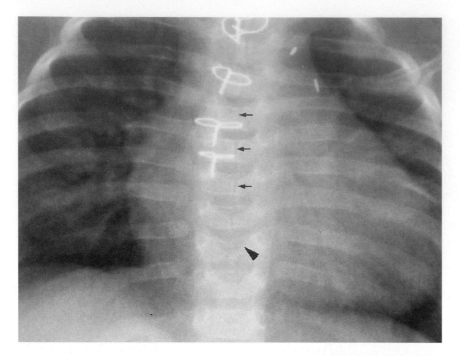

Fig 1-44 Vertebral anomalies. Butterfly vertebrae *(arrowhead)* and sagittal clefts *(arrows)* are associated nonspecifically with congenital heart disease. The large heart reflects left ventricular failure from the left coronary artery arising from the pulmonary artery.

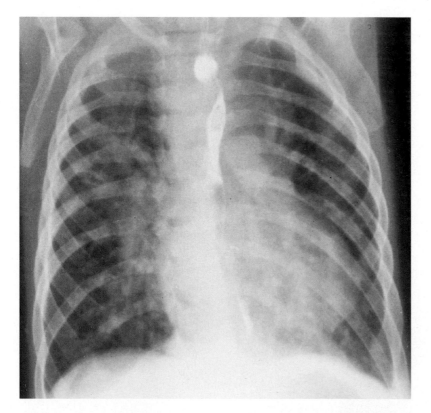

Fig 1-45 Eleven pairs of ribs in Down syndrome. The large heart and the shunt vascularity result from an atrioventricular canal defect. Barium in the esophagus is deviated by a right aortic arch.

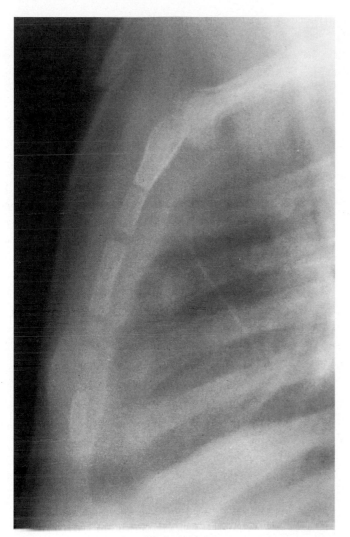

Fig 1-46   Hypersegmentation of the sternum and multiple manubrial ossification centers in Down syndrome.

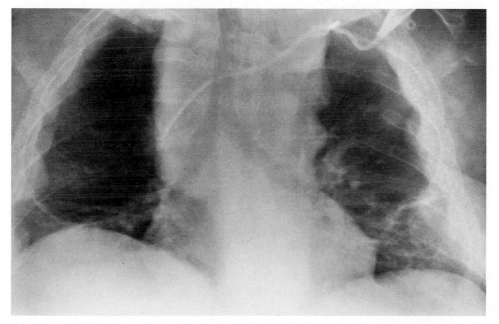

Fig 1-47   Rib notching in neurofibromatosis. Intercostal neurofibroma have notched the ribs bilaterally. Pleural masses, interstitial lung disease at the bases, and the wide mediastinum are other aspects of this disease.

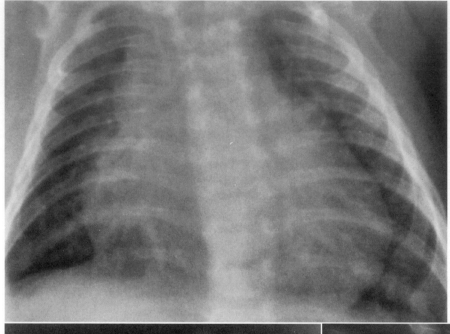

A

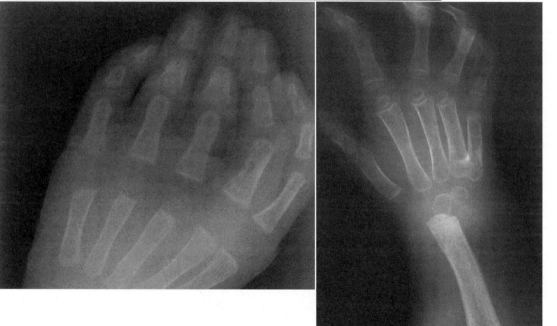

B

C

Fig 1-48   Holt-Oram syndrome. **A,** An atrial septal defect and multiple ventricular septal defects have caused the large heart and the shunt vascularity. **B,** The thumb has three phalanges. **C,** A different patient with an atrial septal defect has an absent radius.

sion of the vertebral end plate, and bony infarcts may be seen in the humeral heads. Thalassemia major also has large lobulated paravertebral masses of marrow hyperplasia and extramedullary hematopoiesis.

Many of the arthritic conditions are associated with fusiform aortic aneurysms, aortic regurgitation, and dissection. Ankylosing spondylitis, Reiter syndrome, and others may cause distinctive abnormalities in the spine. In ankylosing spondylitis, the apophyseal joints are fused

and the posterior spinal ligaments are ossified. Syndesmophyte formation is recognized as a straight line or a smooth curve extending from the middle part of one vertebral body to the adjacent one. In contrast, the osteophytes that bridge the vertebral end plates denote degenerative spondylosis; this pattern has no association with heart disease.

Table 1-1 lists the major syndromes associated with cardiovascular disease.

Table 1-1 Syndromes and metabolic disorders associated with heart disease

Cystic fibrosis	Cor pulmonale
DiGeorge syndrome	Aortic arch interruption, truncus arteriosus, tetralogy of Fallot
Down syndrome	Endocardial cushion defect, mitral valve prolapse
Ellis-van Creveld syndrome	Atrial septal defect, single atrium
Ehlers-Danlos syndrome	Aortic aneurysms, dissection, and rupture; tortuous systemic and pulmonary arteries; congenital heart disease (valvular regurgitation and stenosis); mitral valve prolapse
Friedreich ataxia	Hypertrophic cardiomyopathy
Homocystinuria	Marfan features, coronary thrombosis
Mucopolysaccharidoses	Coronary artery disease, aortic and mitral stenosis and regurgitation
Osteogenesis imperfecta	Aortic regurgitation, aortic aneurysm
Progeria	Accelerated arteriosclerosis, hypertension
Sickle cell anemia	Cardiomyopathy, myocardial infarct, pulmonary infarct, cor pulmonale
Holt-Oram syndrome	Atrial septal defect, ventricular septal defect
Idiopathic hypertrophic subaortic stenosis	Hypertrophic cardiomyopathy, subaortic stenosis
Heterotaxy	Polysplenia or asplenia and congenital heart disease with anomalies of situs and symmetry
Ivemark syndrome	Asplenia and congenital heart disease with anomalies of situs and right-sided symmetry
Kartagener syndrome	Situs inversus with dextrocardia and bronchiectasis
Marfan syndrome	Aortic aneurysm/dissection; aortic, mitral, and tricuspid valve prolapse with regurgitation; mitral annular calcification in young adults
Neurofibromatosis	Aortic and pulmonary stenosis, pheochromocytoma with hypertension, coarctation, aortic aneurysm
Turner syndrome	Coarctation, aortic stenosis, atrial septal defect, pulmonary stenosis, aortic dissection
Noonan (male Turner) syndrome	Pulmonary valve and peripheral stenosis, atrial septal defect, idiopathic hypertrophic subaortic stenosis, ventricular septal defect, patent ductus arteriosus
Rubella	Peripheral and valvular pulmonary stenosis, patent ductus arteriosus, hypoplasia of the aorta, coarctation, atrial septal defect, ventricular septal defect
Treacher Collins syndrome	Atrial septal defect, patent ductus arteriosus, ventricular septal defect
Tuberous sclerosis	Myocardial rhabdomyoma
Williams syndrome	Supravalvular aortic stenosis, peripheral pulmonary stenosis

Data from Taybi H, Lachman RS: *Radiology of syndromes, metabolic disorders, and skeletal dysplasias*, ed 4, St Louis, 1996, Mosby–Year Book.

CORONARY SINUS AND THE LEFT SUPERIOR VENA CAVA

Coronary Sinus

Anatomy and relation to the left superior vena cava

The coronary sinus enters the right atrium anterior to the origin of the inferior vena cava. The eustachian valve of the inferior vena cava and the thebesian valve of the coronary sinus join to form a ridge of tissue between them. The coronary sinus extends behind the heart and becomes the great cardiac vein in the left atrioventricular groove. When a left superior vena cava is present, it joins the great cardiac vein about 2 cm from the right atrium to continue as the coronary sinus.

Location from catheter position

On the frontal chest film a catheter ending in the coronary sinus usually cannot be distinguished from one ending in the body of the right ventricle. For this reason, you should use a lateral as well as a frontal view when placing a catheter or pacing wire into the right ventricle. A power injection suitable for right ventriculography has enough force to rupture the coronary sinus into the pericardium. A lateral view identifies the posteriorly placed coronary sinus line from the right ventricular one (Fig. 1-49).

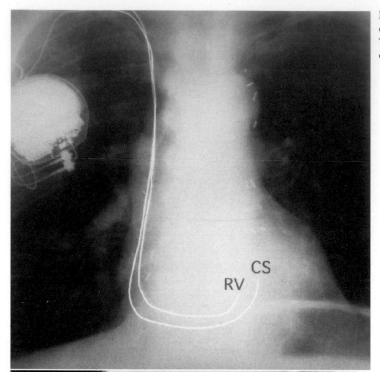

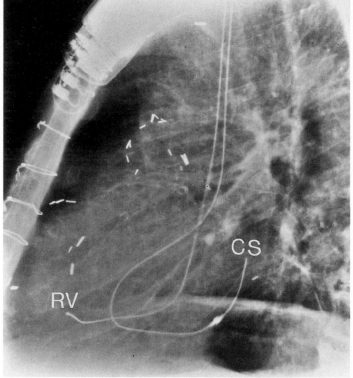

Fig 1-49 Coronary sinus and right ventricular wires. **A,** The dual pacing wires have a similar course on the frontal film. **B,** The lateral view separates the anterior right ventricular *(RV)* electrode from the posterior coronary sinus *(CS)* electrode.

Left Superior Vena Cava

Mediastinal position

A persistent left superior vena cava is a relatively common venous anomaly that usually connects to the right atrium. Rarely, it may connect to the left atrium and then is associated with the heterotaxy syndrome. The left superior vena cava begins at the junction of the left subclavian and jugular veins and descends in front of the aortic arch. It then may pass in front of the left pulmonary artery or go between the pulmonary artery and vein, connect with the left hemiazygos vein, before

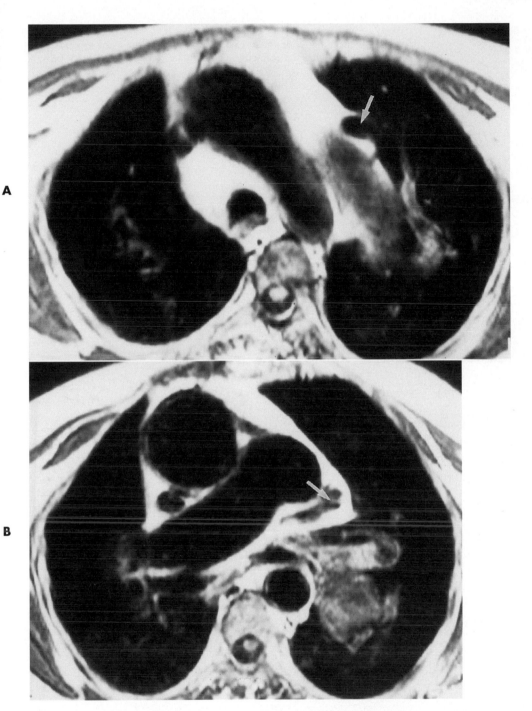

Fig 1-50   Left superior vena cava. **A,** On an MRI image at the level of the aortic arch, the left superior vena cava *(arrow)* is adjacent to the left pulmonary artery in this patient with truncus arteriosus. Although an anomalous pulmonary vein from the left lung may be in this position, lower slices **(B)** show its course *(arrow)* near the left pulmonary artery before it connects to the coronary sinus.

entering the pericardium. The left superior vena cava joins with the great cardiac vein to become the coronary sinus (Fig. 1-50). Right and left superior venae cavae, as with most venous anomalies, have numerous variations. Either the right or left superior vena cava may be absent, or both may persist (Fig. 1-51). The innominate connecting vein rarely is absent.

Catheter course

Although a left superior vena cava usually is discovered inadvertently on a chest film when a left-sided mediastinal catheter is noted, it can be used for central line placement and entry into the heart. The line from the left superior vena cava enters the right atrium and is redirected through the tricuspid valve (Fig. 1-52).

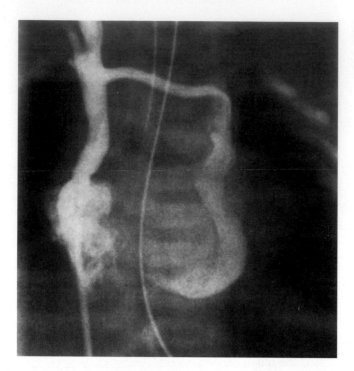

Fig 1-51
Bilateral superior venae cavae. Injection into the right superior vena cava backfills the connecting innominate vein to the left superior vena cava.

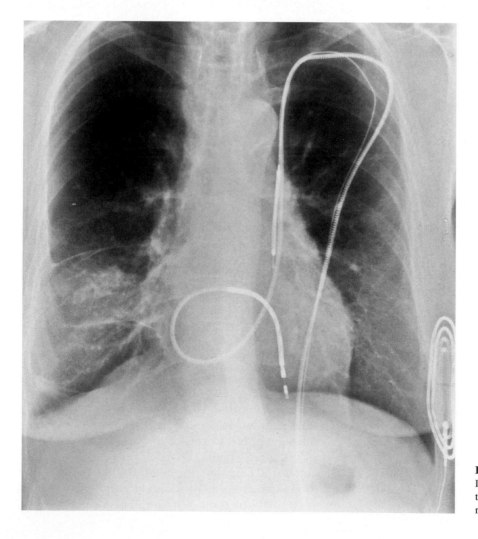

Fig 1-52
Internal cardiovascular defibrillator with electrodes in a left superior vena cava and the right ventricle.

SUGGESTED READINGS

Books

Chen JTT: *Essentials of cardiac roentgenology,* Boston, 1987, Little, Brown.

Elliot LP: *Cardiac imaging in infants, children, and adults,* Philadelphia, 1991, JB Lippincott.

Higgins CB: *Essentials of cardiac radiology and imaging,* Philadelphia, 1992, JB Lippincott.

Keats TE: *Atlas of roentgenographic measurements,* St Louis, 1990, Mosby–Year Book.

Pohost GM, O'Rourke RA: *Principles and practices of cardiovascular imaging,* Boston, 1991, Little, Brown.

Spindola-Franco H, Fish BG: *Radiology of heart, cardiac imaging in infants, children, and adults,* New York, 1985, Springer-Verlag.

Taybi H, Lachman RS: *Radiology of syndromes, metabolic disorders, and skeletal dysplasias,* ed 3, St Louis, 1990, Mosby–Year Book.

Journals

Benjamin EJ, Plehn JF, D'Agostino RB et al: Mitral annular calcification and the risk of stroke in an elderly cohort, *N Engl J Med* 327:374-379, 1992.

Breen JF, Sheedy PF II, Schwartz RS et al: Coronary artery calcification detected with ultrafast CT as indication of coronary artery disease, *Radiology* 185:435-439, 1992.

Chikos PM, Figley MM, Fisher L: Correlation between chest film and angiographic assessment of left ventricular size, *AJR Am J Roentgenol* 128:367-373, 1977.

Comeau WJ, White PD: A critical analysis of standard methods of estimating heart size from roentgen measurements, *AJR Am J Roentgenol* 47:665-677, 1942.

Copel JA, Pilu G, Kleinman CS: Congenital heart disease and extracardiac anomalies: associations and indications for fetal echocardiography, *Am J Obstet Gynecol* 154:1121-1132, 1986.

Danzer CS: The cardiothoracic ratio: an index of cardiac enlargement, *Am J Med Sci* 157:513-521, 1919.

Datey KK, Deshmukh SD, Dalvi CP: Straight back syndrome, *Br Heart J* 26:614-619, 1964.

Edwards DK III, Berry CC, Hilton SW: Trisomy 21 in newborn infants: chest radiographic diagnosis, *Radiology* 167:317-318, 1988.

Eyler WR, Wayne DL, Rhodenbaugh JE: The importance of the lateral view in the evaluation of left ventricular enlargement in rheumatic heart disease, *Radiology* 73:56-61, 1959.

Fallavollita JA, Brody AS, Bunnell IL et al: Fast computed tomography detection of coronary calcification in the diagnosis of coronary artery disease. Comparison with angiography in patients <50 years old, *Circulation* 89:285-290, 1994.

Fleischner FG: The butterfly pattern of acute pulmonary edema, *Am J Cardiol* 20:39-46, 1976.

Gammill SL, Krebs C, Meyers P et al: Cardiac measurements in systole and diastole, *Radiology* 94:115-119, 1970.

Glover L, Baxley WA, Dodge HT: A quantitative evaluation of heart size measurements from chest roentgenograms, *Circulation* 155:1289-1296, 1973.

Henry WL, Morgantroth J, Pearlman AS et al: Relation between echocardiographically determined left atrial size and atrial fibrillation, *Circulation* 53:273-279, 1976.

Henschke CI, Davis SD, Romano PM et al: The pathogenesis, radiologic evaluation, and therapy of pleural effusions, *Radiol Clin North Am* 27:1241-1255, 1989.

Higgins CB, Reinke RT, Jones NE, Broderick T: Left atrial dimension on the frontal thoracic radiography: a method for assessing left atrial enlargement, *AJR Am J Roentgenol* 130:251-255, 1978.

Hoffman RB, Rigler LG: Evaluation of left ventricular enlargement in the lateral projection of the chest, *Radiology* 80:93-100, 1965.

Janowitz WR, Agatston AS, Viamonte M Jr: Comparison of serial quantitative evaluation of calcified coronary artery plaque by ultrafast computed tomography in persons with and without obstructive coronary artery disease, *Am J Cardiol* 68:1-6, 1991.

Keren G, Etzion T, Sherez J et al: Atrial fibrillation and atrial enlargement in patients with mitral stenosis, *Am Heart J* 114:1146-1155, 1987.

Kostuk W, Barr JW, Simon AL, Ross J Jr: Correlations between the chest film and hemodynamics in acute myocardial infarction, *Circulation* 158:624-632, 1973.

Kuriyama K, Gamsu G, Stern RG et al: CT-determined pulmonary artery diameters in predicting pulmonary hypertension, *Invest Radiol* 19:19-22, 1984.

Loecker TH, Schwartz RS, Cotta CW, Hickman JR Jr: Fluoroscopic coronary artery calcification and associated coronary disease in asymptomatic young men, *J Am Coll Cardiol* 19:1167-1172, 1992.

Milne ENC, Pistolesi M, Miniati M, Giuntini C: The radiologic distinction: cardiogenic and noncardiogenic edema, *AJR Am J Roentgenol* 144:879-894, 1985.

Moore EH, Greenberg RW, Merck SH et al: Coronary artery calcifications: significance of incidental detection on CT scans, *Radiology* 172:711-716, 1989.

Petersen P, Kastrup J, Brinch K et al: Relation between left atrial diameters and duration of atrial fibrillation, *Am J Cardiol* 60:382-384, 1987.

Pistolesi M, Milne ENC, Miniati M, Giuntini C: The vascular pedicle of the heart and the vena azygos, *Radiology* 152:9-17, 1984.

Ravin CE: Pulmonary vascularity: radiographic considerations. *J Thorac Imaging* 3(1):1-13, 1988.

Rose CP, Stolberg HO: The limited utility of the plain chest film in the assessment of left ventricular structure and function, *Invest Radiol* 2:139-144, 1982.

Staub NC: New concepts about pathophysiology of pulmonary edema, *J Thorac Imaging* 3(3):8-14, 1988.

Twigg HL, deLeon AC, Perloff JK, Massoud M: Measurement of the straight-back syndrome, *Radiology* 88:274, 1967.

West JB: Regional differences in the lung, *Chest* 74:426-437, 1978.

Woodring JH: Pulmonary artery–bronchus ratios in patients with normal lungs, pulmonary vascular plethora, and congestive heart failure, *Radiology* 179:115-122, 1991.

CHAPTER 2

Echocardiography

MARY ETTA E. KING

STEFAN MARK NIDORF

The Normal Echocardiographic Examination
Left parasternal imaging planes
Apical imaging planes
Subcostal imaging planes
Suprasternal imaging planes
Right parasternal views
Transesophageal imaging
The Normal Doppler Examination
Parasternal long-axis view
Right ventricular inflow view
Apical views
Other views
Evaluation of Cardiac Chambers: Size and Function
Normal linear dimensions
Left ventricular volume
Left ventricular systolic function from two-dimensional images
Left ventricular systolic function from Doppler echocardiography
Left atrium
Right ventricle
Right atrium
Echocardiographic and Doppler Observations in Valvular Heart Disease
Valvular heart disease
Mitral valve disease
Mitral stenosis
Mitral regurgitation
Mitral valve prolapse
Mitral annular calcification
Rheumatic mitral regurgitation
Flail mitral leaflet
Incomplete mitral valve closure
Assessment of mitral regurgitation
Tricuspid valve disease
Aortic valve disease
Aortic stenosis
Aortic regurgitation
Pulmonary valve disease
Prosthetic heart valves

Infective endocarditis
Assessment of Acquired and Congenital Heart Disease
Ischemic heart disease
Assessing left ventricular regional wall motion
Acute complications of myocardial infarction
Silent changes in myocardial structure following myocardial infarction and ventricular remodeling
Cardiomyopathies
Dilated cardiomyopathy
Hypertrophic cardiomyopathy
Restrictive cardiomyopathy
Pericardial disease
Pericardial effusions and pericardial tamponade
Pericardial constriction
Pericardial cysts
Intracardiac masses
Intracardiac tumors
Intracardiac thrombus
Diseases of the aorta
Proximal aortic disease
Disease of the thoracic and abdominal aorta
Congenital heart disease
Atrial septal defects
Ventricular septal defects
Patent ductus arteriosus
Tetralogy of Fallot
Complete transposition of the great arteries
Truncus arteriosus
Double outlet right ventricle
Univentricular heart
Suggested Readings

Over the past decade there has been an enormous increase in the use of echocardiographic imaging in the routine assessment of patients with suspected or proven heart disease. This is not surprising, since echocardiography has a number of advantages compared with other techniques used to evaluate cardiac structure and function. Specifically, it is portable, noninvasive, and does not expose the patient to ionizing radiation. Further, echocardiography allows the structure of each cardiac chamber to be examined in multiple orthogonal planes. Finally, the addition of Doppler technology to ultrasound imaging permits semiquantitative assessment of regurgitant lesions, the accurate assessment of transvalvular gradients, and the estimation of pulmonary artery pressure. As a result, the combined echo-Doppler examination of the heart is now a routine investigation for establishing the presence, severity, and etiologic factors affecting the cardiac valves, as well as the myocardial and pericardial structures.

THE NORMAL ECHOCARDIOGRAPHIC EXAMINATION

During the routine echocardiographic examination, a fan-shaped beam of ultrasound is directed through a number of selected planes of the heart to record a set of standardized views of the cardiac structures for later analysis (Fig. 2-1). These views are designated by the position of the transducer, the orientation of the viewing plane relative to the primary axis of the heart, and the structures included in the image (Weyman et al, 1982).

Left Parasternal Imaging Planes

To obtain parasternal views of the heart, position the ultrasound transducer between the intercostal spaces along the left parasternal border. From this position, it is possible to obtain both long- and short-axis images of the heart and great vessels. In the *long-axis view,* the scanning plane intersects the aortic and mitral valves and comes as close as possible to the ventricular long-axis (Fig. 2-2). A portion of the right ventricle appears anteriorly, and the right (anterior) and noncoronary cusps of the aortic valve are visible. You can appreciate the relative size and mobility of the anterior and posterior mitral leaflets and the insertion of the chordal apparatus onto the anterior mitral leaflet. Finally, while only the base of the interventricular septum and the posterior wall are routinely visible in this view, you may sometimes appreciate the full length of the left ventricle.

Tilting the transducer cranially in the parasternal position allows visualization of the proximal portion of

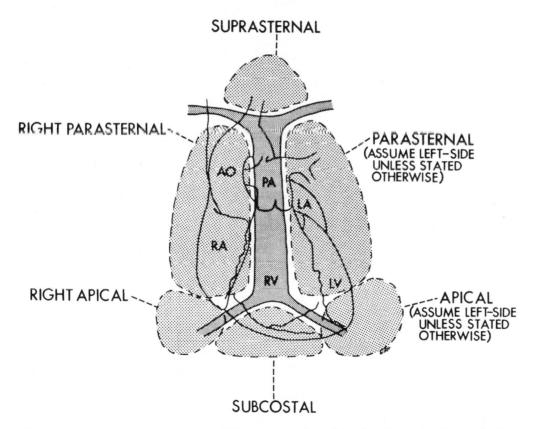

Fig. 2-1   Diagrammatic representation of the anterior surface of the chest illustrating the standard echocardiographic windows (*shaded circles*) and the underlying position of the heart and great vessels. *Ao*=aorta; *LA*=left atrium; *LV*=left ventricle; *RA*=right atrium; *RV*=right ventricle; *PA*=pulmonary artery. (From the *American Society of Echocardiography: Report of the Committee on Nomenclature and Standards in Two-Dimensional Echocardiography.* This figure is reprinted with permission of the American Society of Echocardiography and was originally published in August 1980.)

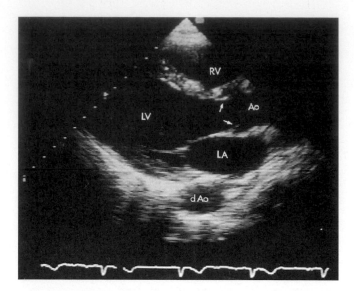

Fig. 2-2 Two-dimensional parasternal echocardiographic view of the long axis of the left ventricle. In this systolic image, the mitral valve leaflets are closed and the aortic valve leaflets *(arrows)* are open. The descending aorta can be seen in cross section as it passes beneath the left atrium. *Ao*=aorta; *dAo*=descending aorta; *LA*=left atrium; *LV*=left ventricle; *RV*=right ventricular outflow tract.

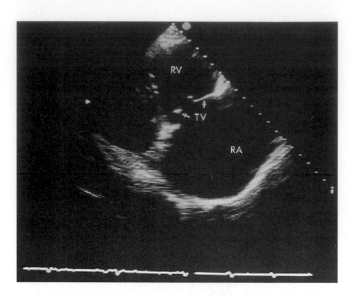

Fig. 2-3 Two-dimensional parasternal echocardiographic view of the long axis of the right heart. The tricuspid valve leaflets *(arrows)* are seen closing in systole. The right atrium is significantly enlarged. *RA*=right atrium; *RV*=right ventricle; *TV*=tricuspid valve.

the aorta. Caudal angulation brings a more complete view of the left ventricular long axis, and rightward angulation allows more complete imaging of the right ventricle. The *right ventricular inflow view* (Fig. 2-3) allows assessment of the right atrium, the proximal portion of the inferior vena cava, and the entry of the coronary sinus, the tricuspid valve, and the base of the right ventricle.

The parasternal short-axis images of the heart are obtained as the transducer is rotated 90 degrees from the long-axis plane and moved from a cranial to a caudal position. In the view at the base of the heart (Fig. 2-4), you can see the right ventricular outflow tract, including the pulmonary valve, the main pulmonary artery, and the right and left pulmonary artery branches. The readily apparent inverted Y in the center of the image is the normal trileaflet aortic valve (in diastole). The left atrium lies posterior to the aorta, and the right atrium, tricuspid valve, and base of the right ventricle lie to the left of the image. With careful scanning in this plane, it is also possible to image the proximal portions of both coronary arteries as they emerge from the aortic root. The right coronary artery usually arises from the right coronary cusp at the 10 o'clock position and the left coronary artery normally arises from the left coronary cusp at the 3 o'clock position.

A series of short-axis images of the left and right ventricles (Figs. 2-5 and 2-6) are created by moving the transducer caudally. In all of these views the heart appears as though viewed from below: the right ventricle is to the

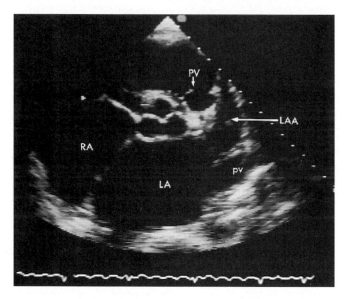

Fig. 2-4 Two-dimensional parasternal short-axis view at the base of the heart. The aortic root with its three aortic sinuses is shown in the center with the left atrium directly posterior to it. A prominent left atrial appendage is present *(long arrow)*, and the left upper pulmonary vein can be seen entering the left atrium. The right ventricular outflow tract lies anterior to the aorta, with the posterior cusp of the pulmonic valve depicted by the *short arrow.* *LA*=left atrium; *LAA*=left atrial appendage; *PV*=pulmonic valve; *pv*=pulmonary vein; *RA*=right atrium.

left of the image and the left ventricle is on the right. The right ventricle appears as a crescentic structure along the right anterior surface of the left ventricle.

The fish-mouthed appearance of the mitral valve characterizes the *short-axis view of the base of the heart*

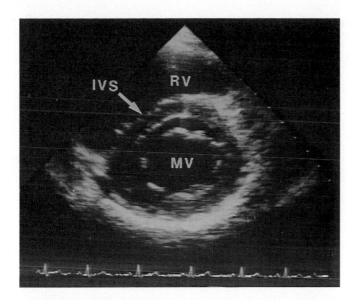

Fig. 2-5 Two-dimensional parasternal short-axis view of the left ventricle at the level of the mitral valve. In diastole, the mitral valve leaflets are open in a "fishmouth" pattern. The left ventricle appears circular and the right ventricle is crescentic in shape. *IVS*=interventricular septum; *MV*=mitral valve; *RV*=right ventricle.

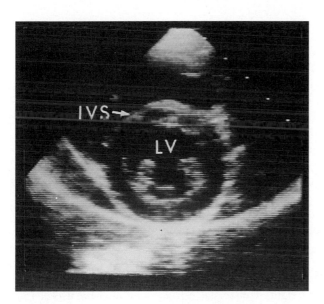

Fig. 2-6 Two-dimensional parasternal short-axis view of the left ventricle at the level of the papillary muscles. Both papillary muscles can be seen projecting into the lumen of the left ventricle. *IVS*=interventricular septum; *LV*=left ventricle.

(see Fig. 2-5). In this view, as at the papillary muscle level, the ventricular myocardium can be divided into segments for the purpose of describing regional function (Fig. 2-7). In the parasternal *short-axis view at the papillary muscle level* you can see both the anterolateral and posteromedial papillary muscles (see Fig. 2-6). Moving the transducer even more caudally allows visualization of the left ventricular apex. The right ventricle is not normally visible at the true apical short-axis level.

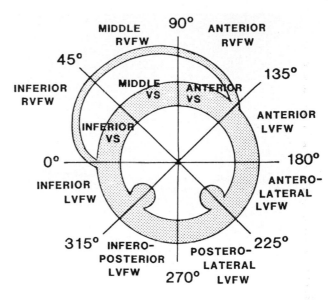

Fig. 2-7 Diagrammatic representation of a cross-sectional view of the heart at the level of the papillary muscles illustrating the subdivision of left and right ventricular myocardium into specific segments. The contractile function of each segment can be evaluated to detect ischemic segmental dysfunction. *LVFW*=left ventricular free wall; *RVFW*=right ventricular free wall; *VS*=ventricular septum. (From Henry WL, et al: *Report of the American Society of Echocardiography Committee on Nomenclature and Standards: identification of myocardial wall segments.* This figure is reprinted with permission of the American Society of Echocardiography and was originally published in 1982.)

Apical Imaging Planes

By placing the transducer at the cardiac apex and orienting the imaging sector toward the base of the heart, it is possible to obtain an *apical four-chamber view of the heart* (Fig. 2-8). This allows visualization of all chambers of the heart, as well as the tricuspid and mitral valves. As the transducer is rotated 45 degrees clockwise to this plane, you can see the apical long-axis view of the heart, and further clockwise rotation of the transducer to a full 90 degrees produces the apical two-chamber view. The *apical two-chamber view* is important because it allows direct visualization of the true inferior and anterior wall of the ventricle. Superficial angulation of the scanning plane from the apical four-chamber view brings the left ventricular outflow tract and aortic valve into view, producing the five-chamber view (Fig. 2-9).

Subcostal Imaging Planes

The subcostal window allows visualization of each of the short-axis images, as well as a four-chamber view of the heart. You can often see the interatrial septum, the inferior vena cava and hepatic veins, the liver, and the abdominal aorta (Fig. 2-10). This window is important because in some instances, as in the intensive care

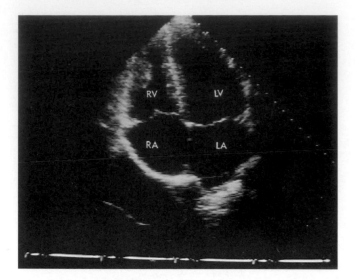

Fig. 2-8 Two-dimensional apical four-chamber echocardiographic view of the heart. To obtain this view, the transducer is placed at the cardiac apex. This produces an image in which the apex and ventricular chambers of the heart are at the top of the image sector and the atria are in the far field of the image. By convention, the left heart structures are positioned to the right of the image. *LA*=left atrium; *LV*=left ventricle; *RA*=right atrium; *RV*=right ventricle.

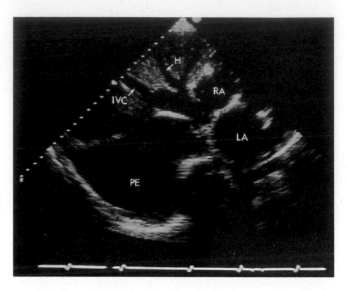

Fig. 2-10 Two-dimensional subcostal view demonstrating the inferior vena cava and hepatic veins entering the right atrium. A portion of the interatrial septum is present between the right and left atrial chambers. This patient has a large pleural effusion. *H*=hepatic vein; *IVC*=inferior vena cava; *LA*=left atrium; *RA*=right atrium; *PE*=pleural effusion.

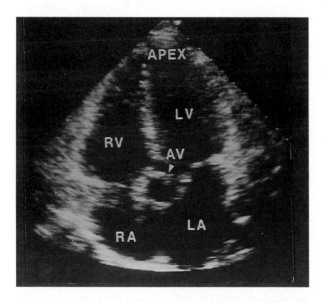

Fig. 2-9 Two-dimensional apical five-chamber echocardiographic view of the heart. From the apical four-chamber view, the transducer is angled superiorly to view the left ventricular outflow tract and aortic valve *(arrowhead)*. *AV*=aortic valve; *LA*=left atrium; *LV*=left ventricle; *RA*=right atrium; *RV*=right ventricle.

unit (ICU) setting, it may be the only viewpoint from which to image the heart in the patient with bandages on the chest wall, lung disease, or pneumothorax. In infants and small children the subcostal window provides excellent images of all cardiac structures (Lange et al, 1979).

Suprasternal Imaging Planes

Suprasternal views are obtained in both longitudinal and transverse planes. The longitudinal plane orients through the long axis of the aorta and includes the innominate, left common carotid, and left subclavian arteries (Fig. 2-11). The transverse plane includes a cross section through the ascending aorta, with the right pulmonary artery crossing behind. Portions of the innominate vein and superior vena cava are visible anterior to the aorta. The left atrium and pulmonary veins are posterior to the right pulmonary artery (Fig. 2-12).

Right Parasternal Views

The right parasternal border may also be useful for viewing the heart in either transverse or longitudinal orientations. These views are particularly helpful with medially positioned hearts, right ventricular enlargement, and rightward orientation of the ascending aorta. By allowing direct visualization of the right atrium, both venae cavae, and the interatrial septum, this view is also of particular value in the assessment of interatrial shunt flow, and in the detection of anomalous pulmonary venous drainage.

Transesophageal Imaging

The esophagus is a valuable "window" to the heart and great vessels, especially in patients in whom transthoracic imaging is limited either by body habitus or lung disease

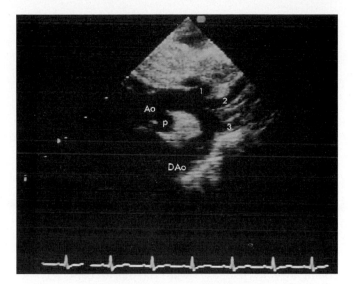

Fig. 2-11 Two-dimensional suprasternal long-axis view of the aortic arch. The proximal portions of the brachiocephalic vessels are demonstrated arising from the aortic arch—*(1)* right brachiocephalic artery, *(2)* left common carotid artery, and *(3)* left subclavian artery. The right pulmonary artery can be seen in cross section as it passes beneath the ascending aorta. *Ao*=ascending aorta; *DAo*=descending aorta; *p*=right pulmonary artery.

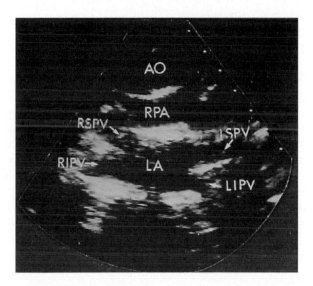

Fig. 2-12 Two-dimensional suprasternal short-axis echocardiographic view of the aortic arch. The right pulmonary artery crosses beneath the aorta and the pulmonary veins enter the left atrium with a "crablike" appearance. *Ao*=aorta; *LA*=left atrium; *LIPV*=left inferior pulmonary vein; *LSPV*=left superior pulmonary vein; *RIPV*=right inferior pulmonary vein; *RPA*=right pulmonary artery; *RSPV*=right superior pulmonary vein.

(Nanda et al, 1990). Further, transesophageal imaging is valuable in the operating room and intensive care setting where it can help assess ventricular function or the adequacy of surgical repair of cardiac defects.

Transesophageal imaging uses a specially designed ultrasound probe incorporated within a standard gastro-

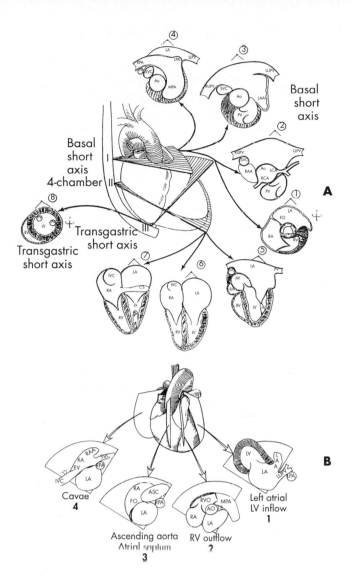

Fig. 2-13 Diagrammatic representation of the standard imaging planes obtained with biplane transesophageal echocardiography. **A** demonstrates the horizontal planes. The transesophageal echo probe is shown following the course of the esophagus behind the heart. Horizontal sections are shown at the base of the heart (level *I*), at the midesophageal level (level *II*), and from within the stomach (level *III*). The corresponding echocardiographic images from each of these levels are depicted around the periphery of the diagram. **B** demonstrates the vertical planes obtained from the transesophageal probe. These planes pass through a more longitudinal axis of the heart. The corresponding echocardiographic images from each of several levels within the esophagus are shown by *arrows*. *Ao*=aorta; *Asc*=ascending aorta; *CS*=coronary sinus; *EV*=eustacian valve; *FO*=foramen ovale; *IVC*=inferior vena cava; *LA*=left atrium; *LAA*=left atrial appendage; *LCA*=left coronary artery; *LLPV*=left lower pulmonary vein; *LPA*=left pulmonary artery; *LUPV*=left upper pulmonary vein; *LV*=left ventricle; *MPA*=main pulmonary artery, *PV*=pulmonary valve; *RA*=right atrium; *RAA*=right atrial appendage; *RCA*=right coronary artery; *RLPV*=right lower pulmonary vein; *RPA*=right pulmonary artery; *RUPV*=right upper pulmonary vein; *RV*=right ventricle; *RVO*=right ventricular outflow tract; *SVC*=superior vena cava. (Modified from Seward JB, et al: Transesophageal echocardiography: technique, anatomic correlations, implementation, and clinical applications, *Mayo Clin Proc* 63:655, 1988; and Seward JB, et al: Biplanar transesophageal echocardiography: anatomic correlations, image orientation, and clinical applications, *Mayo Clin Proc* 65:1197, 1990.)

scope. This semiinvasive procedure requires blind esophageal intubation. Because of the close proximity of the heart to the imaging transducer, high-frequency transducers (5.0-7.5 MHz) are routinely used which allows better definition of small structures than the lower frequencies used transthoracically (2.5-3.5 MHz). Therefore, transesophageal imaging is particularly valuable in the routine clinical setting for the detection of atrial thrombi, small vegetations, diseases of the aorta, atrial septal defects, and the assessment of prosthetic valve function.

Current instrumentation allows imaging of both transverse and longitudinal planes with a biplane or multiplane transesophageal probe. The anteroposterior orientation of images from the esophagus is the reverse of images from the transthoracic window since the ultrasound beam first encounters structures closest to the esophagus (Fig. 2-13).

THE NORMAL DOPPLER EXAMINATION

By applying the Doppler principle to ultrasound, you can analyze the frequency shift of ultrasound waves reflected from moving red blood cells to determine the velocity and direction of blood flow. This can be done with either pulsed Doppler or continuous wave Doppler (Nishimura et al, 1985). While pulsed Doppler allows

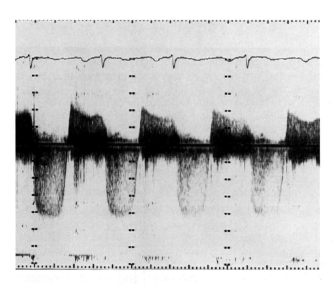

Fig. 2-14 Continuous wave Doppler spectral tracing of flow across the mitral valve from the apical window. In diastole, flow is recorded above the baseline as blood moves toward the transducer at the apex across the mitral valve into the left ventricle. In systole, mitral regurgitant flow is shown below the baseline as it passes away from the apex and into the left atrium. The *dotted lines* are scale markers indicating flow velocity, each demarcation in this case representing 1 m/sec. This patient with rheumatic mitral stenosis has high velocity mitral inflow (2 m/sec) and mitral regurgitation (4.2 m/sec).

analysis of the velocity and direction of blood flow in a particular region, continuous wave Doppler allows resolution and analysis of high-velocity flow along the entire length of the Doppler beam. In both instances the data can be displayed graphically (Fig. 2-14). By convention, flow toward the interrogating transducer is represented as a deflection above, and flow away from the transducer appears as a deflection below the baseline. The x-axis represents time (American Society of Echocardiography, 1984a).

Color-flow mapping also uses pulsed Doppler methodology, but maps flow velocity at multiple sites within an area and overlays this information on a black-and-white two-dimensional image. By convention, color coding for flow velocity toward the transducer is red and flow velocity away from the transducer is blue. Higher velocities are mapped as brighter shades. The addition of yellow and green to the underlying red or blue color map indicates turbulent flow.

Parasternal Long-Axis View

In practice, the routine Doppler examination is integrated with the sequence of imaging described above (Kostucki et al, 1986). Therefore, initial interrogation of the flow patterns associated with the aortic and mitral valves begins in the parasternal long-axis view. In this view, color Doppler is particularly useful because it provides a rapid means of detecting regurgitant flow across the aortic and mitral valves. In this plane, mitral regurgitation usually appears as a discrete blue jet because blood is flowing away from the transducer (Fig. 2-15). Aortic regurgitation may appear as either a blue or red jet emanating from the closed aortic valve in diastole. The color depends on the orientation of the aortic valve and outflow tract relative to the transducer. Small jets of mitral regurgitation are frequent in otherwise normal valves. In contrast, aortic regurgitation of any degree is usually considered abnormal (Choong et al, 1989).

Right Ventricular Inflow View

As the examination proceeds to the right ventricular inflow view, color Doppler can detect flow into the right atrium. Normally, flow from the inferior vena cava is observed as a continuous red jet entering the atrium from below. Pulsed Doppler can confirm the direction and velocity of this flow, which is normally less than 1.0 m/sec. Flow can also be seen to enter the right atrium from the coronary sinus, and frequently some degree of tricuspid regurgitation is also evident. In this view, the jet of tricuspid regurgitant flow appears blue since blood is moving away from the transducer. Small jets of tricuspid regurgitation are considered physiologic and are thought to be due to retrograde flow generated dur-

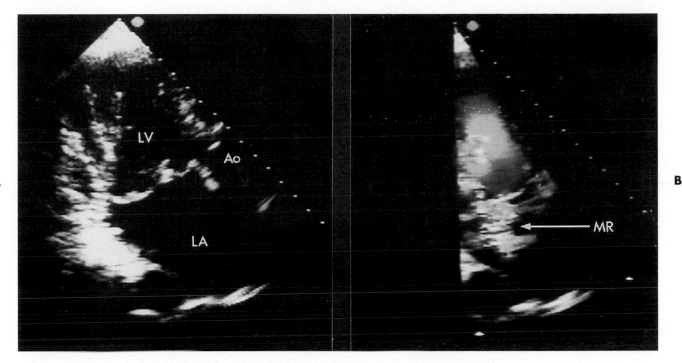

Fig. 2-15   **A** illustrates a two-dimensional apical echocardiographic view of the mitral valve in systole. **B** shows the superimposed color Doppler flow map. A central stream of mitral regurgitation *(arrow)* is shown emerging from the leaflet coaptation point and spreading into the left atrium. The jet is blue (indicating flow away from the transducer) with yellows and greens to reflect turbulent flow. *Ao*=aorta; *LA*=left atrium; *LV*=left ventricle; *MR*=mitral regurgitation. (This figure is reproduced in color before page 1.)

ing valve closure (Choong et al, 1989). Typically, these small jets are of low velocity and may not be pansystolic. Pulsed Doppler can confirm the presence of tricuspid regurgitation, and continuous wave Doppler can assess the peak velocity of regurgitant flow from the right ventricle to the right atrium. Pulsed Doppler can also determine the velocity of antegrade flow across the tricuspid valve in diastole. Normally, the right ventricular inflow Doppler profile is biphasic and of low velocity (<0.6 m/sec) (Kostucki et al, 1986).

From short-axis images at the level of the aortic valve (see Fig. 2-3) it is also possible to assess systolic and diastolic flow across the tricuspid valve. Flow from the inferior vena cava appears as a continuous low-velocity (red) jet emanating from its point of entry into the floor of the right atrium adjacent to the interatrial septum. In children, caval flow can be quite vigorous and may be confused with left-to-right interatrial shunt flow. Interrogation of the pulmonary valve in this plane almost invariably identifies some degree of pulmonary regurgitation, which is visible as a small red jet moving toward the transducer (Choong et al, 1989). Pulsed Doppler can usually confirm the presence of diastolic flow and examine the velocity of flow proximal and distal to the pulmonary valve. The normal velocity of flow across the pulmonary outflow tract is less than 1.5 m/sec (Kostucki et al, 1986).

Values higher than this generally indicate right ventricular outflow obstruction or high flow states.

Apical Views

Further interrogation of valvular flow is performed from apical views. The apical four-chamber view best evaluates flow across the mitral and tricuspid valves, and the apical five-chamber view is useful to assess flow across the aortic valve. These views are of particular value for Doppler assessment of transvalvular flow, since in this plane the Doppler beam is most nearly parallel to the direction of blood flow.

Assessment of diastolic flow across the mitral valve is performed by placing the pulsed Doppler sample volume on the ventricular side of the mitral leaflets, near the valve tips. The normal left ventricular inflow Doppler profile is biphasic (Fig. 2-16). The initial positive deflection (E wave) represents early passive ventricular filling that begins with mitral opening. The subsequent deflection (A wave) reflects the late phase of ventricular filling that occurs as a consequence of atrial contraction. Normally the E wave velocity is less than 1.2 m/sec, and A wave velocity is 0.8 m/sec (Kostucki et al, 1986).

Apical images allow assessment of pulmonary venous inflow and may use either color or pulsed Doppler. In

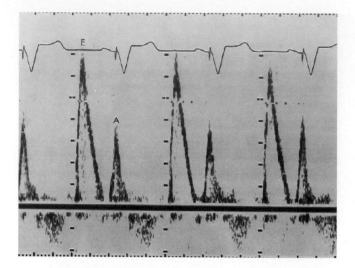

Fig. 2-16 Pulsed Doppler spectral profile of mitral inflow obtained from an apical window. Flow toward the transducer is shown above the baseline in diastole during left ventricular filling. The typical mitral biphasic filling pattern is seen, with a prominent early filling wave (E wave) and smaller late diastolic filling wave (A wave).

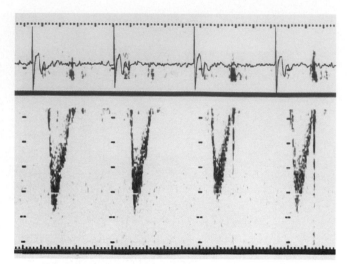

Fig. 2-17 Pulsed Doppler spectral profile of aortic outflow obtained from an apical window. Flow velocities are plotted below the baseline to indicate that the direction of flow is away from the apically positioned transducer. The typical aortic flow profile is a systolic flow with rapid upstroke to a peak velocity in midsystole and rapid decline in velocity during late systole.

order to assess pulmonary inflow by pulsed Doppler, however, it is necessary to place the sample volume 1 to 2 cm into the pulmonary vein. Pulmonary inflow is then biphasic, with accentuated flow toward the transducer in both systole and diastole.

Moving the sample volume to the left ventricular outflow tract enables comparison of flow velocity in this region with that above the aortic valve. From apical views, the aortic outflow Doppler profile appears as a single uniform systolic profile with a peak velocity of less than 1.5 m/sec. In contrast to the mitral inflow signal, aortic flow in this view is a negative deflection, since flow is moving away from the Doppler transducer (Kostucki et al, 1986) (Fig. 2-17).

Other Views

Finally, subcostal views are useful for assessing flow within the inferior vena cava, hepatic veins, and abdominal aorta. The suprasternal window is used for recording flow in the ascending aorta and superior vena cava.

EVALUATION OF CARDIAC CHAMBERS: SIZE AND FUNCTION

Normal Linear Dimensions

By convention, most laboratories report the size of the left atrium, aortic root, and left ventricle from measurement of the linear dimensions of each structure in the parasternal long-axis view of the heart (American

Society of Echocardiography, 1984b) (Table 2-1). All linear dimensions have been shown to bear a direct linear relation to body height (Nidorf et al, 1992). Normal chamber dimensions have also been determined for each of the standard two-dimensional views to allow quantitative assessment of each chamber or great vessel from any view (Triulzi, 1984).

Left Ventricular Volume

There are a number of methods for calculating left ventricular volume from two-dimensional echocardiographic images (Triulzi et al, 1982) (Fig. 2-18). To do this, it is usually necessary to make an assumption about the geometric shape of the left ventricle so that linear measurements can be fitted into the appropriate formulas for the volume of the assumed geometric shape.

The most widely used method employs a standard ellipsoid formula which requires measuring the length of the ventricle and its diameter at the base. Alternatively, Simpson's rule can be used to measure left ventricular volume. This requires measuring of the length of the ventricle from apical views and then determining the volume of a predefined number of disklike cross-sectional segments from base to apex, each of which is assumed to be elliptical. While both methods of volume estimation are valid in normal (symmetric) left ventricles, they are less reliable when there is a distortion of ventricular shape (such as following myocardial infarction). Although not yet commercially available, there are methods for reconstructing the

Table 2-1 Mitral Stenosis Evaluation by Echocardiography

	Grade 1	Grade 2	Grade 3	Grade 4
Leaflet mobility	Highly mobile valve with restriction at the leaflet tips	Midportion and base of leaflets have reduced mobility	Valve leaflets move forward in diastole mainly at the base	No or minimal forward movement of the leaflets in diastole
Subvalvular thickening	Minimal thickening of chordal structures below the valve	Thickening of chordae extending up to one third of chordal length	Thickening extending to the distal third of the chordae	Extensive thickening and shortening of all chordae extending to the papillary muscle
Valvular thickening	Normal (4–5 mm thick)	Midleaflets thickening	Diffuse thickening (5–8 mm)	Marked thickening of all leaflet tissues (>8–10 mm)
Valvular calcification	Single area of increased echo brightness	Scattered areas of brightness confined to leaflet margins	Brightness extending into the midportion of leaflets	Extensive brightness through most of the leaflet tissue

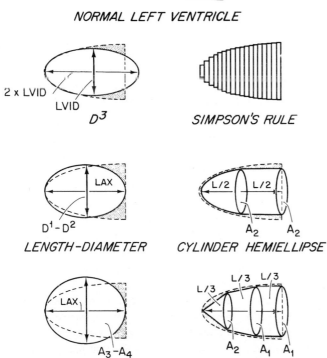

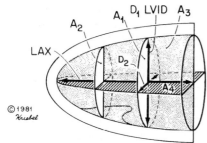

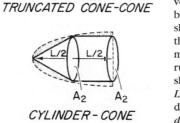

Fig. 2-18 Diagrammatic representation of the left ventricle showing the geometric models that have been used to calculate left ventricular volume. The shaded figure indicates the true chamber volume with the superimposed solid figure demonstrating the geometric shape described by the formula. The Simpson's rule method comes closest to approximating the true shape of the ventricle. A=area; D=diameter; L=length; LAX=long axis length; LVID=left ventricular internal dimension. (From Weyman AE: *Cross-sectional echocardiography*, Philadelphia, 1982, Lea and Febiger.)

three-dimensional shape of the left ventricle from two-dimensional images (Handschumacher et al, 1993). These three-dimensional methods of volume determination make no assumptions about ventricular shape and can accurately determine the volume of both normal and distorted ventricles in invivo models (Siu et al, 1992a,b).

Left Ventricular Systolic Function from Two-Dimensional Images

Real-time echocardiographic assessment of endocardial motion and the degree of wall thickening during systole allows excellent qualitative assessment of global and regional ventricular function (Mann et al, 1986). Using this method, systolic function can be described as either normal or depressed, and regional function is either normal, hyperkinetic, hypokinetic, akinetic, or dyskinetic.

More quantitative assessment of ventricular function is available by estimating the global ejection fraction, determined by calculating either the change in cross-sectional area or change in volume of the ventricle between diastole and systole. In practice, there is good correlation between echocardiographic and both angiographic and radionuclide estimates of ventricular ejection fraction, even when using simple geometric assumptions about ventricular shape (Starling et al, 1981).

By far the simplest method of estimating ejection fraction (EF) is to assume that the change in area at the base of the ventricle is representative of global ventricular function (Quinones et al, 1981). In this way:

$$EF(\%) = \frac{LVIDD^2 - LVISD^2}{LVIDD^2} \times 100$$

Where LVIDD = the internal diameter of the base of the ventricle in diastole; and LVISD = the internal diameter of the ventricle in systole. Since this formula fails to account for apical function, 10% is empirically added if function at the apex is normal, 5% is added if the apex is hypokinetic, and 5% to 10% is subtracted if the apex is dyskinetic (Starling et al, 1981). The development of automated endocardial border detection now makes it possible to obtain an on-line estimate of ejection fraction based on changes in cavity area (Morrissey et al, 1993).

You can also estimate the ejection fraction by assessing the change in ventricular volume during the cardiac cycle using a simple formula which assumes that the left ventricle is spherical:

$$EF(\%) = \frac{LVIDD^3 - LVISD^3}{LVIDD^3} \times 100$$

Methods that estimate ejection fraction based on a single dimension obtained at the base of the heart, however, tend to overestimate global function in patients with apical infarction, and underestimate global function in patients with inferior basal infarctions.

Although more difficult to use, Simpson's rule generally provides a more accurate estimate of ejection fraction because it removes some of the assumptions about ventricular geometry. To perform the Simpson's rule calculation, outline the full ventricular contour from the apical view, and draw a midline between the ventricular apex and the midpoint of the mitral annular plane. Then divide the ventricle into a series of small parallel disks of equal height which run perpendicular to the midline. Since you know the radius and height of each disk, you can calculate its volume. Summing the volume of each disk allows calculation of the ventricular volume. The only limitation is the inability to image the true length of the ventricle in some patients. Nonetheless, this method has been automated for clinical use, and its accuracy can be improved by averaging the estimates of ventricular volume in each systole and diastole from apical four- and apical two-chamber views.

Because all current echocardiographic estimates of ejection fraction make a number of assumptions about ventricular shape, they are most useful in normal or symmetrically dilated hearts. The application of three-dimensional technology, when it becomes commercially available, will have the potential to overcome the problems of estimating left ventricular ejection fraction in distorted ventricles (Handschumacher et al, 1993).

Left Ventricular Systolic Function from Doppler Echocardiography

Doppler echocardiography makes it possible to estimate stroke volume and cardiac output by measuring volumetric flow through the heart (Nishimura et al, 1985). Stroke volume is calculated by measuring the cross-sectional area of a vessel or valve, and then integrating the flow velocities across that specific region in the vessel or valve throughout the period of flow. The product of stroke volume and heart rate then gives an estimate of cardiac output (Fig. 2-19).

While cardiac output can be determined from the pulmonary, mitral, or tricuspid transvalvular flows, the aortic valve diameter and flow velocities are the most accurate and reproducible (Gillam et al, 1985; Labovitz, 1985). Further, there is excellent correlation between Doppler and roller pump estimates of stroke volume (Elkayam et al, 1983). In clinical practice, inaccuracies in measurement of the area of the outflow tract limit the use of Doppler estimates of cardiac output. This technique is successful, however, in following relative changes in cardiac output following pharmacologic intervention, since the area of the outflow tract is assumed to remain constant (Fisher et al, 1983).

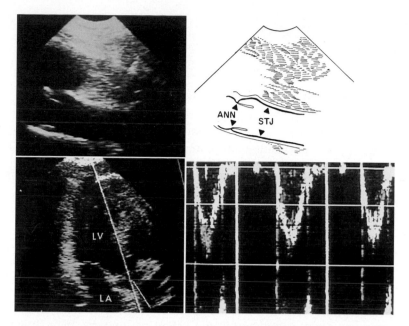

Fig. 2-19 Diagrammatic demonstration of the method for measuring aortic flow by echo-Doppler techniques. The upper left panel is a two-dimensional image of the ascending aorta in systole with the aortic leaflets open. The upper right diagram demonstrates the points of measurement of the aortic annular diameter *(ANN)*. In the lower left panel, the pulsed Doppler sample volume is positioned within the aortic valve leaflets from the apical window in order to record the highest velocity across the aortic valve. The lower right panel depicts the pulsed Doppler profile of aortic flow from which the systolic velocity integral is obtained by tracing the area under the flow envelope. *ANN*=annulus; *D*=diameter; *LA*=left atrium; *LV*=left ventricle. (Reprinted with permission from the American College of Cardiology from Stewart WJ, et al: Variable effects of changes in flow rate through the aortic, pulmonary and mitral valves on valve area and flow velocity: impact on quantitative Doppler flow calculations, *J Am Coll Cardiol* 6:655, 1985.)

Left Atrium

Unlike the left ventricle, the left atrium lacks internal structures that can be used to standardize the measurement of its dimension. Because of this, it is conventional to measure the anteroposterior dimension of the atrium at end-systole in the parasternal long-axis view from a line drawn through the plane of the aortic valve (Triulzi et al, 1984). Atrial enlargement may occur as a consequence of either an increase in atrial pressure (due to mitral stenosis or elevated left ventricular end-diastolic pressure), an increase in volume (as in mitral regurgitation), or as a consequence of primary atrial dysfunction (as in atrial fibrillation).

The left atrial appendage is a "dog ear"-shaped extension of the atrium situated along the lateral aspect of the chamber near the mitral annulus. Although usually inconspicuous, it is easily visible in the parasternal short-axis (see Fig. 2-4) and apical two-chamber views of the atria when there is a dilated left atrium. It is important to realize that the appendage is a trabeculated structure. These trabeculae may be confused with thrombus, which frequently forms within the appendage in patients with mitral valve disease.

Right Ventricle

Morphologically, the right ventricle can be divided into an inflow portion that includes the heavily trabeculated body of the ventricle, and an outflow portion that includes the infundibulum. The inflow portion extends from the tricuspid valve to the apex. The right ventricle generally has a crescentic shape when viewed in short axis, with its medial border formed from the convexity of the interventricular septum. The lateral, or free wall of the right ventricle normally has a radius of curvature approximately equal to the left ventricular free wall. Because of the complex shape of the right ventricle, it is less amenable to geometric modeling than the left ventricle. Therefore, although there are simple, valid two-dimensional echocardiographic criteria for estimating right ventricular volume in nondistorted hearts (Levine et al, 1984), newer sophisticated three-dimensional echocardiographic techniques are more reliable in assessing right ventricular volume (Jiang et al, 1992).

Right ventricular enlargement may occur as a consequence of right ventricular volume loading, right ventricular infarction, or as part of a generalized cardiomyopathic process. In each instance, as dilation progresses the anteroposterior dimension of the ventricle increases and septal motion becomes increasingly abnormal. Specifically, in diastole the septum may appear to flatten, especially at the base, and in early systole the septum may move rightward (paradoxically) rather than leftward.

Pressure loading of the right ventricle results in progressive hypertrophy (Fig. 2-20). This may be difficult to discern with confidence because of the degree of trabeculation of the chamber. A free wall thickness of greater than 5 mm is a quantitative criterion for right ventricular hypertrophy (Weyman et al, 1982). When marked, pressure overloading typically produces systolic flattening of the interventricular septum.

Right Atrium

Assessment of right atrial size is usually made qualitatively by comparing it to the left atrium in the apical four-chamber view. There are several normal structures within the right atrium. These include the eustachian valve, which crosses from the inferior vena cava to the region of the foramen ovale, and the crista terminalis. In the apical four-chamber view, a ridge of tissue that separates the smooth-walled portion of the right atrium from its trabeculated anterior portion is seen frequently as a small mass of echoes located adjacent to the superior border of the right atrium. The right atrial appendage is a broad-based triangular structure that lies anterior to the atrial chamber near the ascending aorta. It is most visible in the parasternal views of the right atrium.

ECHOCARDIOGRAPHIC AND DOPPLER OBSERVATIONS IN VALVULAR HEART DISEASE

Valvular Heart Disease

Mitral valve disease

Mitral stenosis   Although the diagnosis and timing of intervention for mitral stenosis is usually clinical, echocardiographic and Doppler techniques contribute significantly to the assessment of the severity of the valvular disease. Specifically, these techniques provide accurate assessment of valve area, valve morphology, and the degree of pulmonary hypertension.

Acquired mitral stenosis is almost invariably caused by scarring and inflammation of the valve and chordal apparatus from past rheumatic fever (Braunwald, 1992). As a consequence of the disease the mitral leaflets and chordal apparatus become diffusely thickened. Subsequently the valvular apparatus may shorten, fuse together at the commissural margins, and finally calcify. This results in a reduction in leaflet excursion so that the mitral leaflets appear to dome during diastole (Fig. 2-21). As the degree of valvular obstruction increases, flow through the valve decreases, left atrial pressure begins to rise, left atrial size increases (in the apical views, the interatrial septum is seen to bow to the right), and the potential for intraatrial thrombus formation is increased. Typically, the left ventricular size is normal or even small. If there is severe mitral stenosis, there may be paradoxical septal motion

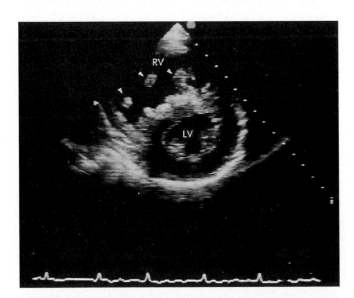

Fig. 2-20 Parasternal short-axis echocardiographic view of the left and right ventricles at the papillary muscle level. The right ventricle is enlarged. Hypertrophy of the free wall and septum and prominent right ventricular papillary muscles *(arrowheads)* are evident. *LV*=left ventricle; *RV*=right ventricle.

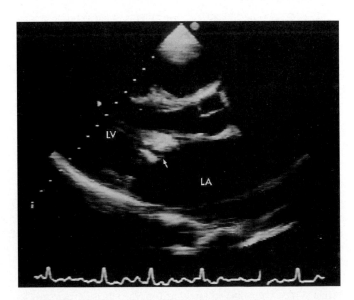

Fig. 2-21 Parasternal long-axis echocardiographic view of the left atrium and left ventricle demonstrating marked calcification of the mitral valve leaflet tips. Instead of opening widely, the leaflets dome in diastole and the mitral orifice is severely restricted *(arrow)*. *LA*=left atrium; *LV*=left ventricle.

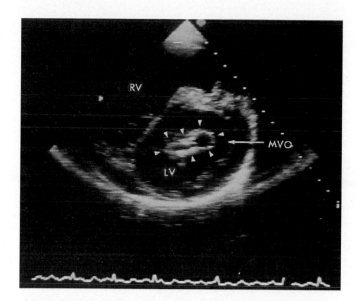

Fig. 2-22 Parasternal short-axis echocardiographic view of the right and left ventricles at the mitral valve level. The mitral valve leaflets are thickened and the valve orifice is eccentrically restricted *(arrowheads)*. The medial commissure is more tightly fused than the lateral commissure resulting in a larger orifice along the lateral aspect of the valve. Enlargement of the right ventricle is also demonstrated. *LV*=left ventricle; *MVO*=mitral valve orifice; *RV*=right ventricle.

as a consequence of slow ventricular filling. Further, if there is pulmonary hypertension, the right heart and the pulmonary arteries may dilate and there may be severe tricuspid regurgitation. Almost all of these morphologic features are evident from the parasternal long-axis view of the heart; however, parasternal short-axis images are essential for planimetry of the mitral valve orifice (Fig. 2-22).

Echocardiographic grading of the severity of mitral stenosis is possible by assessing the degree of leaflet thickening, calcification, and mobility, as well as the degree of chordal thickening and shortening (Weyman et al, 1982) (see Table 2-1). When systematically graded, a low value of 1 to a high value of 4 is given for each of these characteristics. It is then possible to derive a numeric "score" which describes the extent of the mitral valve disease (Abascal et al, 1990). This system is helpful in predicting the likelihood of successful balloon dilatation of the valve, with scores greater than 8 predicting a poor outcome following percutaneous dilatation (Wilkins et al, 1988b).

Direct planimetry of the valve orifice in the short-axis plane can provide an accurate measurement of the mitral valve area (Weyman et al, 1982). This estimate correlates well with the mitral valve orifice measured directly on pathologic study or surgery, and with the estimate of valve area obtained by cardiac catheterization (Martin et al, 1979). It is important to note, however, that measure-

ment of the mitral valve orifice by planimetry is sensitive to gain and depth (which alter the lateral resolution of the image and reduce the ability to accurately define the valve orifice), and to the viewing plane, which may not pass directly through the smallest portion of the mitral valve orifice. Further, in some patients the valve is so calcified that no orifice is readily discernible.

Continuous wave Doppler can help assess the severity of mitral stenosis because it enables calculations of the peak and mean transmitral gradients, and the mitral valve area (Nishimura et al, 1985). For this purpose the apical four-chamber view is best so that the Doppler beam can be directed through to the mitral valve plane, parallel to the direction of left ventricular inflow. In contrast to the Doppler profile through a normal mitral valve, the continuous wave Doppler signal in patients with mitral stenosis demonstrates an increased velocity of flow in early diastole, with a prolonged descent of the early filling (E) wave which may merge into the late filling (A) wave (Fig. 2-23). In patients with atrial fibrillation, the A wave, which reflects atrial contraction, is absent. It is important to note that the degree of prolongation of the phase of early filling relates directly to mitral valve area and to the severity of mitral stenosis.

Once you obtain the continuous wave Doppler profile, it is possible to calculate the transmitral gradient by converting the velocity information provided by the Doppler signal into an estimate of pressure using the simplified Bernoulli equation. In essence, the *Bernoulli theorem* states that the velocity (V) of flow across a stenosis relates to the pressure difference (P) across the stenosis. Specifically, the *simplified Bernoulli equation* predicts that the pressure gradient across a valve approximates a value four times the square of the velocity of flow across the valve ($P = 4 V^2$) (Holen et al, 1976).

Knowing the peak velocity of flow across the mitral valve, therefore, enables calculation of the peak pressure gradient across the valve. Similarly, the average of the velocities throughout all of diastole yields the mean gradient. Most commercial echo-Doppler machines contain software that can automatically integrate the velocity profile once it is traced, and then calculate the mean gradient using the Bernoulli equation. In general, the gradient across the mitral valve obtained by Doppler correlates well with that obtained at catheterization.

Doppler estimates of mitral valve area rely on the observation that the degree of prolongation of early filling (E wave) relates directly to the degree of mitral stenosis. Quantification of this is possible by calculating the time for the pressure gradient across the mitral valve to fall to half its peak value ($P_{1/2}$). To calculate $P_{1/2}$ from the continuous wave Doppler profile you must determine the velocity of flow across the valve when the peak transmitral pressure falls to half its value ($V_{1/2}$). Since peak pressure (P_1) = $4(V_1)^2$, the equation

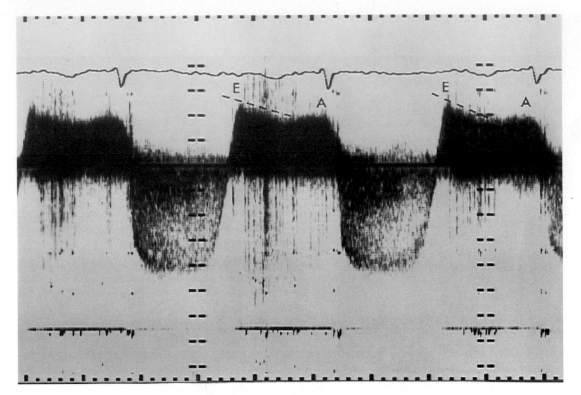

Fig. 2-23 Continuous wave Doppler profile of transmitral flow in mitral stenosis and mitral regurgitation. The transducer is placed at the cardiac apex to interrogate flow across the mitral valve. Flow in diastole is above the baseline, indicating diastolic flow into the ventricle across the valve. Flow in systole is below the baseline as regurgitant flow passes away from the apex into the left atrium. The peak velocity of forward flow *(E)* is increased and the early diastolic slope of the flow velocity *(dotted line)* is delayed. With atrial contraction *(A)*, flow accelerates across the valve and then stops with valve closure in systole. The broad, rounded systolic profile is typical of mitral insufficiency. *E*=early diastolic filling wave; *A*=atrial filling wave.

for *velocity* at the time the pressure gradient has fallen to half its original value is as follows (Hatle et al, 1979; Smith et al, 1986):

Eq. 1 $P_{half} = P_1/2 = 2(V_1)^2$
Eq. 2 $P_{half} = 4(V_{half})^2$
Hence: $4(V_{half})^2 = 2(V_1)^2$
             $V_{half} = V_1/\sqrt{2}$

Once you know P_1 and $V_{1/2}$, you can determine the pressure half-time directly from the Doppler profile (Fig. 2-24). In normal subjects, the pressure half-time is less than 60 ms. In contrast, in patients with mitral stenosis the half-time is usually in excess of 200 ms, with higher values in patients with more severe disease. An empirical formula that relates pressure half-time to the mitral valve area is: Area = $220/P_{1/2}$. This is fairly accurate compared with estimates of valve area determined by catheterization (Hatle et al, 1979; Holen et al, 1976). From this empirical formula, patients with a pressure half-time of greater than 220 ms have a mitral valve area equal to or less than 1.0 cm².

Mitral regurgitation

MITRAL VALVE PROLAPSE Mitral valve prolapse is the most common cause of mitral regurgitation leading to mitral valve surgery in the United States today (Braunwald, 1992). The disease is a degenerative disorder that primarily affects the collagen of the mitral leaflets and chordae; however, it may also affect the aortic and tricuspid valve. Although often diagnosed clinically by the presence of a murmur or click, echocardiography is frequently used to confirm the diagnosis.

Echocardiographically, mitral valve prolapse is suggested by the superior displacement of one or both of the mitral valve leaflets into the atrium during systole. This determination should be made from the parasternal or apical long-axis views and not from the apical four-chamber view. Because of the complex saddle shape of the mitral annulus, minor degrees of superior displacement of the anterior leaflet may normally be recorded from the apical four-chamber view (Warth et al, 1985). Therefore, the diagnosis of mitral valve prolapse should only be made when the long-axis views show leaflet displacement (Levine et al, 1988). In patients with more

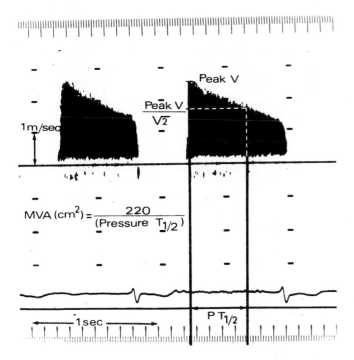

$$MVA\ (cm^2) = \frac{220}{(Pressure\ T_{1/2})}$$

Fig. 2-24 Diagrammatic representation of the continuous wave Doppler flow profile in mitral stenosis. An estimate of the mitral valve area can be made by measuring the time it takes for the transmitral pressure to fall to one half of its initial value—the "pressure half-time." The Doppler equivalent of this principle is the "velocity half-time." The peak velocity across the mitral valve *(Peak V)* is divided by $\sqrt{2}$. The point at which this velocity intersects the slope of the velocity profile *(dotted lines)* is the velocity half-time. The mitral valve area can then be computed by dividing 220 by the velocity half time. *MVA*=mitral valve area; *P*=pressure; $T_{1/2}$= half-time; *V*=velocity. (From Levine RA, et al: Echocardiography: principles and clinical applications, in Eagle KA, et al (eds): *The practice of cardiology*, Boston, 1989, Little Brown.)

advanced disease there is also evidence of leaflet thickening, which relates to the presence of myxomatous infiltration of the valve. There may also be redundant or detached chordae.

There is an important relationship between the appearances of the mitral valve in this condition and both the degree of mitral valve dysfunction and patient prognosis. Specifically, patients with marked displacement, thickening, and deformity of the leaflets (Fig. 2-25) are more likely to have severe mitral regurgitation and to be at greatest risk of valve-related complications including valve surgery and endocarditis (Nidorf et al, 1993).

As in any patient with mitral regurgitation, left atrial size increases with increasing severity of the regurgitant lesion and left atrial dimension can act as an index of the severity and duration of the mitral regurgitation (Reed et al, 1992). Left ventricular size may be normal or dilated. Systolic function is typically hyperdynamic in patients with primary compensated valvular mitral regurgitation of moderate severity. Although no single echocardio-

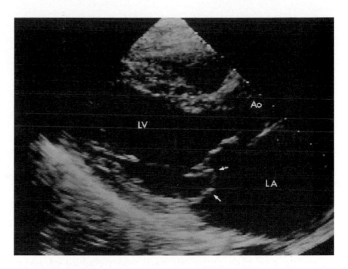

Fig. 2-25 Parasternal long-axis echocardiographic view of the left atrium and left ventricle demonstrating prolapse of the posterior leaflet of the mitral valve. The posterior cusp *(arrows)* bows into the left atrium behind the coaptation point of the mitral leaflets. *Ao*=aorta; *LA*=left atrium; *LV*=left ventricle.

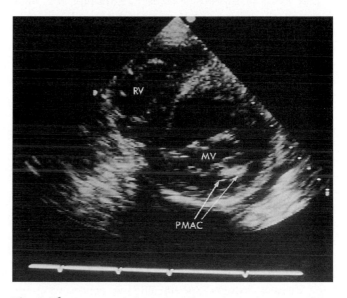

Fig. 2-26 Parasternal short-axis echocardiographic view of the left and right ventricles at the level of the mitral valve. The mitral leaflets *(MV)* form a "fishmouth" pattern in diastole. A focal dense area of calcification is present along the posterior mitral annulus *(arrows)*. *MV*=mitral valve; *PMAC*=posterior mitral annular calcification; *RV*=right ventricle.

graphic index yet accurately predicts the correct timing of mitral valve surgery in patients with primary chronic valvular mitral regurgitation, those with a left ventricular end-diastolic diameter greater than 50 mm tend to have less recovery of ventricular function following surgery (Wisenbaugh et al, 1992).

MITRAL ANNULAR CALCIFICATION   Calcification of the mitral annulus is common in the elderly. It begins as a focal process, affecting the posterior portion of the annular ring (Fig. 2-26), then extends laterally and finally anteriorly. As the process evolves, the base of the mitral leaflets and chordal apparatus thicken and calcify. This impairs the normal mechanism of coaptation leading to mitral regurgitation. It may also result in restriction of mitral inflow with the development of a small transmitral gradient (Braunwald, 1992). Although annular calcification is visible in almost any view, the parasternal short-axis image at the base of the heart is the most useful view for defining the circumferential extent of the disease.

Patients with mitral annular calcification often have nonspecific thickening of the aortic valve, left atrial enlargement, and evidence of left ventricular hypertrophy or regional dysfunction. Annular calcification can be a predictor of systemic embolism, independent of atrial size, cardiac rhythm, and global systolic function (BAATAF, 1990). Mitral regurgitation may lessen the risk of systemic embolism in these patients, indicating that the risk most likely relates to low flow within the atrium.

RHEUMATIC MITRAL REGURGITATION   Although the incidence of rheumatic mitral regurgitation is decreasing, the disease is still prevalent in older patients. Typically, the echocardiogram confirms mitral leaflet and chordal thickening in association with aortic valve disease. As the disease progresses and the leaflets become less mobile, valvular stenosis may also be evident (Weyman et al, 1982). In these cases, echocardiography is most useful in determining whether the valve is predominantly stenotic or incompetent. This information is invaluable for determining the optimal clinical and corrective approach to the valvular lesion.

FLAIL MITRAL LEAFLET   Complete or partial disruption of the support of one or both of the mitral leaflets usually presents suddenly with the development of a new murmur or acute pulmonary edema. In either setting the echocardiogram in association with the clinical picture may provide direct insight into the nature of the underlying disease process. Specifically, the echocardiogram can demonstrate systolic prolapse of the entire leaflet into the left atrium (Erbel et al, 1981) (Fig. 2-27). The clinical picture may help to determine whether the flail leaflet was caused by infective endocarditis, underlying myxomatous mitral valve disease (mitral valve prolapse), or papillary muscle rupture in association with acute myocardial infarction.

INCOMPLETE MITRAL VALVE CLOSURE   In some patients the mitral valve may appear morphologically normal but is clearly incompetent, as evidenced by clinical or echocardiographic signs of moderate to severe mitral regurgitation. In these patients the mitral regurgitation is caused by abnormal (incomplete) closure of the mitral valve caused by either annular dilatation or papillary muscle dysfunction. In both instances, the pattern of leaflet closure appears abnormal in the parasternal and apical views; the mitral leaflets appear to coapt only at their tips, rather than along the distal third of the leaflet. In some instances, there may be complete failure of coaptation. In such cases, you can readily see the ventricular dilatation and global or regional wall motion abnormality that predispose the incomplete mitral valve closure (Godley et al, 1981).

ASSESSMENT OF MITRAL REGURGITATION   Color Doppler readily demonstrates mitral regurgitation. In general it is very sensitive to regurgitant flow through the atrioventricular valves, and small jets of regurgitation are common in normal hearts because of retrograde flow induced by valve closure. Regurgitant jets usually appear as a localized stream of flow emerging from the valve leaflets at valve closure which then expand into the distal chamber. From most sampling windows, the jets of mitral regurgitation are predominantly blue since they are directed away from the transducer. The introduction of yellow and greens in the color flow map indicates high-velocity turbulent flow and results in a pattern referred to as "mosaic." Regurgitation can be confirmed by either pulsed or continuous wave Doppler.

Regurgitant flow characteristically begins at the peak of the R wave on the electrocardiogram (ECG) and continues throughout systole. The peak velocity of these jets reflects the atrioventricular gradient, which you can calculate using the simplified Bernoulli equation (described above). Therefore, the continuous wave Doppler signal in patients with mitral regurgitation usually has a peak velocity of about 5 m/sec, reflecting a peak atrioventricular gradient of 100 mm Hg.

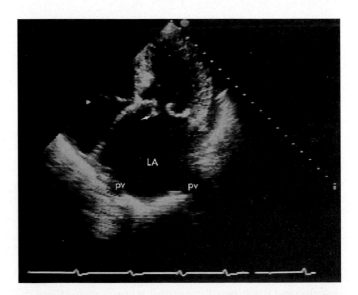

Fig. 2-27   In this apical four-chamber echocardiographic image, the mitral valve leaflets are thickened. A portion of the posterior leaflet is flail and everts into the left atrium (arrow). The left atrium is significantly enlarged secondary to severe mitral regurgitation. LA=left atrium; pv=pulmonary veins.

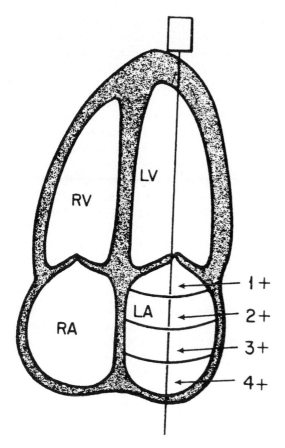

Fig. 2-28 Diagrammatic representation of an apical four-chamber echocardiographic view indicating the method for quantifying the severity of mitral regurgitation. With the transducer placed at the cardiac apex, the mitral insufficiency flow stream is detected within the left atrium either by pulsed Doppler or color flow mapping. The extent of penetration within the atrial chamber is graded from 1 to 4, with the more severe degree of regurgitation reaching the superior wall of the left atrium and into the pulmonary veins. *LA*=left atrium; *LV*=left ventricle; *RA*=right atrium; *RV*=right ventricle. (From Weyman AE: Left ventricular inflow tract I: the mitral valve, in Weyman AE: *Principles and practice of echocardiography, ed 2,* Philadelphia, 1994, Lea & Febiger.)

Semiquantitative assessment of the severity of mitral regurgitation involves integration of many echocardiographic and Doppler variables. Initially, it is helpful to consider the appearance of the valve leaflets, chordae, and the pattern of leaflet coaptation. This may provide insight into both the mechanism and likely severity of regurgitation. It is useful to determine whether the valvular apparatus appears normal or thickened and deformed, and to determine whether the pattern of coaptation is normal, incomplete, or asymmetric (due to complete or partial leaflet flail). With this preliminary assessment, it is possible to gain a sense of whether the degree of regurgitation is likely to be mild, moderate, or severe. For example, it is unlikely that with a normal valvular apparatus and a normal pattern of coaptation there would be more than mild regurgitation, yet it is

highly likely that with a partially flail leaflet there will be moderate to severe mitral regurgitation.

Following assessment of valve morphology and the pattern of coaptation, the pulsed (Abbasi et al, 1980; Esper, 1982) or color Doppler signals may yield further insight into the degree of regurgitation (Ascah et al, 1985; Blumlein et al, 1986). In essence, both forms of Doppler can determine the degree of flow disturbance within the atria (or proximal pulmonary veins). Color flow Doppler has a distinct advantage over pulsed Doppler, since it provides a color map of the net instantaneous velocity of blood flow within the atria at varying time points during systole. From this map it is possible to describe the size (area, length, width at the orifice) and direction (central or eccentric) of the regurgitant jet, without accurate placement of the pulsed Doppler sample volume. Descriptors of jet size relate to the angiographic degree of regurgitation and you can grade the degree of regurgitation semiquantitatively by Doppler (Fig. 2-28) (Miyatake et al, 1986; Helmcke et al, 1987; Spain et al, 1989).

Unfortunately, many factors affect the accurate assessment of the degree of regurgitation. For example, changing either the gain or the PRF (pulse repetition frequency) of the Doppler equipment may alter the relationship between jet size and the degree of regurgitation, resulting in either an artificial increase or decrease in jet size (particularly jet area and length) (Sahn et al, 1988). Further, detection of the regurgitant jet may not be possible in all instances, such as in patients with prosthetic valves which block out or reflect the interrogating Doppler signal and prohibit its passage into the atrium (Sprecher et al, 1987). Finally, the relationship between jet size and severity of regurgitation may be underestimated if the jet is directed eccentrically along the atrial wall, as often occurs with more severe regurgitation.

In an effort to overcome some of the limitations related to analysis of the distal jet, recent research analyzes the size of the flow stream proximal to the valve (i.e., on the ventricular side of the valve) (Recusani et al, 1991). Although this approach is still in its investigative phase, analysis of the size of this proximal flow convergence region may provide accurate assessment of the degree of valvular regurgitation in selected patients (Chen et al, 1993).

Flow reversal in the pulmonary veins by pulsed Doppler offers additional evidence that the degree of mitral regurgitation is likely to be severe (Klein et al, 1991). Since it is the atria that bear the burden of chronic regurgitation, assessment of atrial size may also be valuable in determining its severity and chronicity. However, since other parameters such as atrial fibrillation and left ventricular end-diastolic pressure may also influence atrial size, chamber size alone may be a misleading marker of the severity of regurgitation (Nidorf et al, 1993).

Tricuspid valve disease

Tricuspid regurgitation may occur as a consequence of abnormal development of the valve (Ebstein anomaly), disease affecting the valve leaflets or chordal apparatus (myxomatous degeneration, endocarditis), or of annular dilatation (secondary to right ventricular dilatation).

Assessment of the degree of tricuspid regurgitation is similar to that for mitral regurgitation. In contrast, however, the peak velocity of regurgitant flow across the tricuspid valve is usually 2.5 m/sec, reflecting a peak systolic gradient of 25 mm Hg between the right ventricle and right atrium. In patients without evidence of pulmonary outflow obstruction, accurate assessment of pulmonary artery systolic pressure is possible by adding the estimated right atrial pressure to the estimated systolic atrioventricular gradient. For example, with an atrioventricular gradient of 20 mm Hg, and an estimated right atrial pressure of 10 mm Hg, the estimated pulmonary artery pressure is 30 mm Hg (Berger et al, 1985; Currie et al, 1985a; Dabestani et al, 1987) (Fig. 2-29).

Ebstein's anomaly is a congenital defect characterized by elongation of the anterior leaflet and tethering of the tricuspid valve to the right ventricular endocardium. The septal and posterior leaflet origins are displaced apically, reducing the functional right ventricular size while atrializing the basal portion of the ventricle (Braunwald, 1992). It is easy to diagnose Ebstein's anomaly from the apical four-chamber view (Fig. 2-30). Normally the mitral and tricuspid valves align with slight apical insertion of the tricuspid valve, but in patients with Ebstein's anomaly the septal leaflet of the tricuspid valve is more than 1.0 cm apical to the mitral valve. In most patients tricuspid regurgitation is moderate to severe as assessed by Doppler. Further, color Doppler may detect some degree of right-to-left interatrial shunt flow across either a patent foramen ovale or an atrial septal defect.

Tricuspid stenosis most often occurs as a consequence of rheumatic fever, in which case it invariably occurs with mitral or aortic valve disease (Braunwald, 1992). More rarely, tricuspid stenosis occurs with metasta-

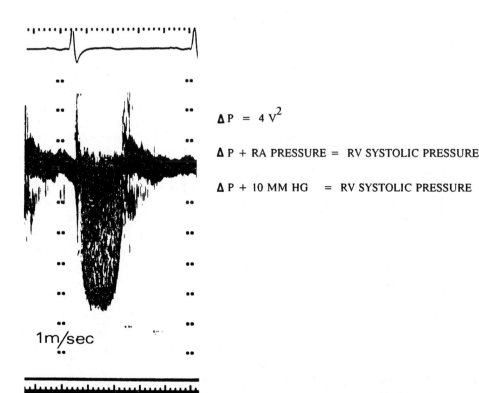

$$\Delta P = 4 V^2$$

$$\Delta P + RA\ PRESSURE = RV\ SYSTOLIC\ PRESSURE$$

$$\Delta P + 10\ MM\ HG = RV\ SYSTOLIC\ PRESSURE$$

Fig. 2-29   The peak velocity of tricuspid regurgitation can be used to predict pulmonary artery pressure. On the left of the figure is a continuous wave Doppler spectral trace of tricuspid regurgitation. The peak velocity of the regurgitant flow is 4.7 m/sec. Using the formula $\Delta P = 4V^2$, the pressure difference between right ventricle and right atrium is 88 mm Hg. Adding an estimated right atrial pressure of 10 mm Hg gives an estimated right ventricular pressure of 98 mm Hg. In the absence of right ventricular outflow obstruction, this right ventricular systolic pressure is identical to pulmonary artery systolic pressure. ΔP=pressure gradient; *RA*=right atrium; *RV*=right ventricle. (From Liberthson RR: Congenital heart disease in the child, adolescent, and adult, in Eagle KA, et al (eds): *The practice of cardiology,* Boston, 1989, Little Brown.)

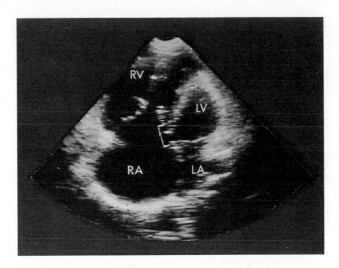

Fig. 2-30 Apical four-chamber echocardiographic view in a patient with Ebstein's anomaly of the tricuspid valve. The anterior leaflet arises normally from the tricuspid annulus but is elongated. The septal leaflet origin is displaced apically more than 13 mm below the mitral leaflet insertion *(bracket)*. Severe tricuspid insufficiency causes right atrial and right ventricular enlargement and dwarfs the left heart chambers. *LA*=left atrium; *LV*=left ventricle; *RA*=right atrium; *RV*=right ventricle. (From Liberthson RR: Congenital heart disease in the child, adolescent, and adult, in Eagle KA, et al (eds): *The practice of cardiology,* Boston, 1989, Little Brown.)

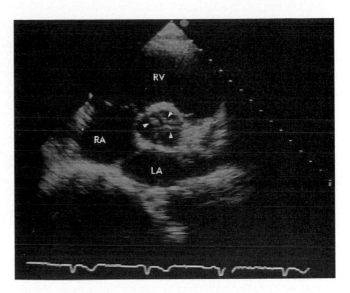

Fig. 2-31 Parasternal short-axis echocardiographic view at the base of the heart in a patient with calcific aortic stenosis. The aortic valve leaflets are calcified highlighting the commissural margins *(arrowheads)*. Immobility of the cusps results in only a slitlike aortic valve orifice in systole. *LA*=left atrium; *RA*=right atrium; *RV*=right ventricle.

tic carcinoid tumors (Howard et al, 1982). In both instances the leaflets and chordae appear thickened, the valve domes during diastole, and as a consequence of the stenosis, there is an increase in right atrial size.

Aortic valve disease

Aortic stenosis   Echocardiographically, aortic stenosis is any abnormality of the aortic valve in which the leaflets restrict the lumen of the outflow tract. The three cardinal features of aortic stenosis are (1) leaflet thickening, deformity, and calcification; (2) decreased mobility or doming of the leaflets, or both; and (3) an absolute decrease in size of the valve orifice due to reduced cusp separation (Weyman et al, 1982) (Fig. 2-31).

Aortic stenosis may be acquired or congenital. In congenital aortic stenosis, the aortic valve may be unicuspid, bicuspid, or rarely, quadricuspid (Fig. 2-32). Typically, the leaflets are thin but appear to dome. This is evident in the parasternal long-axis views in midsystole (Fig. 2-33). Characterization is usually possible by imaging the valve in the short-axis plane to determine the number of cusps and commissures. Although bicuspid valves are by nature stenotic, they may also predispose to significant aortic regurgitation. Identification of a distinctly bicuspid valve may be difficult in older patients, particularly if the valve has begun to calcify.

Unlike congenital aortic valve disease, which usually presents before the fourth decade, acquired calcific aor-

tic stenosis presents in the patient's sixth or seventh decade (Braunwald, 1992). Typically the valve is thickened and calcified and there is reduced cusp separation. Unlike patients with mitral stenosis, it is not usually possible to determine the severity of aortic stenosis from the morphologic features alone. Nonetheless, detection of some residual leaflet motion usually indicates that the valve area is greater than 0.6 cm^2 (Weyman et al, 1982).

None of the typical features of aortic stenosis is necessarily specific for the diagnosis of hemodynamically significant disease. Leaflet thickening is common in the elderly and rarely associated with significant obstruction to outflow. Focal thickening may represent vegetation rather than fibrosis. Although reduced cusp separation and doming of the leaflets are more specific for hemodynamically significant disease, this may also occur in patients with a low cardiac output. Finally, direct measurement of the valve orifice is rarely possible. In patients with significant aortic stenosis, left ventricular size and systolic function are typically normal; however, left ventricular hypertrophy is usually evident (wall thickness ≥12 mm).

Accurate assessment of the degree of stenosis is usually possible using continuous wave Doppler, which allows estimation of the peak and mean aortic gradient and the aortic valve area (Currie et al, 1985b; Hatle et al, 1980). To determine the peak and mean gradient across the valve, you must first obtain accurate profiles of flow emanating from the valve, usually from apical windows. It is also important to interrogate flow through the valve

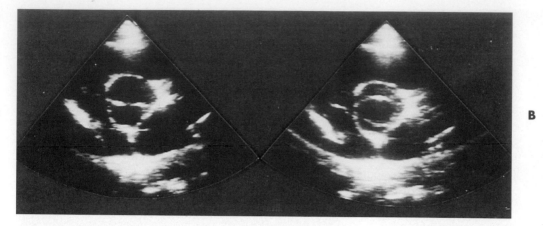

Fig. 2-32 Parasternal short-axis echocardiographic views of the aortic valve in a patient with a bicuspid aortic valve. **A** depicts the valve in diastole with two leaflets and a central commissure. In systole, **(B)**, the commissural opening is elliptical instead of triangular as in the normal trileaflet valve. (From Liberthson RR: Congenital heart disease in the child, adolescent, and adult, in Eagle KA, et al (eds): *The practice of cardiology,* Boston, 1989, Little Brown.)

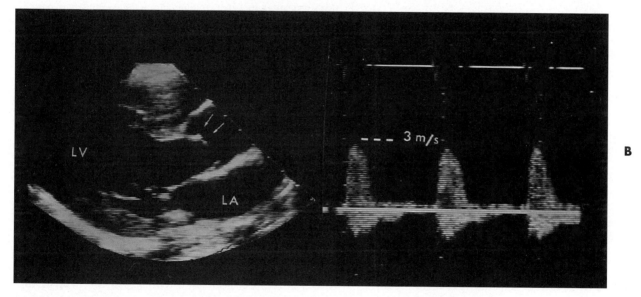

Fig. 2-33 Parasternal long-axis echocardiographic view of the left ventricular outflow tract in a patient with congenital aortic stenosis. In **A**, the aortic leaflets dome into the aortic root in systole *(arrows)*, restricting the flow orifice. **B** is the continuous wave Doppler spectral tracing of transvalvular flow obtained from the suprasternal notch. The peak flow velocity in systole is 3 m/sec, which would predict a 36 mm Hg gradient across the aortic valve. *LA*=left atrium; *LV*=left ventricle. (From Liberthson RR: Congenital heart disease in the child, adolescent, and adult, in Eagle KA, et al (eds): *The practice of cardiology,* Boston, 1989, Little Brown.)

from the right parasternal window because deformation of the aortic leaflets may eccentrically direct the jet of blood flow toward the right sternal border as it enters the aorta. The typical continuous wave Doppler profile of aortic stenosis begins *after* the R wave on the ECG and is not holosystolic. Noting the time of onset and the duration of flow helps to differentiate the aortic stenosis profile from the continuous wave Doppler profile of mitral regurgitant flow.

Once you obtain optimal Doppler profiles, you can use the simplified Bernoulli equation to estimate the aortic gradient (Hatle et al, 1980). In general, estimates of the transaortic gradient by Doppler tend to overestimate the peak-to-peak gradient obtained at catheterization. This is because the Doppler profile provides information about the *instantaneous* gradient through the valve at each point during systole, while the catheterization gradients are derived measurements comparing the peak ventricular systolic pressure to the peak aortic systolic pressure, irrespective of time.

Doppler techniques can also be used to estimate aortic valve area using the continuity equation (Richards et al, 1986). The continuity theorem states that the volume of flow entering a cylinder equals the volume of flow passing through an obstruction within the cylinder, which in turn equals the volume of flow exiting from the cylinder (Fig. 2-34). Since the rate of flow (ml/min) in the cylinder relates to both the velocity (V_1) of flow and to the area of the lumen of the cylinder (A_1), it should be possible to estimate the area of the stenosis (A_2) if you know the velocity of flow through the stenotic region (V_2):

$$(V_1) \times (A_1) = (V_2) \times (A_2)$$
$$A_2 = \frac{(V_1) \times (A_1)}{(V_2)}$$

This concept allows calculation of the area of a stenotic valve (A_2):

- (V_1) = velocity of blood in the outflow tract determined by pulsed Doppler.
- (A_1) = the area of the outflow tract calculated from the direct measurement of its diameter.
- (V_2) = the peak velocity through the valve from the continuous wave Doppler profile across the stenotic valve.

Estimates of aortic valve area by this method relate reasonably well to those obtained from catheterization (Otto et al, 1986). However, they may be subject to error

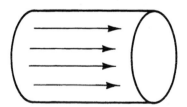

$$\text{Flow (cm}^3/\text{min)} = \text{Area (cm}^2\text{)} \times \text{Vel (cm/min)}$$

Fig. 2-34 Diagrammatic representation of the method for calculating cardiac output by the Doppler technique. Flow is the product of the velocity in centimeters per minute times the cross-sectional area through which the flow passes. This can be applied to flow across any of the cardiac valves, but is most often used for the semilunar valves. The area is calculated by measuring the diameter *(d)* of the aortic or pulmonic annulus and assuming a circular cross-sectional area [A= π (d/2)^2]. *vel*=velocity. (From Ascah KJ, et al: Doppler-echocardiographic assessment of cardiac output, *Radiol Clin North Am* 23:660, 1985.)

due to incomplete ascertainment of the maximal Doppler profile, the presence of atrial fibrillation, and errors in estimating the subaortic diameter.

Aortic regurgitation   Until the addition of Doppler technology, echocardiography could only diagnose aortic regurgitation indirectly. High-frequency diastolic fluttering of one or both of the mitral leaflets suggests the presence of aortic regurgitation. Impingement of the regurgitant jet directly into the leaflets creates this echocardiographic finding. If regurgitation is severe, early diastolic closure of the mitral valve may occur (Botvinick et al, 1975).

Aortic valve abnormalities, such as a bicuspid valve or heavily calcified leaflets, raise the suspicion of associated valve regurgitation. Other morphologic features may indicate the cause of the regurgitant lesion. For example, leaflet prolapse may indicate the presence of a torn leaflet, and the presence of additional mobile echoes adherent to the valve may suggest endocarditis. Further, dilatation of the aortic sinuses or aortic root may indicate Marfan syndrome, ascending aortic aneurysm, or aortic root dissection.

As the severity of aortic regurgitation increases, the left ventricle dilates and hypertrophies. Systolic function is usually preserved. Although the detection of left ventricular dilatation and impairment of systolic function does not imply inoperable disease, patients in whom the left ventricular systolic dimension is greater than 55 mm tend to have a worse outcome following surgery (Bonow et al, 1983). Indeed, there may be significant ventricular remodelling and restoration of systolic function following surgery.

Doppler techniques allow rapid detection of aortic regurgitation by color, pulsed, and continuous wave modalities (Grayburn, 1986) (Fig. 2-35). In the parasternal long-axis views, aortic regurgitation appears as a diastolic red or blue jet emanating from the region of the aortic valve and directed into the left ventricular cavity. Sometimes the jet tracks along the anterior leaflet of the mitral valve. Parasternal short-axis, as well as the apical five-chamber and apical long-axis views may also allow detection of regurgitation, which appears as a red jet because it is directed toward the transducer.

Despite the ready detection of aortic regurgitation by color Doppler, assessing the severity of regurgitation is more difficult and at best only semiquantitative (Diebold et al, 1987; Louie et al, 1987a; Perry et al, 1987). For example, the use of jet length to assess the severity of regurgitation may be misleading as even small jets may coalesce with mitral inflow and appear large (Louie et al, 1987b). An alternative is to consider the cross-sectional area of the jet in the short-axis plane; more severe regurgitation tends to fill a greater portion of the outflow tract in early diastole.

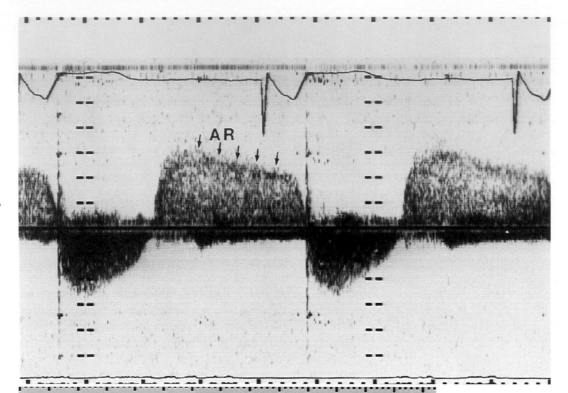

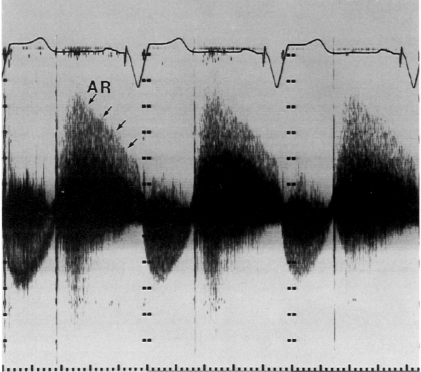

Fig. 2-35 **A** is a continuous wave Doppler spectral trace in a patient with aortic insufficiency. The aortic flow is sampled from the apex with systolic outflow shown below the baseline and diastolic regurgitant flow above the baseline. With normal aortic and left ventricular diastolic pressures, the pressure difference between aorta and left ventricle remains high and the slope of the regurgitant velocities drops off gradually *(arrows)*. In **B,** the aortic insufficiency is severe causing a rapid equilibration of aortic and left ventricular diastolic pressures resulting in a sharp slope in flow velocities *(arrows)*.

Pulsed Doppler can assess the severity of aortic regurgitation by detecting the presence of *late* diastolic flow reversal in the descending aorta which invariably occurs with severe regurgitation (Ciobanu et al, 1982). Finally, measurement of the regurgitant pressure half-time derived from the continuous wave Doppler profile reflects the instantaneous pressure gradient between the aorta and the left ventricle (Teague et al, 1984). Therefore, more rapid pressure half-times reflect rapid increases in diastolic pressure within the left ventricle and reflect more severe regurgitation (see Fig. 2-35). In general, a pressure half-time below 200 ms is indicative of severe aortic insufficiency; however, the utility of this method is limited by the effects of other factors which may raise left ventricular diastolic pressure unrelated to the degree of aortic regurgitation.

Pulmonary valve disease

The pulmonary valve is best visualized in the parasternal short-axis plane, although subcostal views are also useful in children. Patients with rheumatic heart disease may have thickening of the pulmonary valve; however, significant pulmonary stenosis is rare. By far the most common cause of pulmonary stenosis is congenital deformity of the valve (Fig. 2-36). This may occur as a single lesion or in association with other defects (such as tetralogy of Fallot). Typically the valve appears mobile, but the leaflets dome during systole. In routine practice continuous wave Doppler is used to assess the

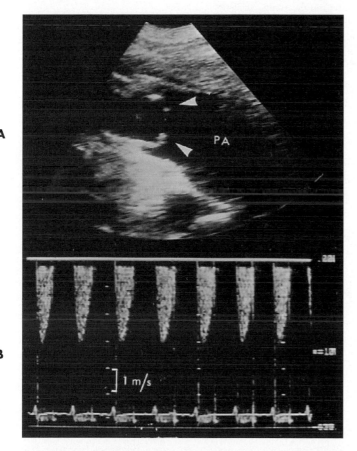

Fig. 2-36 Two-dimensional image and continuous wave Doppler trace in a patient with valvular pulmonic stenosis. **A** is a parasternal long-axis echocardiographic view of the main pulmonary artery. The leaflets are thickened and dome into the pulmonic root in systole *(arrowheads)*. There is poststenotic dilatation of the main pulmonary artery. Doppler velocities across the valve show a peak systolic velocity of 3 m/sec predicting a gradient of 36 mm Hg. *PA*=pulmonary artery. (From Liberthson RR: Congenital heart disease in the child, adolescent, and adult, in Eagle KA, et al (eds): *The practice of cardiology*, Boston, 1989, Little Brown.)

peak velocity across the valve, since this allows peak and mean transvalvular gradient calculation by the modified Bernoulli equation (Lima et al, 1983). There is often associated poststenotic dilatation of the proximal portion of the main pulmonary artery. Further, the right ventricle appears hypertrophied and the interventricular septum flattens during systole as a consequence of the increased pressure load (Weyman et al, 1982).

Color Doppler commonly shows some degree of pulmonary regurgitation as a small red jet directed into the right ventricle toward the transducer. Small jets of regurgitation are physiologic (Choong et al, 1989). More marked degrees of regurgitation occur with pulmonary hypertension, primary valve disease, congenital absence of the pulmonary valve, or after pulmonary valvotomy. There are no formal criteria for Doppler assessment of the severity of pulmonary regurgitation. For clinical purposes, the degree of regurgitation is graded semiquantitatively based on the width and length of the regurgitant jet.

Prosthetic heart valves

Prosthetic heart valves may be either bioprosthetic or mechanical. Bioprosthetic valves, harvested from pig or human hearts, are supported by three struts that connect to a valve ring. Mechanical valve design is more diverse. Some devices have a ball-in-cage design while others have either a single or double disk. Because of the variable nature of these prostheses, it is often possible to determine the specific type of prosthesis by echocardiography, especially since mechanical devices tend to be more reflective. For example, Starr-Edwards valves have a characteristic protrusion of the cage into the left ventricle or aorta, and a unique pattern of ball motion and forward flow around the valve. In contrast, disk valves have a much lower profile, and disk motion may be clearly evident. Finally, bioprosthetic valves are usually recognizable by the supporting strut and by the presence of leaflet motion within the prosthesis (Fig. 2-37).

Not surprisingly, two-dimensional Doppler echocardiography is invaluable in the routine assessment of prosthetic valve function. It allows assessment of the stability of the device and of the degree of stenosis of the prosthesis. Further, echocardiography can also detect regurgitation through or around the valve, vegetation or thrombus within or around the prosthesis, and can assess ventricular function during the postoperative period (Gross and Wann, 1984; Kolter et al, 1983; Sagar et al, 1986; Williams et al, 1985).

Poor seating of the prosthesis may occur as a consequence of paravalvular infection or wear of the sutures supporting the valve ring. As the valve seating becomes unstable, invariably there is some degree of paravalular regurgitation. As the degree of instability increases, the valve is seen to move independently (rock) through the

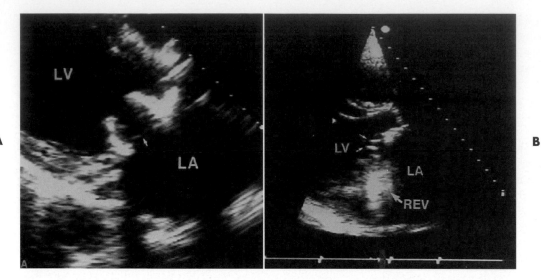

Fig. 2-37   Parasternal long-axis echocardiographic view of the left heart in patients with prosthetic mitral valves. **A** depicts a bioprosthesis with echogenic struts protruding from the mitral annulus into the left ventricle. The bioprosthetic leaflets are thin and faintly seen within the struts *(arrow)*. A St. Jude tilting disk prosthesis is shown in **B**. Two parallel disks are shown in diastole *(arrows)*. Dense reflections from the metallic structures of the valve appear as a bright reverberation in the left atrium. *LA*=left atrium; *LV*=left ventricle; *REV*=reverberation. (From Wilkins GT, et al: Echo-Doppler assessment of prosthetic heart valves, in Weyman AE: *Principles and practice of echocardiography,* ed 2, Philadelphia, 1994, Lea & Febiger.)

cardiac cycle. Marked "rocking" of the prosthesis is a poor prognostic sign because it suggests that at least one third of the valve ring has become unstable. Since infective endocarditis is the most common cause of destabilization, it is important to exclude the presence of paravalvular infection or abscess formation. Although this can occasionally be done from surface imaging, transesophageal imaging is more sensitive and specific.

Continuous wave Doppler can assess the gradient across the prosthesis in the same manner as for native valves. When assessing the significance of the Doppler gradient, however, it is important to bear in mind the following factors:

- The Doppler gradient may overestimate the catheter gradient across both the St. Jude tilting disk and Starr-Edwards valves by up to 40% (Baumgartner et al, 1992).
- Each type of prosthesis has different flow profiles.
- Smaller prostheses will have higher gradients than larger prostheses of the same type.
- The gradient across an aortic prosthesis is critically dependent on ventricular function.

Therefore, in order to make a meaningful statement about the significance of the Doppler gradient across a prosthesis, it is important to consider the size, type, and location of the prosthesis, as well as the left ventricular function.

Detection of a significant increase in gradient across a prosthesis is an important clinical sign because it may indicate valve occlusion or partial obstruction. This may be due either to pannus ingrowth around the sewing ring, or to the presence of a large vegetation or thrombus within the valve apparatus.

To assess the significance of the degree of regurgitation across a prosthetic valve, it is important to consider the type and position of the prosthesis. The type of prosthesis is important since bioprosthetic and Starr-Edwards valves do not normally leak. In contrast, the single disk (Medtronic Hall) valve design allows a small central leak, and the double disk St. Jude valve has small leaks around the disk margins. Therefore, detection of a small central jet of regurgitation is expected in patients with disk valves, is suggestive of valve degeneration in a patient with a bioprosthetic valve, and may indicate either vegetation or pannus ingrowth around the valve ring in a patient with a Starr-Edwards valve (Fig. 2-38). Regardless of valve type, a paravalvular leak would indicate disruption of the valve ring due to either infection or wear of the valve sutures.

Assessment of the degree of regurgitation may be very difficult if not impossible in some patients because the reflectivity of the prosthetic material prevents sufficient penetration of the ultrasound signal beyond the prosthesis. This is particularly a problem in patients with both an aortic and a mitral valve prosthesis. Further, since the regurgitant jets tend to be eccentric, they are easy to miss during a routine examination. Although in some instances these problems can be overcome by imaging the heart in off-axis views, they can be completely over-

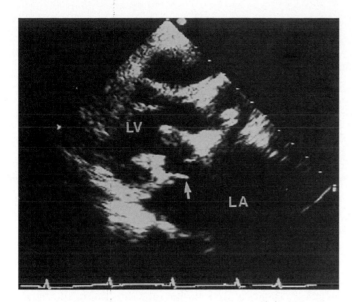

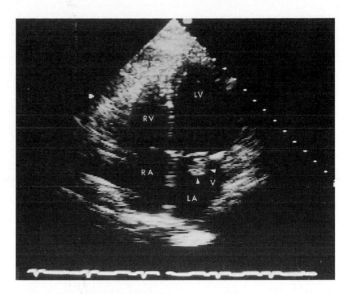

Fig. 2-38 Parasternal long-axis echocardiographic view of the left ventricular inflow tract in a patient with a bioprosthetic mitral valve. The dense struts can be seen extending into the left ventricle from the annulus. The bioprosthetic leaflets have degenerated and one of the cusps is everted and prolapses into the left atrium *(arrow)*, creating severe mitral regurgitation. *LA*=left atrium; *LV*=left ventricle. (From Wilkins GT, et al: Echo-Doppler assessment of prosthetic heart valves, in Weyman AE: *Principles and practice of echocardiography,* ed 2, Philadelphia, 1994, Lea & Febiger.)

Fig. 2-39 Apical four-chamber echocardiographic view of the heart demonstrating a vegetation on the mitral valve. The vegetation is attached on the atrial surface of the anterior leaflet and prolapses into the left atrium *(arrowheads)*. *LA*=left atrium; *LV*=left ventricle; *RA*=right atrium; *RV*=right ventricle; *v*=vegetation.

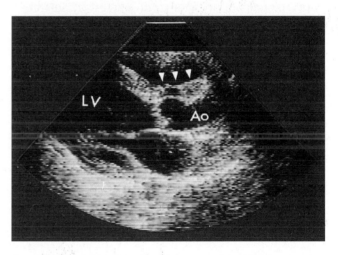

Fig. 2-40 Parasternal long-axis echocardiographic view of the left ventricle in a patient with aortic valve endocarditis and aortic root abscess. The aortic leaflets are thickened. The anterior aortic root wall is also thickened with lucent areas of liquefaction from infection within the wall *(arrows)*. *Ao*=aorta; *LV*=left ventricle. (From Levine RA, et al: Echocardiography: principles and clinical applications, in Eagle KA, et al (eds): *The practice of cardiology,* Boston, 1989, Little Brown.)

come by using the esophageal window since this allows a clear view of both the valve and left atrium (Nanda et al, 1990).

Infective endocarditis

Two-dimensional echocardiography is invaluable in the assessment of patients with a clinical picture of infective endocarditis. Detection of an abnormal mass of echoes on a valve leaflet strongly suggests vegetations (Fig. 2-39). Mitral and tricuspid vegetations are generally on the atrial side of the valve, whereas aortic and pulmonary vegetation tend to form on the ventricular surface. Echocardiography also allows accurate assessment of vegetation morphology (size, mobility, density), detection of extravalvular extension of the infective process, and determination of the degree of valvular dysfunction (Weyman et al, 1982) (Fig. 2-40).

Detection and characterization of such an echogenic mass within a week of presentation in a patient with a suggestive clinical picture has prognostic significance. Specifically, vegetation size, mobility, consistency, and site, all correlate with the risk of in-hospital complications including stroke, heart failure, and valve surgery (Sanfilippo et al, 1991).

Despite the clear value of echocardiography in the assessment of patients suspected of endocarditis, the technique cannot exclude the diagnosis of infective

endocarditis with certainty. There are a number of reasons for this. First, the vegetation may be too small to be resolved, or only be present as focal, nonspecific valvular thickening. Second, the differential diagnosis of a discrete mass of mobile echoes attached to a leaflet includes thrombus, myxoma, fibrin, flail portion of the valve or chordae, old healed vegetation, or aneurysm formation secondary to the infective process (Vuille et al,

1993). Therefore, it is necessary to correlate the echocardiographic findings with the clinical picture in each instance.

ASSESSMENT OF ACQUIRED AND CONGENITAL HEART DISEASE

Ischemic Heart Disease

Because two-dimensional echocardiography is noninvasive and has a high spatial resolution and rapid acquisition time, it is an ideal means of assessing the serial changes in left ventricular structure and function that occur during myocardial ischemia and following myocardial infarction. Further, many studies demonstrate a clear relationship between the location and extent of abnormal wall motion defined echocardiographically and the site of infarction defined by the ECG (Heger et al, 1979) or cineangiogram (Kisslo et al, 1977). The hemodynamic status, the short- and long-term prognosis of the patient (Gibson et al, 1982; Nishimura et al, 1984), and the extent of infarction at autopsy also correlate well with the echocardiographic location and extent of infarction (Wilkins et al, 1988a).

It is not surprising then, that clinical studies demonstrate the value of two-dimensional echocardiography in the immediate diagnosis of ischemia in emergency patients with acute chest pain, and in the early recogni-

tion of the acute mechanical complications of myocardial infarction, including papillary muscle rupture, ventricular septal defect formation, and the late appearance of apical aneurysm and mural thrombosis. Further, early echocardiographic assessment of ventricular and infarct size provides insight into the prognosis of hospital patients with acute myocardial infarction (Mann et al, 1986).

Assessing left ventricular regional wall motion

Echocardiographic assessment of regional wall motion depends on the ability to assess both the degree of endocardial motion and the degree of myocardial thickening. In practice, the assessment of endocardial excursion is simple, but it may be misleading in the presence of noncardiac motion (rotation, translation). Although assessment of myocardial thickening is unaffected by these factors, its use may be limited if visualization of the epicardial and endocardial contours is inadequate (Mann et al, 1986).

Regional wall motion is most frequently described qualitatively as being normal, hypokinetic (moving in the proper direction but at a slower rate and to a smaller extent than normal), akinetic (not moving), or dyskinetic (moving outward in systole). A simple and clinically useful means of quantifying the overall extent of abnormal wall motion is to divide the ventricle into 20 segments of approximately equal size (Fig. 2-41) and to assign a func-

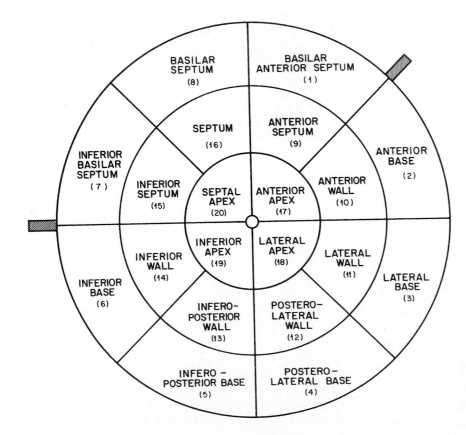

Fig. 2-41 Diagrammatic representation of myocardial segments of the left ventricle as viewed from the cardiac apex. The outer ring is the segments at the base of the heart, the middle ring represents the midventricular circumference of the myocardium, and the central ring is the four portions of the cardiac apex. Thickening and excursion of each of these segments is assessed echocardiographically and can be plotted on this diagram to indicate areas of hypokinesis, akinesis, or dyskinesis. (From Weyman AE: *Cross-sectional echocardiography,* Philadelphia, 1982, Lea & Febiger.)

tional "score" to each segment based on qualitative visual assessment (normal = 0, hypokinesis = 1, akinesis = 2, dyskinesis = 3). In this way, patients with extensive areas of infarction have higher scores. Overall scores derived by this approach correlate with clinical, hemodynamic, and radionuclide indices of infarct severity (Kisslo et al, 1977).

Acute complications of myocardial infarction

The acute mechanical complications of myocardial infarction, including papillary muscle and ventricular septal rupture, are most common after large inferoposterior and inferoseptal infarctions. Clinically, both conditions present with a sudden deterioration in hemodynamic status and the development of a new pansystolic murmur. Although clinical and hemodynamic variables may allow accurate differentiation of these complications, the echocardiographic features of each are specific.

In patients with papillary muscle rupture, one or the other mitral leaflet becomes flail and the head of the ruptured papillary muscle prolapses in and out of the left atrium with each cardiac cycle (Erbel et al, 1981). Further, as a consequence of the acute onset of regurgitation, the noninfarcted myocardium is hyperdynamic and color Doppler confirms a large, usually eccentric jet of mitral regurgitation into a slightly dilated atrium. In contrast, in patients with acute septal rupture, the mitral apparatus is intact and color Doppler can help accurately locate the septal defect. Continuous wave Doppler can determine the peak velocity of interventricular shunt flow, and thus predict the gradient between the left and right ventricles (by using the simplified Bernoulli equation). From this information you can estimate the pulmonary artery pressure.

Rupture of the free wall of the ventricle, which may occur even after small infarctions, is most often rapidly fatal due to acute pericardial tamponade. In some instances, however, pericardial adhesions can limit the extent of pericardial bleeding (either from past pericarditis or prior coronary surgery) and result in a localized pseudoaneurysm. In contrast, true aneurysms usually form after large infarctions affecting either the anterior septal wall, or less commonly, the inferior base of the heart (Fig. 2-42). Aneurysms are characteristically thinned, dyskinetic, and predispose to thrombus formation. Apical thrombus is usually evident as a collection of echogenic material in the region of abnormal wall motion (Visser et al, 1983) (Fig. 2-43). Thrombus may either embolize acutely or become organized, layering along the wall or calcifying with time.

Silent changes in myocardial structure following myocardial infarction and ventricular remodeling

Patients surviving the acute phase of myocardial infarction may develop clinically silent changes in both infarcted and noninfarcted regions (Picard et al, 1990). It is possible for the infarct zone to increase in size either because of infarct expansion (seen as thinning and

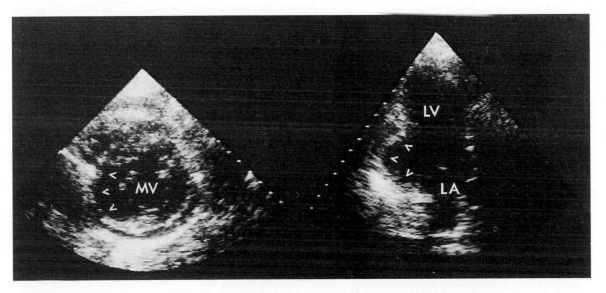

Fig. 2-42 Two-dimensional echocardiographic views of the left ventricle in a patient with an inferobasal aneurysm. In **A,** the left ventricle is viewed in cross section at the mitral valve level. The inferior septum and inferior wall are thinned and bulge out in systole *(arrows)*. In **B,** the left ventricle is viewed from the apex to demonstrate the inferior wall. Again, a "scooped-out" appearance of the inferior wall at the base with thinning of the myocardium can be appreciated *(arrows)*. *LA*=left atrium; *LV*=left ventricle; *MV*=mitral valve. (From Semigram M, Fallon JT: Clinicopathologic correlation, *N Engl J Med* 326:625, 1992, Massachusetts Medical Society. Reprinted by permission of the New England Journal of Medicine.)

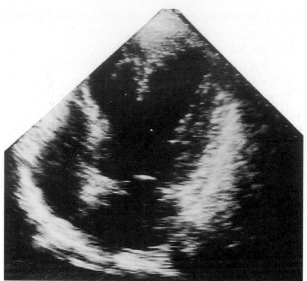

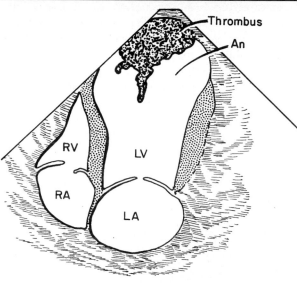

Fig. 2-43 Two-dimensional echocardiographic image and illustrative diagram of a patient with a left ventricular apical aneurysm with thrombus. In the apical view in the upper panel, enlargement and distortion of the left ventricular apex is apparent. An irregular density protrudes into the left ventricular cavity attached broadly along the endocardial surface of the dysfunctional apical myocardium. *An*=aneurysm; *LA*=left atrium; *LV*=left ventricle; *RA*=right atrium; *RV*=right ventricle. (From Siu SCB, Weyman AE: Left ventricle III: coronary artery disease—clinical manifestations and complications, in Weyman AE: *Principles and practice of echocardiography,* ed 2, Philadelphia, 1994, Lea & Febiger.)

bulging of the infarct segment) or infarct extension (seen as infarction of myocardium adjacent to the infarct zone). Further, a global increase in ventricular size proportional to the extent of abnormal wall motion following myocardial infarction may occur because of an increase in the size of the noninfarcted myocardial segments. These otherwise "silent" changes bear independent prognostic information. For example, patients with

evidence of regional infarct expansion are at high risk of early sudden death, while patients with a global increase in ventricular size are at high risk for late cardiac death after myocardial infarction (Braunwald, 1992).

Cardiomyopathies

There are three broad pathologic classifications of cardiomyopathies—dilated, hypertrophic, or restrictive. These categories are based on the morphology of the left ventricle. Echocardiography allows accurate distinction and evaluation of each of these groups.

Dilated cardiomyopathy

Despite the large number of recognized causes of dilated cardiomyopathy, there is rarely a specific etiologic factor and most cases are assumed to be a consequence of viral infection. Typically, all chambers of the heart are dilated and both the right and left ventricles appear diffusely hypokinetic. The feature that most distinguishes idiopathic dilated cardiomyopathy (IDCM) from ischemic cardiomyopathy is the presence of global, rather than regional, dysfunction. In some patients, however, regional dysfunction may be evident because of preservation of systolic function at the base of the left ventricle, or because of the presence of left bundle branch block, which causes paradoxical septal motion. Nonetheless, whereas right ventricular function is often preserved in patients with ischemic cardiomyopathy, this is not typical of other causes.

In most instances, both the mitral and tricuspid valves appear normal. Despite this, there may be significant atrioventricular regurgitation due to incomplete closure of the mitral and tricuspid leaflets consequent to annular dilatation. The regurgitant jets are generally directed centrally, and there may be systolic flow reversal into, and dilatation of, the pulmonary veins.

Patients with IDCM are at risk of systemic embolism. Although identifying those with a particularly high risk is difficult, it is likely that the risk of systemic embolism is greater in patients in atrial fibrillation, as well as in those with identifiable thrombus in the atria or left ventricular cavity (Gottdiener et al, 1983).

Hypertrophic cardiomyopathy

Hypertrophic cardiomyopathies are familial in nature. Pathologically, they are characterized by ventricular hypertrophy, which may be diffuse or localized to the septum, apex, or ventricular free wall (Maron et al, 1981). Patients with septal hypertrophy are classified further into those with or without evidence of dynamic obstruction to left ventricular outflow.

The most common form of hypertrophic cardiomyopathy is associated with septal hypertrophy. Typically, the ratio of septal to posterior free wall thickness is in excess of 1.3:1 (Maron, 1985). The left ventricular cavity usually appears small, and the ventricular apex may be completely obliterated in systole. The mitral valve may be morphologically normal, but there are often subtle anomalies of the mitral apparatus (Braunwald, 1992). These include anterior displacement of the papillary muscles, redundancy of the mitral chordae or leaflets, and in some instances, prolapse of the mitral valve. Mitral regurgitation occurs frequently, and relates to the anatomy of the mitral apparatus and to the degree of outflow tract obstruction.

A hallmark of asymmetric hypertrophic cardiomyopathy with outflow tract obstruction is systolic anterior motion (SAM) of the anterior leaflet of the mitral valve (Gardin et al, 1985) (Fig. 2-44). The interposition of this leaflet tissue causes obstruction to left ventricular emptying in mid- to late systole. This is reflected in aortic valve motion, with a closure pattern in midsystole. Doppler sampling of the left ventricular outflow tract demonstrates increased velocity at the site of leaflet-septal contact, and the continuous wave Doppler profile typically has a late-peaking systolic pattern (Maron et al, 1985) (Fig. 2-45). The peak velocity of this

outflow signal can be used to predict the outflow tract gradient (as previously described for valvular aortic stenosis) (Levine et al, 1987).

Left atrial enlargement is almost invariable. In the presence of atrial fibrillation, both atria are typically dilated. Thickening of the aortic valve, the mitral annulus, anterior mitral leaflet, and upper septum is common, especially in older patients. Although patients with hypertrophic cardiomyopathy are at risk of systemic emboli, rarely are there ventricular and atrial thrombi. Asymmetric septal hypertrophy should be differentiated from discrete upper septal hypertrophy, which is common in elderly hypertensive persons and is not associated with either midseptal hypertrophy or evidence of outflow obstruction.

Restrictive cardiomyopathy

The characteristic morphologic features of restrictive cardiomyopathy are marked ventricular hypertrophy, a small ventricular cavity, and biatrial enlargement. Typically, systolic function is normal or even hyperkinetic. Valvular leaflets may be thickened and there is usually significant mitral and tricuspid regurgitation. The peri-

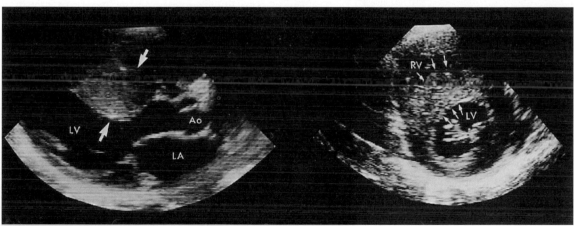

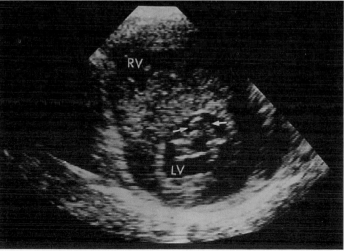

Fig. 2-44 Two-dimensional echocardiographic views of a patient with hypertrophic cardiomyopathy. **A,** Marked asymmetric thickening of the interventricular septum *(arrows)* is notable from both long-axis *(left)* and short-axis *(right)* views of the left ventricle. **B,** An enlarged cross-sectional view of the left ventricle at the level of the mitral valve illustrating the cowl-like shape of the anterior mitral leaflet *(arrows)*. The motion of this portion of the leaflet into the left ventricular outflow tract in systole creates subaortic stenosis. *Ao*=aorta; *LA*=left atrium; *LV*=left ventricle; *RV*=right ventricle.

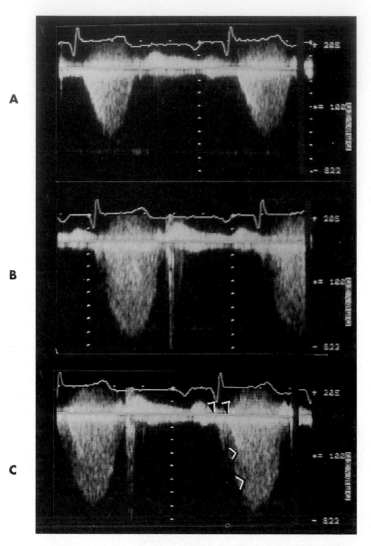

Fig. 2-45 Continuous wave Doppler spectral tracings from the cardiac apex in a patient with hypertrophic cardiomyopathy and dynamic left ventricular outflow obstruction. **A,** Systolic flow below the baseline representing flow out the left ventricular outflow tract. There is a late rise to peak velocity indicating that obstruction occurs as systole progresses. **B,** Mitral regurgitant flow with a broader systolic signal which begins earlier in systole and reaches a higher peak velocity with a rapid early acceleration of flow. **C,** The two Doppler signals are superimposed to demonstrate more clearly the difference in timing and pattern.

cardium also appears normal. The most prominent physiologic derangement is impaired diastolic relaxation reflected in the alteration of the pattern of left ventricular filling on the Doppler profile of mitral inflow. Typically, the initial filling wave (E) is large with rapid deceleration consequent to increased early filling, and the late filling wave (A) is either small or absent owing to a reduced late diastolic filling capacity (Appleton et al, 1988). Although a specific cause is rarely determined, consideration should be given to the possibility of an infiltrative process such as amyloidosis.

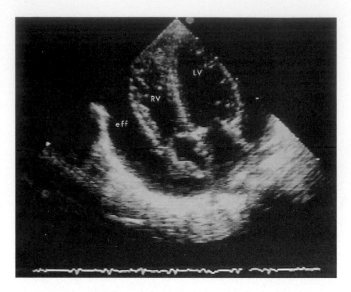

Fig. 2-46 Apical four-chamber echocardiographic view in a patient with a large circumferential pericardial effusion. The borders of the heart are outlined by a dark echolucent space representing fluid within the pericardial sac. *eff*=effusion; *LV*=left ventricle; *RV*=right ventricle.

Pericardial Disease

The pericardium consists of two separate membranous layers, including a visceral layer applied directly to the outer surface of the heart and proximal great vessels and a parietal layer which forms the free wall of the pericardial sac. Because the pericardial sac normally contains only 20 to 50 ml of fluid it is usually seen as a single highly reflective interface. In normal patients with an increased amount of fat overlying the visceral surface of the heart, distinction between the two layers may become evident, particularly anteriorly (Weyman et al, 1982).

Pericardial effusions and pericardial tamponade

Echocardiography is a sensitive technique for the detection and localization of pericardial effusions. Serous pericardial fluid does not reflect ultrasound and therefore appears as an echolucent area within the boundaries of the pericardial sac (Fig. 2-46). The size of the pericardial effusion is usually described semiquantitatively as being small, moderate, or large. When large, the heart swings freely in the pericardial space. In some instances large fluid collections in the pleural space surround the heart and can be difficult to distinguish from fluid within the pericardial space. The distinction is usually evident by noting the relation between the fluid, the posterior surface of the heart, and the descending thoracic aorta. Pericardial fluid extends between the descending thoracic aorta and left atrium (Fig. 2-47). In contrast, the aorta remains closely apposed to the atrioventricular groove in the presence of pleural fluid (Weyman et al, 1982).

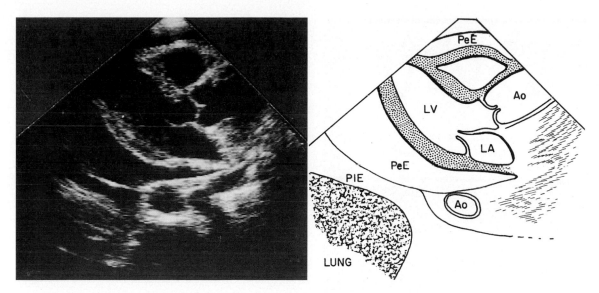

Fig. 2-47   Two-dimensional echocardiographic view and corresponding diagram in a patient with both a pleural and pericardial effusion. The echo-free space anterior and immediately posterior to the heart is pericardial fluid. The parietal pericardial layer divides the posterior pericardial fluid from the pleural fluid. The location of the descending thoracic aorta in relation to the fluid is often helpful in distinguishing pleural from pericardial fluid. The descending aorta is seen in cross section behind the heart. Pericardial fluid lies between the heart and the aorta while pleural fluid is seen posterior to both the heart and the aorta. *Ao*=aorta; *LA*=left atrium; *LV*=left ventricle; *PeE*=pericardial effusion; *PIE*=pleural effusion. (From Sanfilippo AJ, Weyman AE: Pericardial disease, in Weyman AE: *Principles and practice of echocardiography,* ed 2, Philadelphia, 1994, Lea and Febiger.)

In some circumstances the echocardiographic image may suggest the presence of a specific pericardial abnormality such as tumor, fibrin, or organized hematoma. For example, the presence of discrete masses of echoes adherent to the visceral surface of the heart suggests pericardial tumor, whereas discrete strands between the visceral and parietal layers of the pericardium suggest fibrin.

Echocardiography is also useful in determining the hemodynamic significance of pericardial fluid collections. An increase in intrapericardial pressure relative to atrial and ventricular pressure causes inversion of the right atrial free wall at the end of atrial systole (early ventricular diastole), and inversion of the right ventricular free wall in early diastole (Armstrong et al, 1982). Right ventricular inversion is both sensitive and specific for clinically apparent cardiac tamponade (Gillam et al, 1983). In contrast, right atrial inversion is a more sensitive but less specific marker of tamponade. This is not surprising given the thin nature of the right atrial wall and the low pressure within this chamber, which together make the right atrium more sensitive than the right ventricle to subtle changes in pericardial pressure. Nonetheless, when right atrial inversion persists for more than one third of the cardiac cycle, correlation with hemodynamic evidence of tamponade is stronger than for detection of atrial inversion per se (Gillam et al, 1983).

Doppler ultrasound is useful in the assessment of the hemodynamic significance of pericardial effusions. In particular, it is possible to detect exaggerated respiratory phase variation in right and left ventricular inflow and aortic and pulmonary outflow, consequent to the inability of the heart to both fill normally and eject a normal stroke volume in the presence of a tense fluid-filled pericardium (Pandian et al, 1984; Picard et al, 1991). In effect, therefore, the exaggerated respiratory variation in the Doppler profiles is the equivalent of pulsus paradoxus (Fig. 2-48).

Pericardial constriction
The diagnosis of constrictive pericarditis by two-dimensional echocardiography is difficult, but may be suggested by abnormal pericardial thickening or calcification in association with impaired ventricular filling. Typically, pericardial thickening is visible as a thick, uniformly bright echogenic layer surrounding all or part of the left ventricle. In the presence of constriction, ventricular filling occurs early and ceases abruptly in mid-diastole because of the restraining effect of the pericardium, which prevents the ventricular chambers from enlarging as they fill (Chandraratna et al, 1982). This pattern of rapid early diastolic filling and reduced late diastolic filling may also be inferred from the mitral inflow Doppler profile, which typically shows a large early filling (E) wave, and a small or absent late filling (A) wave.

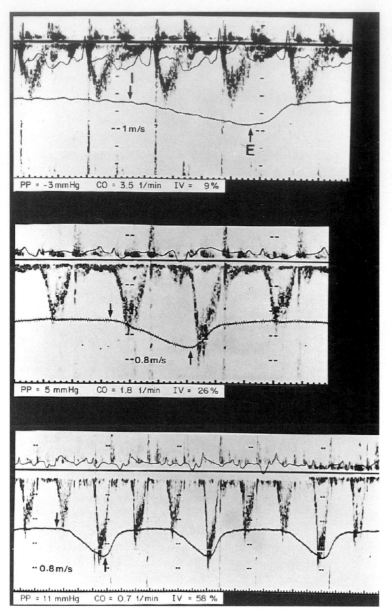

Fig. 2-48 Pulsed Doppler spectral tracings of flow velocity across the pulmonary valve with increasing intrapericardial pressure. The top panel demonstrates the normal degree of variation in pulmonary flow velocity with respiration and normal intrapericardial pressure. The middle panel shows more marked variation in flow velocity when intrapericardial pressure has been raised to 5 mm Hg. In the bottom panel, a 58% increase in flow velocity occurs with inspiration when the intrapericardial pressure is increased to 11 mm Hg. *CO*=cardiac output; *E*=expiration; *IV*=inspiratory variation; *I*=inspiration; *PP*=pericardial pressure. (Reprinted with permission from the American College of Cardiology from Picard MH, et al: Quantitative relation between increased intrapericardial pressure and Doppler flow velocities during experimental cardiac tamponade. *J Am Coll Cardiol* 18:237,1991.)

Other two-dimensional echocardiographic features that may be visible include the lack of respiratory variation in the size of the inferior vena cava, and a specific pattern of motion of the interventricular septum. This "septal bounce" pattern is an initial leftward movement of the septum, which is a consequence of the increased right ventricular inflow during peak inspiration followed by a rapid rightward shift as left ventricular filling begins.

Although none of these signs are either sensitive or specific for the diagnosis of pericardial constriction, with a compatible clinical picture they provide support for the diagnosis. Further, although some Doppler features may prove useful in distinguishing pericardial constriction from restrictive cardiomyopathy (Hatle et al, 1989; von Bibra et al, 1989), the absence of signs of restrictive cardiomyopathy may in itself provide more useful clinical information.

Pericardial cysts

Pericardial cysts are rare benign developmental abnormalities that are usually asymptomatic, but which may come to your attention on a routine chest x-ray. Echocardiographically, they appear as a unilocular fluid-filled thin-walled structure located adjacent to the right atrium or along the lateral border of the right or left side of the heart (Hynes et al, 1983).

Intracardiac Masses

Intracardiac tumors

Intracardiac tumors may be either secondary or primary. Secondary tumors are significantly more frequent than primary tumors and result from aggressive local intrathoracic malignancies which invade the myocardium directly or spread into the atria from the pulmonary

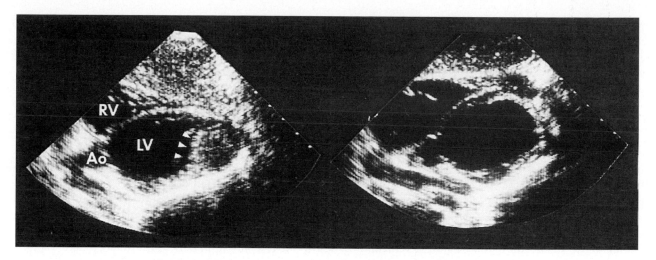

Fig. 2-49 Subcostal long-axis echocardiographic view of the left ventricle demonstrating a cardiac fibroma in the left ventricular apex *(left panel)* and following surgical removal *(right panel)*. *Ao*=aorta; *LV*=left ventricle; *RV*=right ventricle.

vessels. Secondary hematologic spread of disease may also occur from the abdomen, retroperitoneal space, breast, or skin. In keeping with their aggressive nature and means of spread, secondary tumors grow within the myocardium, appearing as distinct, usually brightly echogenic masses. Rarely, secondary tumors may seed the endocardium and appear to grow into the ventricular cavity. Finally, secondary invasion of the pericardium may be visible as discrete regions of thickening of the visceral pericardium in association with a pericardial effusion.

Primary tumors of the heart are distinctly rare and most often benign (Fig. 2-49). The most common tumor is the atrial myxoma. These frequently arise from the left side of the fossa ovalis but may arise anywhere in the atria and occasionally involve the mitral or tricuspid leaflets. They can be either sessile or pedunculated, single or multiple. Myxomas have been associated with other noncardiac conditions including lentiginosis and pituitary tumors (usually familial). Echocardiographically, myxomas are discrete, multilobulated masses. Although usually homogeneous in appearance, they may contain focal areas of lucency due to areas of hemorrhage which occur when the tumor outgrows its blood supply. When large and pedunculated, atrial myxomas may prolapse across the mitral or tricuspid valve in diastole and impair ventricular filling (Salcedo et al, 1983) (Fig. 2-50).

A number of malignant primary tumors may arise in the heart. Rhabdomyosarcomas arise from striated muscle and infiltrate diffusely into the myocardium, particularly the interventricular septum; they may also grow into and obliterate the cardiac chambers. They are more common in children and infants, and are strongly associated with tuberous sclerosis (Braunwald, 1992). In contrast, angiosarcomas are the most common primary cardiac malignancy in adults, and are more common in

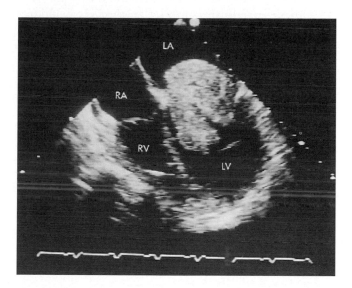

Fig. 2-50 Transesophageal four-chamber echocardiographic view of a large left atrial myxoma prolapsing through the mitral valve. *LA*=left atrium; *LV*=left ventricle; *RA*=right atrium; *RV*=right ventricle.

males. They most commonly arise in the right atrium in the region of the interatrial septum and may be polypoid. Fibrosarcomas arise from endocardial structures, and tend to be large fleshy tumors, which may infiltrate and involve more than one cardiac chamber.

Intracardiac thrombus

Intracardiac thrombus forms as a result of low flow within the heart or as a result of endocardial injury. Thrombus formation most commonly occurs in atrial fibrillation, mitral stenosis, dilated cardiomyopathy, and recent myocardial infarction.

Ventricular thrombi may be laminar, sessile, or independently mobile. They are distinguishable from myocardium because of their discrete nature and distinct echogenicity. Although the degree of echogenicity is variable, older thrombi tend to appear brighter as they become more organized. Ventricular thrombi should be differentiated from false tendons, apical scar, and chest wall artifacts (Asinger et al, 1981). This is usually possible because thrombi are typically seen in at least two views, do not appear as distinct linear midventricular structures, and tend to form in regions of abnormal wall motion. Ventricular thrombi may be detectable within days of myocardial infarction. These thrombi tend to be large and invariably form in the region of abnormal wall motion. The risk of systemic embolism following myocardial infarction is greater in patients with echocardiographic evidence of thrombus, and in these patients the risk relates to the size and mobility of the thrombus.

Atrial thrombi have morphologic characteristics similar to those of ventricular thrombi. They most frequently arise in the atrial appendage, and therefore may be difficult to visualize from transthoracic windows. Transesophageal imaging is often required to confirm or exclude the presence of thrombus with certainty. It is important to differentiate thrombus from the normal trabeculae of the appendage, and from the ridge between the appendage and the lower left pulmonary vein (Nanda et al, 1990).

A number of normal anatomic structures can produce the appearance of a mass lesion in the atria. Specifically, thickening of the tricuspid annulus, prominence of trabeculae along the roof of the atria, and a prominent eustachian valve may all be misdiagnosed as a right atrial tumor. Finally, compression of the atrial wall by an intrathoracic mass or hiatal hernia may also produce the appearance of a left atrial tumor.

Diseases of the Aorta

Transthoracic echocardiography allows routine assessment of the ascending and abdominal portions of the aorta in adults, and variable imaging of the transverse arch and descending thoracic aorta. It is usually possible to obtain complete views of the entire aorta in the pediatric population. Transesophageal imaging aids in more complete examination of the aorta in adults (Nanda et al, 1990).

Proximal aortic disease

An increase in aortic root dimension is typical of proximal aortic root disease. In patients with Marfan syndrome, dilatation typically occurs at the level of the aortic sinuses and the ascending aortic root appears relatively normal. In contrast, in patients with either an atherosclerotic or luetic aortic aneurysm the aorta appears diffusely thickened and dilatation occurs beyond the level of the sinotubular junction; discrete atheromatous

plaques may be seen as irregular thickening of the vessel wall, or as areas of discrete calcification. On occasion, there may be evidence of focal plaque rupture, with linear mobile echodensities attached to the abnormal vessel wall.

Aortic dissection is suggested by aortic root dilatation and a discrete dissection flap, which partitions the aortic lumen (Erbel et al, 1981; Granato and Gibson, 1985) (Fig. 2-51). Typically the true lumen is smaller than the false lumen, increases in size during systole, and has high velocity flow within it (Iliceto et al, 1987). Once aortic dissection is confirmed, it is important to determine whether the dissection involves the ostia of either the coronary or head and neck vessels and whether it has disrupted the aortic valve, resulting in pericardial hemorrhage.

Transesophageal imaging allows the diagnosis of aortic dissection with much higher sensitivity and almost complete specificity (Nienaber et al, 1992). While this is particularly valuable for assessing patency of the proximal left and right coronary ostia, transthoracic imaging is more sensitive for assessing the presence and hemodynamic significance of any pericardial fluid collection. Unfortunately, neither transthoracic nor transesophageal imaging can routinely exclude occlusion of the proximal aortic arch vessels in any given patient.

Finally, a rare but echocardiographically distinct condition of the proximal aorta is the development of an aneurysm of the sinus of Valsalva (Terdjman et al, 1984). This may be clinically silent, but detectable during routine echocardiography as a discrete membranous structure prolapsing into either the right atria (if the aneurysm arises from the noncoronary sinus) or right ventricle (if the aneurysm arises from the right coronary sinus). Rupture of the aneurysm may occur spontaneously or as a consequence of infection, and presents clinically with the development of a continuous murmur. Color Doppler reveals evidence of abnormal aortoatrial or aortoventricular shunt flow. Occasionally, the degree of left-to-right shunt flow may be significant and require surgical correction.

Disease of the thoracic and abdominal aorta

Dissection of the thoracic aorta may occur as a consequence of atheromatous disease or as a result of chest trauma. In cases of suspected dissection, transesophageal imaging is usually required to confirm the diagnosis by echocardiography (Engberding et al, 1987). The features of dissection are the same as those described for the ascending aorta. Abdominal scanning will detect atheromatous disease of the abdominal aorta, including accurate assessment of the size of abdominal aortic aneurysms. Although this is not strictly part of the cardiac ultrasound examination, it is often performed during the routine subcostal assessment of the heart.

The Doppler profile seen in the abdominal aorta may suggest a coarctation; with a significant coarctation, there

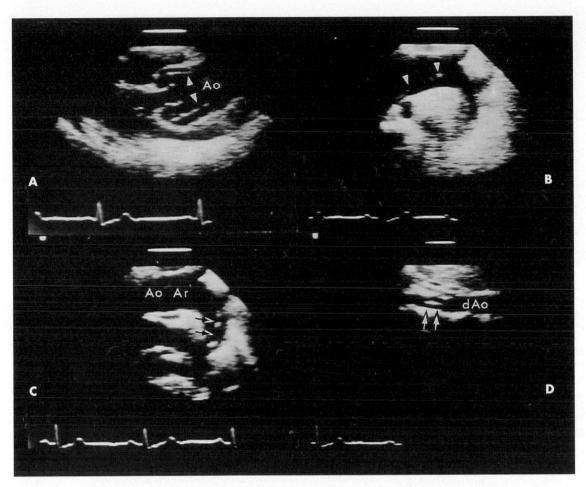

Fig. 2-51   Echocardiographic views of the aortic root depicting an extensive aortic dissection. **A,** Linear echoes within the proximal aortic root are present both anteriorly and posteriorly *(arrows).* Suprasternal views of the ascending and descending thoracic aorta in **B** and **C** continue to demonstrate the dissection flap. **D,** Subcostal imaging of the descending abdominal aorta detects extension of the dissection into the aorta at this level. *Ao*=aorta; *Ao Ar*=aortic arch; *dAo*=descending aorta. (From Weyman AE, Griffin BP: Left ventricular outflow tract: the aortic valve, aorta, and subvalvular outflow tract, in Weyman AE: *Principles and practice of echocardiography,* ed 2, Philadelphia, 1994, Lea & Febiger.)

is continuous systolic and diastolic flow in the aorta. Further, continuous wave Doppler directed through the descending aorta can determine the gradient across the coarctation, and the suprasternal window may allow accurate visualization and location of the coarctation itself, especially in the pediatric patient (Fig. 2-52).

Congenital Heart Disease

Atrial septal defects

Atrial septal defects (ASDs) are among the most common congenital heart lesions. Defects in the interatrial septum are categorized by their location within the septal wall. They include the *ostium secundum* ASD located in the midportion of the atrial septum in the region of the fossa ovalis, the *ostium primum* ASD positioned infe-

riorly near the atrioventricular valves, and the *sinus venosus* ASD located near the entry of the superior or inferior vena cava. Two-dimensional echocardiography can visualize the entire atrial septum and detect an ASD as a discrete absence of echoes in the appropriate area of the septal wall (Fig. 2-53). False-positive dropout of the atrial septum occurs if the ultrasound beam does not strike the atrial septum nearly perpendicularly. However, the acoustic interface between septum and blood at the margin of a true defect creates a particularly dense reflection which helps define the edges of the ASD and distinguishes it from false-positive dropout. Doppler color flow mapping complements two-dimensional imaging by demonstrating flow across the defect as a localized jet from left to right during late systole and diastole (Fig. 2-54). Atrial defects with low right-sided

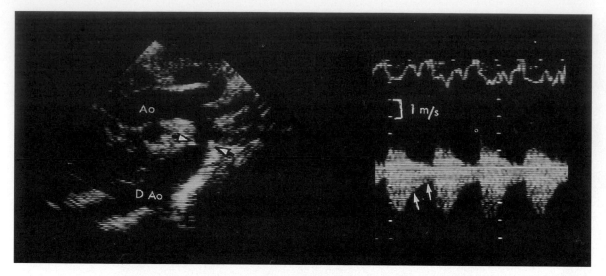

Fig. 2-52 Suprasternal echocardiographic view (left panel) of an aortic coarctation at the isthmus *(arrowheads)*. Mild tubular narrowing of the transverse arch is present as well as poststenotic dilatation of the descending aorta. In the panel on the right, the continuous wave Doppler spectral tracing of flow in the descending aorta is high in velocity (3 m/sec) with a characteristic pattern of continued gradient into early diastole *(arrows)*. *Ao*=aorta; *D Ao*=descending aorta. (From Liberthson RR: Congenital heart disease in the child, adolescent, and adult, in Eagle KA, et al (eds): *The practice of cardiology,* Boston, 1989, Little Brown.)

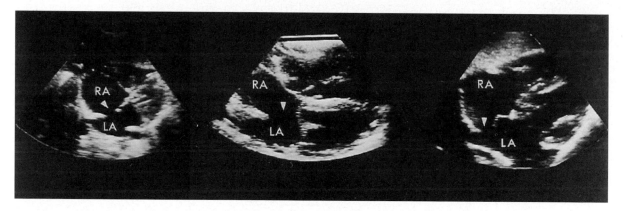

Fig. 2-53 Subcostal echocardiographic views of the heart highlighting the interatrial septum. On the left, a defect in the midatrial septum represents a secundum atrial septal defect. The center panel demonstrates a large area of dropout from the midseptum to the atrioventricular groove indicative of an ostium primum defect. In the panel on the right, a defect is present high in the atrial septum near the roof of the atria *(arrowhead)*, consistent with a sinus venosus defect. *LA*=left atrium; *RA*=right atrium. (From Liberthson RR: Congenital heart disease in the child, adolescent, and adult, in Eagle KA, et al (eds): *The practice of cardiology*, Boston, 1989, Little Brown.)

pressures and predominantly left-to-right shunting are most easily detected. When pulmonary artery hypertension develops, shunt flow is low in velocity and often bidirectional. Thus it may be more difficult to distinguish atrial shunt flow from the other low-velocity flows within the atrium. Pulsed Doppler may confirm the direction and timing of flow across the ASD to supplement the information derived from color flow mapping.

Another noninvasive method for detecting atrial shunts is contrast echocardiography (Gramiak et al,

1969). By rapid intravenous injection of a small volume of agitated saline, the resulting turbulence and dissolved air creates multiple small ultrasound scatterers. This produces a "contrast effect" when compared with the unopacified blood pool, and allows detection of right-to-left shunting by the passage of contrast from the right atrium to the left atrium and ventricle. Left-to-right shunting is visible as a "negative contrast effect" when unopacified left atrial blood enters the contrast-filled right atrium (Weyman et al, 1979) (see Fig. 2-54).

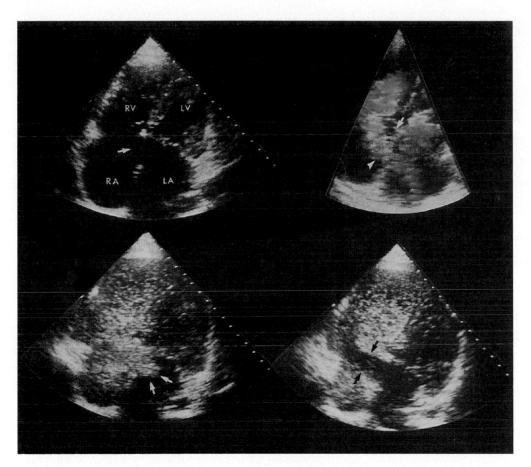

Fig. 2-54   Series of apical four-chamber echocardiographic views in a patient with an ostium primum atrial septal defect. In the upper left panel, the dropout in the lower atrial septum *(arrow)* delineates the defect. Doppler color flow mapping *(upper right)* demonstrates a wide band of flow crossing from the left atrium to the right atrium *(arrows)*. Following intravenous injection of agitated saline, microbubbles are detected as contrast within the cardiac chambers. In the lower left panel, right-to-left shunting can be seen across the defect *(arrows)* and left-to-right negative contrast is shown in the lower right panel *(arrows)* as unopacified blood crosses the atrial defect. *LA*=left atrium; *LV*=left ventricle; *RA*=right atrium; *RV*=right ventricle. (From Levine RA, et al: Echocardiography: principles and clinical applicatons, in Eagle KA, et al (eds): *The practice of cardiology,* Boston, 1989, Little Brown.) (This figure is reproduced in color before page 1.)

When there is an ASD, common associated lesions should be sought. With sinus venosus defects, and less commonly with secundum ASDs, the right pulmonary veins may drain either functionally or anatomically to the right atrium. Two-dimensional imaging and color flow mapping can often demonstrate the entry of all four pulmonary veins. The diagnosis of partial anomalous pulmonary venous return requires careful attention to the superior vena cava and right upper pulmonary vein. Primum atrial septal defects are frequently a part of the spectrum of endocardial cushion defects, which include a deficiency in the atrioventricular septum and anomalies of the atrioventricular valves. Thus, you should look for an associated cleft in the anterior mitral valve leaflet and the presence of a ventricular septal defect (VSD) when a primum ASD is diagnosed (Fig. 2-55).

Estimation of the size of the atrial shunt and its effect on the pulmonary circulation are also important. The atrial defect size can be measured directly from the two-dimensional echocardiogram with high-quality images. However, this may not correlate directly with shunt size since the pulmonary vascular resistance, right ventricular compliance, and intravascular volume all influence the volume of shunt flow. Evidence of right atrial and right ventricular chamber enlargement and paradoxical motion of the interventricular septum are indicative of right ventricular volume overload and generally indicate a pulmonary to systemic shunt ratio of greater than 1.5:1 (Kerber et al, 1973). Doppler estimates of volumetric flow across the pulmonic and aortic valves provides a noninvasive method of measuring the shunt ratio (see Fig. 2-19). The echo-derived shunt ratio ($\dot{Q}p:\dot{Q}s$) corre-

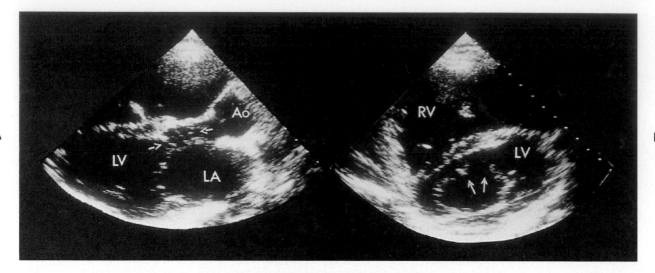

Fig. 2-55   Parasternal echocardiographic views of the mitral valve in a patient with a partial atrio-ventricular canal defect. **A,** Chordal attachments of the anterior leaflet to the septum are seen *(arrows)*. The cross-sectional view of the mitral valve **(B)** shows clearly the cleft in the anterior leaflet *(arrows)*. Right ventricular enlargement and diastolic flattening of the interventricular septum are evidence of right ventricular volume overload from the associated atrial septal defect. *Ao*=aorta; *LA*=left atrium; *LV*=left ventricle; *RV*=right ventricle. (From King ME: Complex congenital heart disease II: a pathologic approach, in Weyman AE: *Principles and practice of echocardiography,* ed 2, Philadelphia, 1994, Lea & Febiger.)

lates well with that obtained at cardiac catheterization (Sanders et al, 1983), but is subject to measurement errors and therefore is used clinically only as a semi-quantitative index of shunt size. There are several methods for quantifying shunt flow by color Doppler, including measurements of the area of shunt flow within the right atrium and of the jet width as it crosses the defect (Pollick et al, 1988). While the latter method correlates more closely with actual shunt size, both methods are still only semiquantitative for clinical purposes.

Ventricular septal defects

The interventricular septum is a complex structure composed of muscular and fibrous tissue. Defects in the septum are extremely common and can occur singly or multiply at many different locations. Figure 2-56 demonstrates the echocardiographic views in which each type of VSD can be recorded. Echocardiographic detection of a VSD depends on echo dropout from the interventricular septum and is further strengthened by the use of pulsed or color flow Doppler to detect turbulent shunt flow across the defect. In Figure 2-57, representative echocardiographic examples of typical VSDs are depicted.

Muscular VSDs occur frequently in young children and the majority of these close spontaneously within the first 2 years of life. Muscular defects near the cardiac apex can be of considerable size and yet be overlooked unless the sonographer closely inspects the apical aspect of the interventricular septum.

The fibrous portion of the interventricular septum, the membranous septum, lies adjacent to the aortic annulus.

Membranous septal defects cause septal dropout beneath the aortic valve. The tricuspid valve septal leaflet and chordal apparatus lie along the right ventricular aspect of the membranous septum. Incorporation of this tissue into a septal aneurysm often causes spontaneous closure of a membranous VSD (Hornberger et al, 1989). The right coronary or noncoronary aortic leaflet occasionally prolapses into a high membranous VSD, effecting defect closure but distorting aortic valve coaptation and causing aortic insufficiency (Fig. 2-58).

Supracristal VSDs occur in that portion of the interventricular septum located above the crista supraventricularis and beneath the pulmonary annulus. Echocardiographic views of the right ventricular outflow tract are best for detecting this type of defect. Prolapse and distortion of the right coronary aortic leaflet also occurs with supracristal VSDs.

Inlet VSDs occur in the region of the septum near the tricuspid and mitral annuli and are often associated with straddling of the tricuspid or mitral valves. *Atrioventricular septal defects* result from the absence of the atrioventricular septum and thus result in a large defect in the center of the heart which has an atrial and an inlet ventricular component. These are also known as "endocardial cushion" or "atrioventricular canal" defects.

When a VSD is restrictive in size and a significant pressure difference exists between left and right ven-

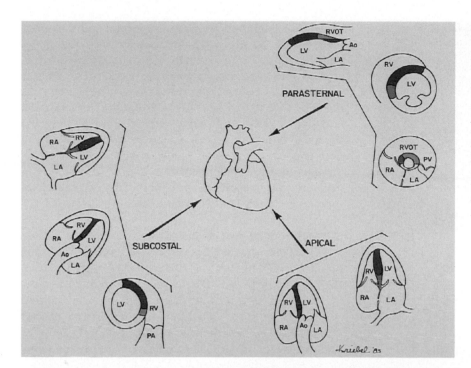

Fig. 2-56 Diagrammatic representation of multiple echocardiographic views of the interventricular septum with color encoding of the subdivisions of the septum. The muscular septum is shown in blue, the inlet septum in green, the infundibular septum in orange, and the membranous septum in red. *Ao*=aorta; *LA*=left atrium; *LV*=left ventricle; *RA*=right atrium; *RV*=right ventricle; *RVOT*=right ventricular outflow tract; *PA*=pulmonary artery; *PV*=pulmonary valve. (From Levine RA, et al: Echocardiography: principles and clinical applications, in Eagle KA, et al (eds): *The practice of cardiology,* Boston, 1989, Little Brown.) (This figure is reproduced in color before page 1.)

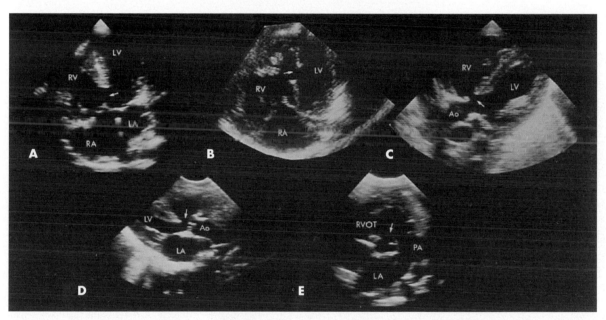

Fig. 2-57   Series of echocardiographic views in patients with ventricular septal defects (VSDs) *(arrows)*. **A,** Apical four-chamber view of a complete atrioventricular canal. **B,** Apical four-chamber view of a muscular defect. **C,** Subcostal view of the left ventricular outflow tract with a membranous VSD. **D,** Parasternal long-axis view of a malalignment VSD with aortic overriding of the septum. **E,** Parasternal short-axis view of the aorta with a supracristal defect. *Ao*=aorta; *LA*=left atrium; *LV*=left ventricle; *RA*=right atrium; *RV*=right ventricle; *RVOT*=right ventricular outflow tract;, *PA*=pulmonary artery. (From Liberthson RR: Congenital heart disease in the child, adolescent, and adult, in Eagle KA, et al (eds): *The practice of cardiology,* Boston, 1989, Little Brown.)

tricles, pulsed and color flow Doppler readily detect the shunt flow across a VSD that may be too small to detect on two-dimensional imaging. A turbulent high-velocity jet enters the right side of the heart adjacent to the defect, and there may be flow within the septal tissue with acceleration along the left ventricular aspect of the communication (Fig. 2-59). When pressures equalize between left and right ventricles, shunt flow is low in velocity and thus may be difficult to discern by color flow mapping.

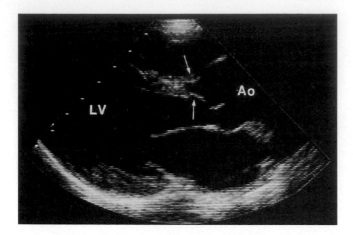

Fig. 2-58 Parasternal long-axis echocardiographic view of the left ventricular outflow tract. The anterior cusp of the aortic valve has prolapsed into a high ventricular septal defect *(arrows)*, effectively closing the interventricular communication but distorting the shape of the aortic valve creating aortic insufficiency. *Ao*=aorta, *LV*=left ventricle. (From Liberthson RR: Congenital heart disease in the child, adolescent, and adult, in Eagle KA, et al (eds): *The practice of cardiology,* Boston, 1989, Little Brown.)

Echocardiography provides important clinical information on shunt size and pulmonary pressure. Significant left-to-right shunting through a VSD enlarges the pulmonary artery, left atrium, and left ventricle. Estimates of Qp:Qs can be made for shunts at the ventricular level, as described for atrial shunts. Using the simplified Bernoulli equation ($P=4V^2$), the systolic pressure gradient between the left and right ventricles can be derived from the peak flow velocity of the left-to-right jet across the VSD. Subtracting this gradient from the aortic systolic blood pressure gives an estimate of the right ventricular and pulmonary artery systolic pressures.

Patent ductus arteriosus

In fetal life, the ductus arteriosus connects the pulmonary artery and aorta to allow passage of blood from the right heart to the systemic circulation without passing through the high resistance pulmonary circuit. Persistence of this channel beyond the first few days or weeks of life is abnormal and is usually an indication for noninvasive or surgical closure. Two-dimensional echo-

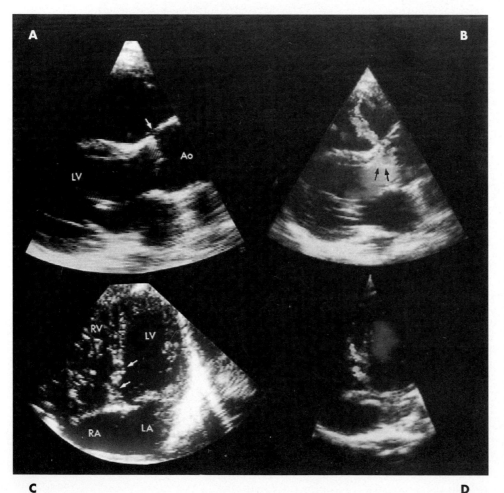

Fig. 2-59 Two-dimensional echo-cardiographic images and color flow Doppler illustration of shunt flow across small ventricular septal defects. **A,** Following repair of a malalignment VSD, a small residual defect is present at the upper edge of the patch *(arrow)*. **B,** The jet of shunt flow is seen as a mosaic-like stream emerging from the right ventricular aspect of the defect. Flow accelerates along the left ventricular septal surface *(arrows)* as it approaches the defect. **C,** Two small defects in the midmuscular septum are present *(arrows)*. Two discrete jets can be detected by color Doppler, shown in **D.** *Ao*=aorta; *LA*=left atrium; *LV*=left ventricle; *RA*=right atrium; *RV*=right ventricle. (This figure is reproduced in color before page 1.)

cardiography can image the ductus arteriosus in the left parasternal and suprasternal views which display the pulmonary artery bifurcation and the descending thoracic aorta (Fig. 2-60). In infants and small children, it is often possible to image this channel throughout its

length and measure its lumen size. Color flow mapping demonstrates the flow within the ductus and main pulmonary artery as a high-velocity jet entering the pulmonary artery. Although shunt flow is usually continuous from the higher-pressure aorta to the lower-pressure pulmonary vessel, the normal systolic forward flow in the pulmonary artery often obscures the systolic shunt flow, and the diastolic flow is the more readily detectable flow signal (Fig. 2-61). With a significant volume of shunt flow, the pulmonary artery will be enlarged, as will the left atrium and left ventricle. There may be retrograde flow in the descending thoracic aorta by pulsed or color flow Doppler, indicating significant runoff from the aorta into the ductus arteriosus.

Tetralogy of Fallot

Tetralogy of Fallot is a well-recognized cyanotic heart defect that results from malalignment and anterior deviation of the parietal band. This creates obstruction to pulmonary outflow and a large subaortic VSD. The pulmonary artery is often underdeveloped and the right ventricle develops hypertrophy in response to the outflow obstruction. Echocardiographically, the deviation of the parietal band is clearly visible as a muscular protrusion into the right ventricular outflow tract. The VSD is usually large and readily imaged beneath the large overriding aortic root (Fig. 2-62). Pulsed and color flow Doppler demonstrate low-velocity flow from the right ventricle passing across the VSD and out the aorta, as

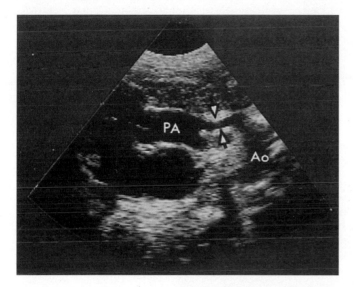

Fig. 2-60 Parasternal long-axis view of the main pulmonary artery in a patient with a large patent ductus arteriosus. The channel highlighted by *arrows* connects the pulmonary artery bifurcation with the descending thoracic aorta. *Ao*=aorta; *PA*=pulmonary artery. (From Levine RA, et al: Echocardiography: principles and clinical applications, in Eagle KA, et al (eds): *The practice of cardiology*, Boston, 1989, Little Brown.)

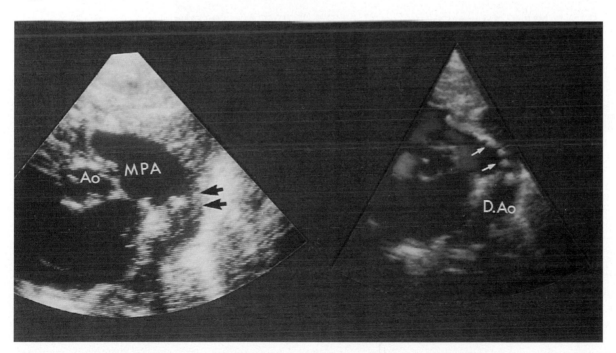

Fig. 2-61   Parasternal short-axis images at the base of the heart depicting a patent ductus arteriosus *(black arrows)* on the left, and the color Doppler appearance of the shunt flow from the descending aorta into the pulmonary artery *(white arrows)* on the right. *Ao*=aorta; *D Ao*=descending aorta; *MPA*=main pulmonary artery. (This figure is reproduced in color before page 1.)

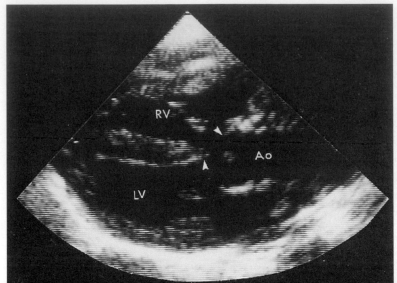

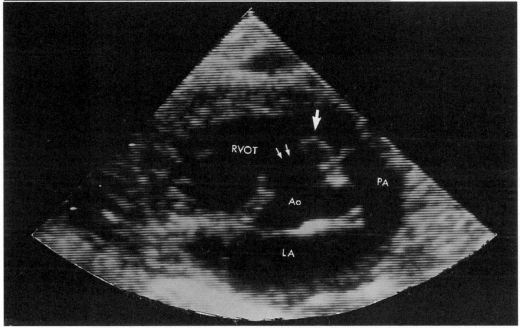

Fig. 2-62 Parasternal echocardiographic images in a patient with tetralogy of Fallot. **A,** A large malalignment ventricular septal defect is present *(arrowheads)* with an overriding aorta. **B,** The hallmark anterior deviation of the parietal band *(large arrow)* narrows the right ventricular outflow tract and leaves the malalignment VSD *(small arrows)*. The main pulmonary artery is small. *Ao*=aorta; *LA*=left atrium; *LV*=left ventricle; *RV*=right ventricle; *RVOT*=right ventricular outflow tract; *PA*=pulmonary artery. (From King ME: Complex congenital heart disease II: a pathologic approach, in Weyman AE: *Principles and practice of echocardiography,* ed 2, Philadelphia, 1994, Lea & Febiger.)

well as high-velocity, turbulent flow in the right ventricular outflow tract. Right ventricular outflow obstruction is usually at multiple sites: the subvalvular muscular ridge, the valvular and annular pulmonary level, and occasionally at the branch pulmonary arteries. Continuous wave Doppler sampling of flow in the right ventricular outflow tract can accurately predict the peak gradient from right ventricle to pulmonary artery (Houston et al, 1986).

Complete transposition of the great arteries

Another common congenital heart defect is complete transposition of the great arteries. In this entity, the aorta arises from the right ventricle and the pulmonary artery has its origin from the left ventricle. Echocardiographically, the great arteries arise in parallel from the base of the heart instead of wrapping around one another. The semilunar valves are visible at roughly the same level relative to the long-axis of the heart and therefore can be imaged simultaneously in the same plane (Fig. 2-63). Following the course of the great arteries, the anterior vessel arches and gives off brachiocephalic vessels, while the posterior artery bifurcates into right and left pulmonary branches. Because the right ventricle supplies the systemic circulation, it is characteristically enlarged and more globular in shape. Complete transposition creates two circulations in parallel, with systemic venous return to the right atrium and ventricle being redirected to the systemic circulation and pulmonary venous flow to the left atrium and left ventricle returning to the lungs. Therefore, some means of mixing of these two circulations is essential. This most often

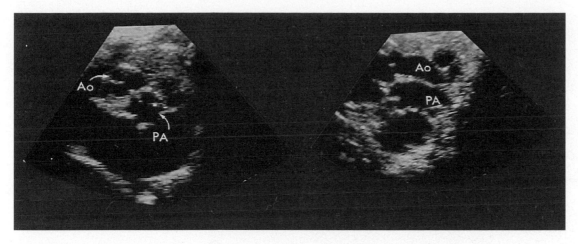

Fig. 2-63 Parasternal echocardiographic images in a patient with complete transposition of the great arteries. **A,** The semilunar valves are both seen in cross section with the aorta lying anterior and to the patient's right: *d*-transposition. The long axis of the great vessels shown in **B** demonstrates their parallel origin from the heart, with the aorta anterior to the pulmonary artery. *Ao*=aorta; *PA*=pulmonary artery. (From Levine RA, et al: Echocardiography: principles and clinical applications, in Eagle KA, et al (eds): *The practice of cardiology,* Boston, 1989, Little Brown.)

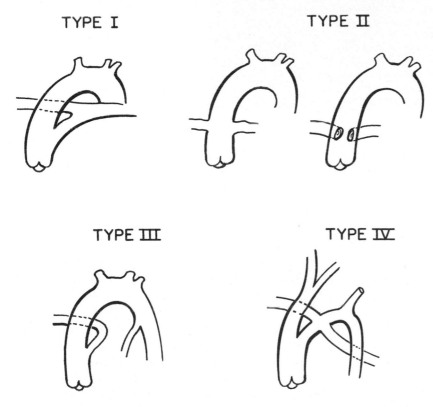

Fig. 2-64 Diagrammatic representation of the classification of truncus arteriosus as proposed by Van Praagh. In type I, there is a short segment of main pulmonary artery arising from the truncus and giving rise to the branch pulmonary arteries. Type II has independent origin of the branch pulmonary vessels directly from the truncus, either to the side or posteriorly. In type III, only one pulmonary artery arises from the ascending trunk with the other lung fed either by a ductus arteriosus or aortopulmonary collaterals. The unusual type IV has a hypoplastic ascending truncus with the pulmonary artery connected to the descending aorta by the ductus arteriosus. (From King ME: Complex congenital heart disease II: a pathologic approach, in Weyman AE: *Principles and practice of echocardiography,* ed 2, Philadelphia, 1994, Lea & Febiger.)

occurs at the atrial level via a patent foramen ovale, but VSDs and a patent ductus arteriosus are also means of intermixing and should be sought during echo-Doppler evaluation. Coronary artery anatomy should also be determined because surgical correction requires translocation of the coronaries from the anterior aorta to the posterior semilunar root. A single coronary artery or an intramural course of a coronary vessel makes translocation more difficult.

Truncus arteriosus

Persistent truncus arteriosus is a rare malformation in which a single arterial trunk arising from the heart supplies the coronary, pulmonary, and systemic circulations. A large VSD is invariably present allowing both ventricles to eject blood into the single arterial vessel. Several patterns of truncus arteriosus are commonly recognized (Van Praagh et al, 1965) (Fig. 2-64). The most frequent patterns are those in which the pulmonary arteries arise

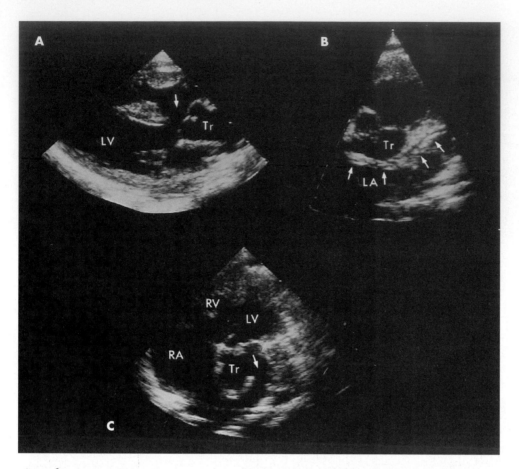

Fig. 2-65 Echocardiographic images of a patient with truncus arteriosus type I. **A,** The large truncal root overrides the interventricular septum with a large outlet ventricular septal defect *(arrow).* **B,** The cross-sectional view at the level of the truncal valve demonstrates the anomalous origin of the left coronary artery from the noncoronary sinus. From the apical five-chamber view **(C)**, the origin of the main pulmonary artery can be seen from the lateral aspect of the truncus *(arrow)* as well as its proximal branching. *LA*=left atrium; *LV*=left ventricle; *RA*=right atrium; *RV*=right ventricle; *Tr*=truncus arteriosus. (From King ME: Complex congenital heart disease II: a pathologic approach, in Weyman AE: *Principles and practice of echocardiography,* ed 2, Philadelphia, 1994, Lea & Febiger.)

from the ascending portion of the truncus, either as a main pulmonary artery, which then branches, or as separate branches from the posterior or lateral walls of the single arterial vessel. Echocardiographic diagnosis is based on demonstrating a large, single great vessel which overrides the interventricular septum above a large VSD, absence of a right ventricular outflow tract and pulmonary valve, and branching of the main pulmonary artery or its independent branches from the large common arterial trunk (Houston et al, 1981) (Fig. 2-65). The truncal valve is often thickened, stenotic, or regurgitant, and may have more than three cusps. Pulsed and color flow Doppler can detect truncal regurgitation and estimate the degree of truncal stenosis.

Double outlet right ventricle

As its name implies, "double outlet right ventricle" is an anomaly in which both great arteries arise entirely or to a major extent from the right ventricle. Left ventricular ejection must perforce pass through a VSD to the right-sided outflow vessels. There is wide variability in the orientation of the great vessels relative to the position of the VSD. The clinical signs and symptoms may be simply those of a large VSD or similar to those in complete transposition. The presence of pulmonary stenosis may create a physiology akin to tetralogy of Fallot or transposition with pulmonary outflow obstruction. The echocardiographic appearance in double outlet right ventricle is of a large outlet VSD and overriding of a great vessel. One key diagnostic feature is the lack of fibrous continuity between the anterior mitral leaflet and the semilunar valve, which is closest to the mitral valve (Macartney et al, 1984). The presence of subarterial conal tissue elevates and displaces the more posterior vessel toward the right ventricle, and it is this conal tissue that is visible as muscle or fibrous tissue separating the mitral valve from its adjacent semilunar valve (Fig. 2-66). Since pulmonary steno-

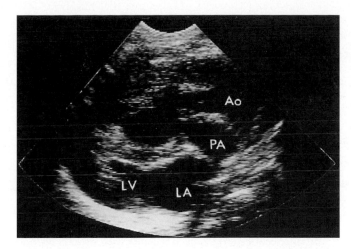

Fig. 2-66 Parasternal long-axis echocardiographic view of the great vessels in a patient with double outlet right ventricle. The aorta and pulmonary artery arise in parallel and both lie anterior to the plane of the interventricular septum. The ventricular septal defect is not imaged in this plane. *Ao*=aorta; *LA*=left atrium; *LV*=left ventricle; *PA*=pulmonary artery. (From Liberthson RR: Congenital heart disease in the child, adolescent, and adult, in Eagle KA, et al (eds): *The practice of cardiology*, Boston, 1989, Little Brown.)

sis is frequent, echocardiographic study should determine its presence and severity.

Univentricular heart

"Univentricular heart" or "single ventricle" occurs when both atrial chambers connect to a single ventricular chamber. Communication between atria and ventricle can be through two atrioventricular valves, a common valve, or a single atrioventricular valve with absence or atresia of the other orifice. The ventricular chamber may be of the right or left ventricular type. When the main chamber is of left ventricular morphology, there is a small anterior outflow chamber which represents the remnant of the right ventricle. In univentricular heart of the right ventricular type, there is a small blind posterior pouch constituting the residual left ventricle. Echocardiographic features of the univentricular heart, then, demonstrate a large single ventricular chamber with no interventricular septum (Huhta et al, 1985) (Fig. 2-67). The small outflow chamber, imaged anteriorly either to the patient's right or left, gives rise to one of the great vessels. If a blind posterior pouch is present, it

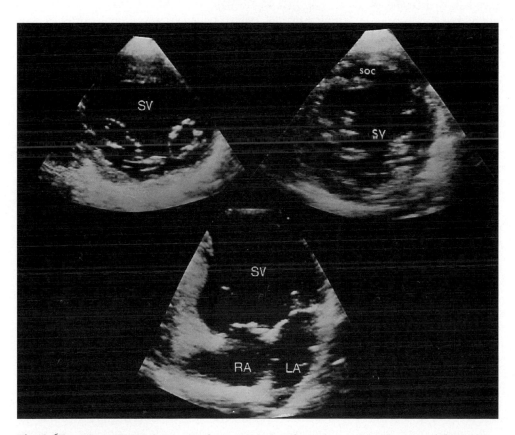

Fig. 2-67 Echocardiographic images from a patient with single ventricle. The upper left panel is a cross-sectional view of both atrioventricular valves entering one ventricle with no interventricular septum between them. The panel on the right shows a small slitlike outlet chamber anterior to the main ventricular cavity. The bottom panel is an apical view demonstrating both atria and atrioventricular valves communicating with one ventricular chamber. *LA*=left atrium; *RA*=right atrium; *soc*=small outlet chamber; *SV*=single ventricle. (From Liberthson RR: Congenital heart disease in the child, adolescent, and adult, in Eagle KA, et al (eds): *The practice of cardiology*, Boston, 1989, Little Brown.)

appears as a small chamber appended to the posterior aspect of the main ventricular chamber, either to the right or left. In the majority of patients with univentricular heart, the great vessels are transposed, with the aorta arising from the outlet chamber and the pulmonary artery arising from the large ventricular chamber.

SUGGESTED READINGS

Books

Braunwald E: *Heart disease: a textbook of cardiovascular medicine*, ed 4, Philadelphia, 1992, WB Saunders.

Feigenbaum H: *Echocardiography*, Baltimore, 1993, Williams & Wilkins.

Snider AR: *Echocardiography in pediatric heart disease*, Philadelphia, 1990, Mosby-Year Book.

Weyman AE: *Principles and practice of echocardiography*, Philadelphia, 1994, Lea & Febiger.

Weyman AE, et al: *Cross sectional echocardiography*, Philadelphia, 1982, Lea & Febiger.

Journals

Abascal VM, et al. 1990. Echocardiographic evaluation of successful outcome in 130 patients undergoing percutaneous balloon mitral valvotomy, *Circulation* 82:448.

Abbasi AS, et al. 1980. Detection and estimation of the degree of mitral regurgitation by range-gated pulse Doppler echocardiography, *Circulation* 61:143.

The American Society of Echocardiography. 1984a. *Recommendations for the terminology and display for Doppler echocardiography*. Raleigh, NC, American Society of Echocardiography, The Doppler Standards and Nomenclature Committee.

The American Society of Echocardiography. 1984b. *Report of the Committee of Nomenclature and Standards in Two-Dimensional Echocardiography*. Raleigh, NC, American Society of Echocardiography.

Appleton CP, et al. 1988. Demonstration of restrictive ventricular physiology by Doppler echocardiography, *J Am Coll Cardiol* 11:757.

Armstrong WF, et al. 1982. Diastolic collapse of the right ventricle with cardiac tamponade: an echocardiographic study, *Circulation* 65:1491.

Ascah KJ, et al. 1985. A Doppler-two-dimensional echocardiographic method for quantification of mitral regurgitation, *Circulation* 72:377.

Asinger RW, et al. 1981. Observations on detecting left ventricular thrombus with two-dimensional echocardiography: emphasis on avoidance of false positives, *Am J Cardiol* 47:145.

BAATAF (The Boston Area Anticoagulation Trial for Atrial Fibrillation Investigators). 1990. Effect of low dose warfarin on the risk of stroke in patients with non-rheumatic atrial fibrillation, *N Engl J Med* 323:1505.

Baumgartner H, et al. 1992. Effect of prosthetic valve design on the Doppler-catheter gradient correlation—an in vitro study of normal St. Jude, Medtronic-Hall, Starr-Edwards, and Hancock valves, *J Am Coll Cardiol* 19:324.

Berger M, et al. 1985. Quantitative assessment of pulmonary hypertension in patients with tricuspid regurgitation using continuous wave Doppler ultrasound, *J Am Coll Cardiol* 6:359.

Blumlein S, et al. 1986. Quantification of mitral regurgitation by Doppler echocardiography, *Circulation* 74:34.

Bonow RO, et al. 1983. The natural history of asymptomatic patients with aortic regurgitation and normal left ventricular function, *Circulation* 68:509.

Botvinick EH, et al. 1975. Echocardiographic demonstration of early mitral closure in severe aortic regurgitation: its clinical implications, *Circulation* 51:836.

Chandraratna PAN, Arnow WS, Imaizumi T. 1992. Role of echocardiography in detecting the anatomic and physiologic abnormalities of constrictive pericarditis, *Am J Med Sci*, 283:141.

Chen C, et al. 1989. Prevalence of valvular regurgitation by Doppler echocardiography in patients with structurally normal hearts by two-dimensional echocardiography, *Am J Cardiol* 117:636.

Chunguang C, et al. 1993. Non-invasive estimation of regurgitant flow rate and volume in patients with mitral regurgitation by Doppler color mapping of accelerating flow field, *J Am Coll Cardiol* 21:374.

Ciobanu M, et al. 1982. Pulsed Doppler echocardiography in the diagnosis and estimation of severity of aortic insufficiency, *Am J Cardiol* 49:339.

Currie PJ, et al. 1985a. Continuous wave Doppler determination of right ventricular pressure: a simultaneous Doppler-catheterization study in 127 patients, *J Am Coll Cardiol* 6:750.

Currie PJ, et al. 1985b. Continuous-wave Doppler echocardiographic assessment of the severity of calcific aortic stenosis: a simultaneous Doppler catheter study in 100 adult patients, *Circulation* 71:1162.

Dabestani A, et al. 1987. Evaluation of pulmonary artery pressure and resistance by pulsed Doppler echocardiography, *Am J Cardiol* 59:663.

Diebold B, et al. 1987. Quantification of aortic insufficiency using color Doppler flow imaging (abstract), *J Am Coll Cardiol* 9:66A.

Elkayam U, et al. 1983. The use of Doppler flow velocity measurement to assess the hemodynamic response to vasodilators in patients with heart failure, *Circulation* 67:377.

Engberding R, et al. 1987. Identification of dissection or aneurysm of the descending thoracic aorta by conventional and transthoracic two-dimensional echocardiography, *Am J Cardiol* 59:717.

Erbel R, et al. 1981. Two-dimensional echocardiographic diagnosis of papillary muscle rupture, *Chest* 79:595.

Erbel R, et al. 1989. Echocardiography in the diagnosis of aortic dissection, *Lancet* 1:457.

Esper RJ. 1982. Detection of mild mitral regurgitation by range-gated pulsed Doppler echocardiography, *Am J Cardiol* 50:1037.

Fisher DC, et al. 1983. The effects of variations on pulsed Doppler sampling site on calculation of cardiac output: an experimental study in open chested dogs, *Circulation* 62:542.

Gardin JM, et al. 1985. Echocardiographic and Doppler flow observations in obstructed and non-obstructed hypertrophic cardiomyopathy, *Am J Cardiol* 56:614.

Gibson RS, et al. 1982. Value of early two-dimensional echocardiography in patients with acute myocardial infarction, *Am J Cardiol* 49:1110.

Gillam LD, et al. 1983. A comparison of right atrial and right ventricular inversion as echocardiographic markers of cardiac tamponade, *J Am Coll Cardiol* 1:738.

Gillam LD, et al. 1985. Which cardiac valve provides the best Doppler estimate of cardiac output in men? *Circulation* 72:(Suppl 3):III-99.

Godley RW, Wann LS, Rogers EW. 1981. Incomplete mitral valve closure in patients with papillary muscle closure with papillary muscle dysfunction, *Circulation* 63:565.

Gottdiener JS, et al. 1983. Frequency and embolic potential of left ventricular thrombus in dilated cardiomyopathy: assessment by two-dimensional echocardiography, *Am J Cardiol* 52:1281.

Gramiak R, et al. 1969. Ultrasound cardiography: contrast studies in anatomy and function, *Radiology* 92:939.

Granato JE, Gibson RS. 1985. Utility of two-dimensional echocardiography in suspected ascending aortic dissection, *Am J Cardiol* 56:123.

Grayburn PA. 1986. Detection of aortic insufficiency by standard echocardiography, pulsed Doppler echocardiography, and auscultation, *Ann Intern Med* 104:599.

Gross CW, Wann LS. 1984. Doppler echocardiographic diagnosis of porcine bioprosthetic cardiac valve malfunction, *Am J Cardiol* 53:1203.

Handschumacher MD, et al. 1993. A new integrated system for three-dimensional echocardiographic reconstruction: development and validation for ventricular volume with application in human subjects, *Am Coll Cardiol* 21:743.

Hatle L, Angelsen B, Tromsdal A. 1979. Non-invasive assessment of atrioventricular pressure half-time by Doppler ultrasound, *Circulation* 60:1096.

Hatle L, Angelsen B, Tromsdal A. 1980. Non-invasive assessment of aortic stenosis by Doppler ultrasound, *Br Heart J* 43:284.

Hatle L, Appleton CP, Popp RL. 1989. Differentiation of constrictive pericarditis and restrictive cardiomyopathy by Doppler echocardiography, *Circulation* 79:357.

Heger JJ, et al. 1979. Cross-sectional echocardiography in acute myocardial infarction: detection and localization of regional left ventricular asynergy, *Circulation* 60:531.

Helmcke F, et al. 1987. Color Doppler assessment of mitral regurgitation with orthogonal planes, *Circulation* 75:175.

Holen J, et al. 1976. Determination of pressure gradient in mitral stenosis with a non-invasive ultra-sound technique, *Acta Med Scand* 199:455.

Hornberger L, et al. 1989. Elucidation of the natural history of ventricular septal defects by serial Doppler color flow mapping studies, *J Am Coll Card* 13:1111-1118.

Houston AB, et al. 1981. Two-dimensional echocardiography in infants with persistent truncus arteriosus, *Br Heart J* 46:492.

Houston AB, et al. 1986. Doppler ultrasound in the estimation of the severity of pulmonary infundibular stenosis in infants and children, *Br Heart J* 55:381.

Howard RJ, et al. 1982. Carcinoid heart disease: diagnosis by two-dimensional echocardiography, *Circulation* 66:1059.

Huhta JC, et al. 1985. Two-dimensional echocardiographic spectrum of univentricular atrioventricular connection, *J Am Coll Cardiol* 5:149.

Hynes JK, et al. 1983. Two-dimensional echocardiographic diagnosis of pericardial cyst, *Mayo Clinic Proc* 58:60.

Iliceto S, et al. 1987. Color Doppler evaluation of aortic dissection, *Circulation* 75:748.

Jiang L, et al. 1992. Three-dimensional echocardiography: in vivo validation for right ventricular volume and function, *Circulation* 86:I-272.

Kerber RE, et al. 1973. Abnormal motion of the interventricular septum in right ventricular volume overload. Experimental and clinical echocardiographic studies, *Circulation* 48:86.

Kisslo JA, et al. 1977. A comparison of real-time, two-dimensional echocardiography and cineangiography in detecting left ventricular asynergy, *Circulation* 55:134.

Klein AL, et al. 1991. Transesophageal Doppler echocardiography of pulmonary venous flow: a new marker of mitral regurgitation severity, *J Am Coll Cardiol* 18:518.

Kolter, MN, et al. 1983. Non-invasive evaluation of normal and abnormal prosthetic valve function, *J Am Coll Cardiol* 2:151.

Kostucki W, et al. 1986. Pulsed Doppler regurgitant flow patterns of normal valves, *Am J Cardiol* 58:309.

Labovitz AJ. 1985. The effects of sampling site on the two-dimensional echo-Doppler determination of cardiac output, *Am Heart J* 109:327.

Lange LW, et al. 1979. Subxyphoid cross-sectional echocardiography in infants and children with congenital heart disease, *Circulation* 59:513.

Levine RAL, et al. 1984. Echocardiographic measurement of right ventricular volume, *Circulation* 69:497.

Levine RAL, et al. 1987. The simplified Bernoulli equation correctly predicts outflow tract pressure gradients in hypertrophic cardiomyopathy (abstract), *J Am Coll Cardiol* 9:237A.

Levine RAL, et al. 1988. Reconsideration of echocardiographic standards for mitral valve prolapse: lack of association between leaflet displacement isolated to the apical four-chamber view and independent evidence of abnormality, *J Am Coll Cardiol* 11:1010.

Lima CL, et al. 1983. Non-invasive prediction of transvalvular pressure gradient in patients with pulmonary stenosis by quantitative two-dimensional echocardiographic Doppler studies, *Circulation* 67:866.

Louie EK, et al. 1987a. Quantitative assessment of aortic insufficiency by color Doppler (abstract), *J Am Coll Cardiol* 9:66A.

Louie EK, et al. 1987b. Early diastolic interaction between the aortic regurgitant jet and mitral inflow: a pulsed Doppler study (abstract), *J Am Coll Cardiol* 9:83A.

Macartney FJ, et al. 1984. Double outlet right ventricle: cross-sectional echocardiographic findings, their anatomical explanation, and surgical relevance, *Br Heart J* 52:164.

Mann DL, Gillam LD, Weyman AE. 1986. Cross-sectional echocardiographic assessment of regional left ventricular performance and myocardial perfusion, *Prog Cardiovasc Dis* 29:1.

Maron BJ. 1985. Asymmetry in hypertrophic cardiomyopathy: the septal to free wall ratio revisited, *Am J Cardiol* 55:835.

Maron BJ, et al. 1981. Patterns and significance of distribution of left ventricular hypertrophy in hypertrophic cardiomyopathy, *Am J Cardiol* 48:418.

Maron BJ, et al. 1985. Dynamic sub-aortic obstruction in hypertrophic cardiomyopathy: analysis by pulsed Doppler echocardiography, *J Am Coll Cardiol* 6:1.

Martin RP, et al. 1979. Reliability and reproducibility of two-dimensional echocardiographic measurement of the stenotic mitral valve orifice area, *Am J Cardiol* 43:560.

Miyatake K, et al. 1986. Semiquantitative grading of severity of mitral regurgitation by real-time two-dimensional Doppler flow imaging technique, *J Am Coll Cardiol* 7:82.

Morrissey RL, et al. 1993. Ventricular volume by echocardiographic automated border detection: on-line calculation without loss of accuracy (abstract), *J Am Coll Cardiol* 21:275A.

Nanda NC, et al. 1990. Trans-esophageal biplane echocardiographic imaging: technique, planes, and clinical usefulness, *Echocardiography* 7:771.

Nidorf SM, et al. 1992. New perspectives in the assessment of cardiac chamber dimensions during development and adulthood, *J Am Coll Cardiol* 19:983.

Nidorf SM, et al. 1993. The relationship between mitral valve morphology and prognosis in patients with mitral valve prolapse: a prospective echocardiographic study of 568 patients, *J Am Soc Echocardiogr* 6:2.

Nienaber CA, et al. 1992. Diagnosis of thoracic dissection, magnetic resonance imaging versus trans-esophageal echocardiography, *Circulation* 85:434.

Nishimura RA, et al. 1984. Role of two-dimensional echocardiography in prediction of in-hospital complications after acute myocardial infarction, *J Am Coll Cardiol* 4:1080.

Nishimura RA, et al. 1985. Doppler echocardiography: theory, instrumentation, technique, and application, *Mayo Clin Proc* 60:321.

Otto CM, et al. 1986. Determination of the stenotic valve area in adults using Doppler echocardiography, *J Am Coll Cardiol* 7:509.

Pandian N, et al. 1984. Flow velocity paradoxus: a Doppler echocardiographic sign of pericardial tamponade: exaggerated respiratory variation in pulmonary and aortic blood flow velocities, *Circulation* 70(Suppl 2):381.

Perry GJ, et al. 1987. Evaluation of aortic insufficiency by Doppler color flow mapping, *J Am Coll Cardiol* 9:953.

Picard MH, et al. 1990. Natural history of left ventricular size and function after acute myocardial infarction: assessment and prediction by echocardiographic endocardial surface mapping, *Circulation* 82:484.

Picard MH, et al. 1991. Quantitative relation between increased intrapericardial pressure and Doppler flow velocities during experimental cardiac tamponade, *J Am Coll Cardiol* 18:234.

Pollick C, et al. 1988. Doppler color flow imaging assessment of shunt size in atrial septal defects, *Circulation* 78:522-528.

Quinones M, et al. 1981. A new, simplified and accurate method for determining ejection fraction with two-dimensional echocardiography, *Circulation* 64:744.

Recusani F, et al. 1991. A new method for quantification of regurgitant flow rate using color flow Doppler imaging of the flow convergence region proximal to a discrete orifice: in vitro study and initial clinical experience in patients with mitral insufficiency, *Circulation* 83:594.

Reed D, et al. 1992. Prediction of outcome after valve replacement in patients with symptomatic chronic mitral regurgitation: the importance of left atrial size, *Circulation* 84:23.

Richards KL, et al. 1986. Calculation of aortic valve area by Doppler echocardiography: a direct application of the continuity equation, *Circulation* 73:964.

Sagar KB, et al. 1986. Doppler echocardiographic evaluation of Hancock and Bjork-Shiley prosthetic valves, *Am J Coll Cardiol* 7:681.

Sahn DJ, et al. 1988. Instrumentation and physical factors related to visualization of stenotic and regurgitant jets by Doppler color flow mapping, *J Am Coll Cardiol* 12:1354.

Salcedo EE, et al. 1983. Echocardiographic findings in 25 patients with left atrial myxoma, *J Am Coll Cardiol* 1:1161.

Sanders SP, et al. 1983. Measurement of systemic and pulmonary blood flow and Qp:Qs ratio using Doppler and two-dimensional echocardiography, *Am J Cardiol* 51:952.

Sanfilippo AJ, et al. 1991. Echocardiographic assessment of patients with infectious endocarditis: prediction of risk for complications, *J Am Coll Cardiol* 18:1191.

Siu SC, et al. 1992a. Three-dimensional echocardiography improves noninvasive left ventricular volume quantitation (abstract), *J Am Coll Cardiol* 19:18A.

Siu SC, et al. 1992b. Three-dimensional echocardiography: in vivo validation for left ventricular volume and function (abstract), *J Am Coll Cardiol* 19:18A.

Smith MD, et al. 1986. Comparative accuracy of two-dimensional echocardiography and Doppler pressure half-time methods in assessing severity of mitral stenosis in patients with and without prior commissurotomy, *Circulation* 73:100.

Spain MG, et al. 1989. Quantitative assessment of mitral regurgitation by Doppler color flow imaging: angiographic and hemodynamic correlations, *J Am Coll Cardiol* 13:585.

Sprecher DL, et al. 1987. In vitro color flow, pulsed and continuous wave Doppler ultrasound masking of flow by prosthetic valves, *J Am Coll Cardiol* 9:1306.

Starling MR, et al. 1981. Comparative accuracy of apical biplane cross-sectional echocardiography and gated equilibrium radionuclide angiography for estimating left ventricular size and performance, *Circulation* 63:1075.

Teague SM, et al. 1984. Doppler half-time index correlates with the severity of aortic regurgitation, *Circulation* 70(suppl):394.

Terdjman M, et al. 1984. Aneurysms of sinus of Valsalva: two dimensional echocardiographic diagnosis and recognition of rupture into the right heart cavities, *J Am Coll Cardiol* 3:1227.

Triulzi MO. 1984. Normal adult cross-sectional echocardiographic values: linear dimensions and chamber areas, *Echocardiography* 1:403.

Triulzi MO, et al. 1982. Normal adult cross-sectional echocardiographic values: left ventricular volumes, *Echocardiography* 2:153.

Van Praagh R, et al. 1965. The anatomy of common aorticopulmonary trunk (truncus arteriosus communis) and its embryologic implications, *Am J Cardiol* 166:406.

Visser CA, et al. 1983. Two-dimensional echocardiography in the diagnosis of left ventricular thrombus: a prospective study of 67 patients with anatomic validation, *Chest* 83:228.

Von Bibra, et al. 1989. Diagnosis of constrictive pericarditis by pulsed Doppler echocardiography of the hepatic vein, *Am J Cardiol* 63:483.

Vuille C, et al. 1993. Natural history of vegetations in successfully treated endocarditis (abstract), *J Am Coll Cardiol* 21:200A.

Warth DC, et al. 1985. Prevalence of mitral valve prolapse in normal children, *J Am Coll Cardiol* 5:1173.

Weyman AE, et al. 1979. Negative contrast echocardiography: a new method for detecting left-to-right shunts, *Circulation* 59:498.

Wilkins GT, et al. 1988a. Correlation between echocardiographic endocardial surface mapping of abnormal wall motion and pathologic infarct size in autopsied hearts, *Circulation* 77:978.

Wilkins GT, et al. 1988b. Percutaneous balloon dilation of the mitral valve: an analysis of echocardiographic variables related to outcome and the mechanism of dilation, *Br Heart J* 60:299.

Williams GA, et al. 1985. Doppler hemodynamic evaluation of prosthetic (Starr-Edwards and Bjorke-Shiley) and bioprosthetic (Hancock and Carpentier-Edwards) cardiac valves, *Am J Cardiol* 56:325.

Wisenbaugh T, et al. 1992. Timing of mitral valve replacement for mitral regurgitation: how soon is too soon and how late is too late? *Circulation* 86:I-497.

Magnetic Resonance Imaging of the Heart

LAWRENCE M. BOXT

JOSE KATZ

KATHLEEN REAGAN

Contraindications
Patient Preparation
   Mental preparation
   Physical preparation
   Patient sedation
   Patient positioning
Electrocardiographic (ECG) Gating
   Lead placement
   Initial ECG assessment
   Peripheral pulse gating
   Respiratory gating
The MR Examination
   Contrast resolution and technique choice
   Effects of the number of excitations
   Slice thickness
   Interslice gaps
   First run scout images
Choosing Imaging Parameters
   Spin-echo acquisition
   Gradient-reversal acquisition
Choosing Gradient Direction
Choosing Imaging Sections
Flow Effects
   Flow-related enhancement
   Echo rephasing
   Diastolic pseudogating
   Echo dephasing
   High-velocity signal loss
Appearance of Flow
Normal and Pathologic Anatomy
Suggested Readings

Magnetic resonance (MR) examination is a noninvasive means of displaying the anatomy of the heart and great arteries in arbitrary tomographic section. It provides imagery of high spatial and contrast resolution, which can be used to evaluate congenital and acquired abnormalities and the results of interventions, either surgical or pharmacologic, for their palliation or cure. In addition, pulse sequences that provide high temporal resolution may be useful to identify and to quantify functional abnormalities. MR examination may be useful as a single imaging modality or as a complement to conventional echocardiography and angiocardiography.

Any commercial MR scanner with an ECG gating system can examine the heart. Interpretation of MR examinations, as in all diagnostic imaging procedures, is based on identifying the abnormal and differentiating it from the normal. The emphasis of this chapter is on the performance of cardiac MR examination and, especially, on the identification and characterization of normal anatomy and function. Rather than provide an atlas of abnormalities as imaged by MR, we supply detailed images of the normal heart supplemented by images of "typical" abnormalities so you can plan, perform, and interpret a cardiac MR examination. The confidence one obtains from having performed an examination will provide impetus to perform another. Soon the value of cardiac MR examination and confidence in the results obtained will percolate among referring clinicians, and more cases will be referred. There is nothing mysterious about imaging the heart. It can be successfully examined by MR if you appreciate cardiac anatomy and basic physiology.

CONTRAINDICATIONS

Contraindications to a cardiac MR examination are the same as those for an MR of any other body part. Absolute contraindications are if the patient has a pacemaker or other implanted electrical stimulator, free particulate iron in the optic globe, or intracerebral aneurysm clips. Mediastinal sutures or clips are not contraindications. With the exception of pre-6000 series Starr-Edwards valves, there are no cardiac prostheses that pose a risk to the patient during or are adversely affected by examination at the magnetic field strengths presently employed (<2 T). There is little data concerning the effect of MR examination on cardiac support hardware, such as implantable ventricular assist devices. Intracoronary and pulmonary artery stents may be safely imaged. The stent appears as a signal void artifact. Thus it is prudent to exclude patients with new instrumentation from MR examination. Pregnancy is a relative contraindication against an MR study. If examination is deemed essential then the unknown risk to the fetus must be weighed against the benefit to the mother.

PATIENT PREPARATION

Mental Preparation

Prior to the procedure you should explain to the patient the general nature of MR examination. Although the study is completely noninvasive, many people become afraid or nervous in the bore of the magnet and the examination cannot be completed. Therefore a pre-examination discussion should emphasize the potential problems of claustrophobia and noise rather than the physics of MR image formation. Take a positive tone. Rather than pointing out how uncomfortable it is to lie still for three quarters of an hour or how nearly one patient in six or seven cannot tolerate the procedure, the examiner should explain that the MR examination provides important anatomic and functional information that can otherwise only be obtained by more invasive methods. Although it is important to explain to patients that they will be lying in tight quarters for the examination and that they should expect to hear a loud clanging noise, it should be pointed out that a technician or attending physician will be in constant contact with them, monitoring their heartbeat.

Physical Preparation

Immediately prior to examination, encourage the patient to empty the bladder. During examination, loud music of the patient's choice aids in keeping his or her attention and in drowning out the noise of gradient changing. An alternative is to use earplugs. Parents can be at the head-end of the magnet during their child's examination, although we discourage the parents from talking to their children (which elicits a response and causes the child to turn his or her head in response to a question). However, reading aloud relaxes the child and aids in acquiring technically adequate imagery. All patients receive a "panic button" that can be used to get your attention during examination. During examination, interact with the patient in a one-way manner rather than engage the patient in conversation between image acqui-

sitions. Let the patient know that all is going well and that they can expect to hear the clanging noise again. Talking to the patient throughout the examination serves to relax and comfort. Some adult patients fall asleep during examination.

Patient Sedation

You should avoid sedation; however, technically adequate examination of children and some adults cannot be performed without medication. Chloral hydrate (up to 100 mg/kg of body weight to a maximum single dose of 1500 mg) may be administered to all children between 18 months and 8 years of age. We do our best to convince parents and clinicians of the need for adequate premedication in small children. We have found no difference in the value of oral versus rectal administration of the drug. Children up to 18 months of age can be studied without medical sedation by withholding the last bottle feeding prior to examination so that the child is brought down to the scanning area hungry. Upon reaching the scanner the child drinks and falls asleep with a full stomach. Adults who have failed previous examination attempts because of claustrophobic symptoms or who have a history of claustrophobia can be given diazepam (Valium) (5 or 10 mg IV, slowly) just prior to entry into the bore of the magnet.

Administration of sedative medication necessitates assignment of adequate facilities for patient monitoring before and after examination. In addition to adequate staffing for supervision of impaired patients, MR facilities should have adequate space where these patients may stay prior to examination and where they may recuperate after completion. Ideally such space should be segregated from nonsedated patients and outpatient areas. Patients with cardiac and pulmonary disease tend to be claustrophobic and often hypoxic and to breathe at a more rapid rate. Therefore functioning ECG and pulse oximetry monitoring devices (and personnel to supervise their output) should be available in MR imaging (MRI) areas. Patients with automated intravenous infusion (IVAC) pumps may be studied in high-field (up to 1.5 T) MR imagers if their pumps are adequately isolated from the magnet. The infusions can either be held immediately prior to entry into the imager or be administered using long extension tubing between the pump and the patient. Patients whose continuous medication must be discontinued for MR examination require close clinical scrutiny.

Patient Positioning

For conventional MR examination of the heart, the patient is usually in the supine position. Examination may be tedious, so it is important that the patient is as comfortable as possible. Although images may be better with the patient's arms elevated above the head, this is clearly not a position that can be maintained and should be avoided. The arms may be crossed over the chest, but be sure that the lateral aspects of the upper arms do not rub against the bore of the magnet because this will trip microswitches and prematurely terminate an examination. If a chest surface coil is used in an examination, then the patient must lie in the prone position, fixing the coil between the chest wall and the patient table. In this circumstance the patient is best able to tolerate examination if lying prone with arms extended in front ("superman position"), and with the head resting on one shoulder.

ELECTROCARDIOGRAPHIC (ECG) GATING

MR examination of the heart requires an adequate ECG tracing to provide a gating signal for timed image acquisition. The quality of cardiac MR images is probably more dependent on the acquisition of an adequate ECG signal than on any other parameter. Furthermore, the effects of a strong magnetic field on the character of any individual patient's ECG tracing are unpredictable.

Lead Placement

It is essential to manipulate the position of ECG leads on the patient's chest and the course of the leads leaving the magnet bore until an adequate tracing is obtained. The position of the leads (anterior, posterior, or lateral chest wall) depends more on personal preference, patient body habitus, and the morphology of the ECG trace, rather than on any cardiac imaging considerations. MR imagers identify the pulse with the greatest amplitude and assign it as the ECG R wave. The ideal ECG tracing is regular and has a tall R wave. Improper choice of leads may produce a tracing that the imager misreads. Assignment of a non-R wave pulse as the R wave results in images that are erroneously labeled as end-diastolic. Furthermore, images obtained at set delays after the first image will all be temporally misaligned with respect to the true ECG R wave. A common version of this phenomenon is found in patients whose ECGs contain very tall P or T waves. In this circumstance, the imager sees the cycle of P and R or R and T waves in these patients as a series of R waves with a very short and irregular RR interval. Thus images are only obtained from a portion of the true RR interval. This produces a series of images from the early (in the case of tall P waves) or late (in the case of tall T waves) portion of the cardiac cycle. Obviously this severely hampers the evaluation of ventricular function. For morphologic image analyses, however, this creates little difficulty for interpretation.

Initial ECG Assessment

The quality of the ECG tracing should be assessed prior to advancing the patient into the bore of the magnet. This preexamination check can save a great deal of preparation time taken by otherwise moving the patient out of and back into the scanner until you obtain an adequate tracing. Anterior chest wall ECG leads usually produce the most consistently useful ECG tracings.

You should ensure that all ECG leads within and exiting the magnet travel parallel to the long axis of the imager and that there are no loops in any of the leads, which would prevent generation of currents. This diminishes potential electrical burn hazard to the patient and improves the quality of the ECG signal. The ECG tracing found on the monitor in the MR control room provides only the length of the RR interval (that is, heart rate) or the occurrence of an extrasystolic cardiac beat. These tracings should never be used to diagnose or to interpret myocardial ischemic changes, the character of the cardiac rhythm, or the nature of such extra beats. Specially shielded ECG leads for this purpose are not commercially available. Therefore, prior to MR examination, you should consider how closely the ECG of a patient with cardiac disease must be monitored.

Peripheral Pulse Gating

The purpose of a gating signal is to provide an electronic landmark for temporal image acquisition. Therefore you can base it on any periodic body function. ECG gating is especially useful because it provides a timing signal related to the electromechanical function of the heart, but other timing signals may also be used. Peripheral pulse gating has the prerequisite characteristic of being periodic and can thus provide regular signals for image acquisition. The time between ventricular systole and the peak of the peripheral pulse, however, depends not only on the distance of the pulse transducer from the heart, but also on the compliance of the arterial tree. Thus, although this technique may provide perfectly adequate images for morphologic examination, its use for quantitative evaluation of cardiac function is untested and may possibly be inaccurate.

Respiratory Gating

Gating image acquisition to the patient's respiratory cycle is not necessary. The up-and-down motion of the heart within the chest during the respiratory cycle does not seem to cause significant artifact either within or immediately adjacent to the heart. Adding this gating signal to the ECG also increases image acquisition time and makes the examination less tolerable for the patient.

THE MR EXAMINATION

Contrast Resolution and Technique Choice

Imaging of the heart requires adequate contrast resolution to differentiate between the cavity and the walls of the cardiac chambers and adequate spatial resolution to identify and to characterize small intracardiac and extracardiac structures. The heart is a periodically moving organ. Thus cardiac MR examination must also provide adequate temporal resolution to differentiate the phases of the cardiac cycle. At minimum the temporal resolution of an acquisition pulse sequence provides images at fixed, known phases in the cardiac cycle. Both conventional spin-echo and gradient-reversal acquisition pulse sequences provide adequate temporal resolution. Spin-echo methods provide the highest contrast between blood-filled cardiac chambers and myocardial wall, but at lowest temporal resolution. With spin-echo techniques you can identify end-diastole by assigning a trigger delay of between 8 and 20 msec after the ECG R wave for the acquisition of the first slice. Each successive anatomic slice is further delayed along the cardiac cycle. Thus conventional spin-echo techniques yield a series of images displaced in time as well as space. If the functional differences among cardiac or extracardiac structures are not important, then this is perfectly adequate for morphologic analysis.

An alternative spin-echo method known as cycled multislice multiphase (CMSMP) spin-echo imaging provides a series of images wherein each image is obtained at comparably incremented temporal and anatomic positions. This technique provides a series of anatomic sections, each obtained at the same various fixed phases in the cardiac cycle. This allows you to compare anatomic slices at the same phases of the cardiac cycle. This method has the advantage of the increased contrast resolution of spin-echo technique. Although temporal resolution is less than that of gradient-reversal methods, you can obtain end-diastolic as well as "most-systolic" images for quantitative analysis.

Although the contrast resolution of gradient-reversal techniques is less than that of spin-echo pulses, its temporal resolution is superior. End-diastolic and end-systolic frames may be obtained for all anatomic sections, and depending on heart rate (which determines length of the RR interval and thus minimum repetition time [TR]), it is possible to obtain up to 24 temporal frame resolution per RR interval for evaluation of diastolic as well as systolic cardiac function.

Effects of the Number of Excitations

Regardless of the pulse sequence you choose, the number of excitations (NEX) chosen to construct an image will effect its spatial resolution. The greater the NEX obtained for signal averaging, the greater the signal-to-noise ratio (SNR) of each image voxel. The SNR of a voxel increases by the square root of the number of NEXs employed to create that voxel (for example, doubling the NEXs from one to two increases the SNR by a factor of 1.4). Increasing the NEX does have its drawbacks. The greater the NEX, the longer the examination time. This decreases patient cooperation, tolerance, and throughput. In addition, it may also degrade image quality. (The greater the NEX, the greater the number of cardiac cycles required for data acquisition. This potentially exposes the examination to more extrasystoles or irregular beats, effectively degrading image quality). Furthermore, prolonging the examination only increases patient restlessness, which results in motion artifact.

One is faced with the problem common to all imaging procedures of paying for higher resolution (and therefore for greater confidence in diagnosis) with prolonged examination time. The latter often leads to greater patient discomfort and decreased patient compliance during examination. Thus increasing the NEX by a factor of four or eight will almost always result in a decrease in image quality by a significant factor. We have found that using four NEX in our conventional spin-echo acquisitions provides superior imagery without unnecessarily prolonging examination time. A compromise between adequate CMSMP and gradient-reversal imagery and examination time is made using two NEXs.

Slice Thickness

The more tissue interrogated during an acquisition, the greater the signal recovered, and thus the greater the SNR of an image voxel. The cost of increasing slice thickness is loss of spatial resolution within that section. Generally, acquiring sections 8 to 10 mm thick in adult patients and 5 to 8 mm thick in children provides sharp images without significant loss of spatial resolution. The increased spatial resolution with thinner sections is rapidly lost in the increased noise. You can increase spatial resolution with spin-echo acquisitions by obtaining a second series of images offset by a fraction (usually one half) of the slice thickness in the direction of the slice encoding gradient. Then, by displaying alternating sections from the two acquisitions (acquisition one, section one; acquisition two, section one; acquisition one, section two; acquisition two, section two; and so on), you can "split the difference" between volume averaged sections, visually interpolate between the alternating acquisitions, and effectively "double" the spatial resolution of the examination.

Interslice Gaps

The morphologic data contained in the interslice gap in an MR examination are lost to interpretation. Thus you should use as small an interslice gap as the imager will allow. You can also apply the split-the-difference technique to those cases in which the information within the gap is important. Slice selection by commercial MR imagers is managed in such a way that cross-talk among adjacent slices is minimized; thus this is not usually a serious problem.

First Run Scout Images

The scout acquisition is designed to provide specific information quickly. You should start with a series of ungated, single NEX spin-echo or gradient-reversal coronal scout images to localize the superior and inferior extent of the heart and aortic arch, and to describe the left-to-right relationships of the lungs and pulmonary arteries. From a coronal scout series, a section through the posterior third of the heart provides imagery containing the tracheal bifurcation, aortic arch, and main pulmonary artery (PA). The top of the first (axial) acquisition may be chosen from the relevant scout section. The number of sections that can be obtained is related to the TR in spin-echo imaging and the number of phases in the cardiac cycle and TR (in the form of the minimum RR interval) when gradient-reversal techniques are employed. Thus one sets the top of an acquisition; the imager "sets" the bottom. Therefore you should usually assume the need for a second acquisition in axial section. This allows you to cover the heart by starting the first acquisition just above the level of the top of the main PA. The second axial acquisition starts slightly less or slightly more than one half the height of the stack of sections, offset caudally. In this way there is overlap of several sections within the heart, as well as coverage above and below.

CHOOSING IMAGING PARAMETERS

Spin-Echo Acquisition

The minimum TR in an ECG-gated spin-echo acquisition is set by the patient's RR interval. When imaging infants and children with very rapid heart rates, the short RR interval results in very short TR, which limits the number of slices. You can overcome this pitfall by gating to every other or every third R wave. This effectively tells the imager that the RR interval is two or three times greater, which increases the number of sections you can obtain per acquisition. It also increases the acquisition time. You get the maximal signal from the shortest echo time (TE); however, shorter TE results in an increased signal from the lung and mediastinal fat, which lowers myocardial contrast. A suggested TE is between 15 and 30 msec.

In adults an 8- to 10-mm slice is sufficient, depending on patient body size and the need for higher resolution imagery. The smallest possible interslice gap (0.5-1.0 mm) is taken using four NEX.

The ratio of the field of view (FOV) to the number of phase encoding steps determines the size of each pixel. Thus for any number of phase encoding steps, the spatial resolution depends on the smallest possible FOV. However, the intensity of "wrap-around" artifacts depends on the amount of tissue outside the FOV. Therefore the chosen FOV is a compromise between increased spatial resolution and overall image quality, which determines confidence in interpretation. When the patient's arms are in the scout section, you should try to keep them outside the FOV; try to image from chest wall to chest wall.

An important parameter with spin-echo sequences is the transverse relaxation time (T2). This measurement describes the rate of dephasing of the transverse magnetization. Calculation of T2 requires image acquisition for two different spin-echoes (for example, 20 and 40 or 30 and 60 msec). From the signal intensities of a given voxel in these two images, you can compute the T2 by dividing the difference between the TEs for the two images by the natural logarithm (ln) of the ratio of the two signal intensities (I):

$$T2=(TE_2-TE_1)/\ln(I_1/I_2)$$

In general T2 depends on the tissue and its characteristics (water content, fibrosis, and degree of perfusion). Furthermore, it depends on motion and it will vary with the different phases of the cardiac cycle. The motion dependence of T2 also depends on the spin-echoes used in the calculation. For example, for constant velocity laminar flow, T2 does not depend on motion when the first and third echoes are used, although it is a strongly varying function of velocity when the first and second echoes are considered. This follows because for laminar flow all protons within a voxel are in phase for even echoes. This phase, however, is different from that of odd echoes for which dephasing occurs. The stronger motion dependence of T2 when the first and second echoes are used in the calculation also appears to occur for pulsatile flow.

The motion dependence of T2 may be valuable in determining whether a given locus of increased signal intensity within a vessel represents a localized nonmoving structure (such as thrombus or an atherosclerotic lesion) or merely a flow artifact. Clearly when T2 is negative or is larger than expected (that is, larger than its baseline value if known or simply just large), this focus of increased signal intensity must represent a flow artifact, not thrombus or an atherosclerotic lesion.

Gradient-Reversal Acquisition

Imaging parameters in gradient-reversal acquisitions depend on imager field strength, gradients, and the temporal and contrast resolution requirements of the examination. The three easily variable parameters are flip angle, TR, and TE. Flip angle choice depends on imager field strength, gradient strength, and desired image contrast. Generally, flip angles in the range of 30 to 45 degrees provide optimum contrast between ventricular chamber blood and myocardial walls of the heart. The hallmark of gradient-reversal imaging is the very short TR and TE employed. These factors are often set arbitrarily by the manufacturer, but may be adjusted by the operator to "tune" acquired images to the tastes of those interpreting the imagery.

Because slice selection is arbitrary in MRI, you need to be aware of potential artifacts that may be produced by the motion of blood through and within the plane of the heart. Improper selection of slice and phase encoding gradient direction will maximize the visualization of the turbulent moving blood at the expense of the interface between the blood and the rhythmically moving myocardium.

Creation of compound-angulated sections, such as the true cardiac axes, requires identification of internal cardiac structures as landmarks. These sections may therefore be more difficult to precisely construct if the examination is performed in a prospective manner using low resolution scout images. For this reason, it is best to construct these sections as you move along in the examination. For example, construction of the true cardiac short axis is performed in the following manner: from the original coronal scout acquisition, choose the section through the body of the left ventricle, and construct a long-axis oblique section through the left ventricle connecting the ventricular apex and aortic valve plane. These long-axis oblique images of the left ventricle are essentially off-axial in orientation. Obtain the true long-axis oblique view of the left ventricle by acquiring off-coronal sections to obtain a ventricular-apex-to-aortic valve-section through the left ventricle.

CHOOSING GRADIENT DIRECTION

The acquisition pulse sequence depends in part on the signal characteristics you want to impart on moving blood. For example, spin-echo techniques result in a relative signal void in regions of rapidly moving blood. Loci of increased signal intensity in such anatomic regions must be differentiated and characterized as flow artifacts, or as real, soft tissue within or adjacent to a chamber or vessel wall. Conversely, blood is bright in gradient-reversal imagery and a relative signal void must be characterized as an intraluminal mass or flow artifact.

The slice selection gradient is perpendicular to the imaging plane, and within this plane you can select the phase and frequency encoding directions. Suitable selec-

tion of these directions can minimize motion artifacts. The frequency encoding gradient allows decomposition of the MR signal into its various frequency components using Fourier analysis. The phase encoding gradient, on the other hand, alters the phase of the MR signal by an amount dependent on its position along the phase encoding gradient.

Two important factors in the selection of the phase encoding direction are FOV and the typical phase encoding banding artifact. If tissue lies outside the FOV then the signal arising from this tissue may confuse interpretation (referred to as wrap-around). Therefore you should select the phase encoding direction that will minimize the amount of tissue outside the FOV.

Motion in the phase encoding direction causes a banding artifact along the direction of the applied gradient. Suitable selection of the phase encoding direction can minimize this banding artifact.

CHOOSING IMAGING SECTIONS

The cardiac axes are not parallel to the body axes. Therefore a significant advantage of MR examination is its ability to select and image in any plane within the chest. The proper choice of section depends on understanding the internal anatomy of the heart as well as the specific questions that need to be answered. Because of ECG gating, cardiac MR examinations usually take longer than examinations of other body parts, and the patients under examination are often sicker and hypoxic, thus more prone to claustrophobia. It is essential to acquire the pertinent information as rapidly as possible. Lovely or exciting images, which do not provide answers to specific questions, are clinically useless. Specific imaging protocols for specific clinical problems limit set-up time for each examination, which enhances patient throughput, puts less strain on each patient, and provides a controlled format for the evaluation of image data.

Imaging parallel to the body axes, for example, in axial, coronal, and sagittal sections, provides no more or less anatomic information than imaging parallel to the true cardiac axes. The advantage of axial cardiac imaging is its ease in set-up and its conventional presentation of image data. It provides information about the internal and external anatomy of the heart in a format that can be easily identified by the cardiac imager; the left-to-right and anterior-to-posterior relations among structures are apparent. This section is necessary in the evaluation of any congenital heart lesion and complements morphologic evaluation of patients with acquired disease. Although standard off-sagittal (LAO or RAO) sectional imaging provides useful morphologic information about the aorta, pulmonary trunk, and main PAs, it has limited value in the assessment of intracardiac anatomy because most intracardiac structures do not lie in such simple planes. Rather, they run in more complex caudocranial as well as sagittal sections. Thus imaging in the compound angulated long and short cardiac axes is very helpful in the evaluation of morphologic changes within the heart, and it is essential when performing quantitative MR examination of the heart. Setting up these views prior to examination of the heart takes experience and may be time consuming because of individual variation in anatomy and changes in cardiac orientation due to chamber dilatation and hypertrophy. The four-chamber view (analogous to the echocardiographic view) demonstrates all four cardiac chambers as well as the AV and semilunar valves. The "horizontal long-axis left ventricular" view demonstrates the segments of left ventricular myocardium for analysis of wall motion disturbances. The "cardiac short-axis oblique" view provides visualization of the left and right ventricular myocardium as well as the interventricular septum in a section normal to the long axis of the left ventricle. This view allows evaluation of the cross-sectional chamber area to assess chamber volume. Cine-mode sequential display of images shows the beating heart and wall thickening and thinning. Akinetic wall segments in myocardial infarctions can easily be identified.

FLOW EFFECTS

Proper interpretation of MR images of the heart and cardiovascular system requires an understanding of the principles of flow, otherwise erroneous image interpretation may occur. For example, if care is not taken, a flow artifact may be wrongly interpreted as a thrombus because both structures may appear as focal regions of increased signal intensity within a cardiac chamber.

Quite generally, flow effects may lead to an increase or decrease in signal intensity. Flow effects leading to an increase in signal intensity include flow-related enhancement, echo rephasing, and diastolic pseudogating. On the other hand, flow effects leading to a decrease in signal intensity include echo dephasing, turbulence, and high-velocity signal loss.

Flow-Related Enhancement

Flow-related enhancement refers to the phenomenon that when slowly moving blood enters the first slice (entry slice) of a multislice imaging volume, its signal intensity will be stronger than that of stationary blood. This increase in signal intensity of slowly moving blood relative to stationary blood arises because protons in slowly moving blood are unsaturated (that is, fully magnetized) while those in stationary blood are partially saturated (that is, demagnetized). Hence the signal obtained from these latter protons is weaker, depending on the TR

(the time between 90-degree pulses) and the longitudinal relaxation time (T1) (the parameter used to estimate the time required for the equilibrium magnetization [Mz] to return to its original value after administration of a 90-degree pulse) of the blood itself.

Echo Rephasing

Echo rephasing is the process by which populations of protons with random phase are brought into phase coherence for either odd (the first, third, fifth, and so on) (odd-echo rephasing) or even (second, fourth, sixth, and so on) (even-echo rephasing) spin echoes. After a 90-degree pulse is applied to flip the Mz of the tissue to the transverse (xy) plane, the angle (phase) that each of the various spins subtends with the x-axis will generally be different for each of these spins because of magnetic field inhomogeneities. This condition is referred to as phase incoherence. In the presence of constant (time independent) flow and for the usual magnetic field gradients, all the proton spins within a voxel for any given even echo will have the same phase (that is, they have been refocused and are now in a state of phase coherence) because of the 180-degree pulse applied in the spin-echo sequence. Thus quite generally, for the usual employed gradients, whenever blood is moving at constant velocity, even echoes have a higher signal intensity than odd echoes. It should be mentioned, however, that because blood flow is pulsatile (that is, flow velocity is time dependent in a periodic manner), rephasing may also occur for odd echoes in certain circumstances. The presence (or absence) of even-echo rephasing may be of considerable value in distinguishing whether a focal region of increased signal intensity in a cardiac chamber represents thrombus or flow artifact. In particular, a thrombus (or any other nonmoving structure) will generally be characterized by a decrease in signal intensity of even echoes relative to odd echoes (that is, signal intensity of the first echo is greater than that of the second echo). On the other hand, an increase in signal intensity of the even echoes relative to the odd echoes (that is, signal intensity of the second echo is greater than that of the first echo) represents a flow artifact and is merely a consequence of even-echo rephasing.

Diastolic Pseudogating

Diastolic pseudogating refers to the phenomenon that there may be an increase in signal intensity of blood whenever the cardiac and MR cycles become synchronized, even when image acquisition is not ECG gated. That is, if the ratio between the TR and the ECG RR interval (the cardiac period) is an integer, images will always be obtained at the same point within the cardiac cycle. Whenever these points occur in diastole, the moving spins within a blood vessel will all be in phase and have a brighter signal than those in blood moving at a faster velocity.

Echo Dephasing

Echo dephasing refers to the phenomenon of a decrease in signal intensity within a voxel depending on the proton velocity distribution within the voxel. For laminar flow with constant velocity, odd-echo dephasing will always occur within a voxel. However, for plug flow (for which all spins across a vessel have the same constant velocity), odd-echo dephasing does not occur because all protons are in phase for both odd and even echoes and the signal intensity of odd echoes cannot then be lower than that of even echoes. Even-echo dephasing may not occur for constant velocity flow for the usual gradients. However, for pulsatile blood flow, even-echo dephasing may occur under certain circumstances as described earlier.

There are other frequent effects of spin dephasing. In particular, blood turbulence will cause signal loss because of the rapidly varying velocities within a voxel. Furthermore, a dark ring at the interface between vessel wall and blood frequently occurs because of the large change in velocity (that is, a large velocity gradient) near the vessel wall, with subsequent signal cancellation.

High-Velocity Signal Loss

High-velocity signal loss occurs when blood appears dark because it moves through the imaging volume before it was possible to apply all the pulses necessary to form a spin-echo. Although this is an important mechanism of signal loss for motion perpendicular to the imaging plane, it is seldom a contributing factor for signal loss of blood moving within the imaging plane (that is, for moving blood perpendicular to the slice selection gradient).

APPEARANCE OF FLOW

MR images are frequently acquired using gradient-reversal sequences. In contrast to spin-echo techniques, gradient-reversal sequences do not employ a 180-degree pulse but, rather, expose tissue in the imaging plane to a rapid change in gradient direction. Hence, high-velocity signal loss does not occur because a gradient is being applied at each instant in time between the 90-degree pulse and the time at which the echo is acquired. Furthermore, dephasing mechanisms are not important because a rephasing gradient is applied before echo detection. Flow-related enhancement, on the other hand, occurs in both spin-echo and gradient-reversal sequences; however, it is more prominent on gradient-reversal sequences.

In general, because of flow-related enhancement and absence of the factors that cause signal loss in a spin-echo sequence, blood appears bright in gradient-reversal sequences. Furthermore, because of the short TR and the low flip angles employed in gradient-reversal sequences, every slice acquired by gradient-reversal technique is essentially an entry slice. By definition, the flip angle denotes the angle by which the Mz is rotated by a radiofrequency pulse. In addition, the short TR reduces the signal due to stationary tissue and further increases the contrast between moving blood and stationary tissue.

NORMAL AND PATHOLOGIC ANATOMY

Evaluation of a cardiac MR examination is a rigorous routine of interpreting images in anatomic sequence through the heart and in temporal sequence within the cardiac cycle. In this way you can identify structures by analysis of their relative position within or adjacent to the heart, and evaluate possible abnormalities by comparing them with an assumed normal position or configuration. Evaluation of serial sections will help you to visualize the object in a three-dimensional manner. There is no better method for evaluating cardiac function than to watch it contract and relax in cine mode.

The following description of the normal heart and great vessels is intended to help the operator appreciate the appearance of normal cardiac structures and begin to understand the three-dimensional relations of these structures. The emphasis is on identification of normal. Illustrations of common examples of abnormal structures are provided for comparison. For detailed discussion of specific findings in specific lesions, see the short reference list at the end of the chapter.

High in the chest the three branches of the aortic arch, the left innominate vein, the trachea, and the esophagus are surrounded by mediastinal fat (Fig. 3-1, A). At this level the innominate, left common carotid, and left subclavian arteries are related obliquely from anterior and right to posterior and left. The left innominate vein begins to course caudally and towards the right, running anterior and slightly superior to the arteries of the aortic arch. Nestled between the left subclavian artery and the midline trachea, you can identify the relatively muscular esophagus. Immediately caudal to this, behind the manubrium sternum, the left innominate vein continues its course toward the right innominate vein, passing anterior to the origin of the innominate artery (Figs. 3-1, B and C). You can now identify the left-sided aortic arch. The left innominate vein usually joins the right innominate vein to form the superior vena cava (SVC) at the level of the top of the aortic arch (Fig. 3-2, A). The left-sided aortic arch courses from anterior to posterior and medial to lateral as it leaves the middle mediastinum to

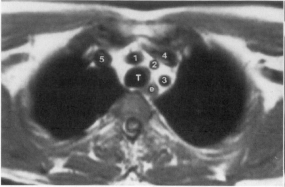

A

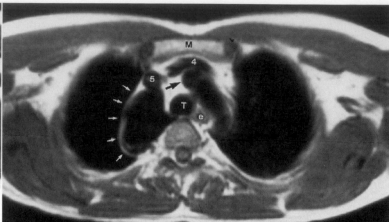

B

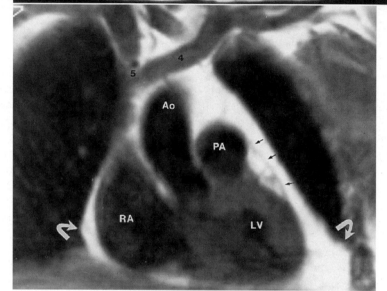

C

Fig. 3-1 **A,** Axial spin-echo section just caudal to the pulmonary apices. TR=835 msec, TE=30 msec, slice thickness=10 mm. The midline trachea *(T)*, the innominate artery *(1)*, the left common carotid artery *(2)*, the left subclavian artery *(3)*, the esophagus *(e)*, the left innominate vein *(4)*, and the right innominate vein *(5)* are encased in mediastinal fat. **B,** Axial spin-echo image obtained 1 cm caudal to Figure 3-1, *A.* TR=835 msec, TE=30 msec, slice thickness=10 mm. Just posterior to the manubrium of the sternum *(M)*, the left innominate vein *(4)* continues its course inferiorly and towards the right to join the right innominate vein *(5)*. The origin of the innominate artery from the aortic arch *(arrow)* is identified. Fat in an azygos fissure *(small arrows)* is an incidental finding. The trachea *(T)* and esophagus *(e)* are labeled. **C,** Coronal spin-echo image from another patient. TR=840 msec, TE=30 msec, slice thickness=10 mm. The left innominate vein *(4)* crosses cephalad to the aortic arch *(Ao)* to join with the right innominate vein *(5)* just posterior to the plane of the superior vena cava *(not seen)*. The pericardial reflection *(small arrows)* on the main pulmonary artery *(PA)* can be seen within the mediastinal fat. The right heart-border-forming right atrium *(RA)* and the apex of the left ventricle *(LV)* are surrounded by epicardial fat pads *(curved arrows)*.

enter the posterior mediastinum (Fig. 3-2, *B*). After the takeoff of the left subclavian artery, the thoracic aorta descends behind the heart to the left of the spine (Fig. 3-2, *C*). Cases of right aortic arch (Figs. 3-3, *A* and *B*) may be diagnosed by the characteristic course and appearance of the aorta. A tubular retrotracheal locus of signal void (Fig. 3-3, *B*) should alert the observer to the presence of an aberrant (left) subclavian artery.

Immediately caudad to the confluence of the innominate veins at the level of the tracheal carina is the entry of the azygos vein into the SVC (Fig. 3-4, *A*). The azygos vein courses to the right of the descending thoracic aorta until about the level of the left atrium, where it begins to head towards the right, behind the right hilum (Fig. 3-4, *B*). It then passes over the right main bronchus to enter the SVC (Fig. 3-4, *C*). At about this level, below the inferior aspect of the aortic arch, you can identify the top of the main and proximal left PA. As the main PA courses from anterior to posterior, it gradually passes to

the left to enter the left hilum as the left PA. The left PA descends into the parenchyma of the left lung anterior to the descending thoracic aorta. Coarctation of the thoracic aorta may be diagnosed by identifying a focal narrowing of the descending thoracic aorta just distal to the origin of the left subclavian artery with narrowing of the aortic isthmus, the portion of the aortic arch just proximal to the left subclavian artery (Fig. 3-5, *A*). Spin-echo MR technique may be used to identify dilated intercostal collateral vessels in relation to the poststenotic proximal descending aorta (Fig. 3-5, *B*).

The right PA takes off from the main PA at a sharp angle to pass behind the ascending aorta (Fig. 3-6, *A*). As the right PA courses from left to right it moves caudally, passing behind the ascending aorta and SVC to enter the right hilum. The right hilum is inferior to the left hilum. The pulmonary valve is not often demonstrated in axial section, but it may be visualized in the sagittal section (Fig. 3-6, *B*). The pulmonary valve is supported by the

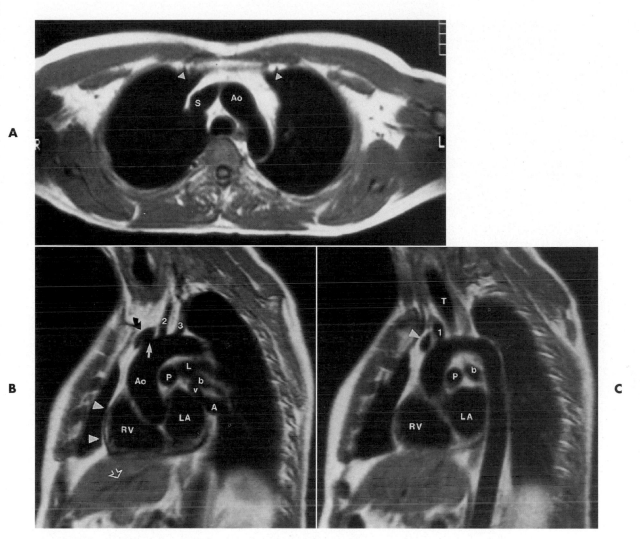

Fig. 3-2 A, Axial spin-echo image obtained 1 cm caudal to Figure 3-1, *A.* TR=835 msec, TE=30 msec, slice thickness=10 mm. The left innominate vein has joined the right innominate vein to form the superior vena cava *(S)* just slightly posterior to the anterior aspect of the ascending aorta *(Ao).* The left and right internal mammary arteries *(arrowheads)* are embedded in anterior chest wall fat. **B,** LAO off-sagittal image obtained to the left of the thoracic spine. TR=835 msec, TE=30 msec, slice thickness=10 mm. The ascending aorta *(Ao)* becomes the aortic arch with the origin of the innominate artery *(arrow),* which lies just behind the left innominate vein *(curved arrow).* The proximal portions of the left common carotid *(2)* and left subclavian *(3)* arteries are displayed. The transverse pulmonary artery *(P)* travels along the top of the left atrium *(LA).* The left pulmonary artery *(L)* is the continuation of the main pulmonary artery, and it crosses over the top of the left mainstem bronchus *(b).* A segment of the left lower lobe pulmonary vein *(v)* lies adjacent to a segment of the descending thoracic aorta *(A).* The right ventricular sinus *(RV)* is enveloped by the pericardium *(arrowheads).* A hepatic vein *(open arrow)* is found heading towards the right atrium. **C,** LAO sagittal spin-echo image obtained 2 cm to the right of figure 3-2, *B.* TR=835 msec, TE=30 msec, slice thickness=10 mm. The midline is identified by the trachea *(T).* Anterior and to the right of the trachea is the innominate artery *(1)* and vein *(arrowhead).* The transverse right pulmonary artery *(P)* is anterior and slightly caudad to the right mainstem bronchus *(b).* The left atrium *(LA)* and right ventricle *(RV)* are again demonstrated.

right ventricular infundibulum and lies anterior, cephalad, and to the left of the aortic valve. You can differentiate between the main PA and the right ventricular outflow tract by observing the thickness of the wall. The right ventricular infundibulum is a muscular structure and therefore appears thicker than the aorta, an adjacent large artery. The transverse right PA passes directly over the top of the left atrium, lying anterior to the plane of the tracheal bifurcation. By the time it reaches the right hilum, it lies inferior and anterior to the right main

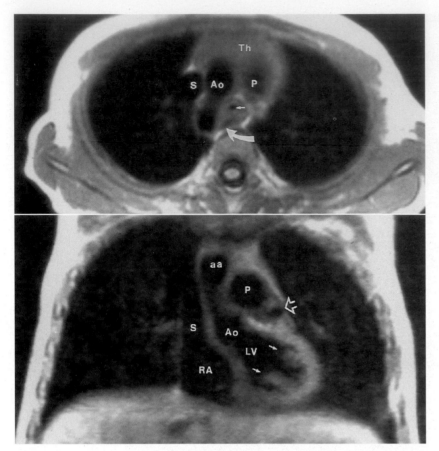

Fig. 3-3 Examination of a 15-month-old girl with respiratory stridor. **A,** Axial spin-echo image. TR=435 msec, TE=30 msec, slice thickness=6 mm. The aortic arch *(Ao)* is to the right of the trachea *(small arrow)*. The superior vena cava *(S)* is lateral to the aortic arch. An aberrant left subclavian artery *(curved arrow)* is seen posterior to the trachea traveling towards the left shoulder. The tops of the main pulmonary artery *(P)* and thymus *(Th)* are seen. **B,** Coronal spin-echo image of the same patient. TR=435 msec, TE=30 mscc, slice thickness=6 mm. The superior vena cava *(S)* drains into the right heart-border-forming right atrium *(RA)*. The aorta *(Ao)* takes its usual origin from the left ventricle *(LV)*. However, the course of the aorta is unusual in that the aortic arch *(aa)* comes to lie to the right of the midline. The main pulmonary artery *(P)* and left atrial appendage *(open arrow)* are seen. The two left ventricular papillary muscles *(small arrows)* are identified.

bronchus (Figs. 3-6, *C* and *D*). Just beyond its passage in front of the right main bronchus, the right upper lobe PA (truncus anterior) originates. In general the caliber of the main PA is not much greater than that of the aorta just above the aortic annulus. Therefore when the caliber of the main PA is greater than that of the aorta and this increase in caliber extends into the proximal left and right PA branches, you should consider an abnormality such as increased PA pressure or blood flow (Fig. 3-6, *E*).

The course of the transverse right PA is oblique with respect to the conventional axial imaging section, therefore the entire right PA is often not visualized in a single axial image. You can find the relations among the distal right PA, SVC, and right bronchus in axial section in images obtained caudal to those containing the bifurcation of the main PA (Fig. 3-7, *A*) or the steep sagittal long-axis section (Fig. 3-7, *B*). Slightly inferior and lateral to the proximal left PA lie the left upper lobe pulmonary vein and the long fingerlike left atrial appendage. The left upper lobe pulmonary vein enters the left atrium just posterior to the orifice of the left atrial appendage. The orifice of the left atrial appendage is slightly anterior to the entry of the vein. In the axial or coronal section the two structures may not be separable; however, you can identify and characterize the two structures in the sagittal long-axis section (Fig. 3-7, *C*).

By the level of the transverse right PA you should be able to see the pericardium (Fig. 3-7, *A*). MR is an excellent means of visualizing the pericardium and pericardial space. Sandwiched between the epicardial and pericardial fat, the pericardial space (the two leaves of pericardium containing the small amount of pericardial fluid) appears as a pencil-thin curvilinear signal void surrounding the heart, proximal ascending aorta, and main PA. However, because of motion artifacts or little adjacent fat, the entire pericardium may not be visualized in any single section. To evaluate the pericardium it may be necessary to acquire images in multiple oblique sections. Small pericardial effusions often collect behind the heart or adjacent to the right atrial border (Fig. 3-8, *A*). Inflammatory pericardial disease manifests itself as diffuse thickening of the pericardial tissue itself, often involving the entire cardiac perimeter (Fig. 3-8, *B*).

The right upper lobe pulmonary vein courses posteriorly and caudally to enter the left atrium behind the SVC drainage into the right atrium (Figs. 3-9, *A* and *B*). The left lower lobe pulmonary vein may be seen at this same level ascending towards the posterior aspect of the left atrium, anterior to the descending thoracic aorta. Imaged in axial section, the proximal ascending aorta appears ovoid in shape as it approaches the aortic root. Anterior to and wrapping around the ascending aorta is

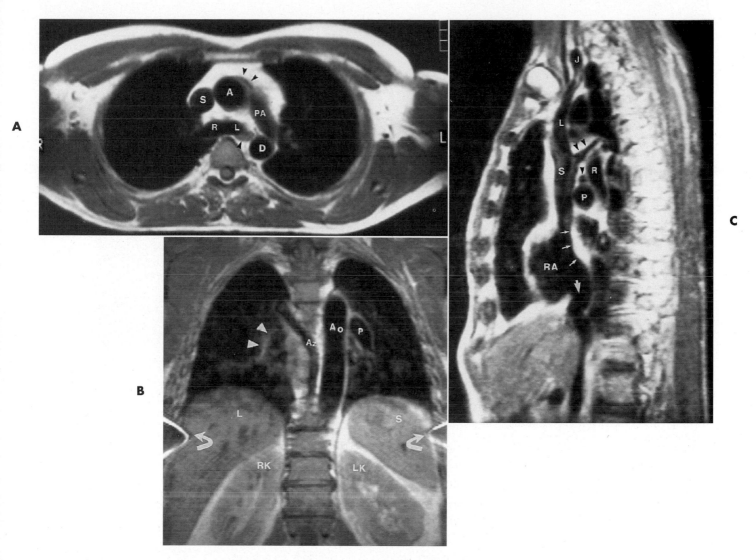

Fig. 3-4 **A,** Axial spin-echo image obtained 1 cm caudad to Figure 3-2, *A.* TR=835 msec, TE=30 msec, slice thickness=10 mm. Just to the left of the plane of the ascending *(A)* and descending *(D)* aorta lies the top of the main pulmonary artery *(PA).* The proximal left *(L)* and right *(R)* mainstem bronchi of the tracheal carina are seen. Just posterior and to the left of the left bronchus is the collapsed esophagus *(arrowhead).* The superior vena cava *(S)* lies to the right of the ascending aorta. An anterior superior pericardial recess *(arrowheads)* lies anterior to the ascending aorta, adjacent to the pulmonary artery. **B,** Coronal spin-echo image of the same patient. TR=835 msec, TE=30 msec, slice thickness=10 mm. The azygos vein *(Az)* ascends parallel to the descending thoracic aorta *(Ao)* in front of and then to the right of the spine above the level of the right hilum *(arrowheads).* The descending left pulmonary artery *(P)* is seen. The liver *(L),* spleen *(S),* and right *(RK)* and left *(LK)* kidneys are labeled. Note the wrap-around artifact *(curved arrows)* caused by choice of too small an image FOV. **C,** LAO sagittal spin-echo image of a different patient through the right hilum. TR=730 msec, TE=30 msec, slice thickness=8 mm. The azygos vein is seen *(arrowheads)* coming over the right bronchus *(R),* right upper lobe pulmonary vein *(arrowhead),* and right pulmonary artery *(P)* to enter the superior vena cava *(S)* from its posterior aspect. The left internal jugular vein *(J)* drains into the left innominate vein *(L)* and then into the superior vena cava. The superior vena cava enters the right atrium *(RA)* slightly anterior to the entrance of the inferior vena cava *(arrow).* The increased signal intensity of fat within the interatrial septum *(small arrows)* is evident.

the right atrial appendage. The appendage itself is contained within the pericardium and pericardial fluid, and may be found between it and the ascending aorta (Fig. 3-10, *B*). This broad-based, triangular-shaped extension of the morphologic right atrium may appear to contain

intermediate signal. This signal is caused by a volume-averaging effect between the pectinate muscles of the wall and the cavity of the appendage.

The tricommissural aortic valve contains three sinuses of Valsalva (Figs. 3-10, *A-C*). The superior-most sinus is the

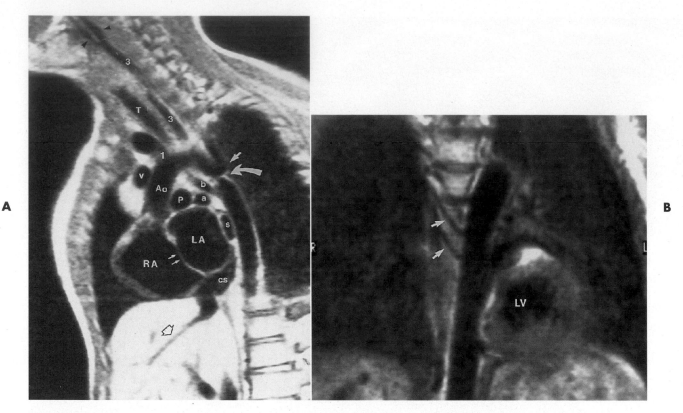

Fig. 3-5   A, LAO sagittal spin-echo image from a 7-year-old boy referred for differential upper and lower extremity pulses. TR=425 msec, TE=30 msec, slice thickness=7 mm. The aortic coarctation *(curved arrow)* is seen just distal to the unusual origin of the left subclavian artery *(arrow).* The innominate artery just proximal to the origin of the right common carotid artery *(1),* the midline trachea *(T),* and portions of the left common carotid artery *(3),* including the bifurcation into external and internal carotid arteries *(arrowheads)* are seen. The innominate vein *(v)* is found anterior to the aortic arch *(Ao).* The distal portion of a left-sided superior vena cava *(s)* just prior to its emptying into the dilated coronary sinus *(cs)* is seen. A hepatic vein *(open arrow)* drains into the inferior vena cava prior to its entry into the right atrium. The wall of the right atrium *(RA)* is sectioned obliquely, giving the impression of myocardial thickening. The interatrial septum *(small arrows)* appears to thin in the region of the foramen ovale. The right pulmonary artery *(P)* in this oblique section lies anterior to the left atrial appendage *(a)* and left main bronchus *(b).* **B,** Coronal spin-echo image of the aorta in a 9-year-old patient with coarctation of the aorta. TR=350 msec, TE=30 msec, slice thickness=7 mm. Dilated right intercostal arteries *(arrows)* enter the descending thoracic aorta beyond the coarctation segment. The cavity of the left ventricle *(LV)* is seen.

anterior sinus, which contains the origin of the right coronary artery. The intermediate-position sinus is the posterior left sinus, from which the left main coronary artery originates. The inferior-most sinus is the posterior right (noncoronary) sinus. During ventricular diastole you can identify the commissures of the valve by their characteristic tripod appearance. In the axial section (Fig. 3-10, *A*) the oblique orientation of the valve annulus distorts its round shape. Abnormalities of the aortic valve manifest themselves by producing jets of turbulent blood flow either in the antegrade (as in aortic stenosis) or retrograde (as in aortic insufficiency) direction. These fan-shaped loci of turbulent blood flow are well demonstrated using gradient-reversal imaging techniques (Figs. 3-11, *A* and *B*).

By the level of the aortic annulus the SVC has entered the right atrium and you can identify the superior-most portion of the interatrial septum, the sinus venosus portion. The interatrial septum is usually flat or bulges toward the right atrium, and it contains fat, which makes it easy to identify. The surface of the septum wraps around the posterior and left superior aspects of the right atrium and the right lateral and inferior aspects of the left atrium. The left atrium is superior to, posterior to, and to the left of the right atrium. Thus in the axial and sagittal section, the interatrial septum may have an off-coronal (Fig. 3-10, *A*), off-axial (Fig. 3-10, *C*), and off-sagittal (Fig. 3-10, *D*) orientation.

Atrial septal defects may be confused with an intact but thin septum. This is due to the problem of imaging the complex geometry of the septum in tomographic section, and the paucity of signal-producing protons in such a thin structure. Thus MR diagnosis of atrial septal

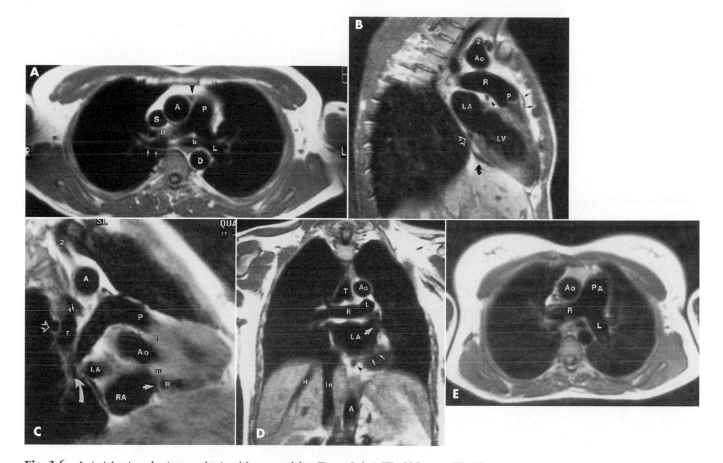

Fig. 3-6 **A,** Axial spin-echo image obtained 1 cm caudal to Figure 3-4, *A.* TR=835 msec, TE=30 msec, slice thickness=10 mm. The relationship of the superior vena cava *(S)*, ascending aorta *(A)*, main pulmonary artery *(P)*, and descending aorta *(D)* is typical. The anterior pericardial recess *(arrowhead)* is continuous with the space in the cephalad section (Fig. 3-4, *A*). The left pulmonary artery *(L)* is viewed lateral to the proximal left main bronchus *(b)* as it crosses over the more distal segment. The right main bronchus *(small arrows)* lies posterior to the right pulmonary artery *(R)*. **B,** RAO sagittal long-axis spin-echo image in a different patient through the sinuses of Valsalva of the pulmonary artery *(P)*. TR=740 msec, TE=30 msec, slice thickness=8 mm. In this obliquity the right pulmonary artery *(R)* is an extension of the main pulmonary artery, and it courses beneath the aortic arch *(Ao)* at the level of the origin of the left common carotid artery *(2)* and the left atrium *(LA)*. The signal void of the left main coronary artery viewed in cross section *(arrowhead)* and of the coronary sinus *(open arrow)* define the superior and inferior portions of the posterior atrioventricular ring. The mitral apparatus (not visualized in this section) is contained by this ring and separates the left atrium from the left ventricle *(LV)*. The reflection of the pericardium on the main pulmonary artery *(small arrows)* and the inferior pericardial space *(curved arrow)* may be seen. **C,** RAO sagittal long-axis spin-echo image 2 cm to the right of Figure 3-5, *B.* TR=740 msec, TE=30 msec, slice thickness=8 mm. The infundibular interventricular septum *(i)* separates the pulmonary artery *(P)* from the aortic root *(Ao)*. The membranous interventricular septum *(m)* is superior to the tricuspid valve *(arrow)*, which separates the right atrium *(RA)* from the inflow portion of the right ventricle *(R)*. The right lateral aspect of the left atrium *(LA)* is just below the right pulmonary artery. This far to the patient's right, the tracheal bifurcation *(small arrows)*, right mainstem bronchus *(r)*, and right lower lobe bronchus *(curved arrow)* are seen. The azygos vein *(open arrow)* is seen as it crosses the right mainstem bronchus. The proximal left common carotid artery *(2)* is seen leaving the aortic arch *(A)*. **D,** Coronal spin-echo image in the plane of the tracheal bifurcation *(T)*. TR=835 msec, TE=30 msec, slice thickness=10 mm. The left-sided aortic arch *(Ao)* displaces the trachea to the right. The main pulmonary artery divides in this plane to form the right pulmonary artery *(R)* and the left pulmonary artery *(L)*. The right pulmonary artery travels along the superior aspect of the left atrium *(LA)*. The left atrial appendage and left upper lobe pulmonary vein are volume averaged *(short arrow)* and cannot be differentiated. The mitral apparatus *(small arrows)* is contained within the posterior atrioventricular ring. Also within the inferior aspect of the ring is the coronary sinus *(arrowhead)*. A hepatic vein *(H)* and the intrahepatic inferior vena cava *(In)* are viewed just proximal to their entry into the right atrium. A portion of the upper abdominal aorta *(A)* may be seen. **E,** Axial spin-echo image of a 23-year-old woman with primary pulmonary hypertension. TR=800 msec, TE=30 msec, slice thickness=10 mm. The main pulmonary artery *(PA)* and both the left *(L)* and right *(R)* pulmonary arteries are dilated out to the left and right hila. The ascending aorta *(Ao)* is smaller in caliber than the main pulmonary artery.

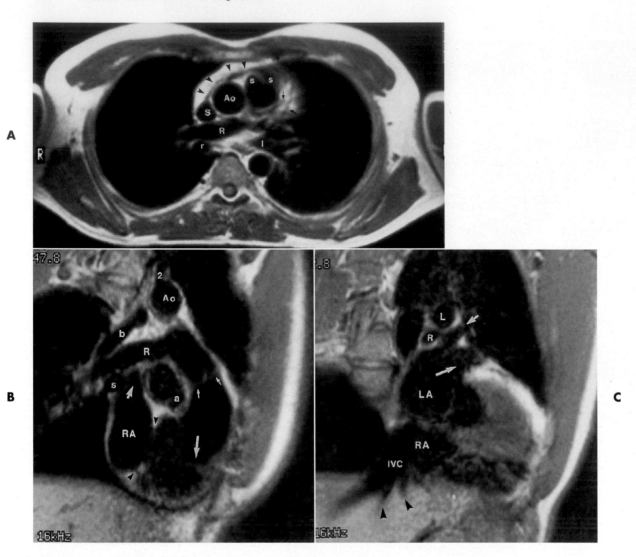

Fig. 3-7 **A,** Axial spin-echo image obtained 1 cm caudad to Figure 3-6,*A.* TR=835 msec, TE=30 msec, slice thickness=10 mm. Two of the sinuses of Valsalva of the pulmonary artery *(s)* may be appreciated. The superior vena cava *(S),* ascending aorta *(Ao),* and proximal main pulmonary artery are enveloped by the pericardium *(arrowheads).* The transverse right pulmonary artery *(R)* passes anterior to the right main bronchus *(r)* and behind the superior vena cava to enter the right hilum. The left main bronchus *(l)* is poorly visualized as it enters the left pulmonary parenchyma. Serpiginous, bifurcating loci of signal void *(small arrows)* are the epicardial branches of the left coronary artery. **B,** RAO sagittal long-axis spin-echo image just to the left of the section in Figure 3-6, *C.* TR=740 msec, TE=30 msec, slice thickness=10 mm. Leaflets of the pulmonary valve *(small arrows),* which is cephalad, anterior and to the left of the aortic valve (anterior sinus of Valsalva *[a]*) are seen. The right pulmonary artery *(R)* courses posterior and superior to the ascending aorta, anterior and slightly inferior to the right mainstem bronchus *(b)* to enter the right hilum. The ostium of the right atrial appendage *(short arrow)* lies medial to the entry of the superior vena cava *(s)* into the right atrium *(RA).* The tricuspid annulus is contained within the fat of the anterior atrioventricular ring *(arrowheads).* A right ventricular papillary muscle extending from the free wall may be seen *(long arrow).* The left common carotid artery *(2)* originates from the aortic arch *(Ao).* **C,** RAO sagittal long-axis spin-echo image 4 cm to the left of the section in **B.** TR=740 msec, TE=30 msec, slice thickness=10 mm. The interatrial septum separates the left atrium *(LA)* from the right atrium *(RA).* Hepatic vein branches *(arrowheads)* join the inferior vena cava *(IVC)* just prior to its entry into the right atrium. The left upper lobe pulmonary vein *(short arrow)* enters the left atrium obliquely, just posterior to the orifice of the left atrial appendage *(long arrow).* The left pulmonary artery is seen in cross section *(L);* a segment of the right pulmonary artery *(R)* is viewed in tangent.

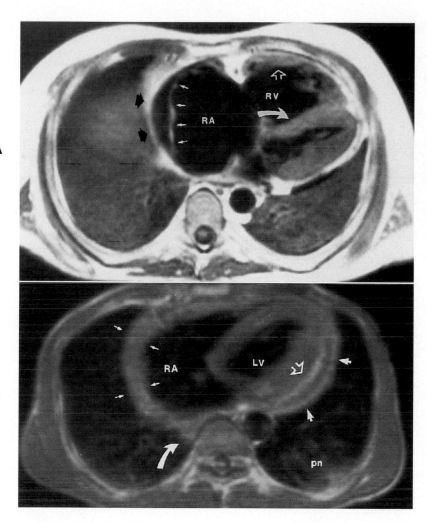

Fig. 3-8 A, Axial spin-echo image through the tricuspid valve annulus of a patient with idiopathic pulmonary fibrosis. TR=900 msec, TE=30 msec, slice thickness=10 mm. The lateral border of the right atrial wall *(small arrows)* is displaced medially by a signal void apparently contained within the epicardial fat *(broad black arrows)*, which is a small pericardial effusion. Note the thickened right ventricular free wall *(open arrow)*, straightening of the interventricular septum *(curved arrow)*, and increased signal intensity of both lungs. **B,** Axial spin-echo image in a patient with tuberculous pericarditis. TR=650 msec, TE=30 msec, slice thickness=10 mm. There is diffuse, nearly homogeneous increase in the thickness and signal intensity of the pericardium. The increase in thickness can be seen by inspection of the distance between the cavity and the lateral wall of the right atrium *(RA, small arrows)*, and between the epicardial fat of the free wall of the left ventricle *(LV, open arrow)* and the pericardial fat exterior to the pericardium *(short arrows)*. An enlarged right-sided lymph node *(curved arrow)* and left lower pneumonia *(pn)* are evident.

defect depends not only on demonstration of the defect in the atrial septum, but also on characterization of findings secondary to the shunt, including chamber dilatation secondary to volume overload and identification of associated abnormalities, such as anomalous pulmonary venous drainage (Figs. 3-12, *A-C*).

The posterior right (noncoronary) sinus of Valsalva relates to both the right and left atrium and to the interatrial septum (Fig. 3-13, *A*). Fibrous continuity between the anterior leaflet of the mitral valve and the annulus of the aortic valve, involving the posterior left and/or posterior right sinuses of Valsalva, may be identified in axial or horizontal long-axis images of the heart (Fig. 3-10, *B*). At this level in the heart you can identify the fat of the anterior atrioventricular ring, which separates the right heart-border-forming right atrium from the right ventricle. Contained within the ring is the signal void of the descending portion of the right coronary artery. Due to its orientation and its paucity of signal-generating tissue, the membranous interventricular septum may not be identified in the axial section. Commonly there is a void between the crest of the muscular interventricular sep-

tum and the posterior right sinus of Valsalva. In the oblique section (Fig. 3-13, *B*) the membranous septum may be identified and characterized. In true ventricular septal defects (VSD), as with atrial septal defects, there are cardiac changes associated with the hemodynamic sequelae (such as right ventricular hypertrophy or dilatation) and other morphologic lesions associated with the VSD itself (such as in tetralogy of Fallot) (Fig. 3-14).

The anterior atrioventricular ring contains the tricuspid valve, which guards the right ventricular inflow. Thus at this level within the heart, the relation of the right and left ventricular inflows may be appreciated; in the D-looped heart, the right ventricular inflow is to the right of the left ventricular inflow. The right ventricular free wall myocardium is thinner than that of the left ventricle. Normally it can be barely differentiated from anterior pericardial fat. Trabeculations of the right ventricle may not always be spatially resolved by MRI. Frequently, however, you can find a locus of increased signal intensity interposed at the apex of the right ventricle, between the free wall and the interventricular septum, which represents the moderator band. As mentioned, the free wall of

A

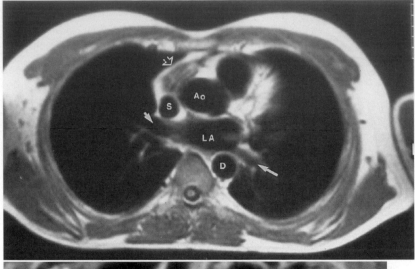

B

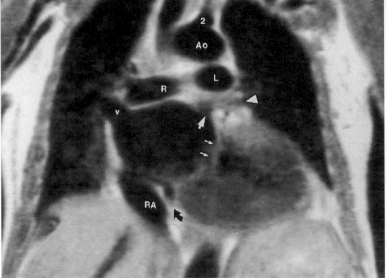

Fig. 3-9 **A,** Axial spin-echo image obtained 1 cm caudad to Figure 3-7, *A.* TR=835 msec, TE=30 msec, slice thickness=10 mm. The proximal aorta *(Ao)* ascends obliquely to the imaging plane, causing its apparent oval cross section. The left atrium *(LA)* lies posterior to the aortic root. The right upper lobe pulmonary vein *(short arrow)* enters the left atrium behind the superior vena cava *(S).* The left lower lobe pulmonary vein *(long arrow)* enters just anterior to the descending thoracic aorta *(D).* The right atrial appendage *(open arrow)* lies anterior and to the right of the ascending aorta. **B,** Coronal spin-echo image from another patient obtained through the right pulmonary artery *(R).* TR=740 msec, TE=30 msec, slice thickness=10 mm. The left-sided aortic arch *(Ao)* displaces the trachea to the right. The origin of the left common carotid artery *(2)* is seen. Just caudad to the proximal left pulmonary artery *(L)* is the left atrial appendage *(arrowhead).* The ostium of the left atrial appendage *(short arrow)* is just cephalad to the mitral valve *(small arrows).* The right upper lobe pulmonary vein *(v)* is large. Just caudad to the left atrium, within the fat of the posterior atrioventricular groove, is the coronary sinus *(curved arrow).* The posterior aspect of the right atrium *(RA)* lies just inferior to the left atrium.

the right ventricle is only about 3 mm thick and may not be visually separated from the epicardial fat. In cases of right ventricular hypertrophy, the right ventricular free wall thickness is increased and the trabecular pattern of the free wall and right ventricular side of the interventricular septum may be more apparent (Fig. 3-15). Furthermore, the increase in right ventricular afterload, which results in hypertrophic myocardium, also results in right ventricular hypertension. The normal convexity of the interventricular septum towards the right ventricular cavity is straightened or even reversed so that the septum bows toward the left ventricular cavity (Fig. 3-15).

Left ventricular myocardium in spin-echo MR images should be homogeneous in texture, but may look slightly mottled. Nevertheless it should be of nearly uniform thickness around the contour of the left ventricle. Ventricular myocardium thickens during ventricular systole and relaxes and thins during diastole. In the axial section there may appear to be increased myocardial

thickness at the ventricular apex; however, this is a result of oblique sectioning with respect to the axis of the left ventricle. Left ventricular hypertrophy is identified as thickening of the ventricular myocardium at the expense of the ventricular cavity (Fig. 3-16). Image acquisition in the axial section may be entirely adequate for identification of this condition. Tumors of the heart may be identified as loci of abnormal signal intensity within the normal myocardium and cardiac structures. MR may dramatically display distortion of adjacent structures caused by the growing mass (Figs. 3-17 and 3-18).

Left ventricular dilatation may be identified in any imaging plane (Fig. 3-19). The dilated ventricle produces extrinsic compression of the right atrium and ventricle, and often of the descending thoracic aorta. Although images acquired oblique to the long and short axes of the left ventricle may be useful in judging the status of the ventricle, short-axis image acquisition should be used for quantitation of left ventricular volume.

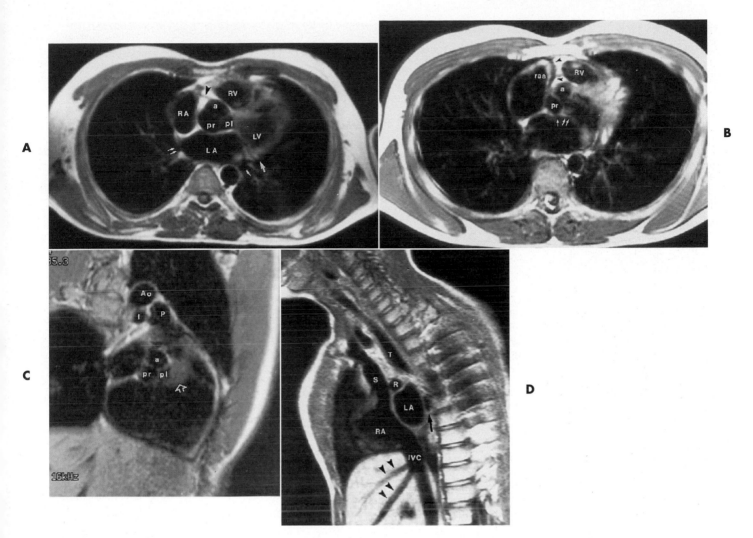

Fig. 3-10 A, Axial spin-echo image obtained 1 cm caudad to figure 3-9, *A*. TR=835 msec, TE=30 msec, slice thickness=10 mm. The three sinuses of Valsalva—the posterior left *(pl)*, the posterior right *(pr)*, and the anterior *(a)*—are seen. The proximal right coronary artery *(arrowhead)* originates from the anterior sinus of Valsalva and then acutely turns towards the fat of the anterior atrioventricular ring. The right ventricular outflow tract *(RV)* can be characterized by the thickness of the right ventricular free wall. To the left of the posterior atrioventricular ring *(short arrow)* lies the left ventricle *(LV)*. The left lower lobe *(small arrow)* and right lower lobe *(small arrows)* pulmonary veins may be seen entering the left atrium *(LA)*. Note the relationship among the posterior right (noncoronary) sinus of Valsalva and both the right *(RA)* and left atria *(LA)*. **B,** Axial spin-echo image obtained from another patient at nearly the same anatomic level as in **A.** TR=720 msec, TE=20 msec, slice thickness=8 mm. The apex of the right atrial appendage *(raa)* is surrounded by fat and contained within the pericardial sac *(arrowheads)*. Note the anterior *(a)* and posterior right *(pr)* sinuses of Valsalva. The fibrous continuity between the aortic ring and the anterior mitral leaflet *(small arrows)* is identified as a locus of increased signal intensity at this junction. The sinus of the right ventricle *(RV)* lies directly anterior to the aortic ring. **C,** RAO sagittal long-axis spin-echo image obtained from a third patient through the aortic root. TR=750 msec, TE=20 msec, slice thickness=10 mm. The orientation of the anterior *(a)*, posterior left *(pl)*, and noncoronary posterior right *(pr)* sinuses of Valsalva is exaggerated in this section (see Figs. 3-8, *A* and *B*). The posterior border of the right ventricular outflow tract is formed by the crista supraventricularis *(open arrow)*. The main pulmonary artery *(P)* lies caudad and to the left of the aortic arch *(Ao)*, and anterior and to the left of the left bronchus *(l)*. **D,** LAO sagittal spin-echo image just to the left of midline. TR=785 msec, TE=30 msec, slice thickness=8 mm. The interatrial septum separates the left atrium *(LA)* from the right atrium *(RA)*. The transverse right pulmonary artery *(R)* travels across the top of the left atrium, posterior to the superior vena cava *(S)*. The proximal right main bronchus tapers as it moves to the right, away from the plane of the trachea *(T)*. Proximal to the entrance of the inferior vena cava *(IVC)* into the right atrium, it is joined by hepatic veins *(arrowheads)*. A portion of the left lower lobe pulmonary vein *(arrow)* is seen behind the left atrium.

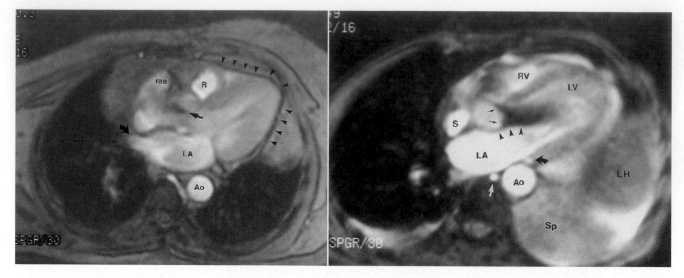

Fig. 3-11 **A,** Horizontal long-axis gradient-reversal image obtained through the left ventricular outflow during ventricular systole. TR=35 msec, TE=16 msec, slice thickness=10 mm. A fan-shaped signal void *(small arrow)* caused by the stenotic aortic valve extends from the aortic plane into the proximal ascending aorta. The left ventricular myocardium is thickened. The right ventricular outflow tract *(R)* and descending aorta *(Ao)* have high signal because of rapidly flowing blood. The right upper lobe pulmonary vein *(curved arrow)* is seen entering the left atrium *(LA)*. The right atrial appendage *(raa)* is superior and anterior to the ascending aorta. Notice the pencil-thin signal void of the pericardial space surrounding the heart *(arrowheads)*. **B,** Horizontal long-axis gradient-reversal image obtained from a different patient through the left ventricular outflow during ventricular diastole. TR=32 msec, TE=16 msec, slice thickness=10 mm. A broad signal void extends from the aortic valve *(short arrows)* into the dilated left ventricle *(LV)* along the anterior mitral leaflet *(arrowheads)* representing the flow of blood from the aorta in this case of aortic regurgitation. The right ventricle *(RV)*, left atrium *(LA)*, superior vena cava *(S)*, and descending aorta *(Ao)* contain high-signal rapidly flowing blood. The coronary sinus *(curved arrow)* and azygos vein *(white arrow)* are seen as well. In this oblique section the left hemidiaphragm *(LH)* and spleen *(Sp)* are found posterior to the heart. The band of increased signal intensity surrounding the ventricular myocardium is a hemmorhagic pericardial effusion.

Left and right ventricular myocardial function may be assessed qualitatively in the axial or horizontal long axis section, but quantitative analysis of ventricular volume, myocardial mass, and systolic shortening should be performed in the cardiac short-axis section, normal to the long axis of the left ventricle (Fig. 3-20). Whether studied using gradient-reversal or spin-echo technique, short-axis cardiac MRI provides accurate depiction of myocardial wall thickness and cavitary size. Summing cross-sectional ventricular chamber and myocardial area over all slices and multiplying by the slice thickness (Simpson rule) provides right and left ventricular chamber volume and myocardial volume measurements. Multiplying myocardial volume by the density of myocardium (1.05 g/cc) yields myocardial mass. Furthermore, evaluation of short-axis imagery allows estimation of right ventricular volume and pressure loading conditions. That is, throughout the cardiac cycle the interventricular septum should appear to be a continuation of the left ventricular myocardium, and to bow somewhat toward the right ventricular cavity. The left ventricular papillary muscles may be identified as soft tissue signal extending from the

free wall of the left ventricle into the left ventricular cavity (Fig. 3-13, *A*). In short-axis images of the heart, the papillary muscles may be identified in cross section (Figs. 3-20 and 3-21) as intracavitary filling defects or soft tissue masses.

The inferior aspect of the interatrial septum may not contain adequate tissue to generate a signal in an MR image (Fig. 3-22, *A*). You should be careful not to confuse this paucity of signal with a true atrial septal defect. In the absence of associated findings of a right-sided cardiac volume load, such a diagnosis is unlikely. In any event, a defect in this portion of the interatrial septum may be identified or excluded by examination in orthogonal section (Fig. 3-22, *B*). The crista terminalis, the remnant of the right valve of the sinus venosus, separates the pectinate muscles of the right atrial appendage from the smooth wall of the right atrium. It may be identified as a round locus of increased signal intensity along the lateral wall of the right atrium (Fig. 3-23).

Depending on the choice of TE used in spin-echo examination, the signal of increased pulmonary basilar interstitial water content may be enhanced in MR images

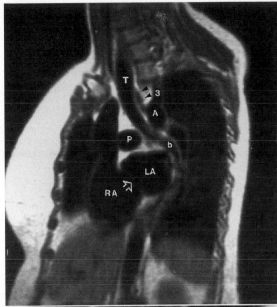

B

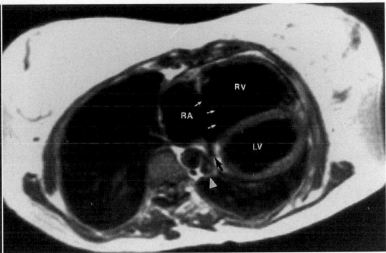

A

C

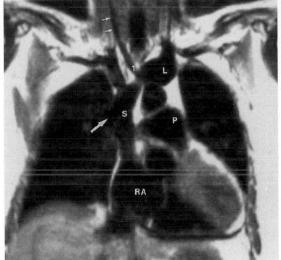

Fig. 3-12 **A,** LAO sagittal spin-echo image of a 40-year-old woman with atrial septal defect, bilateral partial anomalous pulmonary venous return, and left aortic arch with aberrant right subclavian artery. TR=800 msec, TE=30 msec, slice thickness=10 mm. The trachea *(T)*, tracheal bifurcation, and left mainstem bronchus *(b)* are seen. The interatrial septum is incomplete *(open arrow)*; the right atrium *(RA)* and right pulmonary artery *(P)* are dilated. The superior vena cava is enlarged because of the increased flow from the anomalous pulmonary veins (not in this section). The left subclavian artery *(3)* takes its typical vertical origin from the distal aortic arch *(A)*. The proximal portion of the aberrant right subclavian artery *(arrowheads)* travels behind the trachea. **B,** Axial spin-echo image of a 47-year-old woman with atrial septal defect. TR=825 msec, TE=30 msec, slice thickness=10 mm. The right atrium *(RA)* and right ventricle *(RV)* are dilated, and the heart is rotated in a clockwise manner into the left chest. The tricuspid valve leaflets bow towards the right ventricle *(small arrows)*. The coronary sinus *(black arrow)* is normal in caliber indicating normal right atrial pressure. The esophagus *(arrowhead)* lies to the left of the aorta and just behind the posterior atrioventricular ring of the heart. **C,** Coronal spin-echo image of the woman in **A.** TR=800 msec, TE=30 msec, slice thickness=10 mm. The left upper lobe pulmonary vein (not shown) drains into the left innominate vein *(L)* which is dilated. The right upper lobe pulmonary vein (not shown) drains into the lateral aspect *(arrow)* of the midsuperior vena cava *(S)*. The main pulmonary artery *(P)* and right atrium *(RA)* are enlarged. The innominate artery *(1)* becomes an isolated common carotid artery *(small arrows)*.

(Fig. 3-22, *A*). That is, the gravity-dependent posterior accumulation of interstitial lung water in a patient who has been supine for 30 to 60 minutes will be identified as increased signal, and this signal will be enhanced by using shorter TE. Therefore the increased signal identified may not necessarily represent the result of a pathologic process.

The coronary sinus is contained within fat on the right side of the posterior atrioventricular groove. It enters the right atrium along its posterior medial aspect, just inferior and medial to the tricuspid annulus (Fig. 3-24). Coronary sinus blood flow is segregated from inferior vena caval blood flow by the eustachian valve. The signal void of the distal right coronary artery travels in the inferior aspect of the anterior atrioventricular groove towards the intersection of the atrioventricular ring and inferior interventricular septum, the crux of the heart.

The anterior pericardial space is identified on this and other sections as a pencil-thin line of signal void contained within the epicardial and pericardial fat (Figs. 3-2, *B*; 3-4, *A*; 3-6, *A*; 3-7, *A*; 3-11, *A*; 3-24, *B*).

The tricuspid valve apparatus (Fig. 3-25) is not always demonstrated in axial section. When present it appears as a thin locus of increased signal within the signal void of the right atrioventricular junction. More often, however, the tricuspid valve may be demonstrated in the off-axial or off-sagittal section. The superior aspect of the tricuspid annulus lies just inferior to the membranous interventricular septum. In cases of valvular atresia and, in particular, in tricuspid atresia, there is increased fat deposition in the atretic valve ring (Fig. 3-14, *C*).

Thus spin-echo and gradient-reversal MR pulse sequences may be used to display normal and abnormal cardiac anatomy and to provide a means of demonstrat-

Text continued on page 122

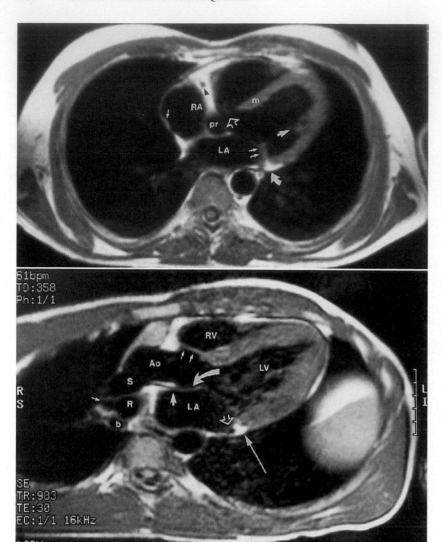

Fig. 3-13 **A,** Axial spin-echo image obtained 1 cm caudad to Figure 3-10, *A.* TR=835 msec, TE=30 msec, slice thickness=10 mm. The right coronary artery is a signal void *(arrowhead)* within the fat of the anterior atrioventricular ring. The locus of increased signal intensity on the wall of the right atrium *(RA)* is the crista terminalis *(small arrow).* The gap in the posterior aspect of the interventricular septum *(open arrow)* is occupied by the thin, membranous portion of the septum. The muscular interventricular septum *(m)* and papillary muscle *(short arrow)* are evident. The posterior right (noncoronary) sinus of Valsalva *(pr)* abuts both the left atrium *(LA)* and the right atrium. Portions of the mitral apparatus *(small arrows)* may be seen. The fat demarcating the posterior atrioventricular groove *(curved arrow)* and posterior attachment of the mitral valve *(small arrows)* contained within the ring are identified. **B,** Horizontal long-axis spin-echo image obtained from a different patient. TR=983 msec, TE=30 msec, slice thickness=10 mm. The membranous interventricular septum *(small arrows)* separating the left ventricle *(LV)* from the right ventricle *(RV)* is well displayed. The anterior mitral leaflet *(curved arrow)* is in fibrous continuity with the aortic valve *(short arrow).* The superior vena cava *(S)* is volume averaged with the ascending aorta *(Ao)* and anterior to the right pulmonary artery *(R).* The right upper lobe pulmonary artery *(small arrow)* and right bronchus *(b)* are demonstrated. The coronary sinus *(open arrow)* is just to the right of the fat of the posterior atrioventricular groove *(long arrow).*

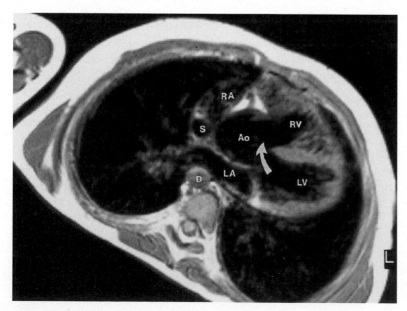

Fig. 3-14 Axial spin-echo image of a 7-year-old boy with tetralogy of Fallot and right aortic arch (not shown). TR=520 msec, TE=30 msec, slice thickness=7 mm. The dilated aorta *(Ao)* overrides the large interventricular septal defect *(curved arrow)* between the left ventricle *(LV)* and the hypertrophied, trabeculated right ventricle *(RV).* To the right of the fat of the anterior atrioventricular groove lies the right atrium *(RA),* into which drains the superior vena cava *(S).* The small left atrium *(LA)* is typical of patients with tetralogy of Fallot. The descending thoracic aorta *(D)* is to the right of the spine.

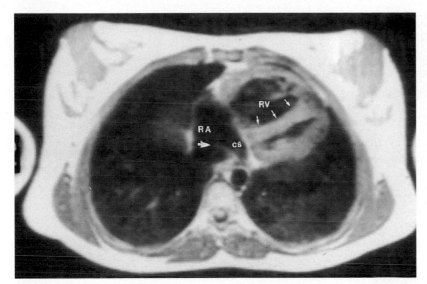

Fig. 3-15 Axial spin-echo image of a 24-year-old woman with primary pulmonary hypertension. TR=620 msec, TE=30 msec, slice thickness=8 mm. The free wall of the right ventricle *(RV)* is markedly thickened. The interventricular septum *(small arrows)* bows toward the left ventricle. The right atrium *(RA)* and coronary sinus *(cs)* are dilated. The eustachian valve *(short arrow)* is seen.

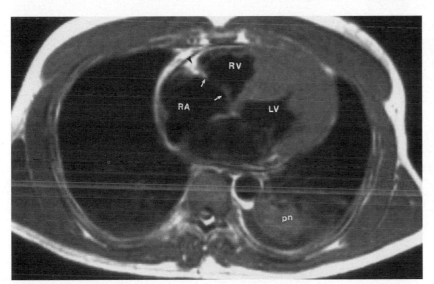

Fig. 3-16 Axial spin-echo image from a 32-year-old man with hypertrophic obstructive cardiomyopathy. TR=820 msec, TE=30 msec, slice thickness=8 mm. The marked thickening of the left ventricular *(LV)* myocardium is evident. The right ventricle *(RV)* appears small. The tricuspid valve *(small arrows)* separating the right atrium *(RA)* from the right ventricle is contained within the anterior atrioventricular groove *(arrowhead)*. Incidentally noted is left lower lobe pneumonia *(pn)*.

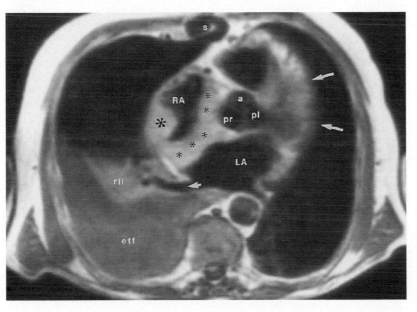

Fig. 3-17 Axial spin-echo image of a 56-year-old man with a cardiac lymphoma obtained through the aortic sinuses of Valsalva *(a, pr, pl)*. TR=640 msec, TE=30 msec, slice thickness=10 mm. The right atrial *(RA)* nodular mass *(*)* and infiltration *(*)* of the right atrial wall, interatrial septum, and space between the right atrium and aortic sinuses are homogeneous and of different signal intensities than the left ventricular myocardium *(long arrows)*. There is right lower lobe collapse *(rll)* and a large right pleural effusion *(eff)*. The right lower lobe pulmonary vein *(short arrow)* drains into the left atrium *(LA)*. The signal void *(s)* caused by a wire sternal suture is evident.

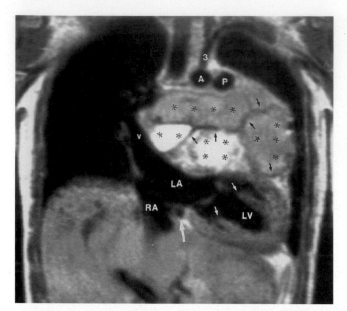

Fig. 3-18 Coronal spin-echo image of a 13-year-old girl with fibrous histiocytoma of the pericardium. TR=560 msec, TE=30 msec, slice thickness=7 mm. The bulky, septated *(small arrows)* inhomogeneous mass *(*)* compresses the left atrium *(LA)* and left ventricle *(LV)* from above, and displaces the aortic arch *(A)* and main pulmonary artery *(P)* from below. The left ventricular papillary muscles *(small arrows)* and left subclavian artery *(3)* are seen. The coronary sinus *(long arrow)* lies inferior to the left atrium and medial to the posterior aspect of the right atrium *(RA)*. The right upper lobe pulmonary vein *(v)* is widely patent.

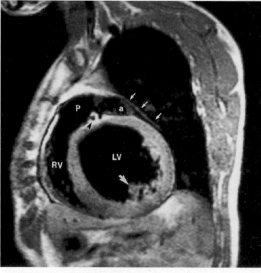

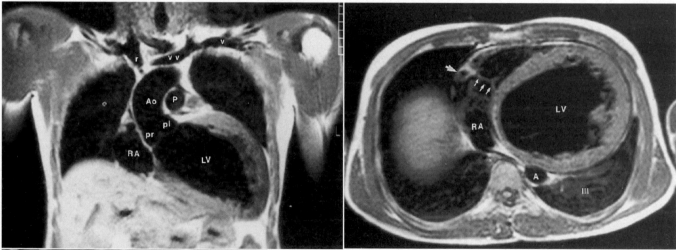

A

B

C

Fig. 3-19 Spin-echo images of a 52-year-old man with chronic rheumatic aortic regurgitation. **A,** Coronal image through the aortic valve. TR=800 msec, TE=30 msec, slice thickness=10 mm. The left ventricle *(LV)* and ascending aorta *(Ao)* are dilated. The posterior right *(pr)* and posterior left *(pl)* sinuses of Valsalva are seen. The left ventricular myocardium is markedly hypertrophied. The main pulmonary artery *(P)* and right atrium *(RA)* are normal. The left subclavian vein *(v)* drains into the left innominate vein *(vv)*, which has not yet joined with the right innominate vein *(r)*. **B,** Axial image through the tricuspid valve. TR=800 msec, TE=30 msec, slice thickness=10 mm. The dilated left ventricle *(LV)* compresses the right atrium *(RA)* and descending aorta *(A)*. The tricuspid valve *(small arrows)* may be seen. The right coronary artery *(short arrow)* is embedded within the fat of the anterior atrioventricular groove. Note the increased signal of the compressed left lower lobe *(lll)*. **C,** LAO sagittal image through the pulmonary valve. TR=800 msec, TE=30 msec, slice thickness=10 mm. The inferior left ventricular papillary muscle *(short arrow)* originates from the free wall of the dilated and hypertrophied left ventricle *(LV)*. The left atrial appendage *(a)* is enveloped within the pericardium *(small arrows)*. The left main coronary artery *(arrowhead)*, embedded in epicardial fat, passes behind the main pulmonary artery *(P)*. The right ventricle *(RV)* is normal.

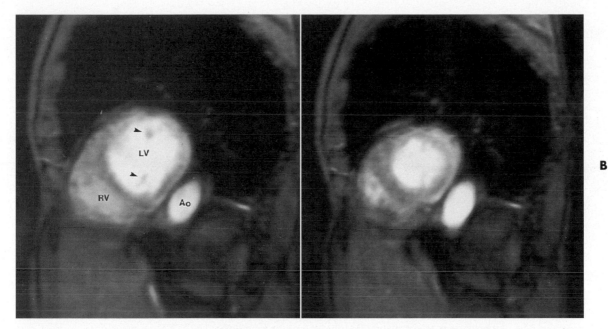

Fig. 3-20 Short-axis gradient-reversal images obtained from a 52-year-old male patient with emphysema. **A,** End-diastolic image obtained 18 msec after the ECG R wave. TR=34 msec, TE=15 msec, slice thickness=8 mm. The lungs are hyperinflated. The increased signal intensity of the blood within the left ventricle *(LV)*, right ventricle *(RV)*, and descending thoracic aorta *(Ao)*, is typical of this type of acquisition sequence. The contrast between the blood-filled ventricular cavities and myocardial walls is less than in spin-echo technique. The two left ventricular papillary muscles *(arrowheads)* appear as loci of decreased signal intensity within the cavity. The interventricular septum bows towards the right ventricle in this normal heart. **B,** End-systolic image obtained 300 msec after the ECG R wave. TR=34 msec, TE=15 msec, slice thickness=8 mm. The myocardium has thickened and the ventricular cavities have decreased in size. The inhomogeneity of signal in the right ventricular cavity results from the muscular trabeculations.

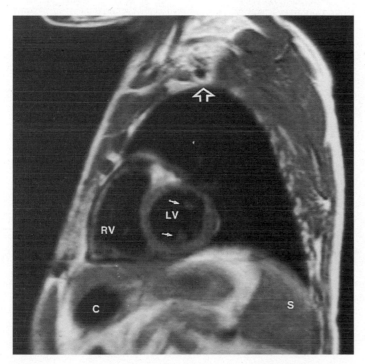

Fig. 3-21 Short-axis end-diastolic spin-echo image obtained 18 msec after the ECG R wave. TR=840 msec, TE=30 msec, slice thickness=10 mm. Compare the contrast between left ventricular *(LV)* and right ventricular *(RV)* blood and myocardium with Figure 3-20. The left ventricular papillary muscles *(small arrows)* are seen in cross section. The signal void of the left subclavian artery *(open arrow)* may be seen. Below the diaphragm the transverse colon *(C)* and spleen *(S)* are identified.

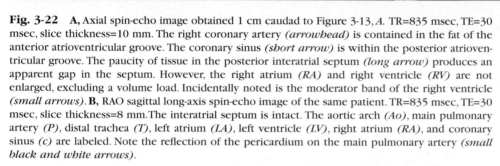

Fig. 3-22   **A,** Axial spin-echo image obtained 1 cm caudad to Figure 3-13, *A*. TR=835 msec, TE=30 msec, slice thickness=10 mm. The right coronary artery *(arrowhead)* is contained in the fat of the anterior atrioventricular groove. The coronary sinus *(short arrow)* is within the posterior atrioventricular groove. The paucity of tissue in the posterior interatrial septum *(long arrow)* produces an apparent gap in the septum. However, the right atrium *(RA)* and right ventricle *(RV)* are not enlarged, excluding a volume load. Incidentally noted is the moderator band of the right ventricle *(small arrows)*. **B,** RAO sagittal long-axis spin-echo image of the same patient. TR=835 msec, TE=30 msec, slice thickness=8 mm. The interatrial septum is intact. The aortic arch *(Ao)*, main pulmonary artery *(P)*, distal trachea *(T)*, left atrium *(LA)*, left ventricle *(LV)*, right atrium *(RA)*, and coronary sinus *(c)* are labeled. Note the reflection of the pericardium on the main pulmonary artery *(small black and white arrows)*.

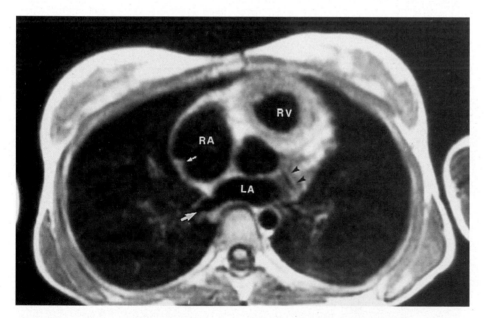

Fig. 3-23   Axial spin-echo image of a 20-year-old woman with valvular pulmonic stenosis. TR=920 msec, TE=20 msec, slice thickness=7 mm. The crista terminalis is a locus of increased signal intensity *(small arrow)* on the lateral wall of the right atrium *(RA)*. The right lower lobe pulmonary vein *(large arrow)* drains into the left atrium *(LA)*. Note the thickening of the myocardium of the right ventricular outflow tract *(RV)*. The left circumflex coronary artery *(arrowheads)* passes over the posterior atrioventricular ring.

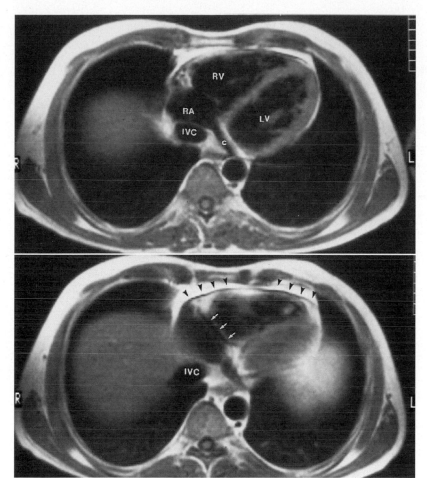

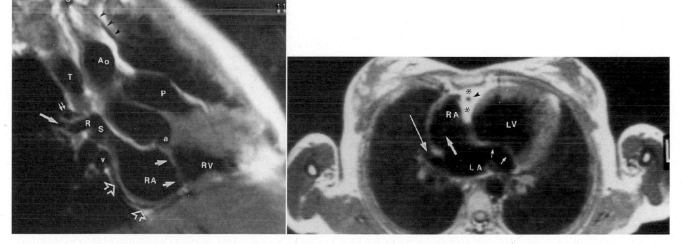

Fig. 3-24 Axial spin-echo images. **A,** Image obtained 1 cm caudad to Figure 3-22, *A.* TR=835 msec, TE=30 msec, slice thickness=10 mm. Blood enters the right atrium *(RA)* from the inferior vena cava *(IVC)* and coronary sinus *(c).* **B,** Image obtained 1 cm caudad to **A.** TR=835 msec, TE=30 msec, slice thickness=10 mm. A hepatic vein joins with the inferior vena cava *(IVC)* prior to its entry into the heart. The signal void of the distal right coronary artery *(small arrows)* traveling in the inferior aspect of the anterior atrioventricular ring is seen. The anterior pericardial space is clearly identified *(arrowheads).*

Fig. 3-25 **A,** RAO sagittal long-axis spin-echo image. TR=780 msec, TE=20 msec, slice thickness=8 mm. The left internal mammary artery *(arrowheads)* is seen descending from the left subclavian artery *(3).* The aortic arch *(Ao)* and trachea *(T)* have a normal relationship. The distal transverse right pulmonary artery *(R)* and right upper lobe pulmonary artery branch *(long arrow)* are superimposed on the superior vena cava *(S).* The azygos vein *(small arrows)* is immediately superior to the right pulmonary artery. The right atrium *(RA),* tricuspid valve *(short arrows),* and right ventricular inflow *(RV)* are labeled. The right lower lobe pulmonary vein *(v)* is below, at the level of the entrance of the superior vena cava into the right atrium. Note the pericardial space *(open arrows)* just lateral to the right atrial wall. The anterior aortic sinus of Valsalva *(a)* and proximal main pulmonary artery *(P)* are identified. **B,** Axial spin-echo image of a 22-year-old woman with tricuspid atresia. TR=680 msec, TE=30 msec, slice thickness=7 mm. The increased fat in the anterior atrioventricular ring *(*)* is characteristic of an atretic valve. The signal void of the right coronary artery *(arrowhead)* is seen within the fat in the atrioventricular groove. The right upper lobe pulmonary vein *(long arrow)* empties into the left atrium. The gap *(short arrow)* between the right atrium *(RA)* and the left atrium *(LA)* is an atrial septal defect. The mitral valve *(small arrows)* protects the dilated left ventricle *(LV).*

ing a wide range of congenital and acquired conditions. Interaction with referring clinicians will define the specific questions to be answered by the MR examination. Getting a good ECG pulse tracing will aid greatly in acquiring a diagnostic image. Understanding the anatomy of the heart is critical in order to make cardiac diagnoses. Following these three tenets will allow you to fully exploit MR techniques for the diagnosis and investigation of patients with heart disease.

SUGGESTED READINGS

Book

Higgins CB, Silverman NH, Kersting-Sommerhoff BA, Schmidt K: *Congenital heart disease: echocardiography and magnetic resonance imaging,* New York, 1990, Raven Press.

Journals

Boxt LM, Katz J, Kolb T et al: Direct quantitation of right and left ventricular volumes with nuclear magnetic resonance imaging in patients with primary pulmonary hypertension, *J Am Coll Cardiol* 19:1508-1515, 1992.

Katz J, Boxt LM, Sciacca RR et al: Motion dependence of myocardial transverse relaxation time in magnetic resonance imaging, *Magn Reson Imaging* 8:449-458, 1990.

Mirowitz SA, Lee JKT, Gutierrez FR et al: Normal signal-void patterns in cardiac cine MR images, *Radiology* 176:49-55, 1990.

Nazarian GK, Julsrud PR, Ehman RL, Edwards WD: Correlation between magnetic resonance imaging of the heart and cardiac anatomy, *Mayo Clin Proc* 62:573-583, 1987.

Yoo S-J, Lim T-H, Park I-S et al: Defects of the interventricular septum of the heart: En face MR imaging in the oblique coronal plane, *AJR Am J Roentgenol* 157:943-946, 1991.

CHAPTER 4

Cardiac Angiography

Techniques
   Indications
   Catheterization techniques
   Cineangiography
   Projection positions
   Radiation exposure and protection
Coronary Artery Anatomy
   Right coronary artery
      Sinoatrial nodal artery
      Conus artery
      Distal right coronary artery
   Left coronary artery
      Left circumflex artery
      Left anterior descending artery
   Cardiac veins
Cardiac Chambers
   Right atrium
   Right ventricle
   Left atrium
   Left ventricle
Cardiac Valves
   Tricuspid valve
   Mitral valve
   Pulmonary valve
   Aortic valve
Suggested Readings

TECHNIQUES

The imaging of the cardiac chambers and coronary arteries is fundamental to the accurate diagnosis of heart diseases that are characterized by morphologic abnormality. Although cross-sectional techniques are increasingly used to diagnose many cardiac diseases, the standard imaging examination, at least for the coronary arteries, remains cineangiography. Cardiac catheterization is performed to provide hemodynamic information, to visualize the interior of the heart, and to perform interventional procedures.

Indications

The Committee on the Indications for Coronary Arteriography of the American Heart Association has proposed that coronary arteriography should be used "to establish if significant coronary arterial disease is present or absent in a patient whose diagnosis is otherwise uncertain, or in whom a diagnosis is considered essential for management." The final decision must ultimately be based on an analysis of the expected benefits of the procedure balanced against the risks of the technique. Patients who undergo cardiac surgery are usually catheterized first, although with evolving noninvasive techniques, some aspects of the catheterization may be modified or omitted. The clinical variables that can be determined by cardiac catheterization include measurement of chamber pressures, detection of intracardiac shunts, characterization of myocardial performance, quantitation of valvular stenoses and regurgitation, and imaging of cardiac anatomy. When such information is essential for a management decision, a catheterization is warranted. In children, clinical indications include cyanosis of cardiac origin; heart failure that responds poorly to medical management; a deteriorating clinical course in a patient with heart disease under medical management; and the need to define parameters that are difficult to obtain without catheterization, such as the pulmonary vascular resistance, the severity of valvular stenosis, or the anatomy of the malformation.

There are few contraindications to cardiac catheterization if the information to be obtained is critical to the patient's care. Patients who are liable to have arrhythmias (Ebstein anomaly) or who are in cardiogenic shock have been thought too unstable to undergo catheriza-

123

tion. However, with the availability of transvenous cardiac pacemakers and intraaortic balloon pumps, these patients are now expected to have low morbidity when undergoing invasive procedures. If medical therapy can improve the patient's hemodynamic status, some conditions warrant postponement of cardiac catheterization. Patients in congestive heart failure usually benefit from medical therapy to alleviate pulmonary edema before coronary angiography and left ventriculography are done. Correction of abnormal bleeding and prothrombin times is essential to produce hemostasis; abnormal values frequently occur when anticoagulants or aspirin is not stopped long enough for the drug to be cleared. In a similar fashion, blood sugar and serum potassium levels should be corrected before catheterization. Other conditions such as digitalis intoxication, severe hypertension, poor renal function, and febrile illnesses, should be controlled before elective catheterization. Acute myocardial infarction is a relative contraindication unless angioplasty or emergency surgery is planned.

See Box 4-1 for relative contraindications to coronary angiography.

Catheterization Techniques

The technique of routine radiologic visualization by selective injection of the coronary arteries was first developed in 1959 by Mason Sones, a pediatric cardiologist who only the year before had successfully performed intracardiac angiography in children. In the Sones technique a single catheter is inserted through a brachial arteriotomy. The catheter can then be directed into each coronary artery.

Ricketts and Abrams extended the concept of selective coronary catheterization by devising two catheters, one for each coronary artery, that could be introduced percutaneously into the femoral artery by the Seldinger technique. The concept of a preshaped catheter for selective catheterization was refined by Amplatz and others; various shapes were devised to surmount the difficulties of different aortic sizes and ectopic locations of coronary arteries (Fig. 4-1). In 1967 radiologist Melvin Judkins designed preshaped catheters for both the right and left coronary arteries. The left coronary catheter, if properly aligned, needed only to be advanced around a normal aortic arch to fall into the ostium; whereas the right coronary catheter needed a 180-degree twist after it had passed around the arch (Fig. 4-2). Different catheter shapes and other refinements were introduced by Bourassa and associates, Schoonmaker, and others.

Cineangiography

Because cineangiography yields images with resolution of 0.1 mm, this technique is the best way to visual-

Box 4-1 Relative Contraindications to Coronary Angiography

a. Recent stroke (within 1 month).
b. Progressive renal insufficiency.
c. Active gastrointestinal bleeding.
d. Fever possibly due to infection.
e. Active infection.
f. Short life expectancy due to other illnesses such as cancer or severe pulmonary, hepatic, or renal disease.
g. Severe anemia.
h. Severe uncontrolled systemic hypertension.
i. Severe electrolyte imbalance.
j. Severe systemic or psychologic illness in which prognosis is doubtful or behavior is unpredictable producing undue risk of cardiac catheterization.
k. Very advanced physiologic (not chronologic) age.
l. Patient refusal to consider definitive treatment such as angioplasty, coronary artery bypass surgery, or valve replacement.
m. In unstable patients, lack of a cardiac surgical team in the hospital. (Patients refractory to maximal medical therapy should generally be transferred to a center where surgical backup is immediately available.) Under special circumstances, such as when the condition of a hospitalized patient can be readily stabilized by balloon counterpulsation, coronary angiography can be undertaken in the hospital without a cardiac surgical team. However, well-defined mechanisms must be in place for rapid referral and acceptance of such patients by a hospital in which emergency surgery or angioplasty can be carried out with minimal delay.
n. Digitalis intoxication.
o. Documented anaphylaxis during previous exposure to angiographic contrast material. In most patients with a history of immediate generalized anaphylactoid reaction to contrast material, the reactions do not constitute anaphylaxis, and these individuals can safely undergo coronary angiography using premedication with corticosteroids and antihistamines.

Reprinted with permission from the American College of Cardiology from Ross J et al: Guidelines for coronary angiography: a report of the American College of Cardiology/American Heart Association Task Force on assessment of diagnostic and therapeutic cardiovascular procedures, *J Am Coll Cardiol* 10(4):935-950, 1987.

ize accurately coronary anatomy and stenoses. However, the proximal 2 cm of the coronary arteries can be seen with a resolution of 1 to 2 mm using ultrasound and magnetic resonance imaging (MRI) (Fig. 4-3). Heart motion so far has precluded accurate imaging of the middle and distal segments of the coronary arteries by techniques other than angiography.

Angiographic rooms for cardiac evaluation are outfitted in a similar fashion to rooms used for other vascular techniques. Rapid film changer programs are used for pulmonary arteriography, venacavography, and aortogra-

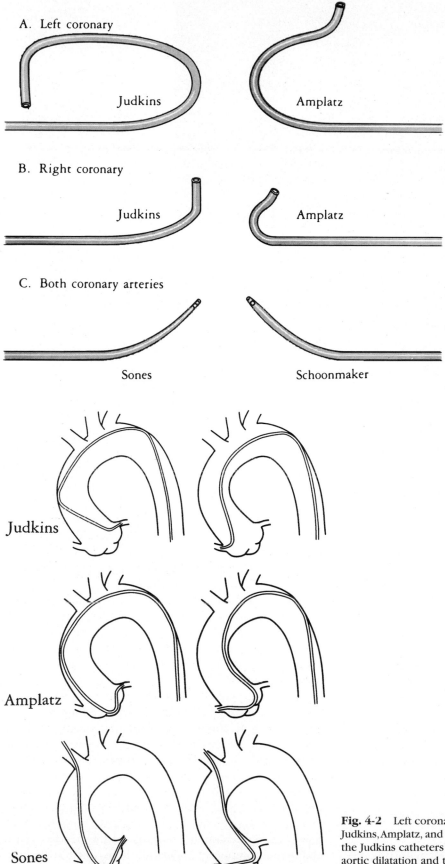

A. Left coronary

Judkins   Amplatz

B. Right coronary

Judkins   Amplatz

C. Both coronary arteries

Sones   Schoonmaker

Judkins

Amplatz

Sones

Fig. 4-1 Coronary catheters. **A** and **B**, The Judkins and Amplatz series of catheters have a different shape for the right and left coronary arteries. **C**, The Sones and Schoonmaker catheters can be directed by the operator into either coronary artery.

Fig. 4-2 Left coronary and right coronary catheter positions for the Judkins, Amplatz, and Sones techniques. Because the second curve of the Judkins catheters touch the ascending aorta, they are affected by aortic dilatation and tortuosity. The Amplatz and Sones catheters rest on the aortic valve and are easier to control with a dilated root.

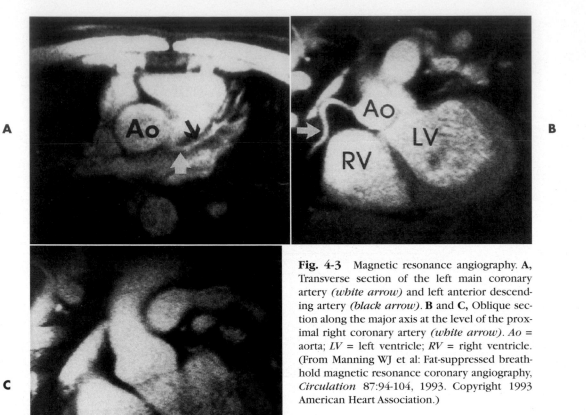

Fig. 4-3 Magnetic resonance angiography. **A,** Transverse section of the left main coronary artery *(white arrow)* and left anterior descending artery *(black arrow)*. **B** and **C,** Oblique section along the major axis at the level of the proximal right coronary artery *(white arrow)*. *Ao* = aorta; *LV* = left ventricle; *RV* = right ventricle. (From Manning WJ et al: Fat-suppressed breath-hold magnetic resonance coronary angiography, *Circulation* 87:94-104, 1993. Copyright 1993 American Heart Association.)

phy. The major difference is that coronary angiography is recorded on cine film. Many laboratories also use cine filming for recording details of the central pulmonary arteries and for thoracic aortography.

Because processing of cine film takes 20 to 30 minutes, video recording on tape or disk is done at the time of cine fluorography so that the result can be viewed quickly. The image intensifiers may be chosen for single, double, or triple mode operation. The single mode operation is less costly and theoretically offers a higher resolution; the double and triple modes of operation offer more flexibility and allow both magnification (for coronary angioplasty) and a larger field of view (FOV) for large heart evaluation or aortography.

Video recording also allows stop-frame techniques and slow-motion analysis. Digital subtraction angiography is useful in imaging the aortic arch where the background frame has little motion.

Projection Positions

Most cardiac angiography is performed with projections that align the x-ray beam with the axis of the heart.

The right anterior oblique (RAO) view profiles the long axis of the right and left ventricles parallel to the interventricular septum. The mitral and tricuspid valves are in tangent so that regurgitation is projected in the plane of the film. In the left anterior oblique (LAO) view the interventricular and interatrial septa are aligned perpendicular to the film plane. In this view the tricuspid and mitral valves are seen in their frontal projections. Ventricular septal defects, aortic root to right heart fistulas, and systolic anterior motion of the mitral valve project in the plane of the film.

Compound angulation is frequently used to align the x-ray beam orthogonal to the heart. In addition to RAO and LAO projections, the image intensifier is tilted toward the head or the foot of the patient. In a cranial projection the image intensifier angles toward the head of the patient, whereas in a caudal projection the image intensifier angles toward the patient's feet. You can identify a cranial projection by an unusually high diaphragm. In a caudal angulation the diaphragm is generally not visible. Cranial angulation also projects the heart over the abdomen. Compound angulation is part of the standard evaluation of the coronary arteries to project each branch and its bifurcation so that no overlap is present. Diseases in which compound angulation is necessary include ventricular septal defects and systolic anterior motion of the anterior leaflet of the mitral valve in hypertrophic cardiomyopathy, where the cranial LAO projection is employed. Examples of compound projections are listed in Box 4-2 along with typical examples for which they are used.

Box 4-2   Axial Projections in Congenital Heart Disease

SITTING PROJECTION (40-DEGREE CRANIAL)

Pulmonary arteries in tetralogy of Fallot
Pulmonary arteries in pulmonary atresia with
    ventricular septal defect
Pulmonary sling
Vascular ring (double aortic arch)
Supravalvular pulmonary stenosis

LONG-AXIAL OBLIQUE PROJECTION (70-DEGREE LAO AND 20-DEGREE CRANIAL)

Ventricular septal defects
    Membranous
    Malalignment (tetralogy)
    Muscular
    Subpulmonary (with reciprocal RAO view)
Subaortic stenosis
Subpulmonary stenosis in transposition of the great
    arteries
Atrial septal defect, secundum
Straddling tricuspid valve
Coronary artery distribution in tetralogy of Fallot
Mitral valve in idiopathic hypertrophic subaortic
    stenosis

FOUR-CHAMBER PROJECTION (40-DEGREE LAO AND 40-DEGREE CRANIAL)

Atrioventricular canal defects
Ventricular septal defect, atrioventricular canal type
Single ventricle
Tricuspid atresia
Patent ductus arteriosus
Straddling tricuspid or mitral valve

COMPOUND 40-DEGREE CRANIAL AND 20-DEGREE LAO

Left ventricular right atrial shunt

COMPOUND 40-DEGREE CRANIAL AND 30-DEGREE RAO

Fontan shunt (right atrium to pulmonary artery
    conduit)

COMPOUND 15-DEGREE CAUDAL AND 20-DEGREE LAO

Mustard interatrial baffle (postoperative
    d-transposition)

Because an angiogram is a projection image rather than a tomogram, the picture of the coronary arteries, cardiac chambers, and valves is a summation of many overlapping structures. Biplane orthogonal projections are required to evaluate cardiac structures completely.

The catheter techniques, injection rates, and other technical factors are summarized in Tables 4-1 and 4-2. Power injection techniques are used for all types of cardiac angiography except for coronary arteriography in which injection is by hand. When high flow exists in the coronary arteries, such as in arteriovenous fistulas and in aortic regurgitation, a power injection can be used safely with the same techniques used to inject small arteries in other parts of the body.

Radiation Exposure and Protection

Radiation exposure to both the patient and the operating personnel has been the focus of numerous studies. The amount of radiation received varies widely among laboratories and depends on the type of equipment employed, the operating techniques, the length of the procedure, the administrative procedures concerning the placement of personnel, and the shielding of the x-ray beam.

Exposure from fluoroscopy alone results in a skin dose to the patient of about 2 R/min. Fluoroscopy time for adult coronary arteriography usually ranges from 10 to 20 minutes. Exposure during cinefluorography depends on the radiation dose per frame and the length of filming time. Exposure per frame, when surveyed over many types of equipment, ranges from 10 to 100 μR/frame. At the usual frame rate of 30 frames/sec and with an attenuation factor for the adult heart ranging between 500 and 1000, the skin exposure rate for a radiation dose of 50 μR/frame ranges from 45 to 90 R/min. The trade-off with lowering the radiation dose per frame is a poorer image. The "grain" on a cine film mainly represents quantum mottle, which is a statistical fluctuation in the spatial distribution of x-ray photons on the film. The minimum amount of radiation necessary to produce an acceptable image is 20 μR; therefore, a dose of 20 to 25 μR/frame represents a balance of diagnostic picture quality and minimum radiation exposure to the patient. Most cine equipment is adjusted by the manufacturer to have an output of 50 to 75 μR/frame.

The hazards of ionizing radiation are well known to many radiologists and should be understood by all physicians who use x-ray equipment. Guidelines for a maximum limit on the yearly occupational exposure have been established by the National Council on Radiation Protection (NCRP) (Table 4-3). The NCRP is considering lowering the total body limit to 1 to 2 rem annually. Lead eyeglasses and thyroid shielding help to diminish the dose received by the angiographer.

Table 4-1 Technical factors for angiography in adults

Procedure site	Contrast injection Rate (ml/sec)	Volume (ml)	Rapid Film Changer (films/sec for number of films)
Intracardiac			
Right atrium	20	40	3/sec for 3; 1/sec for 6
Left atrium	20	40	3/sec for 3; 1/sec for 4
Right ventricle	15	50	4-6/sec for 3; 1/sec for 6
Left ventricle	13	50	4-6/sec for 3; 1/sec for 3
Coronary arteries	Hand injection	RCA-6	Cinefluorography at 30/sec
		LCA-8	
	Power injection		
	4	8	
Pulmonary arteries			
Main	30-35	60-70	3/sec for 3; 1/sec for 10
Right or left	20	40	
Vena cava	20	40	2/sec for 10
Thoracic aorta	30	60	3/sec for 3; 1/sec for 6
Aneurysmal aorta	35-40	70-80	4/sec for 3; 1/sec for 6

Table 4-2 Technical factors for thoracic angiography in children

Procedure site	Contrast injection Volume (ml/kg)	Delivery Time (sec)	Comments
Intracardiac	1-1.5	1-1.5	Volume is adjusted to the size of the vascular bed and the flow through it.
Right atrium			
Right ventricle			Delivery time is roughly that of two heartbeats; for example, at heart rate of 120 beats/sec, inject contrast over 1 sec.
Left atrium			
Left ventricle			
Pulmonary artery	2	1.5	Absolute maximum contrast dose is 5 ml/kg/day adjusted downward if renal function is decreased and if baby is less than 1 month old.
Thoracic aorta	2	1.5	

Table 4-3 Summary of recommendations for maximum x-ray dose

Occupational exposure for people working with radiation	
Annual	50 mSv (5 rem)
Cumulative	10 mSv (1 rem) times age
Public exposure	
Annual	1 mSv (100 mrem)
Lens of eye	15 mSv (1.5 rem)
Skin	50 mSv (5 rem)
Embryo/fetus during gestation	0.5 mSv (50 mrem)

Note: Average annual background radiation from natural sources: 3 mSv (300 mrem). Adapted with permission from National Council on Radiation Protection and Measurements: Limitation of exposure to ionizing radiation, Report No 116, Bethesda, MD, 1993.

Operator radiation exposure during interventional procedures is much higher than that for diagnostic angiography. Mikalason and colleagues surveyed interventional angiographers from 17 institutions and calculated a mean annual effective dose to the angiographer of 0.3 to 1 rem (3 to 10 mSv). Dash and colleagues found that d uring percutaneous angioplasty operator radiation exposure is nearly doubled compared to routine coronary angiography.

Radiation exposure to the patient undergoing cardiac catheterization is higher than that for any other type of radiologic examination but has been justified because the information gained is considered to be necessary for clinical management (Table 4-4). Repeated catheterizations, particularly in critically ill children, may give a very large radiation dose over a relatively short time span.

Table 4-4   Summary of mean radiation exposure during cardiac catheterization to patient and physician

	Mean dose (mrem)	
Site	Patient	Physician
ADULTS		
Eye	—	20
Thyroid	250	16
Chest	1100	500
Chest (inside apron)	—	50
Hand	—	10-30
Gonads	12	<10
Skin (direct beam)	25,000-50,000 (25-50 R)	
CHILDREN		
Eye	25	
Thyroid	430	
Chest	7500	
Abdomen	150	
Gonads	10	
COMPARISON EXPOSURES		
1-year cumulative background from natural sources	100	
Chest radiograph	10	
Upper gastrointestinal series	3000	
Lumbar spine series	3000	
Pulmonary angiography	15,000	
Chest fluoroscopy	1-2 rad/min	

Reprinted with permission of *American Journal of Cardiology* from Miller SW, Castronovo FP Jr: Radiation exposure and protection in cardiac catheterization laboratories, *AM J Cardiol* 55:171-176. Copyright 1985 by Excerpta Medica, Inc.

Radiation reduction involves the three classic parameters of time, shielding, and distance, and can be individually adapted by each laboratory to make the x-ray exposure to both the patient and the physicians as low as possible. The time an operator is exposed can be reduced in several ways. About half of the cardiac catheterization exposure occurs during fluoroscopy and the remainder during cineangiography. The fluoroscopy time can be considerably reduced by using short bursts of the fluoroscope rather than a prolonged, continuous exposure. In addition, by prolonging the time between catheterizations, the operator can lessen the amount of radiation received per unit of time. For example, Dash and colleagues have calculated that it is necessary to limit the number of coronary angioplasty procedures to five cases per week to meet the occupational exposure guidelines of 100 mrads/week. Nurses and technicians can be rotated to other duties so that they are not continuously present in the angiography room.

Additional local lead shielding should be considered to help limit scattered radiation. The smallest x-ray beam

possible will help to reduce the exposure rate of both the patient and the operator. Movable shields or drapes are available for most of the current angiographic units. Side drapes between the patient and the operator reduce scatter passing through the patient that would ordinarily be received by the operator. Cranial and caudal angulations considerably increase the x-ray tube output, the radiation received by the patient, and the secondary scatter received by the angiographer.

Because radiation decreases as the square of the distance, all personnel who are not needed in the room should be located elsewhere. For instance, the electrophysiologic data collection can be performed from a remote location rather than beside the fluoroscopy table. Those nurses and technicians staying in the room should remain as far as practical from the x-ray tube. The radiation physicist can monitor the radiation burden, evaluate the fluoroscopy techniques for each angiographer, and periodically measure the radiation output at various places in the room.

CORONARY ARTERY ANATOMY

Coronary angiography is performed in at least two projections because it is a projectional technique and atherosclerotic lesions are typically eccentric. The initial RAO and LAO angiograms project the coronary arteries away from the spine (Fig. 4-4). The stenoses are then defined and overlapping branches eliminated with compound views by adding cranial and caudal angulation.

Right Coronary Artery

The right coronary artery originates from the right sinus of Valsalva and continues in the right atrioventricular groove to the crux of the heart. Its ostium is usually in the upper two thirds of the sinus but may be ectopically located from slightly below the aortic valve leaflets in the left ventricle to a few centimeters superiorly in the ascending aorta. In bicuspid aortic valves in which the two sinuses of Valsalva are placed anteriorly and posteriorly, the right coronary artery may go anterior from the sinus as compared to the more common angulation of 30 degrees to the right of the sternum in patients with tricuspid aortic valves. The right coronary artery in the LAO view has a "C"-shape and is conveniently divided into proximal, middle, and distal segments (Fig. 4-5). The proximal right coronary segment lies beneath the right atrial appendage.

Sinoatrial nodal artery

The sinoatrial nodal artery branches from the proximal right coronary artery in roughly 50% of patients (Fig. 4-6). When it does not come from the right coronary

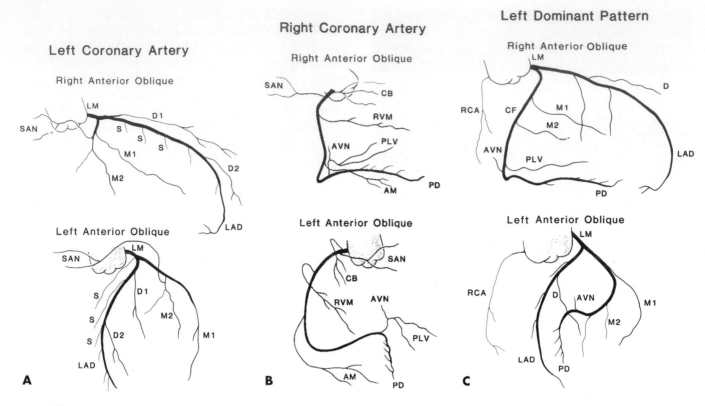

Fig. 4-4 Coronary arteries. *LM* = left main artery; *LAD* = left anterior descending artery; *D1, D2* = diagonal branches; *S* = septal branches; *M1, M2* = circumflex marginal branches; *SAN* = sinoatrial artery; *CF* = left circumflex artery; *PD* = posterior descending artery; *AVN* = atrioventricular node artery; *RCA* = right coronary artery; *CB* = conus branch; *RVM* = right ventricular marginal branch; *AM* = acute marginal branch; *PLV* = posterior left ventricular artery.

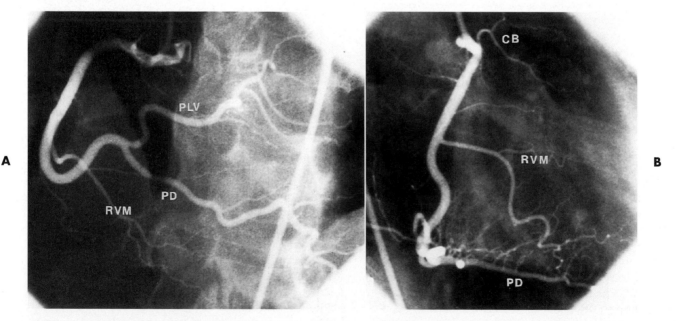

Fig. 4-5 The right coronary artery. **A,** Cranial LAO projection. **B,** RAO projection in a different patient. *CB* = conus branch; *RVM* = right ventricular marginal artery; *PD* = posterior descending artery; *PLV* = posterior left ventricular artery.

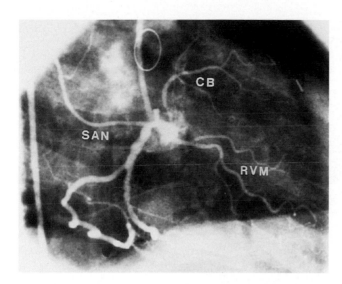

Fig. 4-6 Sinoatrial nodal artery. In the RAO projection the sino-atrial nodal artery goes posteriorly to the right atrium to wrap around the superior vena cava. *CB* = conus branch; *RVM* = right ventricular marginal artery; *SAN* = sinoatrial nodal artery.

artery, a longer atrial artery originates from the left circumflex artery and terminates in the same location by sending an anterior and posterior branch around the superior vena cava at the right atrial junction.

Conus artery

The conus artery is the first ventricular branch of the proximal right coronary artery. This artery has a separate origin from the sinus of Valsalva in about half of all angiograms (Fig. 4-7). The conus artery goes anteriorly around the right ventricular conus or infundibulum and frequently ends in three short branches that resemble a pitchfork. This artery is a common collateral channel to the left anterior descending artery and is then called the "circle of Vieussens." The conus artery may also go inferiorly over the right ventricular free wall to form a distal marginal branch. Other right ventricular branches from the middle and distal segments of the right coronary artery are called marginal branches. The acute marginal artery is a large right ventricular marginal artery near the bend in the artery between the middle and distal segments (the acute margin of the heart). Any right ventricular marginal branch may continue along the diaphragmatic wall of the right ventricle to become a short posterior descending artery (Fig. 4-8).

In about 3% of patients a small artery originates near the conus artery, which supplies the superior portion of the interventricular septum. The right superior septal perforator artery goes deeper into the myocardium than is usually the case with the conus artery and ends with several straight branches parallel to the interventricular septum (Fig. 4-9).

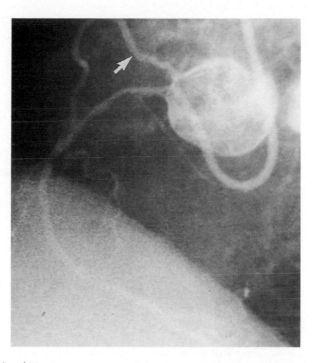

Fig. 4-7 Separate origin of the conus artery *(arrow)* from the right sinus of Valsalva is shown.

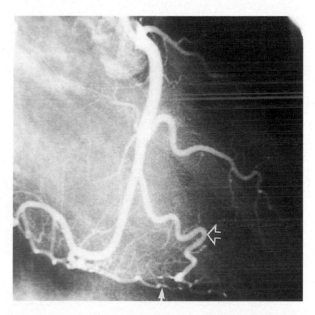

Fig. 4-8 The right coronary artery. In the right oblique projection the inferior septum is supplied by both the posterior descending artery *(arrow)* and the acute marginal branch *(open arrow)*.

Distal right coronary artery

The distal right coronary artery has so many variations that the naming of small branches is at times difficult. The distal right coronary artery typically ends by dividing into a posterior descending artery and a posterolateral left ventricular artery (Fig. 4-10). In about

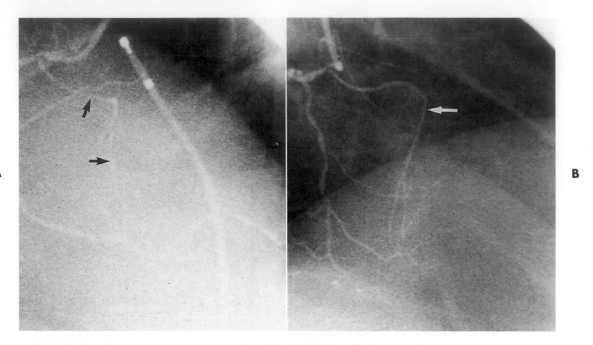

Fig. 4-9 Right superior septal perforator artery *(arrows).* **A,** LAO projection. **B,** RAO projection.

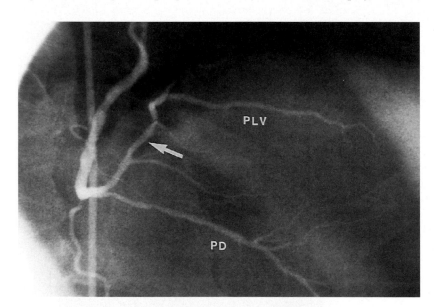

Fig. 4-10 Distal right coronary artery. The cranial right oblique projection spreads the posterior descending artery away from the posterior left ventricular artery, which is a continuation of the posterolateral left ventricular artery *(arrow). PD* = posterior descending artery; *PLV* = posterior left ventricular artery.

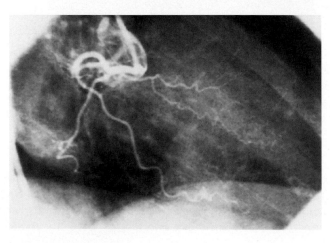

Fig. 4-11 Nondominant right coronary artery. Several vestigial right ventricular marginal branches supply the anterior wall of the right ventricle in this RAO projection.

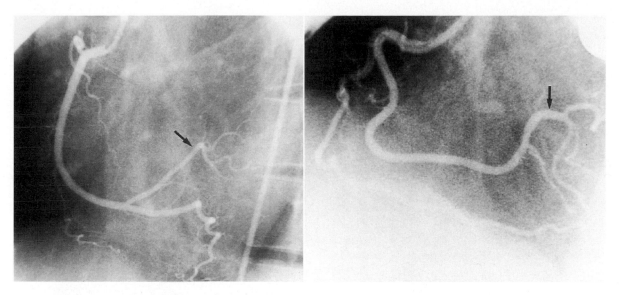

Fig. 4-12   Two variations of the U-bend *(arrow)* in the posterior left ventricular branch of the right coronary artery are shown.

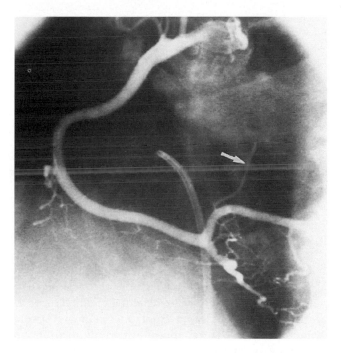

Fig. 4-13   Atrioventricular nodal artery. The U-bend of the posterior left ventricular artery is the origin of the atrioventricular nodal artery *(arrow)* as seen on this LAO view.

90% of people the right coronary artery ends in the posterior descending artery and is therefore named the "dominant" artery. When the left circumflex artery ends in the posterior descending artery, the right coronary artery is "nondominant" and the left circumflex artery is then the dominant blood supply inferiorly (Fig. 4-11). There are many variations in the vascular pattern of the inferior part of the ventricular septum. A codominant

pattern is when either a posterior descending artery originates from both the distal right coronary and the left circumflex arteries, or when the posterior descending artery comes from the right coronary artery and a long left circumflex artery supplies the posterior left ventricular wall. There may be one to five posterior descending arteries, some of which begin as either right ventricular marginal arteries or left circumflex marginal arteries. The posterolateral left ventricular artery lies in the distal atrioventricular groove and supplies several posterior left ventricular arteries over the posterolateral wall of the left ventricle. This segment frequently has a middle part that is shaped like an inverted "U"-bend at the crux of the heart (Fig. 4-12). The atrioventricular nodal artery originates near this "U"-bend and goes superiorly for about 1 cm to the region of the atrioventricular node (Fig. 4-13).

Left Coronary Artery

The left sinus of Valsalva is the origin of the left coronary artery. The left main artery does not taper and typically is about 1 cm long (Fig. 4-14). However, there may be no left main artery with the left anterior descending artery and left circumflex arteries originating separately from the left sinus. The left main coronary artery may trifurcate into a left anterior descending artery, an intermediate artery or ramus medianus (Fig. 4-15), and the left circumflex artery. The caudal LAO (also called the "spider" view because of the arachnoid shape of the proximal left coronary artery) puts the left main and proximal circumflex arteries in the plane of the film, but it foreshortens the left anterior descending artery (Fig. 4-16).

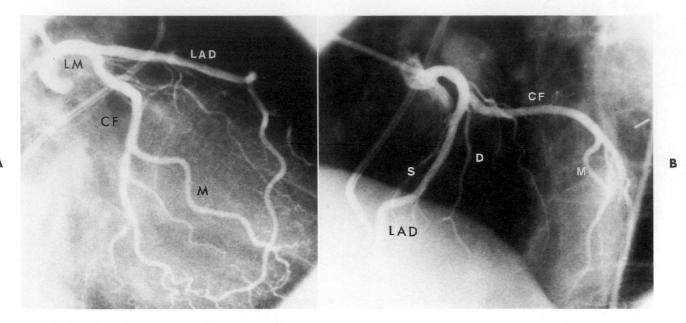

Fig. 4-14   Left main coronary artery. **A,** Caudal RAO projection. **B,** Cranial LAO projection. Abbreviations as in Figure 4-4.

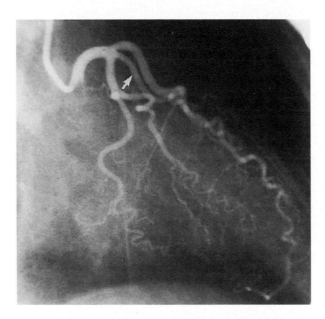

Fig. 4-15   Intermediate artery *(arrow)* between the left anterior descending and the left circumflex arteries is shown.

Left circumflex artery

The left circumflex artery lies in the left atrioventricular groove and may exist only as a vestigial twig or may be so long that it ends by becoming the left posterior descending artery (Fig. 4-17). Its major branches are called left circumflex marginal arteries and are numbered first, second, and so on. Because the inferior and left side of the heart is the obtuse border, marginal branches in this location may be called obtuse marginal arteries (Fig. 4-18). Late filming of a left coronary artery

injection shows the coronary veins. The great cardiac vein, which becomes the coronary sinus, is in the left atrioventricular groove and serves as a landmark for the left circumflex artery.

Left anterior descending artery

The left anterior descending artery lies in the interventricular groove and supplies two distinctive types of branches, septal and epicardial (Fig. 4-19). Septal branches go to the interventricular septum, usually along the right ventricular side of the septum, and originate from the left anterior descending artery in a nearly perpendicular direction. The septal branches may themselves have branches, and commonly the first septal branch may have a broomlike appearance. Epicardial branches over the anterolateral wall are called diagonal arteries and they number from one to many. Several characteristics of the left anterior descending artery are unique and help to identify this artery on a coronary angiogram. The anterior descending artery is usually the longest branch of the left coronary artery and it ends at the cardiac apex or occasionally continues to supply most of the inferior septum. The termination characteristically looks like an inverted "Y" (Fig. 4-20). Unlike other branches of the left coronary artery, the left anterior descending artery has numerous septal branches throughout its length (Fig. 4-21). A rare septal branch may come from the left main, a diagonal, or a circumflex marginal artery proximally. There is little motion of the left anterior descending artery in contrast to the 1-cm excursion of the left circumflex artery adjacent to the left atrium.

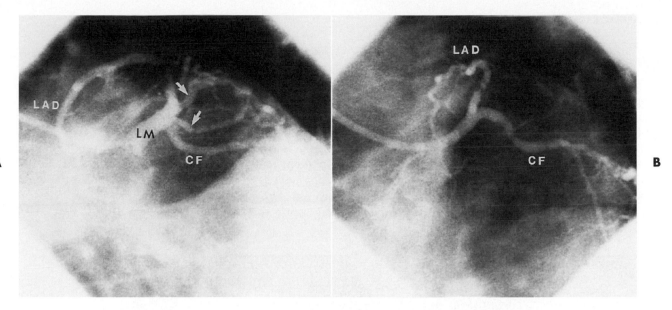

Fig. 4-16 "Spider" projection. **A,** The caudal LAO projection separates the left anterior descending artery from two ramus branches *(arrows)* and the left circumflex artery. **B,** A severe stenosis is present in the left anterior descending artery. *LM* = left main coronary artery; *LAD* = left anterior descending artery; *CF* = left circumflex artery.

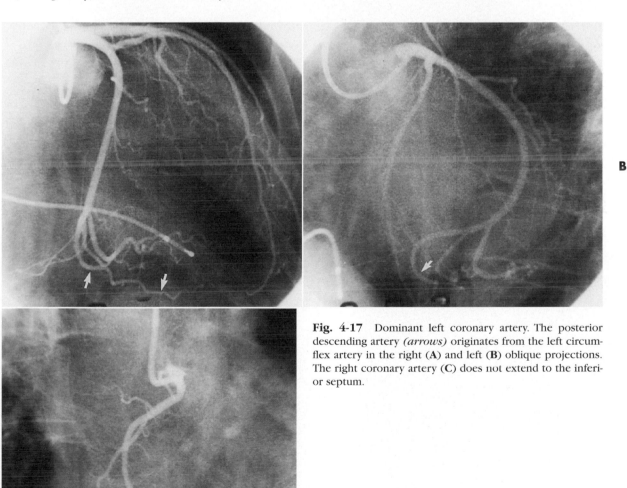

Fig. 4-17 Dominant left coronary artery. The posterior descending artery *(arrows)* originates from the left circumflex artery in the right (**A**) and left (**B**) oblique projections. The right coronary artery (**C**) does not extend to the inferior septum.

Cardiac Veins

Identification of the cardiac veins is useful in angiography because they mark the atrioventricular and interventricular boundaries of the chambers. Occasionally they demonstrate anomalies such as persistent left superior vena cava terminating in the coronary sinus, absence of the coronary sinus, or anomalous pulmonary venous connection to the coronary sinus. Veins are distinguished from coronary arteries because the veins opacify several seconds after arterial injection, have less opacification than the corresponding adjacent arteries, are generally larger than the adjacent arteries, and drain into the coronary sinus or a cardiac chamber.

The coronary sinus begins at its opening into the right atrium with its Thebesian valve and extends along the left atrioventricular sulcus to the bifurcation with the oblique vein of Marshall. In a normal heart this latter vein is obliterated, but when it remains patent it continues as a left superior vena cava. The continuation of the coronary sinus beyond this vein of Marshall is the great cardiac vein. This vein extends beneath the left atrial

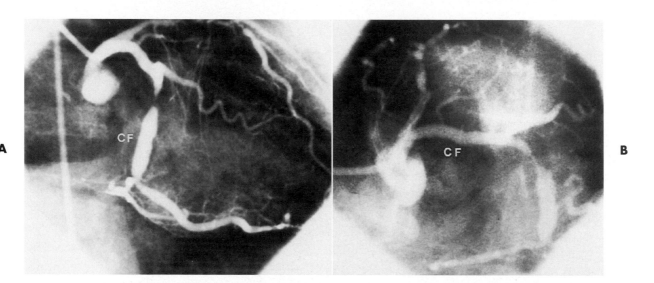

Fig. 4-18 Arteritis in the left circumflex artery. **A,** Caudal RAO view shows a stenosis proximal to a segmental ectasia in a left dominant circumflex artery. **B,** Spider view. *CF* = left circumflex artery.

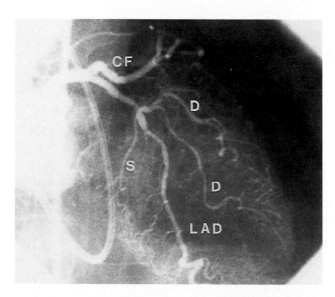

Fig. 4-19 Left anterior descending artery. Cranial RAO view projects the left circumflex artery over the left anterior descending artery. This compound view separates the diagonal arteries from the septal branches. Abbreviations as in Figure 4-4.

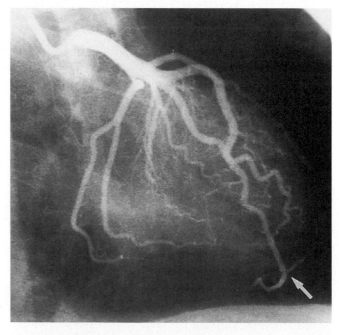

Fig. 4-20 Typical Y-shaped termination of the left anterior descending artery *(arrow)* is shown.

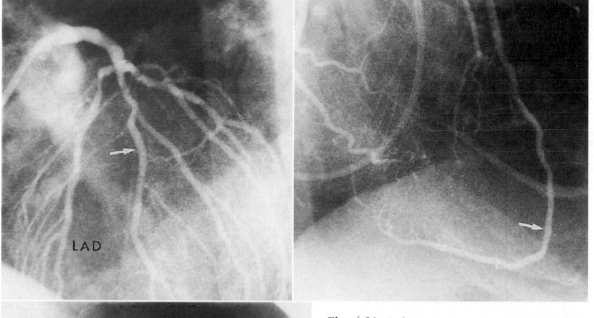

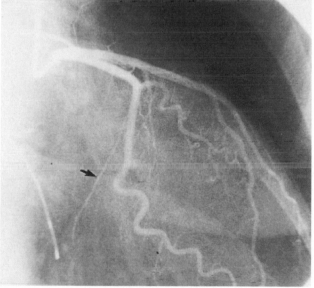

Fig. 4-21 Left coronary artery variations. **A,** LAO view shows trifurcation of the left main artery into the left anterior descending, intermediate, and circumflex arteries. There are two septal branches arising from the intermediate artery *(arrow)*. *LAD* = left anterior descending artery. **B,** The left anterior descending artery *(arrow)* in the RAO view goes around the apex to supply the entire inferior septum. **C,** The left circumflex artery gives off two marginal branches, then continues as a vestigial vessel *(arrow)* in the atrioventricular groove.

appendage and becomes the anterior interventricular vein beside the left anterior descending artery.

The left ventricle has veins that lie roughly beside the major arteries (Fig 4-22). The anterior interventricular vein lies adjacent to the left anterior descending artery; it extends superiorly from the apex to pass beneath the left atrial appendage and joins the great cardiac vein beside the left circumflex artery.

The posterior interventricular vein, also called the middle cardiac vein, runs beside the posterior descending artery from the apex to the crux and either drains into the coronary sinus or separately enters the right atrium.

The small cardiac vein lies in the right atrioventricular sulcus beside the distal right coronary artery and drains into the posterior interventricular vein, the coronary sinus, or directly into the right atrium. Right atrial veins are rarely seen during injection into the right coronary artery, but they may be visible if the catheter is obturated and the injection is made under pressure.

CARDIAC CHAMBERS

Each of the four cardiac chambers has distinctive features that aid in its identification in all but the most primitive hearts (Box 4-3).

Right Atrium

The right atrium has an appendage that is larger than the left atrial appendage and has a broad-based connec-

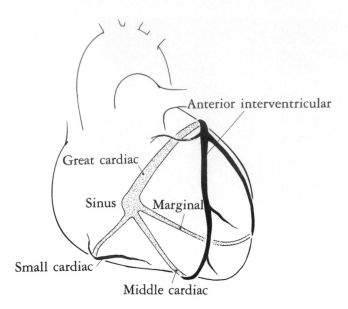

Fig. 4-22 Cardiac veins connecting to the coronary sinus are shown.

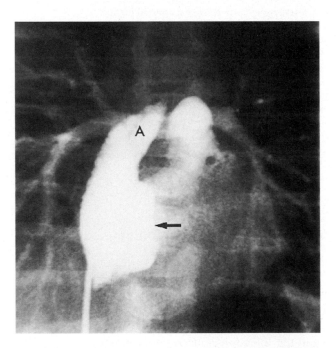

Fig. 4-23 The right atrium. The wide atrial appendage (*A*) projects over the right pulmonary artery. The tricuspid valve *(arrow)* is closed.

Box 4-3   Angiographic Characteristics of the Cardiac Chambers*

RIGHT ATRIUM

Connects with the inferior vena cava
Has an appendage with a broad opening
Receives thebesian veins
Has a roughly cylindrical shape except for the
    inflow region of the tricuspid valve
Crista terminalis and pectinate muscles
Lies on the same side as the trilobed lung and liver,
    and on the opposite side of the stomach
(Connects with the superior vena cava)
(Connects with the coronary sinus)

LEFT ATRIUM

Has an ellipsoidal shape
Lies in the midline or slightly to the side of the
    bilobed lung
Has a smooth wall except for the appendage
Has a slender appendage with a narrow opening
(Connects with the pulmonary veins)

RIGHT VENTRICLE

Has a triangular shape on the posteroanterior view
    and a crescentic shape on the lateral view
Coarse, deep trabeculations, including the septum
Conus (crista supraventricularis) between the tricus-
    pid and pulmonary valves
Tricuspid atrioventricular valve
Occasionally a well-defined septal papillary muscle
    (moderator band)

LEFT VENTRICLE

Has an oval shape in diastole in most projections
Fine, shallow trabeculations
Mitral-aortic continuity (absence of a subaortic
    conus)
Bicuspid atrioventricular valve
Absence of septal papillary muscles; smooth septal
    surface
(Usually two well-defined papillary muscles on the
    free wall)

*These features are usually found in normal hearts. Those in parentheses may be lacking if congenital anomalies are present. Some characteristics need modification if congenital heart disease is present; for examples, in transposition of the great vessels, there is mitral-pulmonary continuity in the left ventricle.

tion to the main chamber (Fig. 4-23). The inflow structures of the right atrium are the inferior vena cava, the superior vena cava, and the coronary sinus. The internal structures are difficult to identify angiographically, but MRI usually shows the fossa ovalis, crista terminalis, and the pectinate muscles.

Right Ventricle

The right ventricle has a complex shape consisting of a triangular body and a cylindrical outflow tract. Its three parts are the inflow segment, the body, and the outflow segment (Fig. 4-24). The inflow region is the tricuspid valve and its apparatus including the papillary muscles. The anterior, posterior, and septal leaflets of the tricuspid valve are easily identified on an echocardiogram and frequently can be separately distinguished during angiography and MRI. Compared to the left ventricle, the right ventricle has larger trabeculations that extend onto the septum. The moderator band usually is the largest trabeculation near the septum. The walls of the right ventricle are named according to their location: anteroseptal, apical, and diaphragmatic in the RAO view, and septal and anterior in the LAO view. The outflow tract of the right ventricle is the infundibulum or conus and is cylindrical (Fig. 4-25). The pulmonary valve is separated from the tricuspid valve by the infundibulum—a landmark difference from the left ventricle in which the aortic and mitral annuli join poste-

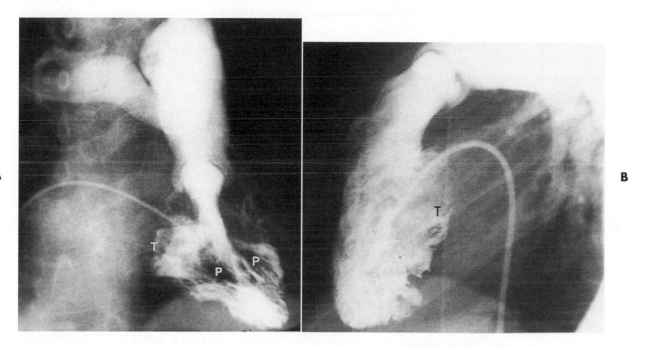

Fig. 4-24 The right ventricle. **A,** RAO cranial projection. **B,** Lateral projection. Systolic images of valvular pulmonic stenosis show a domed pulmonic valve and poststenotic dilatation of the main and left pulmonary arteries. *T* = tricuspid valve; *P* = papillary muscles.

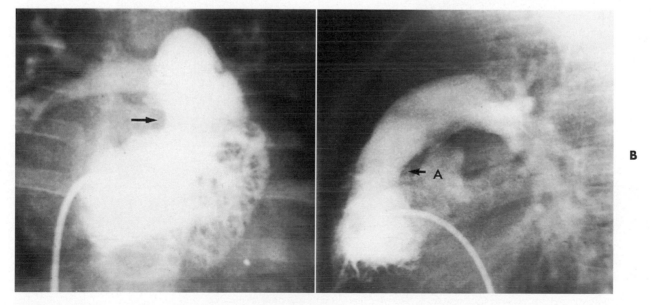

Fig. 4-25 The right ventricular infundibulum. The parietal band *(arrow)* is the muscle medial **(A)** and posterior **(B)** to the right ventricular outflow tract. Faint opacification of the left ventricle in the lateral projection occurred through a ventricular septal defect *(arrow). A* = aorta.

riorly. This conal segment has normal contractions and may narrow considerably in systole in right ventricular hypertrophy.

Left Atrium

The left atrium is behind and to the left of the right atrium. The pulmonary veins connect with this chamber either as four individual vessels or, occasionally, the superior and inferior pulmonary veins on each side have joined before connecting to the heart. The body of the

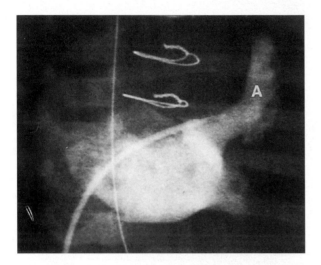

Fig. 4-26 The left atrium. The catheter enters the left atrium across a patent foramen ovale. The appendage (A) is narrow and unusually long.

left atrium has no trabeculations, but the interior of the left atrial appendage may be finely striated. In contrast to the right atrium, the left atrial appendage has a narrow neck and normally contains less volume (Fig. 4-26).

Left Ventricle

The left ventricle has an oval shape and finer trabeculations than the right ventricle (Fig. 4-27). The mitral valve (considered part of the left ventricle) consists of anterior and posterior leaflets. The anterior or septal leaflet covers about one third of the mitral circumference and has a smoothly rounded border. The posterior leaflet typically has several scallops and covers two thirds of the mitral circumference. The chordae occasionally can be seen as thin lucencies on a left ventriculogram. The papillary muscles may have single or multiple heads and connect about one half of the distance between the base and the apex of the left ventricle. Because the papillary muscles look like filling defects on the left ventriculogram, they occasionally are confused with thrombus. However, the papillary muscles contract during systole as the adjacent wall also contracts, a criterion that distinguishes thrombus or tumor from papillary muscles. A major landmark of the left ventricle is the continuity of the mitral and aortic valves. Unlike the right ventricle, there is no muscle between the aortic and mitral valves.

The walls of the left ventricle are arbitrarily divided into five segments in the RAO projection and into four segments in the LAO view (Fig. 4-28). The septum and the

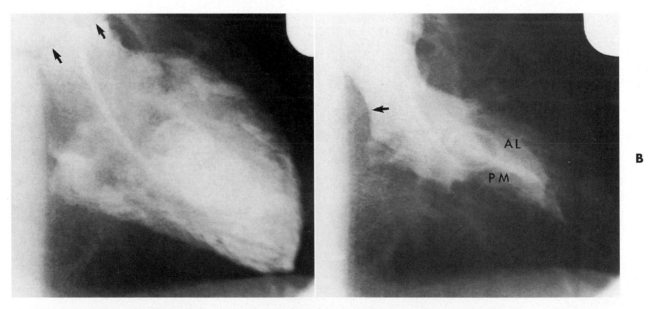

Fig. 4-27 The left ventricle in diastole and systole. **A,** The 30-degree RAO projection in diastole demonstrates the closed aortic valve *(arrows)* and the inflow of unopacified blood through the open mitral valve. **B,** In systole the mitral valve is closed *(arrow).* The anterolateral *(AL)* and posteromedial *(PM)* papillary muscles are larger and nearly touch.

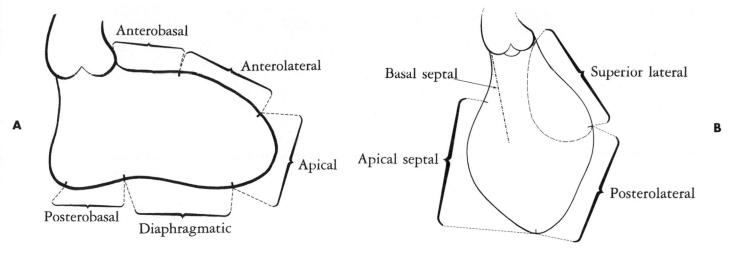

Fig. 4-28   Left ventricular wall segments. **A,** RAO view. **B,** LAO view.

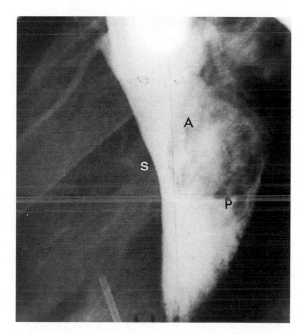

Fig. 4-29   The left ventricle in the cranial LAO projection. The interventricular septum (*S*) is abnormally bowed toward the left ventricle because an atrial septal defect has caused right ventricular enlargement. This diastolic frame shows the open anterior (*A*) and posterior (*P*) leaflets of the mitral valve.

anterior leaflet of the mitral valve are better seen if cranial angulation is added in the LAO projection (Fig. 4-29).

CARDIAC VALVES

Tricuspid Valve

The tricuspid valve (occasionally the normal tricuspid valve has only two cusps) is considered part of the right ventricle and consists of three leaflets: septal, pos-

terior, and anterior. The septal leaflet is the smallest and is attached through small chordae to the septum. Because this leaflet is being derived from endocardial cushion tissue, it is malformed when endocardial cushion tissue is deficient. The anterior and posterior leaflets are attached to the anterior and posterior walls, respectively. On frontal projections these leaflets form the medial boundary of the right ventricle during systole, but they are usually invisible in diastole except for occasional segments, which appear as thin, lucent streaks. The chordal attachments of the tricuspid leaflets insert into several papillary muscles on both the septal surface and the free wall.

Mitral Valve

The mitral apparatus consists of five related structures (Fig. 4-30): (1) the leaflets; (2) the chordae tendineae; (3) the annulus; (4) the papillary muscles; and (5) the left ventricular wall. Disorders in any of these structures may result in dysfunction of the valve. Furthermore, abnormalities in the left ventricular wall adjacent to the papillary muscles, such as infarct or aneurysm, may also cause mitral regurgitation.

The mitral annulus serves as a fulcrum for the leaflets. The muscle adjacent to the fibrous portion of the mitral annulus causes this region to contract during systole. In disease states that lead to left ventricular enlargement, the mitral annulus can dilate proportionately. Radiographically, this structure when calcified serves as a marker for the adjacent left circumflex artery and the coronary sinus. The plane of the attachment of the mitral leaflets to the annulus is the posterior extent of the leaflets during systole; leaflet motion beyond this plane is abnormal and is encountered in the prolapsing mitral leaflet syndrome.

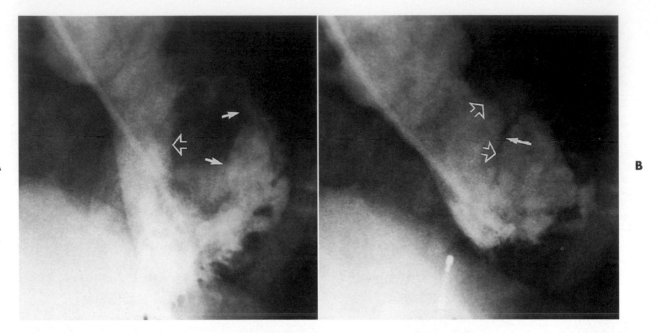

Fig. 4-30   The mitral valve in diastole (**A**) and systole (**B**) in the LAO projection. The anterior leaflet (*open arrows*) is adjacent to the septum and aortic valve. The posterior leaflet (*solid arrows*) lies beside the superolateral left ventricle.

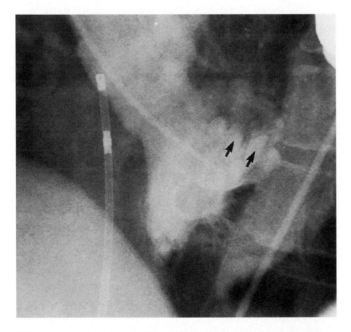

Fig. 4-31   Multiple small scallops *(arrows)* of the posterior mitral leaflet, which are slightly prolapsed into the left atrium, are shown.

The posterior left atrial wall continues as the posterior leaflet of the mitral valve. In severe dilatation of the left atrium the posterior wall of the atrium may pull the posterior mitral leaflet superiorly, contributing in a small way to mitral regurgitation.

The anterior mitral leaflet subtends about one third of the circumference of the mitral ring and is adjacent mainly to the posterior and left aortic cusps. The anteri-

or leaflet has a longer base-to-margin length compared with the posterior leaflet, but the surface area of both leaflets is equal. The anterior leaflet is identified on the left ventriculogram as the posterior straight line of contrast material extending inferiorly from the aortic valve. The posterior mitral leaflet has three and occasionally up to five scalloped segments. When three segments are present, they are the middle, posteromedial, and anterolateral segments, and they correspond to the adjacent left ventricular papillary muscles. In the RAO view the mitral leaflets are well defined in systole when the valve is closed but are normally not seen in diastole. The reverse happens in the LAO projection in which the mitral leaflets are seen mainly in diastole.

The chordae tendineae extend from the heads of the anterolateral and posteromedial papillary muscles, branch into several divisions, and then insert both onto the leaflets and into the subjacent left ventricular endocardium. The chordae from one papillary muscle extend to both mitral leaflets so that a rupture of the papillary muscle leads to severe instability in both valve leaflets during systole. Chordae originating from a papillary muscle typically split into three smaller chords before inserting into the leaflet (however, the division is inconstant). The clinical significance of this split is that rupture of a single chorda usually has no effect on mitral valve competency, and rupture of several chordae may produce only mild mitral regurgitation. Chordae are usually not seen on a normal left ventriculogram, but they may become visible if thickened because of a rheumatic process or if stretched and elongated as in the prolapsing mitral leaflet syndrome (Fig. 4-31).

Normally the papillary muscles contract before the adjacent left ventricular wall does, which brings the leaflets back into position for the ensuing rise in the left ventricular systolic pressure. When this sequence is altered, for example during a premature ventricular con-

traction, the mitral valve becomes slightly incompetent. In systole, as the left ventricular apex moves toward the base of the heart, the papillary muscles tense and counterbalance the shortened distance between the chordal insertions and the mitral leaflets, thus preventing regurgitation. In the papillary muscle dysfunction syndrome, the area around a papillary muscle is infarcted or ischemic, which prevents contracting of this muscle. Mitral regurgitation then ensues and the leaflets can occasionally be seen prolapsing into the left atrium.

Pulmonary Valve

The sinuses and cusps of the pulmonary valve are designated as anterior, left, and right. The cusps of the pulmonary valve are visible on an angiogram during diastole; however, during the ejection phase the leaflets are very thin and are positioned against the main pulmonary artery such that they are usually not visible (Fig. 4-32). The attachments of the pulmonary cusps serve as an important landmark for identifying the upper portion of the right ventricular conus. On a lateral projection (Fig. 4-33) the angle of the blood flow through the pulmonary valve follows a vertical line roughly parallel to the sternum. In pathologic conditions such as tetralogy of Fallot the angle of blood flow becomes more horizontal. The practical implication is that in a normally formed heart the pulmonary valve is roughly in tangent in the posteroanterior view, but in the patient with tetralogy of Fallot a steep cranial angulation is necessary to profile the valve.

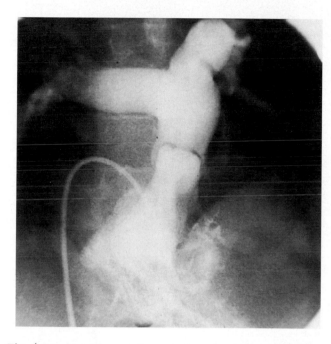

Fig. 4-32 Cranial angulation puts the pulmonary annulus in tangent and elongates the outflow region from the infundibulum to the left pulmonary artery. The pulmonary valve is stenotic.

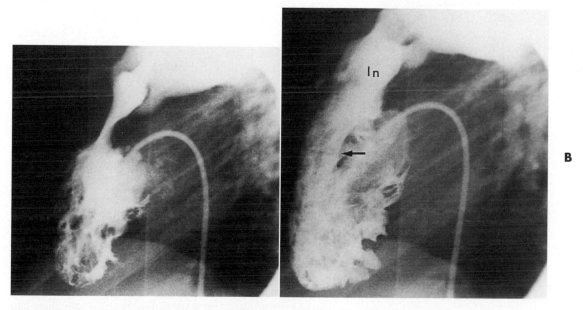

A

B

Fig. 4-33 The pulmonary and tricuspid valves in the lateral projection. **A,** In systole the pulmonary valve is domed with a jet through it, indicating stenosis. **B,** The infundibulum (*In*) is larger in diastole so that a dynamic subvalvular infundibular stenosis is present. Note the anterior leaflet of the tricuspid valve (*arrow*).

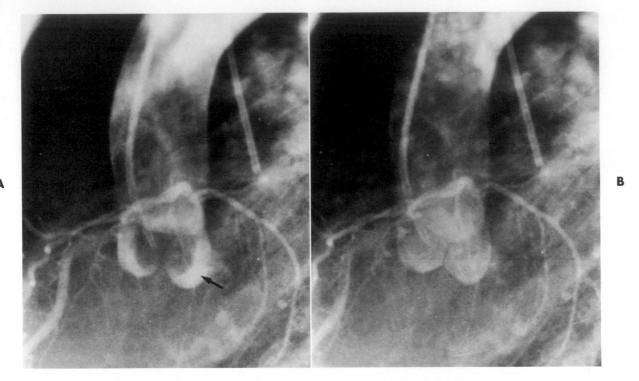

Fig. 4-34 Aortic valve in diastole (**A**) and systole (**B**) in the lateral projection. The *arrow* indicates the noncoronary sinus. The left coronary artery originates superiorly from the left sinus, and the right coronary artery originates anteriorly from the right sinus.

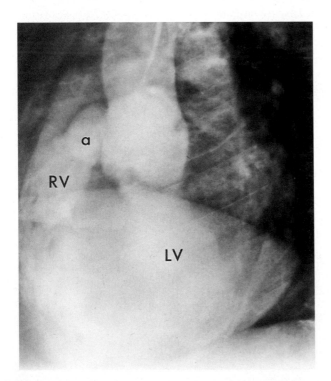

Fig 4-35 Rupture of the right sinus of Valsalva into the right ventricle. An aortic root abscess (*a*), which caused aortic regurgitation into the left ventricle (*LV*), later eroded into the right ventricle (*RV*).

Aortic Valve

The aortic sinuses of Valsalva and their cusps are named the right, left, and posterior or noncoronary (Fig. 4-34). The sinuses of Valsalva extend to the sinotubular ridge, which marks their junction with the aorta. The coronary arteries usually originate in their respective sinuses about two thirds of the distance superiorly between the aortic valve and the sinotubular ridge. The posterior sinus is next to the atrial septum so that a rupture of this sinus could extend into either atrium. The right sinus of Valsalva is adjacent to the right atrium and the right ventricle (Fig. 4-35), and the left sinus of Valsalva is next to the left atrium and the left ventricle. On the lateral projection of an ascending thoracic aortogram, the plane of the aortic valve is tilted so that the caudal extension of a line perpendicular to this plane goes posteriorly. When the aorta is "untucked," which occurs in truncus arteriosus and in transposition of the great vessels, a line perpendicular to the plane of the aorta is more anterior (Fig. 4-36). Like the pulmonary valve leaflets, the aortic leaflets are difficult to see during systole, but during diastole they mark the boundary of the left ventricle and the sinuses of Valsalva. The leaflets may occasionally flutter in a person with a high cardiac output or in an elderly patient, possibly related to turbulence immediately beyond the cuspal attachments.

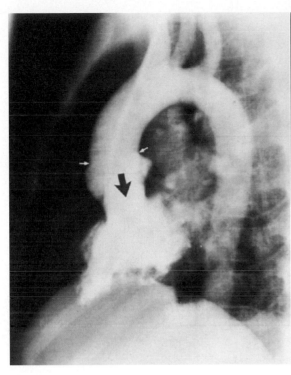

A

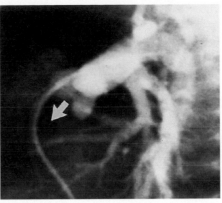

B

Fig 4-36   The tilt of the aortic root. **A,** Normally a line *(large arrow)* through the plane of the sinotubular ridge *(small arrows)* points posteriorly. **B,** In truncus arteriosus in which both the aorta and the pulmonary arteries originate from the truncal valve, a line *(arrow)* through the "untucked" valve points anteriorly.

SUGGESTED READINGS

Books

Grossman W, Baim DS: *Cardiac catheterization, angiography and intervention,* Philadelphia, 1991, Lea & Febiger.

Mettler FA Jr, Upton AC: *Medical effects of ionizing radiation,* Philadelphia, 1995, WB Saunders.

Miller SW: *Cardiac angiography,* Boston, 1984, Little, Brown.

Journals

Amplatz K, Formanek G, Stanger P, Wilson W: Mechanics of selective coronary artery catheterization via femoral approach, *Radiology* 89:1040, 1967.

Basic radiation protection criteria, National Council on Radiation Protection and Measurements, Rep No 60, Washington, DC, 1991.

Bristow WJD, Burchell HB, Campbell RW et al: Report of the Ad Hoc Committee on the indications for coronary arteriography, *Circulation* 55:969A, 1977.

Cousin AJ, Lawdahl RB, Chakraborty DP, Koehler RE: The case for radioprotective eyewear/facewear: practical implications and suggestions, *Invest Radiol* 22:688-692, 1987.

Dash H, Leaman DM: Operator radiation exposure during per cutaneous transluminal coronary angioplasty, *J Am Coll Cardiol* 4:725-728, 1984.

Davis K, Kennedy JW, Kemp HG et al: Complications of coronary arteriography from the collaborative study of coronary artery surgery (CASS), *Circulation* 59:1105, 1979.

Edwards M: Development of radiation protection standards, *Radiographics* 11:699-712, 1991.

Elliott LP, Bargeron LM, Soto B et al: Axial cineangiography in congenital heart disease, *Radiol Clin North Am* 18:515, 1980.

Gertz EW, Wisneski JA, Gould RG et al: Improved radiation protection for physicians performing cardiac catheterization, *Am J Cardiol* 50:1283, 1982.

Johnson W et al: Coronary angiography 1984-1987: a report of the Registry of the Society for Cardiac Angiography and Interventions. I. Results and complications, *Cathet Cardiovasc Diagn* 17:5, 1989.

Judkins MP: Selective coronary arteriography, a percutaneous transfemoral technique, *Radiology* 89:815, 1967.

Kohn HI, Fry RJM: Radiation carcinogenesis, *N Engl J Med* 310:504-511, 1984.

Lozner E et al: Coronary arteriography 1984-1987: a report of the Registry of the Society for Cardiac Angiography and Interventions. 2. An analysis of 218 deaths related to coronary angiography, *Cathet Cardiovasc Diagn* 17:11, 1989.

Miller RA, Warkentin DL, Felix WG et al: Angulated views in coronary angiography, *AJR Am J Roentgenol* 134:407, 1980.

Miller SW, Castronovo FP: Radiation exposure and protection in cardiac catheterization laboratories, *Am J Cardiol* 55:171-176, 1985.

Niklason LT, Marx MV, Chan HP: Interventional radiologists: occupational radiation doses and risks, *Radiology* 187:729-733, 1993.

Pattee PL, Johns PC, Chambers RJ: Radiation risk to patients from percutaneous transluminal coronary angioplasty, *J Am Coll Cardiol* 22:1044-1051, 1993.

Perloff JK, Roberts WC: The mitral apparatus. Functional anatomy of mitral regurgitation, *Circulation* 46:227, 1972.

Richman AH, Chan B, Katz M: Effectiveness of lead lenses in reducing radiation exposure, *Radiology* 121:357, 1976.

Roberts WC, Cohen LS: Left ventricular papillary muscles. Description of the normal and a survey of conditions causing them to be abnormal, *Circulation* 46:138, 1972.

Roberts WC, Perloff JK: Mitral valvular disease. A clinicopathologic survey of the conditions causing the mitral valve to function abnormally, *Ann Intern Med* 77:939, 1972.

Ross J, Brandenberg RO, Dinsmore RE et al: Guidelines for coronary angiography: a report of the American College of Cardiology/American Heart Association Task Force on assessment of diagnostic and therapeutic cardiovascular procedures, *J Am Coll Cardiol* 10(4):935-950, 1987.

Rueter FG: Physician and patient exposure during cardiac catheterization, *Circulation* 58:134, 1978.

Waldman JD, Rummerfield PS, Gilpin EA et al: Radiation exposure to the child during cardiac catheterization, *Circulation* 64:158, 1981.

Webster EW. On the question of cancer induction by small x-ray doses, *AJR Am J Roentgenol* 137:647, 1981.

Wholey MH: Clinical dosimetry during the angiographic examination: Comments on coronary arteriography, *Circulation* 50:627, 1974.

Wold GJ, Schelle RB, Agarwal SK: Evaluation of physician exposure during cardiac catheterization, *Radiology* 99:188, 1971.

Wyman RM, Safian RD, Portway V et al: Current complications of diagnostic and therapeutic cardiac catheterization, *J Am Coll Cardiol* 12:1400, 1988.

SPECIFIC DISEASES

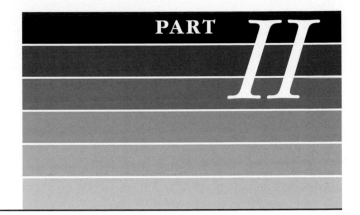

PART

II

CHAPTER 5

Valvular Heart Disease

Valvular Aortic Stenosis
  Chest film findings
  Imaging features
  Congenital valvular aortic stenosis
  Acquired valvular aortic stenosis
Subvalvular Aortic Stenosis
  Pathologic abnormalities
  Angiographic findings
  Unusual subaortic obstruction
Supravalvular Aortic Stenosis
  Classifications
  Associated lesions
Aortic Regurgitation
  Chest film findings
  Angiographic technique
  MRI technique
  Imaging findings
  Specific causes of aortic regurgitation
  Prosthetic aortic valves
Mitral Stenosis
  Chest film findings
  Imaging approach to mitral stenosis
  Rheumatic mitral stenosis
  Congenital abnormalities causing left ventricular inflow obstruction
    Cor triatriatum
    Congenital mitral stenosis—hypoplastic left heart syndrome
Mitral Regurgitation
  Chest film findings
  Angiographic evaluation
  Rheumatic mitral regurgitation
  Mitral valve prolapse
  Chordal rupture
  Papillary muscle rupture
  Papillary muscle dysfunction
  Imaging complications of mitral valve replacement
Pulmonary Stenosis and Regurgitation
  Chest film findings

  Valvular pulmonary stenosis
  Subvalvular pulmonary stenosis
  Supravalvular pulmonary stenosis
  Pulmonary regurgitation
Tricuspid Valve Disease
  Tricuspid stenosis
  Tricuspid regurgitation
  Ebstein anomaly
  Other imaging findings
Suggested Readings

Cardiac imaging in suspected valvular disease determines the involvement of the valves, the extent of the stenosis or regurgitation, and the hemodynamic consequence of the pressure or volume overload on the heart. It also evaluates associated conditions, such as aortic dissection or aneurysm, and ventricular contractility and enlargement.

The chest film serves not only as the initial imaging examination to detect valvular disease but also is the main procedure to visualize any complications such as pulmonary edema and cardiac or aortic dilatation. Imaging the heart chambers with echocardiography, magnetic resonance imaging (MRI), or angiography then follows. Noninvasive Doppler techniques or invasive measurements by catheter allow quantitative hemodynamic evaluations.

See Figure 5-1 for anatomic positions of the heart valves.

VALVULAR AORTIC STENOSIS

As with any valvular stenosis, aortic stenosis can exist at the valvular, subvalvular, or supravalvular level (Box 5-1).

A number of features of aortic stenosis at the valvular level are common to several types of pathologic condi-

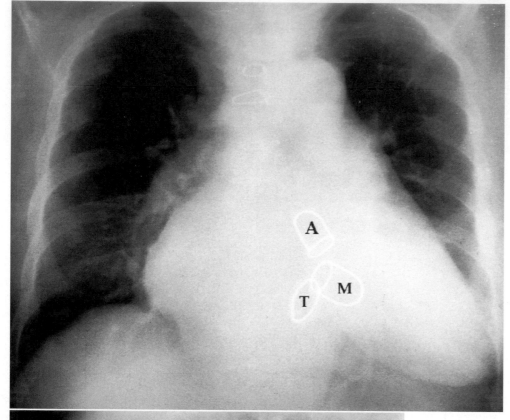

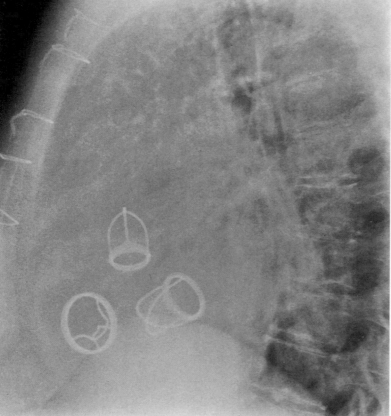

Fig. 5-1 Anatomic position of the heart valves. **A,** Frontal projections of aortic (*A*), mitral (*M*), and tricuspid (*T*) prosthetic valves demonstrate that these three valves frequently overlap one another. **B,** The lateral projection identifies the tricuspid valve as anterior to the mitral valve. The direction of blood flow through the prosthetic valves as indicated by the ball or disk is another marker to identify each valve.

tions; these differ only in the age of the patient and in the degree of severity. The signs include:

• Calcification of the leaflets
• Thickened leaflets
• Decreased amplitude of excursion
• Leaflet deformity and doming
• A narrow orifice marked by a jet of contrast media or blood through it
• Poststenotic dilatation of the ascending aorta
• Left ventricular abnormalities, namely, hypertrophy

Chest Film Findings

The chest film abnormalities depend on the age of the patient as well as the severity of the stenosis. In infancy, pulmonary edema with generalized cardiomegaly is the typical appearance of obstruction to blood flow at any point between the pulmonary veins, left heart, and aorta (Fig. 5-2). The adult heart has normal size and the lungs are clear because left ventricular failure and dilatation occur only in terminally ill patients (Fig. 5-3). Calcification in the aortic valve over age 40 years occurs in all types of aortic stenosis and clinically marks the stenosis as severe. Dilatation of the ascending aorta is frequent in aortic stenosis but correlates rather poorly with severity or with the site of the stenosis (one third of patients with subvalvular aortic stenosis have dilated aortas).

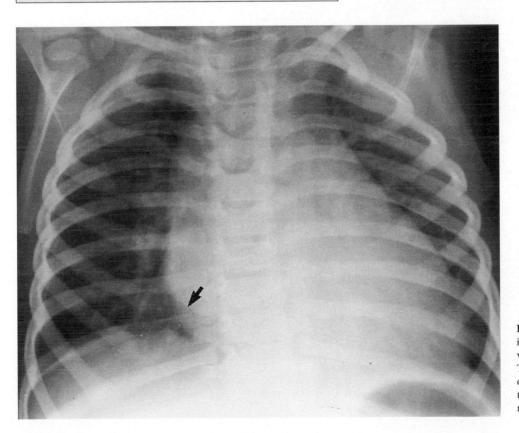

Fig. 5-2 Aortic stenosis in the infant. The heart is globally enlarged with leftward dilatation of the apex. The large left atrium has a double density *(arrow)* which projects into the lung. The pulmonary hila have mild edema.

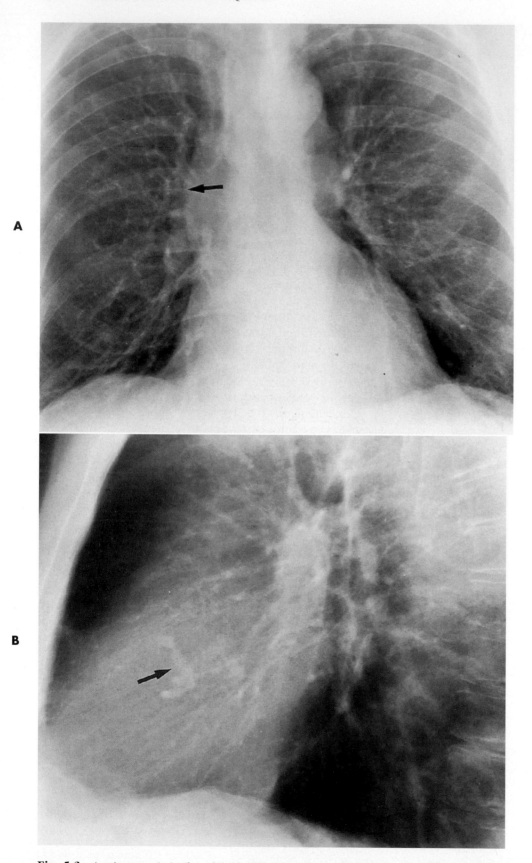

Fig. 5-3   Aortic stenosis in the adult. **A,** The heart size is normal and the lungs are clear. The ascending aorta *(arrow)* is mildly dilated. **B,** The aortic valve *(arrow)* is irregularly calcified.

Imaging Features

Leaflet motion, as seen during angiography, will be abnormal if there is deformity, fibrosis, or calcification. The mildest form of abnormal motion is often visible during left ventriculography for mitral stenosis; the aortic leaflets appear thickened, signifying involvement with rheumatic process, but there is no aortic pressure gradient. A slow opening and closing of the leaflets, and rarely, even doming, may be visible in the absence of an aortic gradient. In general, complete visibility of the leaflets in systole indicates an abnormality because normal leaflets, if visible, are less than 1 mm in width.

A narrow orifice to the aortic valve is visible either as a jet through the valve on a left ventriculogram or as a negative effect during supravalvular aortography. You can roughly estimate the degree of aortic stenosis by comparing the width of the jet with the diameter of the aortic annulus. When the jet is less than 15% of the diameter of the annulus there is severe aortic stenosis. However, it may also be present when the width of the column of blood through the valve appears to be the same size as the annulus. This latter finding is typical of calcific aortic stenosis in the elderly and in many cases of rheumatic involvement of the aortic valve. In the former, the valve orifice is irregularly eccentric without commissural fusion, allowing the stream of contrast material adjacent to the three commissures to project over the entire width of the aorta. Calcification may be so extensive that the leaflets are akinetic.

Poststenotic dilatation of the ascending aorta results from the jet through the valve striking the lateral aortic wall. The lateral wall of the aorta becomes both dilated and elongated, further accentuating the rightward displacement of the aorta into the right lung. Poststenotic dilatation occurs in 25% of patients with subvalvular aortic stenosis. By its nature, supravalvular stenosis does not have dilatation of the aorta. As a rule, you can correlate poststenotic dilatation with the location (i.e, valvular) but not with the severity of the aortic stenosis. Poststenotic dilatation happens in all age groups, even neonates.

In most children and adults with pure, severe aortic stenosis, the left ventricle has a small cavity that is hypercontractile and has the usual signs of hypertrophy. In the absence of other anomalies, left ventricular dilatation in pure aortic stenosis is direct evidence of heart failure, a complication that is particularly critical in neonates. In this condition, the left ventricle usually exhibits diffuse hypokinesis with an increased end-diastolic volume and low ejection fraction. In severe heart failure, segmental wall motion abnormalities occur in the absence of coronary disease, particularly in the anterior and lateral segments.

Congenital Valvular Aortic Stenosis

The bicuspid aortic valve is the most common congenital cardiac malformation, occurring in 0.5% to 2.0% of the population. This malformation is usually not stenotic during infancy (although it may be so) but may become stenotic as fibrosis and calcification occur. Bicuspid valves can be either stenotic, regurgitant, or both. There is infective endocarditis in 75% of those with pure regurgitation.

Distinctive calcifications on the lateral chest film characterize the congenital bicuspid aortic valve. Calcium is visible in the raphe of the valve and in the line of insertion of the shallow conjoint leaflet and the convex nonfused leaflet (Fig. 5-4). A noncongenital cause of a bicuspid valve occurs from fusion of the commissures of the aortic leaflets in rheumatic heart disease.

The angiographic appearance of a congenital bicuspid valve is two sinuses of Valsalva and two leaflets (Fig. 5-5). The valve orifice may be oriented in either an anteroposterior direction, which divides the leaflets into right and left cusps, or in a right-left direction, dividing the valve into anterior and posterior leaflets. If the cusps are on the right and left, there may be a raphe in the right cusp, and each sinus of Valsalva gives origin to a coronary artery. If the cusps are anterior and posterior, a raphe, if present, occurs in the anterior cusp, and both the coronary arteries arise from the anterior sinus of Valsalva. The normal aortic valve may acquire a bicuspid appearance when one commissure fuses as a result of rheumatic heart disease. In general, the congenital bicuspid valve will have one of the sinuses of Valsalva and its leaflet occupy half the circumference of the aortic annulus, while the acquired bicuspid valve with one fused commissure still demonstrates three sinuses of Valsalva of nearly equal size. In diastole the congenital bicuspid valve may appear to have three sinuses of Valsalva because the raphe is visible and divides one of the two leaflets in half.

The congenital bicuspid aortic valve is recognizable most accurately during systole. The systolic appearance of a noncalcified congenital bicuspid valve typically includes domed and thickened leaflets (Fig. 5-6). The jet through the valve is usually slightly eccentric in direction but appears through the central part of the aortic annulus. In contrast, the jet through the rare unicommissural valve is quite eccentric.

Bicuspid aortic valves are associated with many types of congenital heart disease. Half of those with coarctation of the aorta have a bicuspid aortic valve (Fig. 5-7). More generally, any malformation of the aorta, such as aortic arch atresia or interruption or the hypoplastic left heart syndrome, has a high incidence of bicuspid aortic valve.

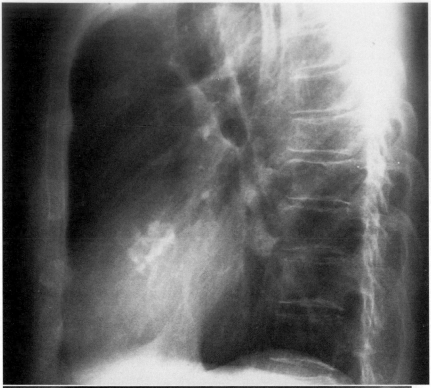

A

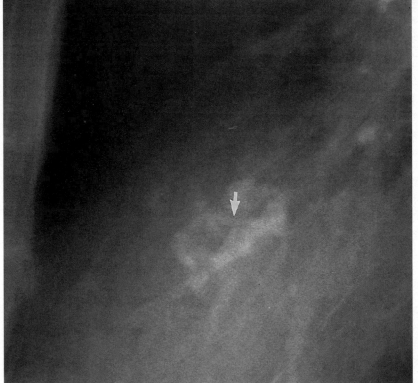

B

Fig. 5-4 Calcified bicuspid aortic valve. **A,** Dense calcifications in the heart lie on a line drawn between the sternodiaphragmatic angle and the carina locating the calcium to be in the aortic valve. **B,** Magnification view shows the ring of calcium and the central raphe *(arrow)*.

The congenital unicuspid aortic valve is intrinsically stenotic and may at times be incompetent. This valve may exist with no lateral attachments and appear as a diaphragm with a central opening. A second type of unicuspid valve has one lateral attachment to the aortic annulus with the commissure appearing as a raphe between the central point and the aortic wall. Both types of valve are rare. In systole there is an eccentric jet against the posterior wall of the aorta with no leaflet tissue posteriorly. In diastole a sinus of Valsalva may appear anteriorly but not posteriorly.

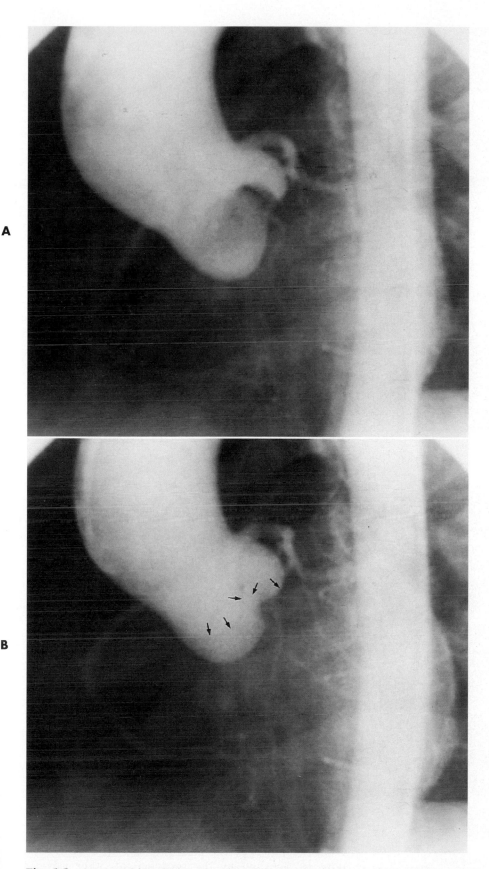

Fig. 5-5   Congenital bicuspid aortic valve. **A,** In systole, the two leaflets and their sinuses of Valsalva are best visualized in the left anterior oblique projection. **B,** In diastole, three sinuses of Valsalva are visible, one of these actually representing a single sinus with a raphe *(arrows)*.

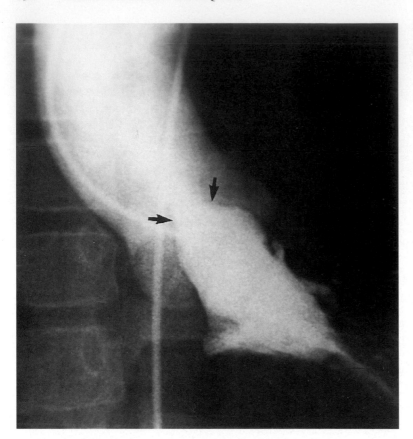

Fig. 5-6   Congenital aortic stenosis. The aortic leaflets *(arrows)* are domed and have a jet of contrast medium through them. More than half of the left ventricular cavity is obliterated. The aortic gradient was 90 mm Hg.

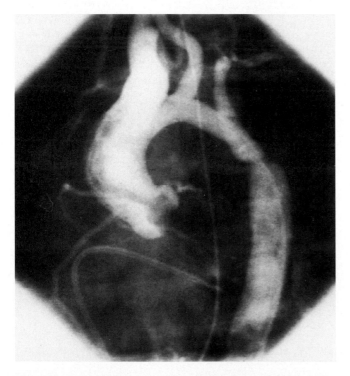

Fig. 5-7   Coarctation of the aorta and bicuspid aortic valve. The narrow jet through the valve indicates severe stenosis. Note the jet hits the opposite wall of the ascending aorta, a cause for later post-stenotic dilatation.

Acquired Valvular Aortic Stenosis

The aortic valve that is not stenotic at birth may become so in two ways: (1) the congenitally malformed valve, typically bicuspid, may become fibrotic and calcify: with gradual obstruction of its orifice; or (2) a normal tricuspid aortic valve may develop commissural fusion or leaflet thickening and fibrosis, or both. The endstage of any of these processes is a severely calcified valve, and it may be impossible to determine the initial process. In the extreme, the leaflets may be so thickened as to be akinetic. Unlike the congenital, non-calcified bicuspid aortic valve, these endstage valves usually do not have a jet through them (Fig. 5-8). The stream of contrast medium or blood through the distorted and curved linear orifice is turbulent. Doming of the leaflets is always seen in the noncalcified congenital aortic stenosis, but is an inconstant feature in an endstage aortic valve.

Calcific aortic stenosis in the adult results from rheumatic heart disease, occurs on a congenital bicuspid aortic valve, and occurs in the elderly. Although some overlap occurs, you can differentiate these three conditions by age and by the presence of other valvular lesions. The congenital bicuspid aortic valve begins to calcify in the fourth decade, while degenerative aortic

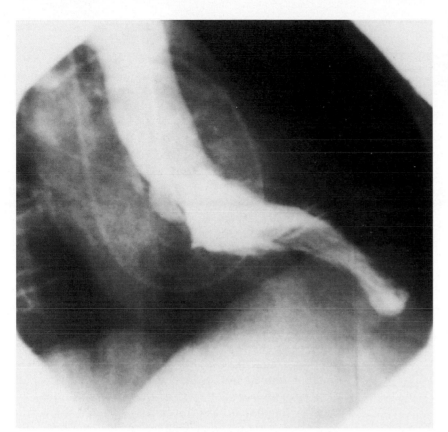

Fig. 5-8 Calcific aortic stenosis. Severe aortic stenosis exists, although the leaflets are poorly seen and no jet of contrast media passes through the valve. The large papillary muscles and distorted cavity represent moderate left ventricular hypertrophy.

stenosis affects those over 65 years of age. In the Third World countries, calcification in rheumatic aortic stenosis may appear in the late teens but is unusual in the United States until the fourth decade. With the aortic stenosis of rheumatic heart disease, mitral stenosis does not occur for at least 7 to 10 years after an episode of acute rheumatic fever, and aortic stenosis may develop about 7 years after that.

An important clue to the diagnosis of rheumatic disease in the aortic valve is the presence of mitral stenosis or regurgitation and calcification or thickening in the mitral leaflets in an otherwise functional valve. One characteristic of rheumatic aortic stenosis is the fusion of the commissures adjacent to the aortic wall. In general, these valves have either the usual appearance of a tricuspid valve or have one distorted sinus of Valsalva that occupies more than half the aortic annular circumference. When there is fusion of multiple commissures, the leaflets are usually so thickened and distorted that valve morphology is indistinguishable from other types of aortic stenosis.

Aortic stenosis in the elderly results from degeneration of the valve leaflets with subsequent thickening and calcification. Some patients have coronary calcification and calcification in the mitral annulus, as well as in the aortic arch. These aortic valves are tricuspid and have clumps of calcium within the webs of the leaflets. In contrast to rheumatic valves, the commissures are not fused (Fig. 5-9).

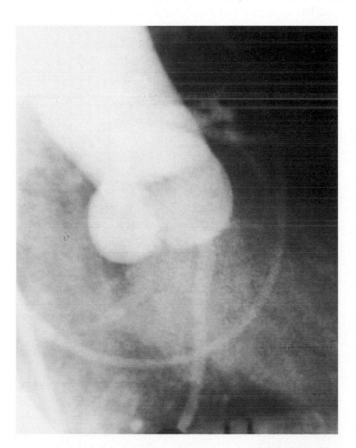

Fig. 5-9 Aortic stenosis in the elderly without a jet through the valve. Supravalvular aortogram in systole shows a tricuspid valve without commissural fusion. Moderate calcium was present in the leaflets. The left ventricle is faintly outlined by mild aortic regurgitation.

SUBVALVULAR AORTIC STENOSIS

Pathologic Abnormalities

Subvalvular aortic stenosis, or subaortic stenosis, consists of a heterogeneous group of abnormalities, several of which are associated with other types of cardiac malformation. These obstructions include:

- A discrete fibrous membrane
- Fibromuscular tunnel
- Redundant mitral valve tissue with accessory endocardial cushion tissue
- Conoventricular malalignment
- Hypoplasia of the aortic valve region in the hypoplastic left heart syndrome
- Obstruction to the outlet chamber of a primitive ventricle
- Hypertrophic cardiomyopathies, particularly idiopathic hypertrophic subaortic stenosis

Angiographic Findings

Optimal visualization of the angiographic features of most of these conditions is possible with biplane left ventriculography with cranial angulation in the left oblique projection. Since several of these malformations may be quite subtle (particularly discrete membranous subaortic stenosis), standard ventriculography may not demonstrate a lesion that is quite evident on pressure tracings. In these instances, an aortic root injection is useful since many of these valves are incompetent and the regurgitant stream outlines the subaortic chamber (Fig. 5-10). A magnetic resonance scan in planes aligned to the cardiac axis can sort out subaortic complexities with tomographic imaging (Fig. 5-11).

About 15% of patients with congenital obstruction to left ventricular outflow have discrete membranous subaortic stenosis. This consists of a 1- to 4-mm-thick membrane below the aortic valve. The membrane varies in position from just below the aortic valve to about 4 cm beneath it. The membrane may attach to the anterior leaflet of the mitral valve and strands from this membrane may extend to the aortic cusps (Fig. 5-12). About one third to one half of these patients have aortic insufficiency and less than 5% have mild mitral insufficiency.

In membranous subaortic stenosis, the true aortic leaflets usually have an abnormal appearance and motion. Unless there is also valvular stenosis, the leaflets are not domed but usually are mildly thickened and may have an irregular surface. The jet through the subvalvular membrane also must pass through the aortic leaflets generating considerable turbulence. The aortic leaflets typically have an incomplete opening and may partially close in midsystole before finally attaining the maximum orifice size. In general, you will often see a subvalvular jet extending through the aortic leaflets if the obstruction is just beneath the aortic valve. It

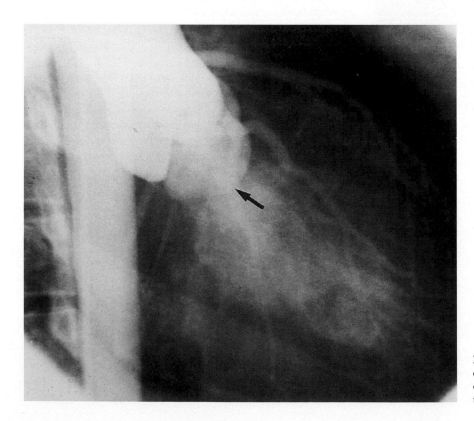

Fig. 5-10   Subaortic membrane demonstrated with an aortogram. The aortic regurgitation outlines the membrane *(arrow)* as well as fills the left ventricle.

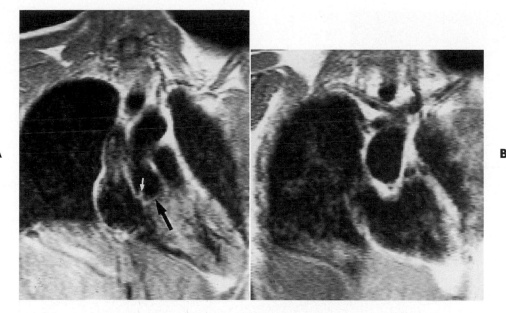

Fig. 5-11   Membranous and fibromuscular subaortic stenosis. **A,** A thin membrane *(black arrow)* is present about 1 cm below the right aortic cusp *(white arrow).* **B,** A subaortic conical narrowing represents the fibromuscular component. (From Miller SW, et al: Cardiac magnetic resonance imaging: The Massachusetts General Hospital experience, *Radiol Clin North Am* 23:745-764, 1985.)

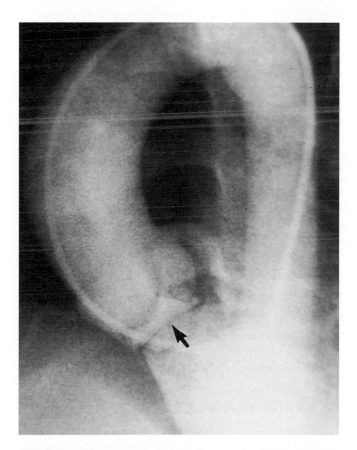

Fig. 5-12   Discrete membranous subaortic stenosis. Cranial angulation in the left anterior oblique projection outlines a linear lucency *(arrow)* below the aortic leaflets, extending from the septum to the mitral valve.

becomes less visible or may be absent if the obstruction lies at a lower level.

In tunnel subaortic stenosis, the obstruction extends 1 to 3 cm below the aortic annulus. One type is a fibromuscular bar extending near or onto the anterior leaflet of the mitral valve. Another type has a long conical narrowing in the subaortic region with little change between systole and diastole (Fig. 5-13). The left ventricle shows the usual signs of hypertrophy, but occasionally this overgrowth of muscle may produce bizarre shapes.

Idiopathic hypertrophic subaortic stenosis (discussed in Chapter 8) is a dynamic form of subaortic stenosis. The obstruction occurs in systole with the abnormal anterior systolic motion of the anterior leaflet of the mitral valve. During diastole, the stenosis disappears as the mitral leaflet resumes its normal position. A similar dynamic subvalvular stenosis may be seen in transposition of the great arteries. Here the mitral leaflet creates a subpulmonary stenosis as the left ventricle is connected to the pulmonary artery.

Unusual Subaortic Obstruction

Subaortic obstruction may rarely result from valve abnormalities or malalignment defects in complex congenital heart disease. Accessory mitral valve tissue, anomalous attachment of the mitral valve and its chordae tendineae, or a displaced annular insertion of the anterior leaflet result in outflow obstruction. The angiographic

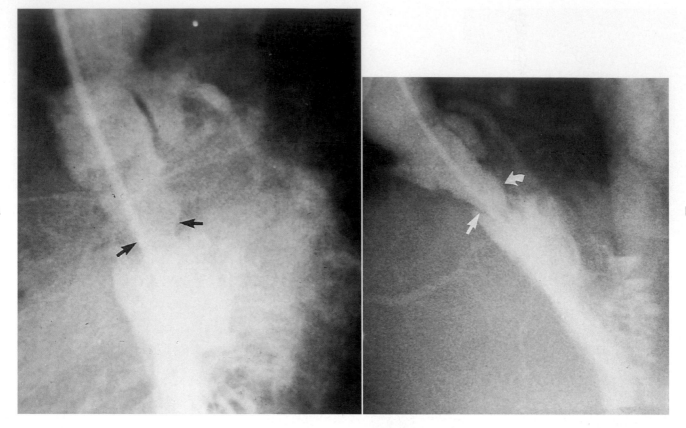

Fig. 5-13   Tunnel subaortic stenosis. **A,** A conical narrowing *(arrows)* in the long axial oblique projection persisted unchanged throughout the cardiac cycle. The aortic leaflets are thick. Moderate supravalvular stenosis is also present. **B,** A fibromuscular subaortic stenosis *(arrows)* is complicated anteriorly by a membrane and posteriorly by slight systolic anterior motion of the anterior leaflet of the mitral valve.

findings with each of these abnormalities varies; however, an asymmetric filling defect that moves into the subaortic region during systole and returns to a more posterior and inferior location during diastole is often visible during left ventriculography. Other complex congenital malformations have subaortic obstruction with conoventricular malalignment (e.g., aortic atresia and ventricular septal defect and in transposition with the aorta originating above an infundibular chamber).

SUPRAVALVULAR AORTIC STENOSIS

The least common type of left ventricular outflow obstruction occurs in the ascending aorta immediately above the sinuses of Valsalva and coronary arteries. More distal stenoses in the aortic arch and isthmus, such as interruption of the aortic arch, coarctation, Takayasu's aortitis, and other types of true aortic stenosis are usually classified as aortic rather than cardiac pathologic conditions, although associated anomalies frequently coexist.

Classifications

There are three types of supravalvular stenosis. The hourglass type consists of a narrow segment of the ascending aorta just distal to the origin of the coronary arteries (Fig. 5-14). The second type is a membrane or fibrous diaphragm at the sinotubular aortic junction (Fig. 5-15). The least common is hypoplasia of the entire ascending aorta from the sinotubular junction to the origin of the brachiocephalic artery. In actual practice, these three forms overlap and are alternatively classified as discrete or diffuse stenoses, categories that correspond to the alternatives in surgical treatment.

Associated Lesions

Associated cardiac lesions occur in two thirds of patients with supravalvular aortic stenosis. Common abnormalities are hypoplastic aortic valve annulus and valvular aortic stenosis (Fig. 5-16). Some of these patients are part of a generalized disorder associated

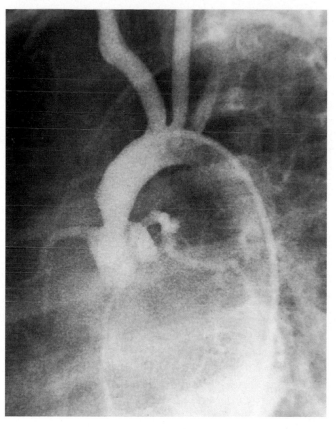

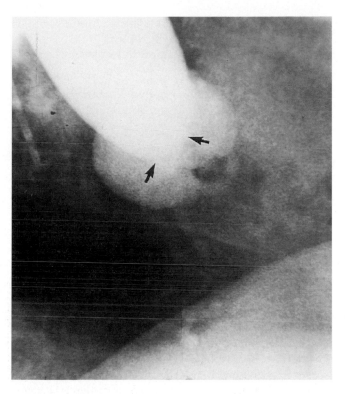

Fig. 5-15 Supravalvular aortic stenosis. A discrete stenosis *(arrows)* is seen at the junction of the aorta and the sinuses of Valsalva.

Fig. 5-14 Hourglass type of supravalvular aortic stenosis shows large sinuses of Valsalva and large coronary arteries.

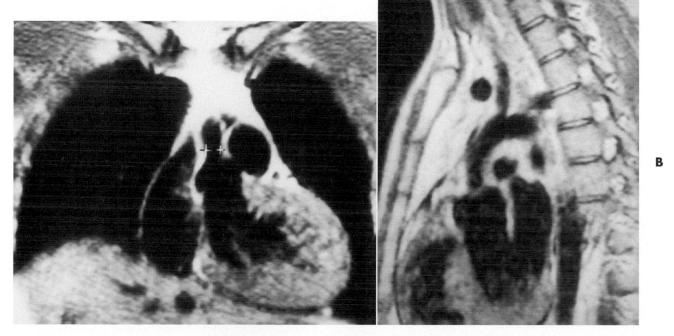

A

B

Fig. 5-16 Supravalvular aortic stenosis. **A,** Coronal MRI shows the hypoplastic aorta *(crosses)* beginning above the aortic root. **B,** The hypoplastic left heart syndrome has a ventricular septal defect with absence of the inferior half of the septum.

with hypercalcemia in infancy, elfin facies, and stenoses in other arteries (Williams syndrome).

Associated findings in supravalvular aortic stenosis are:

- Valvular and peripheral pulmonary stenosis
- Hypoplasia of thoracic and abdominal aorta
- Isolated stenoses in
    Aortic arch arteries
    Renal arteries
    Celiac axis
    Superior mesenteric artery

The coronary arteries are proximal to the obstruction and are subject to elevated left ventricular systolic pressure from birth, making them both dilated and tortuous.

AORTIC REGURGITATION

Aortic regurgitation results from a cusp abnormality, distortion of the aortic root, or dilatation of the aorta. Aortic valves that have stenosis generally also have some regurgitation. When the leaflets are abnormal, the regurgitation frequently is from rheumatic disease, infective endocarditis, or a bicuspid valve. When the ascending aorta is the cause of regurgitation, common causes are Marfan syndrome, aortic dissection, aortitis,

ankylosing spondylitis, systemic hypertension, and syphilis (Box 5-2).

Chest Film Findings

If the aortic regurgitation is both chronic and severe, the chest film hallmarks are left ventricular enlargement and dilatation of the entire aorta (Fig. 5-17). This pattern follows the principle that regurgitation of any of the heart valves enlarges structures on both sides of the insufficient valve. If the regurgitation is acute, signs of left ventricular failure are present—pulmonary edema and pleural effusions. Then, after several days, the left ventricle is visibly dilated.

Angiographic Technique

The angiographic examination should demonstrate the insufficient valve, allow quantitation of the regurgitant volume, and demonstrate the pathologic changes. If there is moderate regurgitation, you may also compute left ventricular volume and the ejection fraction.

The typical examination is a biplane supravalvular aortogram performed in both oblique projections. The injection rate varies, depending on patient age, the size of the ascending aorta, and the clinical judgment of the severity of the runoff. For example, in the adult with suspect-

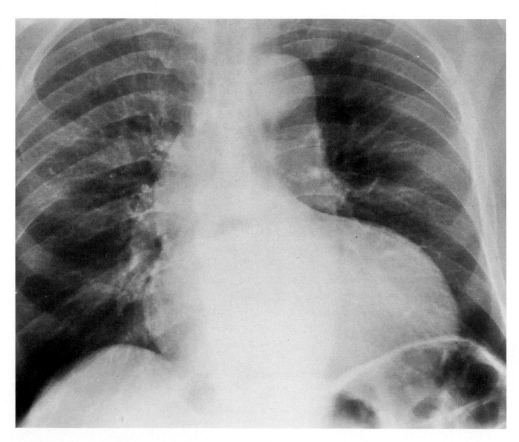

Fig. 5-17 Chest film in chronic severe aortic regurgitation. Structures on both sides of the regurgitant valve are large, reflecting the high output state—the left ventricle and the entire thoracic aorta.

Box 5-2   Causes of Aortic Regurgitation

LEAFLET ABNORMALITY

Rheumatic with fused commissures
Endocarditis with perforation or vegetations
Bicuspid aortic valve
Syphilis with rolled leaflet edges
Secondary to any type of aortic stenosis
Prolapsing leaflets from
    Marfan syndrome
    Ventricular septal defect

AORTA DILATATION

Hypertension
Aortitis
    Ankylosing spondylitis
    Reiter syndrome
    Rheumatoid arthritis
    Relapsing polychondritis
    Giant cell aortitis
    Relapsing polychondritis
Annuloaortic aneurysm (Marfan syndrome)
Osteogenesis imperfecta
Ehlers-Danlos syndrome
Pseudoxanthoma elasticum

DISTORTED ROOT

Dissection
Trauma
Sinus of Valsalva aneurysm

---

ed severe aortic regurgitation, an injection rate of 35 to 40 ml/sec over 2 seconds gives good visualization with large films and a serial rapid film-changer. The standard 30 ml/sec usually suffices with cineangiography. During the test injection you should take care to position the catheter tip freely in the ascending aorta at the sino-tubular ridge. Analysis of cuspal motion necessitates the cine technique.

MRI Technique

Cine MRI as well as color flow Doppler ultrasound can identify and quantitate valvular regurgitation. On both techniques, the imaging plane is rotated to include the aortic root and the regurgitant jet. Cine MRI (gradient refocused MRI), a "white blood" technique, is set up to provide repetitive loops of a cardiac cycle with both magnitude and phase reconstruction. Aortic regurgitation is identified as a discrete area of signal loss coming from the aortic valve into the left ventricle during diastole.

Subjective assessment of the amount of regurgitation is clinically useful to plan therapy. Medical treatment with afterload reducing agents are commonly prescribed for mild to moderate regurgitation, whereas surgical valve replacement is needed for severe regurgitation. Under these circumstances, the following grading system is the standard of practice to assess aortic regurgitation:

Grade 1 (trace): Slight regurgitation with opacification only of the ventricle adjacent to the aortic and mitral valves
Grade 2 (mild): Moderate opacification of the entire left ventricle usually with clearing on the succeeding beat
Grade 3 (moderate): Dense opacification of the left ventricle for two to three beats before clearing begins
Grade 4 (severe): Left ventricular opacification more dense than the aorta and lasting several beats after the end of the injection

Imaging Findings

Stenotic valves, vegetations, and prolapse of one of the cusps are easy to identify, while perforation of a cusp is rarely visible directly. The regurgitant jet into the left ventricle is visible on an MRI (Fig. 5-18), ultrasound, or angiographic study. Aortic root abscesses and aortic dissection in the root produce an unstable aortic annulus, but may leave the leaflets intact. A paravalvular regurgitation around a prosthetic valve can result from endocarditis in the aortic root or with dehiscence of part of the valve ring. Dilatation of the aorta itself may enlarge the aortic annulus so that the leaflets do not coapt. Giant cell aortitis and connective tissue diseases typically dilate the aorta so that mild regurgitation ensues. Severe regurgitation more commonly results from cystic medial necrosis where both the aortic root and ascending aorta have an aneurysmal pear shape with obliteration of the sinotubular junction.

Specific Causes of Aortic Regurgitation

When the aortic valve is incompetent, the differential diagnosis is either a condition that primarily affects the aortic valve or one that secondarily results from a disease in the ascending aorta.

Fibrosis from the valvulitis in rheumatic heart disease is the most common aortic valve abnormality that causes regurgitation. These valves have thickened cusps which are shortened by the fibrotic process and may have some commissural fusion. Depending on the severity of the rheumatic process, the leaflets may have no visible calcium or, conversely, they may be reduced to irregular lumps with poor motion. The regurgitant jet is usually central unless the valve commissures are fused asymmetrically. In degenerative aortic valve disease, which occurs in persons over age 65, the cusps are thickened

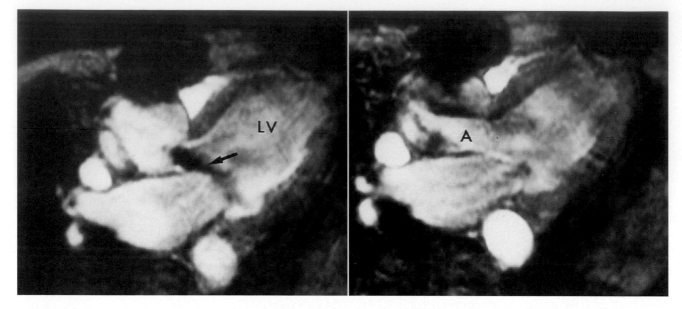

Fig. 5-18   Aortic regurgitation imaged with cine MRI. **A,** The signal void *(arrow)* in the diastolic frame is the jet of aortic regurgitation into the left ventricular (LV) outflow region. **B,** In the systolic frame, the aortic valve (A) region has normal forward flow, but the leaflets are thick. The linear lucency in the aortic root is an intimal flap of a dissection.

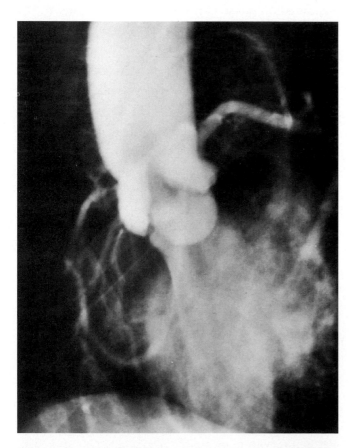

Fig. 5-19   Aortic regurgitation in degenerative aortic valve disease of the elderly. Supravalvular aortogram shows three leaflets without commissural fusion. The valve is moderately calcified. The aortic regurgitation is moderate (grade 3).

and immobile but without commissural fusion. Then regurgitation occurs over a broad front that is essentially the same diameter as the aortic annulus (Fig. 5-19). Fine fluttering of the anterior leaflet of the mitral valve is occasionally visible if the aortic regurgitation is severe.

Infective endocarditis can lead to aortic regurgitation with either perforation of a cusp (Fig. 5-20) or prolapse of an aortic cusp from destruction of the adjacent annulus (Fig. 5-21).

Common consequences of aortic valve infective endocarditis are:

- Aortic regurgitation
- Vegetations of bacterial endocarditis
- Systemic emboli
- Left ventricular failure from aortic regurgitation or coronary emboli
- Aortic root and myocardial abscesses
- Peripheral manifestations: mycotic aneurysms, splenomegaly and infarction, renal failure

Prolapse of one or more cusps appears in several acquired and congenital lesions. The aortic cusps in Marfan syndrome (rarely, in other diseases of elastic tissue) are large with deep sinuses of Valsalva and laxity in their supporting structures. Eversion of an aortic cusp into the left ventricle occurs in about 5% of ventricular septal defects in which the right or the noncoronary leaflet becomes adherent to the superior margin of the septal defect (Fig. 5-22). In a traumatic tear of the aortic root and in aortic dissection, the supporting points of the

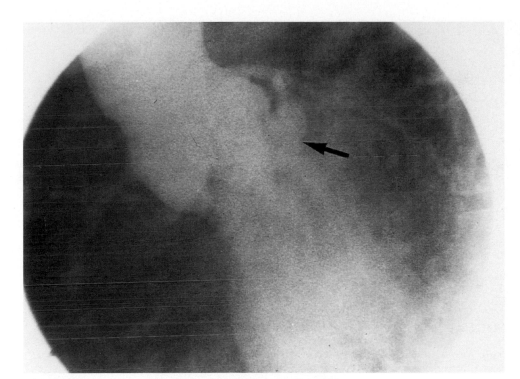

Fig. 5-20 Aortic root abscess. Left anterior oblique aortogram shows a small collection of contrast media *(arrow)* in the subaortic region. The aortic regurgitation is severe.

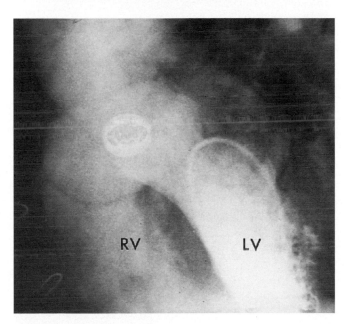

Fig. 5-21 Ventricular septal defect resulting from an abscess in the aortic root extending into the interventricular septum. Note the prosthetic aortic valve in the middle of the large aortic root abscess which has destroyed the upper ventricular septum. Regurgitation occurs into both the right *(RV)* and left *(LV)* ventricles.

leaflets may become unhinged from the annulus and then prolapse. With more severe loss of support, the leaflets can be flail with coarse vibrations in the regurgitant stream.

Most stenotic valves usually have an element of regurgitation. The congenital bicuspid aortic valve may be the

cause of severe regurgitation with or without stenosis. Infective endocarditis is a prime concern in patients with known bicuspid valves and new onset–aortic regurgitation.

Primary diseases of the ascending aorta that cause dilatation, such as ankylosing spondylitis and rheumatoid arthritis, may also enlarge the orifice of the aortic valve. Cystic medial necrosis of the aorta produces regurgitation by similar mechanisms, with or without annuloaortic ectasia and dissection (Fig. 5-23). In syphilitic aortitis, the cause of regurgitation may be purely the result of the rolled and thickened edges of the aortic valve, or from aneurysms of the sinuses of Valsalva or other adjacent structures. (See Chapter 10 for other causes of aortic regurgitation.)

Prosthetic Aortic Valves

Regurgitation after cardiac valve replacement may be of two kinds: valvular or paravalvular. Growth of scar tissue into the valve may prevent the ball or disk from seating completely, thereby causing regurgitation through the valve. In the porcine valves, the leaflets may degenerate or perforate. The regurgitant jet occurs through the prosthesis with an eccentric jet. Paravalvular regurgitation is seen as contrast material beside the sewing ring (Fig. 5-24). The usual cause of late paravalvular regurgitation, and in fact a possibility at any time after valve replacement, is prosthetic endocarditis. When this occurs, the angiographic findings are a fistula between the sinuses of Valsalva and the left ventricle and pseudo-

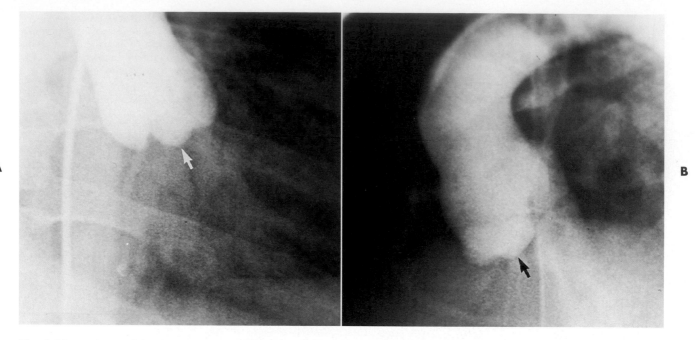

Fig. 5-22 Prolapse of the right aortic cusp *(arrow)* resulting from fibrous adhesions pulling the leaflet into a closing ventricular septal defect. Mild aortic regurgitation is present. The cineangiogram in the right **(A)** and left **(B)** anterior oblique projections shows faint aortic regurgitation and opacification of the pulmonary artery from passage of contrast across the ventricular septal defect.

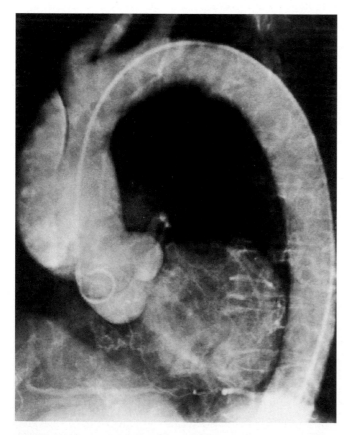

Fig. 5-23 Torn leaflet from a dissection. The intimal flap of the aortic dissection has ripped a cusp from the aortic annulus and caused moderate regurgitation.

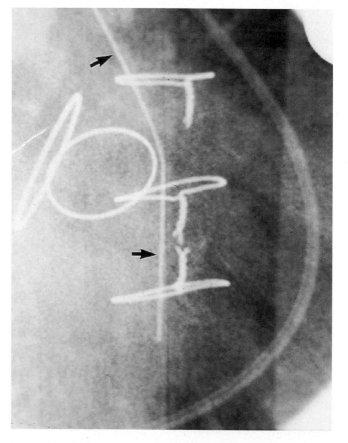

Fig. 5-24 Paravalvular leak. A catheter *(arrows)* has been passed from the aorta beside the Hancock valve into the left ventricle.

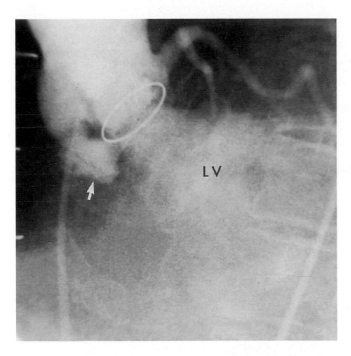

Fig. 5-25 Pseudoaneurysm *(arrow)* in the aortic root after valve replacement. In the left anterior oblique projection a pseudoaneurysm is seen near the anterior aspect of the aortic root; this abscess is in the upper part of the ventricular septum. The left ventricle *(LV)* is mildly opacified by both valvular and paravalvular regurgitation.

aneurysms adjacent to the prosthesis (Fig. 5-25). Vegetations may extend into the valve and cause decreased motion of the leaflets.

MITRAL STENOSIS

Most mitral stenosis is acquired and results from rheumatic carditis that occurred 5 to 10 years previously. Less common is a left atrial myxoma, thrombus, or a tumor which may prolapse through the mitral orifice during diastole and create stenosis. Rarely, the calcium in a mitral annulus may be so extensive that the leaflets become thickened and stenotic. Infective endocarditis with a large vegetation and congenital mitral stenosis are unusual causes of an obstructive mitral valve.

Early in the course of rheumatic mitral stenosis in the adult, the pulmonary blood flow redistributes to the upper lobes. Later, the pulmonary arteries enlarge as pulmonary arterial hypertension develops. Later still, the right ventricle fails both from a pressure overload from pumping into hypertensive pulmonary arteries and from pulmonary regurgitation from a dilated annulus. In the late stage of rheumatic mitral stenosis, tricuspid regurgitation may develop from the dilated right ventricle or rarely from intrinsic rheumatic disease on the tricuspid valve.

Box 5-3   Causes of Mitral Stenosis

ACQUIRED

Rheumatic (predominant cause)
Prolapse of left atrial tumor or thrombus
Leaflet deposits from amyloid or carcinoid or mucopolysaccharidoses

CONGENITAL

Hypoplastic left heart syndrome
Parachute deformity
Obstructing papillary muscles
Ring of connective tissue on left atrial side of mitral annulus

---

Time course of mitral stenosis in the adult is:

- Left atrium enlarges and pulmonary blood flow redistributes to the upper lobes (Fig. 5-26)
- Interstitial lung disease with Kerley B lines
- Pulmonary arteries enlarge as pulmonary arterial hypertension develops (Fig. 5-27)
- Right ventricular enlargement from pressure overload from hypertensive pulmonary arteries
- Pulmonary regurgitation from a dilated pulmonary artery
- Right ventricular failure
- Tricuspid regurgitation (Fig. 5-28)

See Box 5-3 for a summary of causes of mitral stenosis.

Chest Film Findings

The chest film in mitral stenosis physiologically reflects the left atrial hypertension. There are signs of left atrial enlargement, but the left ventricle has normal size. In the child with a hypoplastic left heart syndrome and congenital mitral stenosis, there is an enlarged heart and pulmonary edema. In the adult with rheumatic heart disease, the onset of mitral thickening and chordal scarring and retraction occurs over such a long interval that the lungs have made adaptive changes in the walls of the pulmonary arteries and veins. The lungs have an interstitial pattern which is probably part fibrosis and part edema. Pulmonary edema is visible as an interstitial pattern but not as an acinar pattern, unless there is a complication such as an infected or thrombosed valve. Patients with severe mitral stenosis rarely may have hemoptysis. The site of bleeding is probably in the engorged plexus of vessels around the middle to smaller bronchi. A late sequela of the bleeding is the development of hemosiderosis (Fig. 5-29). These deposits may ossify.

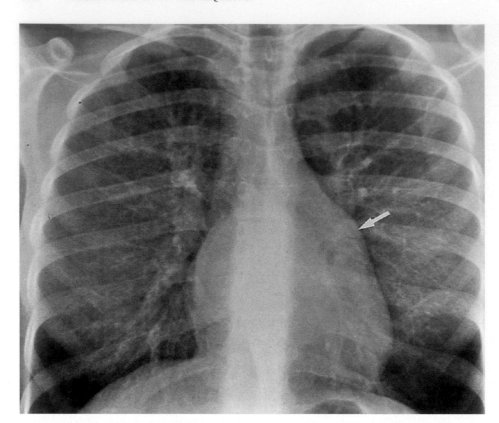

Fig. 5-26 Mitral stenosis. The large left atrial appendage *(arrow)* is rather specific for rheumatic mitral stenosis. The left ventricle has normal size, and the upper lobe vessels are dilated indicating pulmonary venous hypertension.

Calcification in the mitral valve is nodular and amorphous. The amount of calcium roughly correlates with the degree of mitral stenosis, but, unlike the aortic valve, the mitral valve may be severely stenotic and have no radiologically visible calcification (Fig. 5-30). As a late sequela to the inflammatory carditis in acute rheumatic fever, the left atrium may calcify (Fig. 5-31). These patients have long-standing atrial fibrillation and are at risk for left atrial thrombus and emboli.

Imaging Approach to Mitral Stenosis

You will usually use echocardiography to evaluate abnormalities of the mitral valve. As discussed in Chapter 2, the area of the mitral orifice is measured by ultrasound, and the salient characteristics of mitral stenosis are graded: calcification and mobility in the valve, submitral scarring, and leaflet thickening. Left ventriculography (Fig. 5-32) is needed before percutaneous mitral valvuloplasty (PMV) to grade mitral regurgitation, as moderate to severe regurgitation precludes PMV. Occasionally, pulmonary arteriogram or a left atrial injection through a patent foramen ovale helps evaluate suspected abnormalities on the left atrial side of the mitral valve. Of course, you should not use a left atrial injection from a transseptal approach if you suspect a myxoma or a thrombus because the procedure can dislodge emboli.

Rheumatic Mitral Stenosis

The hallmarks of mitral stenosis are the calcified, hypokinetic, and domed mitral leaflets. In severe mitral stenosis, the left atrium is always large and the left ventricle is smaller than normal with a slightly decreased ejection fraction. The doming of the leaflets signals a stenotic valve. Fusion of the commissures is not directly visible, but the leaflet doming and the jet of unopacified blood in the left ventricle are indirect signs of the stenotic orifice. The leaflets are thickened and slightly nodular and appear to attach directly to the papillary muscle.

Retraction and scarring of the chordae tendineae may result in a subvalvular mass which mimics vegetations. The subvalvular scarring, particularly that involving the posteromedial papillary muscle, appears to pull this muscle toward the base of the left ventricle (Fig. 5-33). Subvalvular scarring itself can produce substantial mitral stenosis.

Less common causes of obstruction about the mitral valve include left atrial myxomas and "ball valve" thrombi, which originate in the left atrium and prolapse through the mitral valve during diastole and thereby obstruct it. Processes outside the heart (constrictive pericarditis or adjacent mediastinal masses) can press on and distort the mitral valve and cause extrinsic mitral stenosis.

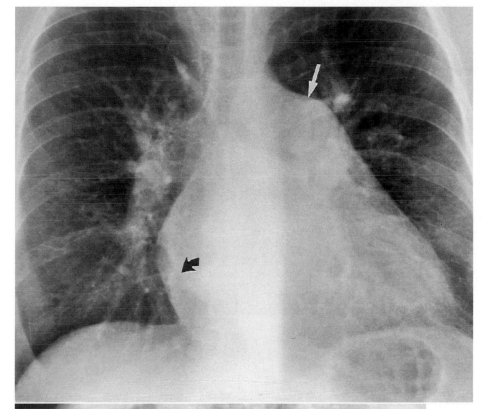

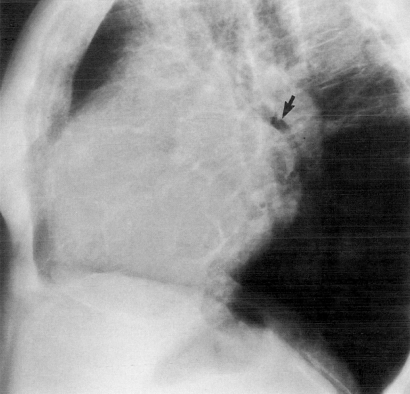

Fig. 5-27 Pulmonary artery hypertension in mitral stenosis. **A,** Large main *(white arrow)* and hilar pulmonary arteries plus dilated upper lobe vessels resulting from pulmonary arterial and venous hypertension. The left side of the heart-lung interface is mainly the large right ventricle which has rotated the normal-sized left ventricle posteriorly. Note the double density of the left atrium *(black arrow).* **B,** Lateral view shows the large right ventricle touching the sternum and the left mainstem bronchus *(arrow)* displaced posteriorly by the large left atrium.

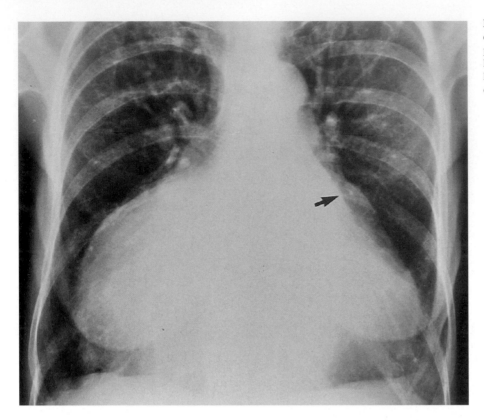

Fig. 5-28 Endstage rheumatic heart disease. The huge right atrium reflects tricuspid stenosis and regurgitation and right heart failure. Note the left lower lobe collapse *(arrow)* from compression by the dilated heart.

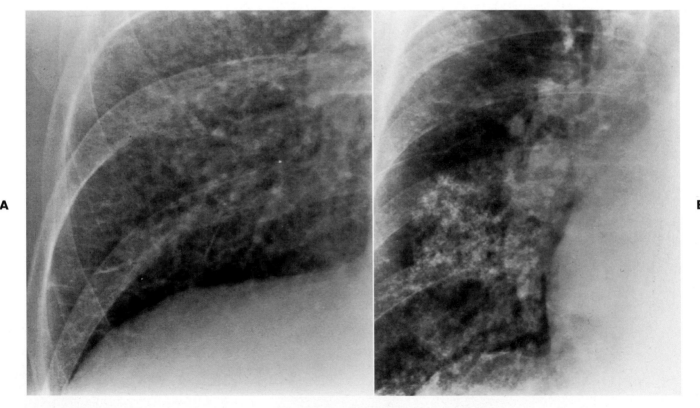

A   B

Fig. 5-29 Hemosiderosis in mitral stenosis. **A,** Nodular pattern with Kerley B lines. **B,** Segmental dense acinar opacities.

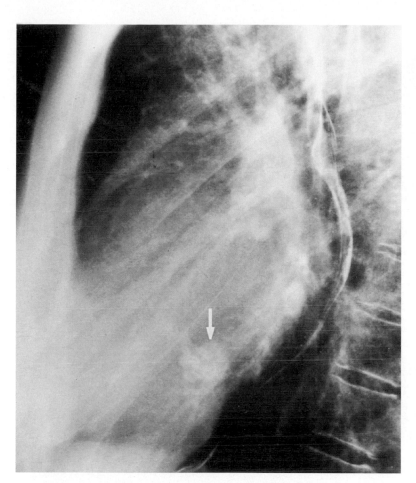

Fig. 5-30 Mitral leaflet calcification *(arrow)* in mitral stenosis. This calcification is more easily seen on the lateral chest film because it overlaps the spine on the posteroanterior film. Note barium in the esophagus is pushed posteriorly by the enlarged left atrium.

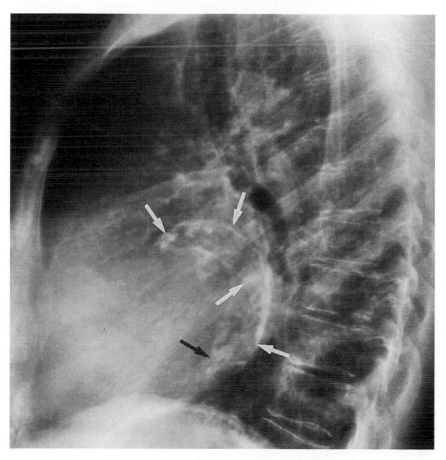

Fig. 5-31 Left atrial calcification *(white arrows)*. The mitral valve *(black arrow)* is calcified and the left bronchus is displaced posteriorly.

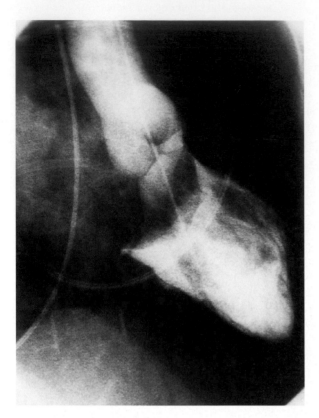

Fig. 5-32   Rheumatic mitral stenosis. The mitral valve in diastole is incompletely opened (domed) from commissural fusion. The rounded anterolateral wall and flat inferior wall are typical of right ventricular dilatation that compresses the left ventricle.

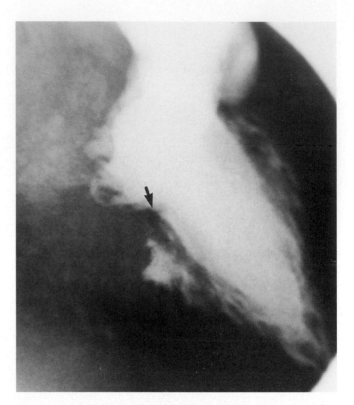

Fig. 5-33   Subvalvular fibrosis in mitral stenosis. Moderate retraction of the tip of the papillary muscle *(arrow)* toward the mitral leaflets. Severe fibrosis has caused a tumorlike mass consisting of matted chordae tendineae and the posteromedial papillary muscle. There is moderate mitral regurgitation into a large left atrium.

Congenital Abnormalities Causing Left Ventricular Inflow Obstruction

Congenital types of left ventricular inflow obstruction result from malformations in the mitral valve, the left atrium (cor triatriatum), or, rarely, in the pulmonary veins (pulmonary venous hypoplasia or atresia). When associated with other abnormalities of the left ventricle, aortic valve, and aorta, the term *hypoplastic left heart syndrome* is appropriate.

Cor triatriatum

Cor triatriatum is an anomaly in which the left atrium and the mitral valve are divided from the confluence of pulmonary veins by a constriction. The communication between the accessory chamber, which is the confluence of pulmonary veins and the true left atrium, is a diaphragm or membrane containing either single or multiple orifices. A tubular constriction between the common pulmonary veins and the left atrium may also be found in cor triatriatum.

In most patients with this anomaly, the mitral valve, left atrial appendage, and fossa ovalis (secundum atrial septal defect) are associated with the true left atrial cavity. A catheter entering the right atrium would pass

through an atrial septal defect into the true left atrium adjacent to the mitral valve. Exceptions exist, however, so that the foramen ovalis may connect the right atrium with the accessory chamber receiving the pulmonary veins. Partial anomalous pulmonary venous connections are frequent. Cor triatriatum can occur as an isolated anomaly but occurs frequently with ventricular septal defects, coarctation of the aorta, or a common atrioventricular canal defect.

The chest film shows pulmonary venous hypertension and an enlarged heart. An angiogram with the catheter through the patent foramen ovale shows a distorted, small atrial chamber without visualization of the pulmonary veins or their connections with the heart (Fig. 5-34).

Congenital mitral stenosis—Hypoplastic left heart syndrome

Congenital mitral stenosis is an uncommon malformation and comprises several anatomic types. Typical congenital mitral stenosis consists of obstruction by the leaflets and their chordal attachments. The leaflets are thickened and bulge into the left ventricular cavity during diastole (Fig. 5-35). There are two papillary muscles that have reduced interpapillary distance; the left ventricle has normal size. Another type of mitral obstruction is

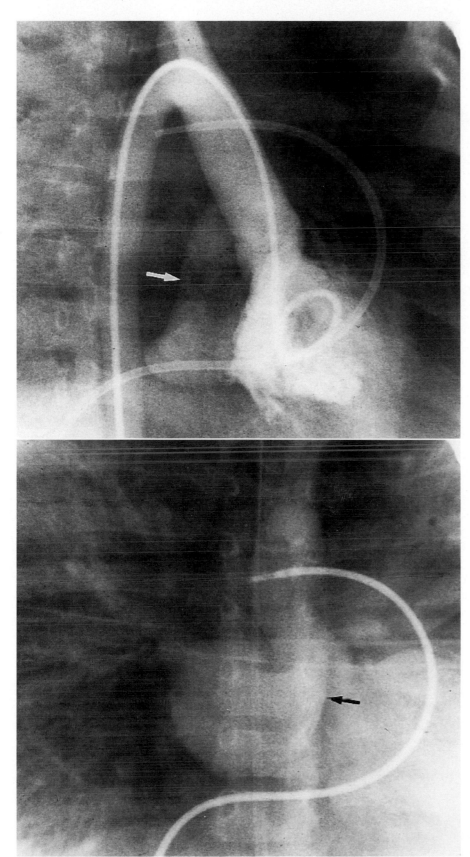

Fig. 5-34   Cor triatriatum. **A,** Mitral regurgitation during a left ventriculogram outlines the left side of the membrane *(arrow)* of the cor triatriatum and the appendage of the left atrium. **B,** The venous phase of a right pulmonary arteriogram shows the right side of the membrane *(arrow)* and the connection with the pulmonary veins.

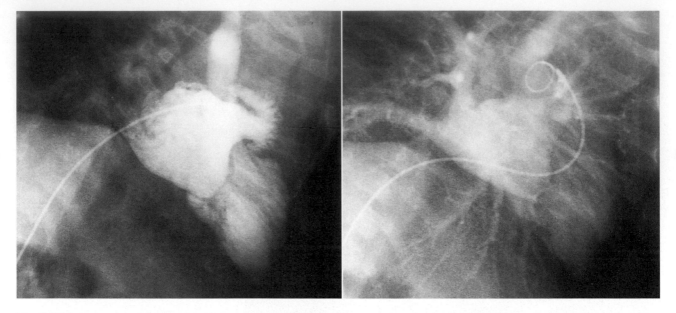

Fig. 5-35   Congenital mitral stenosis. Two angiographic techniques to visualize the stenotic mitral valve or exclude a cor triatriatum are **A,** a left atrial injection with the catheter through the foramen ovale, and **B,** a pulmonary artery injection. The transit of contrast through the lungs is prolonged with unusually good visualization of the pulmonary veins.

a supramitral ring that originates on the left atrial side of the mitral valve as accessory tissue above and adjacent to the mitral orifice. In the parachute mitral valve, a single papillary muscle is present that receives all of the chordae. This single papillary muscle is visible as a filling defect within the left ventricle on its inferior surface. The mitral leaflets are thickened and deformed and may show eccentric doming. The Shone syndrome consists of the parachute mitral valve, supravalvular ring of the left atrium, subaortic stenosis, and coarctation of the aorta. A hypoplastic mitral valve associated with hypoplasia of the remainder of the left side of the heart characterizes the hypoplastic left heart syndrome. You can distinguish this from other congenital forms because this type has hypoplasia of all parts of the mitral valve: the leaflets, chordae, papillary muscles, and annulus.

MITRAL REGURGITATION

Malfunction of any part of the mitral apparatus may lead to regurgitation. Mitral apparatus consists of:

- Mitral leaflets
- Chordae
- Papillary muscles
- Mitral annulus
- Adjacent left ventricular wall

Leaflet abnormalities include thickening in rheumatic disease and perforation in infective endocarditis. Mitral

valve prolapse has abnormalities in all parts of the mitral apparatus that can cause regurgitation. These include redundant valve leaflets with more than the usual number of scallops, elongated chordae, annular dilatation, and enlargement of the left ventricle. Rupture of the *chordae* typically causes acute severe pulmonary edema and may have its onset after lifting heavy objects. Flail mitral leaflets usually develop from the rupture of multiple chordae. They result in an erratic motion of the mitral leaflets with prolapse into the left atrium. *Papillary muscle* rupture is a complication of myocardial infarction and typically has ischemia of the adjacent left ventricular wall. Less severe ischemia of the ventricle can lead to papillary muscle dysfunction, which you can recognize by akinetic or hypokinetic segments with resultant mitral regurgitation. Left ventricular enlargement will dilate the *mitral annulus* and not allow the leaflets to coapt. An aneurysm of the *left ventricular wall* may distort the papillary muscles and change the geometric alignment so that mitral regurgitation ensues.

See Box 5-4 for a summary of causes of mitral regurgitation.

Chest Film Findings

The detection of mitral regurgitation on the plain chest film depends on the chronicity and severity of the disease. Acute, severe mitral regurgitation causes pulmonary venous hypertension and pulmonary edema, but little cardiac dilatation. After several days, as the heart

Box 5-4   Causes of Mitral Regurgitation

LEAFLET

Rheumatic
Prolapse syndrome
Endocarditis
Trauma
Systemic lupus erythematosus
Left atrial myxoma
Cleft leaflet in atrioventricular canal defect
Tumor deposit

CHORDAE

Rupture from trauma, infection, congenital malformation, or cystic medical necrosis

PAPILLARY MUSCLE

Rupture from ischemia or infarct
Parachute mitral valve (single papillary muscle)

ANNULUS

Left ventricular dilatation from any cause

LEFT VENTRICULAR WALL

Papillary muscle dysfunction from ischemia, infarct, or aneurysm
Idiopathic hypertrophic subaortic stenosis

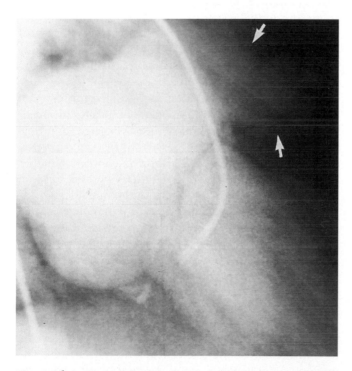

Fig. 5-36   Mitral regurgitation in acute rheumatic fever. The left atrium is more densely opacified than the left ventricle. Note the large left atrial appendage *(arrows)*.

begins to dilate, the lungs also begin to adapt with intimal hyperplasia and muscular hypertrophy in the arterial and venous walls so alveolar pulmonary edema regresses and an interstitial pattern appears. After weeks to months of chronic mitral regurgitation, the left atrium and left ventricle are enlarged. The pulmonary pattern is quite variable and may range from a normal vascular pattern, to cephalization of flow, to signs of interstitial lung disease. There are occasionally Kerley B lines. In long-standing mitral regurgitation, particularly from a rheumatic cause, the pulmonary pattern has a poor correlation with the actual amount of regurgitation.

Angiographic Evaluation

The object of imaging in mitral regurgitation is to identify its cause and to grade the severity. Echocardiography is the method of choice to look at the valve leaflets. Echocardiography and MRI can detect mitral regurgitation with great sensitivity, but left ventriculography mainly is used to grade the severity. Angiographic assessment is based on how much contrast flows into the left atrium and how long it takes to flow out:

Grade 1: Mild regurgitation with opacification only of the left atrium adjacent to the mitral valve
Grade 2: Moderate opacification of the entire left atrium, usually with clearing on the succeeding beat
Grade 3: Dense opacification of the left atrium for two to three beats before clearing begins
Grade 4: Left atrial opacification more dense than the left ventricle, going into the pulmonary veins, and taking several beats to clear

Rheumatic Mitral Regurgitation

In acute rheumatic fever with carditis, the major valve lesion is mitral regurgitation; there is no stenosis (Fig. 5-36). The regurgitation may resolve and reappear 5 to 10 years later when mitral stenosis becomes symptomatic. The mitral valve then has calcified, domed leaflets; fusion of the commissures; and short, retracted papillary muscles.

Mitral Valve Prolapse

At first glance mitral prolapse appears to be a leaflet abnormality, but it may encompass all parts of the mitral apparatus. Mitral regurgitation occurs when the cusps and chordae have redundant and exuberant valve tissue. Floppy valves show multiple scallops on the posterior leaflet with elongation of the chordae. Annular dilatation, chordal elongation and rupture, and occasionally, left ventricular contraction abnormalities occur.

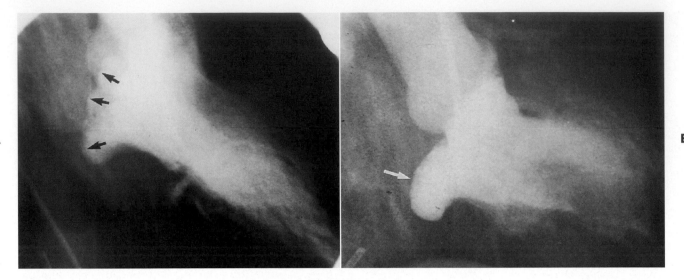

Fig. 5-37 Intrinsic and geometric types of mitral prolapse *(arrows)*. **A,** The mitral leaflets in Marfan syndrome have an abnormal number of multiple scallops. **B,** The mitral prolapse associated with atrial septal defect has no scallops *(arrow)* but is related to the shape of the left ventricle, which is distorted from right ventricular dilatation. After repair of the atrial defect, the prolapse was no longer present.

There is a roughly 5% incidence of mitral valve prolapse in the general population. There may be mild prolapse in normal hearts, or mitral prolapse associated with severe mitral regurgitation, subacute bacterial endocarditis, chest pain, or, rarely, sudden death. Intrinsic mitral prolapse is present from birth, such as that in Marfan syndrome in which both the mitral and tricuspid valves have redundant atrioventricular leaflets. Geometric distortion of the left ventricle, such as right ventricular enlargement that bows the interventricular septum to the left in atrial septal defect, can create moderate prolapse (Fig. 5-37).

The angiographic hallmark of mitral prolapse during left ventriculography is the passage of the mitral leaflets behind the plane of the mitral annulus into the left atrium (Fig. 5-38). The leaflet motion may begin in any scallop of the posterior leaflet or of the anterior leaflet. Then, as systole continues, the prolapse proceeds as a posterior curling of the central and free edge of the leaflet. Occasionally, the chordae tendineae are visible as linear lucencies of unusually long length. The onset of prolapse occurs early in systole and becomes more severe toward the middle and end of systole.

The degree of mitral regurgitation is obviously a function of the severity of the prolapse. Of those who have severe mitral regurgitation, most have prolapse of the entire posterior leaflet or of both the anterior and posterior leaflets. Prolapse of only one scallop of the posterior leaflet is generally associated only with mild mitral regurgitation. When there is severe regurgitation, particularly with prolapse of an entire leaflet, ruptured chordae are probably present.

Chordal Rupture

In addition to the chordal abnormalities seen in mitral valve prolapse and Marfan syndrome, primary rupture of the chordae tendineae is a common cause of acute mitral regurgitation. Less common malformations include anomalous mitral arcade and other congenital malformations associated with atrioventricular valves. Bacterial endocarditis and rheumatic fever account for roughly half of patients with ruptured chordae. Chordae in the posterior leaflet have a greater propensity to rupture than do those in the anterior leaflet. Since the chordae themselves are rarely visible angiographically, the major features are those of mitral regurgitation and abnormal leaflet motion. The degree of mitral regurgitation depends on the number of ruptured chordae; whether they are primary, secondary, or tertiary chordae; and on the remaining structural support of the mitral leaflet.

Mitral prolapse or flail leaflets occur in more than half of left ventriculograms performed in the clinical setting of chordae rupture (Fig. 5-39). Which leaflet prolapses depends on the location of the ruptured chordae, but in general the posterior leaflet, often the posteromedial scallop, is the more frequent location. A flail leaflet implies rupture of numerous chordae and suggests the possibility of detachment of the head of the papillary muscle. When a flail leaflet occurs, there is an erratic motion of one of the leaflets into the left atrium. The motion of the leaflet is different from beat to beat and frequently has a superimposed high-frequency whipping motion. There is always severe mitral regurgitation.

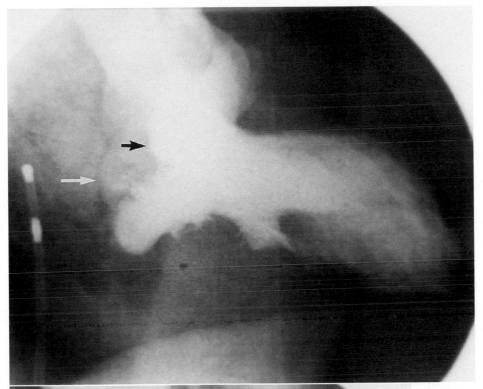

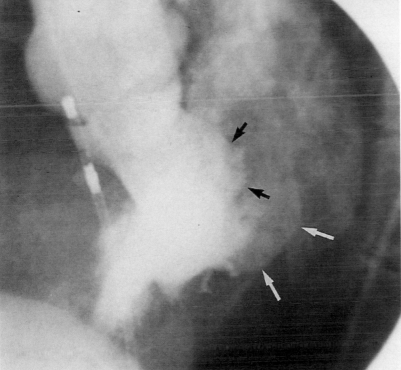

Fig. 5-38   Mitral valve prolapse. **A** and **B,** Both the anterior leaflet *(black arrows)* and posterior leaflet *(white arrows)* in these midsystolic frames are on the left atrial side of the mitral annulus. Moderately severe mitral regurgitation outlines the posterior left atrial wall. The left ventricle has an unusual shape in the right anterior oblique view with a concave inferior wall and large posteromedial papillary muscle.

Papillary Muscle Rupture

Rupture of the head of the papillary muscle commonly results from acute myocardial infarction, although chest trauma, endocarditis, and primary left ventricular muscle diseases may also be culprits. It more frequently involves the posteromedial muscle, possibly because the anterolateral muscle has better collateral circulation. Since each papillary muscle supplies chordae tendineae to both mitral leaflets, rupture of a head of the papillary muscle produces instability in both anterior and posterior leaflets and leads to

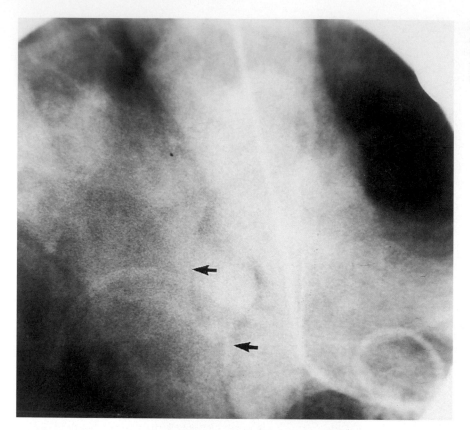

Fig. 5-39   Ruptured chordae tendineae with flail leaflets *(arrows)*. Both anterior and posterior mitral leaflets prolapse into the left atrium with resultant severe regurgitation. The posterior leaflet shows erratic motion.

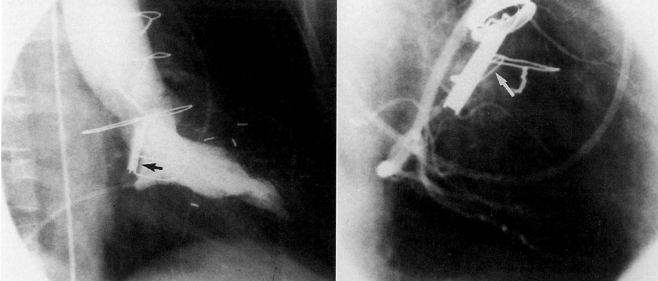

A

B

Fig. 5-40   Prosthetic mitral stenosis. **A,** A thin layer of thrombus *(arrow)* on the valve seat limits the mobility of the poppet in the Starr-Edwards valve. **B,** The tilting disk *(arrow)* in diastole should open about 80 degrees but thrombus prevents it from moving beyond 15 degrees.

severe mitral regurgitation. Since the infarct that produces the rupture usually involves a large area of myocardium, the left ventriculogram shows segmental wall motion abnormalities adjacent to the abnormal papillary muscle. These motion abnormalities are conspicuous and range from severe hypokinesis to dyskinesis. The motion of the mitral leaflets ranges from moderate prolapse to flail. The clinical problem is to distinguish this catastrophe from rupture of the interventricular septum.

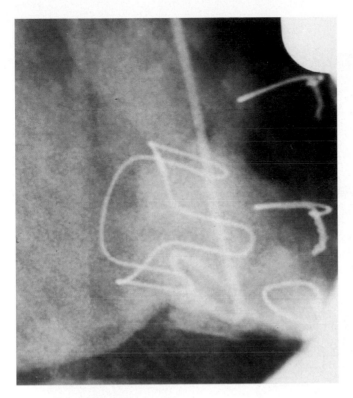

Fig. 5-41 Paravalvular mitral regurgitation. Contrast medium flows inferior to the Carpentier-Edwards mitral valve and into the large left atrium.

Papillary Muscle Dysfunction

A myocardial infarct or ischemia in the region of a left ventricular papillary muscle causes a segmental wall abnormality. Akinesis is common but hypokinesis from a non-Q-wave infarct or dyskinesis from an aneurysm is not rare. When these abnormalities involve the segment of the wall with the papillary muscle, the mitral apparatus is maligned and regurgitation occurs. This regurgitation is usually mild unless the papillary muscle is infarcted.

Imaging Complications of Mitral Valve Replacement

Prosthetic valve stenosis, regurgitation, and dysfunction are general indications for postoperative catheterization. Bleeding, tamponade, and myocardial infarction are usually diagnosed by clinical criteria. Prosthetic mitral stenosis is diagnosed by measuring the transvalvular gradient with a catheter in the left ventricle and another in the left atrium. The valve leaflet or disk may not have a full range of motion or may be stuck half-opened (Fig. 5-40). Prosthetic mitral regurgitation, depending on the type of valve, may be through the valve or beneath it (Fig. 5-41).

PULMONARY STENOSIS AND REGURGITATION

Pulmonary stenosis is an obstruction to right ventricular emptying and can occur at the valvular, subvalvular,

Box 5-5   Causes of Pulmonary Stenosis

VALVULAR

Congenital
   Diaphragm with central hole
   Bicuspid
   Dysplastic with thickened immobile cusps (seen in Noonan syndrome)
Acquired
   Carcinoid
   Rheumatic heart disease (very rare)

SUBVALVULAR

Congenital
   Hypoplastic crista supraventricularis in tetralogy of Fallot
   Discrete membranous
   Double-chambered right ventricle (anomalous muscle bar)
Acquired
   Right ventricular hypertrophy
   Tumor

SUPRAVALVULAR

Congenital
   Williams syndrome
   Tetralogy of Fallot
Acquired
   Carcinoid
   Rubella
   Tumor or thrombus
   Surgical banding
   Takayasu's aortoarteritis
   Behçet disease

Box 5-6   Causes of Pulmonary Regurgitation

Dilatation of annulus secondary to pulmonary hypertension
Endocarditis
Congenitally stenotic pulmonary valve
Congenitally absent pulmonary valve
After pulmonary valve surgery
Trauma

or supravalvular level. Most causes are congenital and occur in the valve.

See Boxes 5-5 and 5-6 for a summary of the causes of pulmonary stenosis and regurgitation.

Chest Film Findings

The chest film findings in pulmonary stenosis are variable and depend on the age of the patient and on associated abnormalities. In the infant, the large thymus may

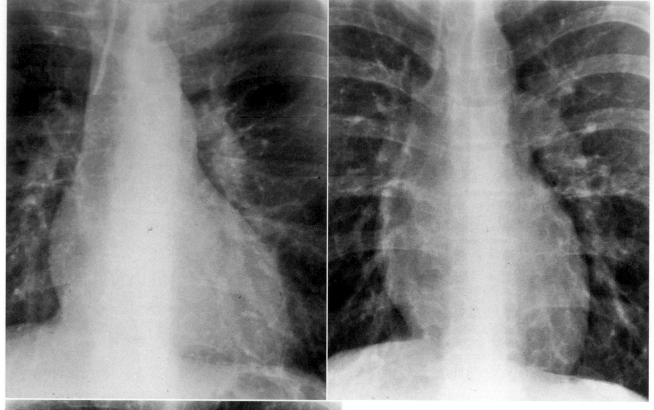

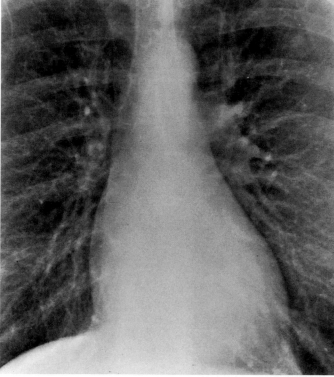

Fig. 5-42 Variations in the pulmonary arteries in valvular pulmonary stenosis. **A,** Typical appearance is a normal cardiothoracic ratio, convex main pulmonary artery segment, and a dilated left pulmonary artery. **B,** The main pulmonary artery is not enlarged with a straight segment. The left pulmonary artery is dilated and tapers rapidly. Occasionally, the large left hilum can be mistaken for lymphadenopathy. **C,** An atrial septal defect and pulmonary stenosis create a mixed pattern of shunt vascularity plus a large left pulmonary artery. The pulmonary annulus is hypoplastic causing the main pulmonary artery segment to be straight.

obscure the mediastinum so you can detect the disease only if there is decreased pulmonary flow. In the older child and adult, the classic film of valvular pulmonary stenosis shows mild enlargement of the right ventricle and moderate enlargement of the main and left pul-monary artery (Fig. 5-42). The right pulmonary artery has normal size (Fig. 5-43). In congenital pulmonary stenosis, particularly with hypoplasia of the main pulmonary artery, the pulmonary artery segment is concave. Unless the pulmonary obstruction is so severe as to reduce car-

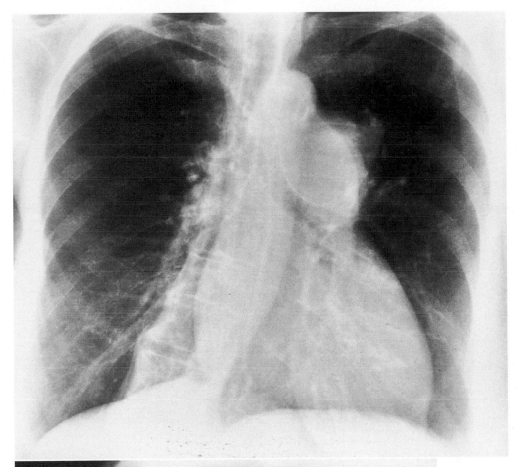

A

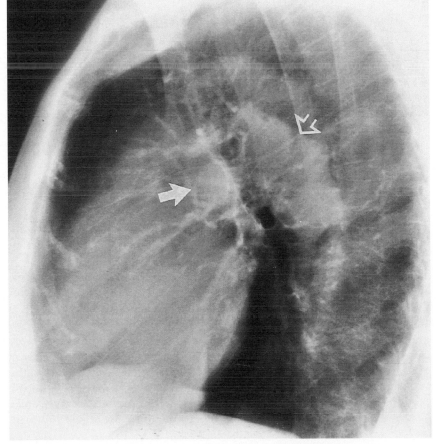

B

Fig. 5-43 Different size of the right and left pulmonary arteries in valvular pulmonary stenosis. **A,** The convex large main pulmonary artery partially hides the left pulmonary artery. **B,** The right pulmonary artery *(white arrow)* has normal size in relation to the width of the trachea. The dilated left pulmonary artery *(open arrow)* is visible into the distal lung.

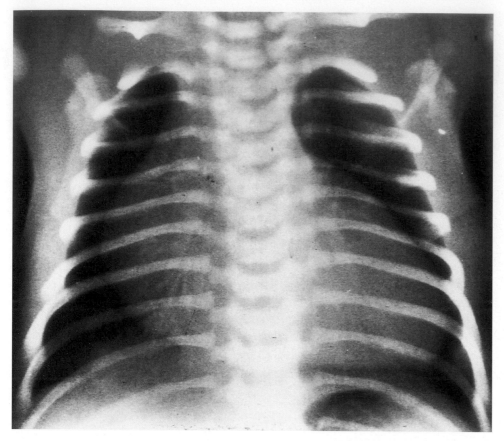

Fig. 5-44   Pulmonary atresia. The lungs have decreased flow and are hyperlucent. The heart is overall enlarged, particularly the right atrium, from blood flowing right to left through a foramen ovale.

diac output, the overall heart size is normal. In pulmonary valve atresia, with or without an intact ventricular septum, the heart is enlarged, and the cardiac contour is distinctive with right atrial dilatation (Fig. 5-44). The chest film in supravalvular pulmonary stenosis typically shows a straight main pulmonary artery segment and small hilar structures.

Valvular Pulmonary Stenosis

The most frequent cause of valvular pulmonary stenosis is a congenital defect. The valve usually is a membrane with a central hole but can be bicuspid or tricuspid. When this lesion calcifies, there has been previous endocarditis. Rare forms of pulmonary stenosis include tumor, thrombi, and aneurysms of the aortic sinus of Valsalva that prolapse through a membranous ventricular septal defect. Roughly 50% of patients with a carcinoid tumor that metastasized to the liver have pulmonary and tricuspid valve lesions. This tumor, with its vasoactive amines, causes endocardial thickening which leads to pulmonary stenosis, regurgitation, and tricuspid regurgitation.

Angiographically, the pulmonary valve is evaluated with a right ventriculogram. The leaflets have a domed appearance in systole yet form the normal sinuses of Valsalva in diastole (Fig. 5-45). The jet of contrast through the lesion is in the center of the valve and points toward the main and left pulmonary arteries, producing poststenotic dilatation of these structures and sparing the right pulmonary artery. Although there is usually poststenotic dilatation of the pulmonary artery, the degree of dilatation does not correlate well with the severity of the gradient. When other lesions are present, as in tetralogy of Fallot, the pulmonary artery segment is concave.

In some patients with valvular pulmonary stenosis, the infundibulum may be hyperkinetic with extreme narrowing in systole but a normal diastolic diameter (Fig. 5-46). The hyperkinetic systolic narrowing of the infundibulum occurs in its middle portion during contraction of the septal and parietal bands of the crista supraventricularis, giving an hourglass appearance to the infundibulum. After surgical or angioplasty repair of the stenotic valve, this subvalvular infundibular stenosis may be accentuated more because of the decreased afterload,

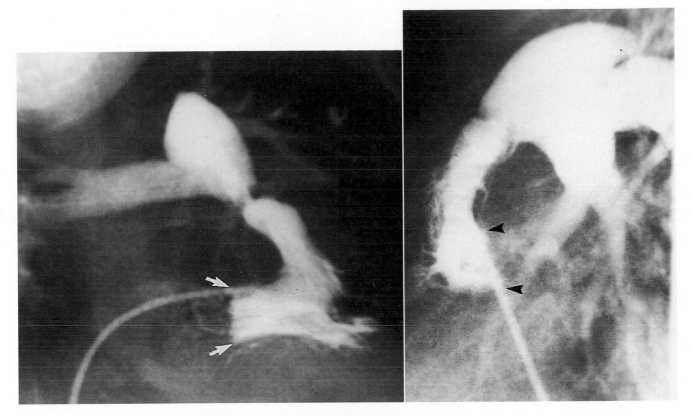

Fig. 5-45   Valvular pulmonary stenosis. **A,** Slight cranial angulation in the right anterior oblique projection places the plane of the pulmonary valve tangential to the x-ray beam and also demonstrates the origin of the right pulmonary artery. In general, a steeper cranial angulation is preferred since most congenitally malformed pulmonary valves have a vertical tilt. In this patient, the poststenotic dilatation of the main pulmonary artery is so massive that the left pulmonary artery could be seen only on the lateral projection. **B,** The symmetric doming of the pulmonary valve is confirmed in the lateral view. A small jet through the orifice attests to the severe stenosis. Note the small tricuspid annulus *(arrows)*.

and, in rare instances, fatal right ventricular failure happens because of complete occlusion of the hyperdynamic outflow tract: the suicidal right ventricle.

The dysplastic pulmonary valve and the bicuspid valve represent less common types of valvular stenosis. The dysplastic pulmonary valve, which occurs in 15% of hearts with isolated pulmonary stenosis, has three cusps which are thickened with unfused commissures. The bases of the sinuses of Valsalva are deformed and small as a result of excess tissue at the base of the leaflets (Fig 5-47). The dysplasia also includes the pulmonary annulus, which is hypoplastic, as is the main pulmonary artery adjacent to the sinuses. Because the leaflets are stiff and thick, there is little change in their position throughout the cardiac cycle. This motion is in contrast to that in typical valvular stenosis with fused commissures, which shows a flexible domed membrane in systole and rounded sinuses of Valsalva in diastole. The sinuses in the dysplastic pulmonary valve are irregular and narrow in diastole; the thick leaflets produce an asymmetrically orient-

ed orifice in systole. The recognition of the dysplastic pulmonary valve is important, because unlike other types of valvular stenosis it responds poorly to percutaneous valvuloplasty.

The bicuspid pulmonary valve appears similar to the bicuspid aortic valve, namely, unequal sinuses of Valsalva with fusion of one of the leaflets with a raphe, and a sinus of Valsalva occupying about half the valve circumference. Bicuspid pulmonary valves are present in about 50% of patients with tetralogy of Fallot. As part of this malformation, the annulus is often small and the supravalvular region of the main pulmonary artery is hypoplastic. This combination of abnormalities produces an angiographic appearance that has been likened to an "open clamshell engulfing the infundibulum" (Fig. 5-48). In addition to the other features of tetralogy of Fallot, the areas of obstruction include the infundibular and supravalvular narrowing. There is usually no poststenotic dilatation of the distal main pulmonary artery.

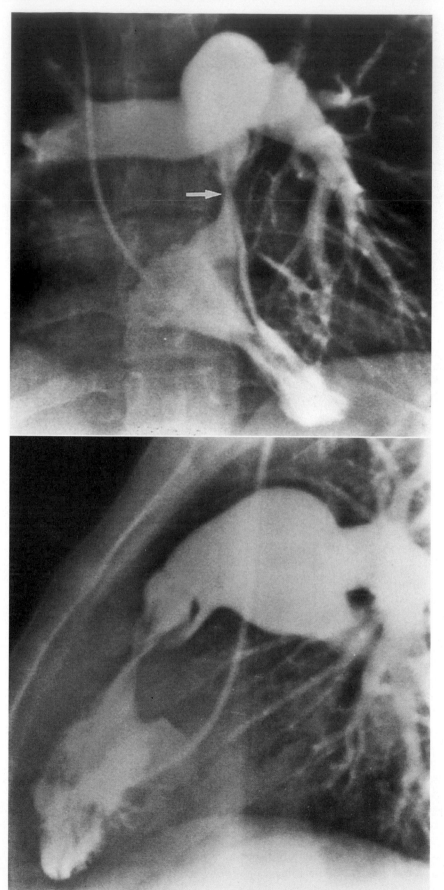

Fig. 5-46 Dynamic subvalvular stenosis secondary to valvular stenosis. **A,** In late systole the infundibular stenosis almost occludes the region below the pulmonary valve *(arrow)*. **B,** The lateral view shows the domed pulmonary valve, the infundibular stenosis, and the dilated main and left pulmonary arteries. In diastole there was no infundibular stenosis.

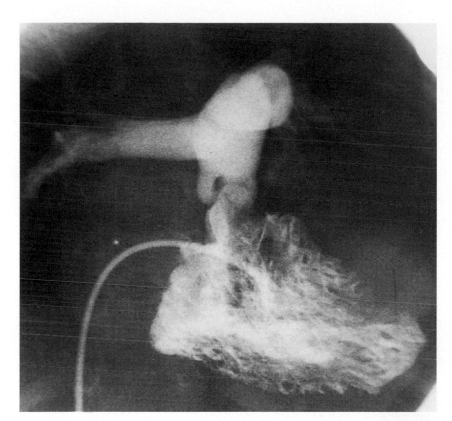

Fig. 5-47 Dysplastic pulmonary valve. The sinuses of Valsalva are mildly deformed and eccentric in diastole. The annulus and infundibulum are slightly hypoplastic. The leaflets had little change in systole.

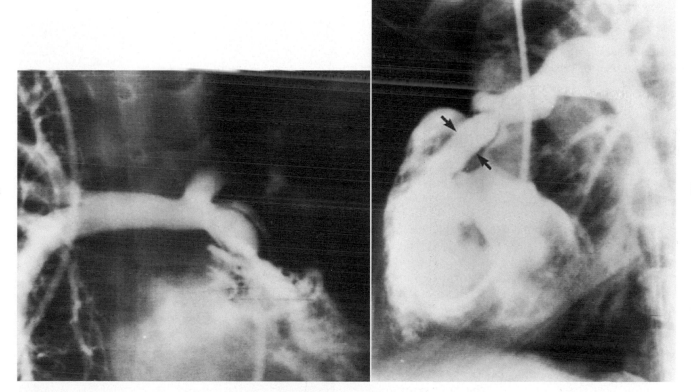

A

B

Fig. 5-48 Bicuspid pulmonary valve in tetralogy of Fallot. **A,** The length of the leaflets of the pulmonary valve appears greater than the width of the annulus. In addition to the doming of the leaflets, the infundibulum is hypoplastic. The left pulmonary artery is not seen because of competing flow through a left Blalock-Taussig shunt. **B,** On the lateral view, the hypoplastic infundibulum *(arrows)* is below the domed pulmonary valve. The left ventricle is opacified through the ventricular septal defect.

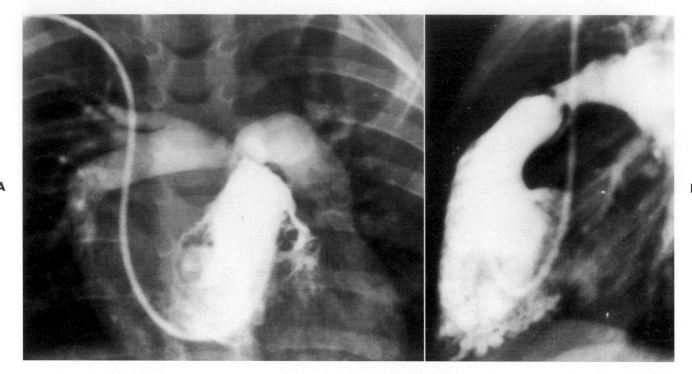

A

B

Fig. 5-49   Pulmonary valve annulus stenosis. **A,** The right ventriculogram shows narrowing at the pulmonary valve and supravalvular stenosis involving the bifurcation of the right and left pulmonary arteries. A large trabeculation is seen laterally. **B,** On the lateral view in systole, the leaflets of the stenotic valve are domed and the annulus is small. The main pulmonary artery is mildly hypoplastic.

The annulus of the pulmonary valve may be hypoplastic. The leaflets of the valve and the adjacent main pulmonary artery are usually small and form part of the stenosis (Fig. 5-49).

Congenital absence of the pulmonary valve is usually associated with a ventricular septal defect, annular pulmonary stenosis, and aneurysmal dilatation of the main pulmonary artery and the central part of both the right and left pulmonary arteries. This lesion can occur as an isolated entity but is associated with tetralogy of Fallot. The syndrome may also include a right aortic arch and peripheral pulmonary artery stenoses. The hilar pulmonary arteries may compress the bronchi leading to hyperinflated lungs.

In Noonan syndrome, many have a dysplastic pulmonary valve. Hypertrophic cardiomyopathy commonly accompanies the pulmonary stenosis as part of the autosomal dominant syndrome.

Subvalvular Pulmonary Stenosis

Subpulmonary obstruction may occur either in the infundibulum or at the junction of the right ventricular body with the infundibulum. Primary infundibular obstruction is a rare malformation which may appear as either a fibrous band or a threadlike cavity through the infundibulum (Fig. 5-50). Discrete narrowing at the level of the crista supraventricularis divides the right

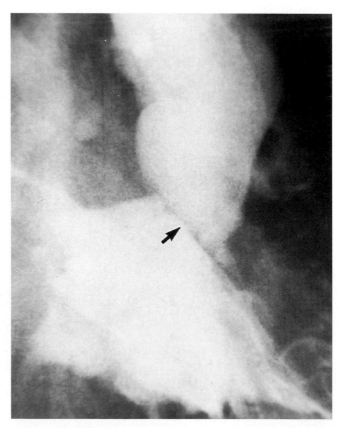

Fig. 5-50   Discrete infundibular pulmonary stenosis. A thin membrane is seen as a lucency between the body of the right ventricle and the infundibulum *(arrow)*.

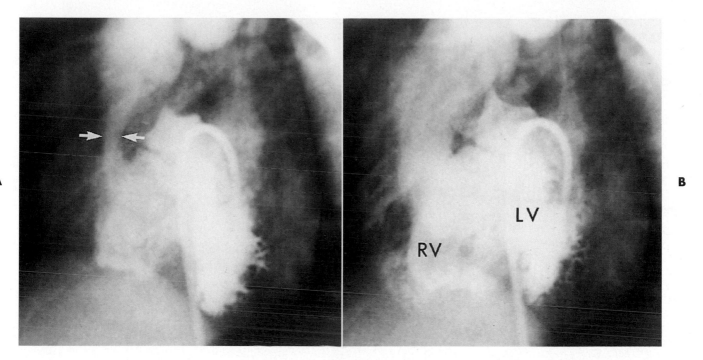

Fig. 5-51 Gasul phenomenon. **A** and **B,** The catheter has crossed the patent foramen ovale to enter the left ventricle (*LV*). In this lateral projection the body of the right ventricle (*RV*) has become opacified through the ventricular septal defect. In systole (**A**), the infundibulum (*arrows*) is markedly narrow, while in diastole (**B**), no subvalvular stenosis exists.

ventricle into a main cavity and an infundibular chamber. In this situation, there is contraction of the infundibular chamber during systole, leading to more severe obstruction in addition to its fixed, discrete narrowing. The pulmonary valve may be normal but usually shows slight thickening, presumably because of the turbulence created by the obstruction.

Other types of subpulmonary obstruction result from the muscular hypertrophy of the hypertrophic cardiomyopathies. The right ventricular outflow tract can show dynamic narrowing in idiopathic hypertrophic subaortic stenosis.

Infundibular stenosis frequently coexists with valvular stenosis. This type is not seen until after the patient is several months old, when other signs of right ventricular hypertrophy also becomes visible. Dynamic infundibular stenosis during systole may appear with a ventricular septal defect. This hypertrophy in the outflow tract decreases the left-to-right flow across the ventricular septal defect (Gasul phenomenon) and may cause stenosis that increases with age (Fig. 5-51).

Hypoplasia of the crista supraventricularis is the main element in the infundibular stenosis in tetralogy of Fallot. The underdevelopment of the infundibulum is associated with displacement of the crista above the ventricular septal defect. About half of patients with tetralogy of Fallot also have valvular pulmonary stenosis, in which case the pulmonary annulus is also small.

Obstructing muscular bands of the right ventricle, an abnormality that has also been called double-chambered right ventricle, may cause an obstruction either in the body of the right ventricle or higher in the infundibular region. These muscle bundles are seen as filling defects in the right ventricle which may not contract. When the anomalous muscle occurs in the true right ventricular cavity, its location is variable; it may extend from the apex as a triangular mass on the posteroanterior projection or from the tricuspid valve to the junction of the infundibulum as a diagonal or wedge-shaped filling defect (Fig. 5-52).

Supravalvular Pulmonary Stenosis

In supravalvular pulmonary stenosis, the pulmonary arteries are hypoplastic and may have segmental focal stenoses. In tetralogy of Fallot, there frequently is mild focal stenosis at the origin of the left and occasionally of the right main pulmonary artery. Occasionally the left pulmonary artery is absent. Rare causes of supravalvular pulmonary stenosis include Williams syndrome, carcinoid syndrome from an abdominal tumor with liver metastases, extrinsic stenoses from mediastinal fibrosis or tumor, and rubella.

These stenoses have a wide spectrum of morphologic appearance, from a short, discrete area of narrowing to long, diffuse hypoplastic segments involving several

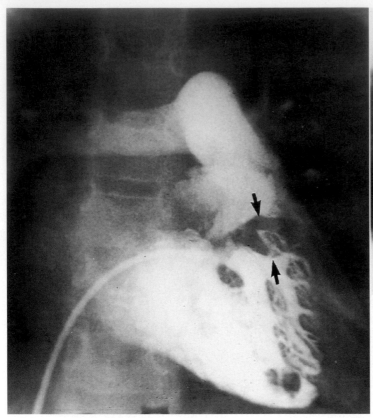

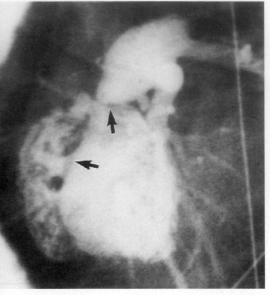

Fig. 5-52 Double-chambered right ventricle. **A,** A muscular bar *(arrows)* extends horizontally from near the tricuspid annulus to the anteroseptal wall and separates the body and infundibular sections of the right ventricle. **B,** A second type of obstructing muscular band *(arrows)* runs vertically on the free wall of the right ventricle and angles across the bottom of the infundibulum.

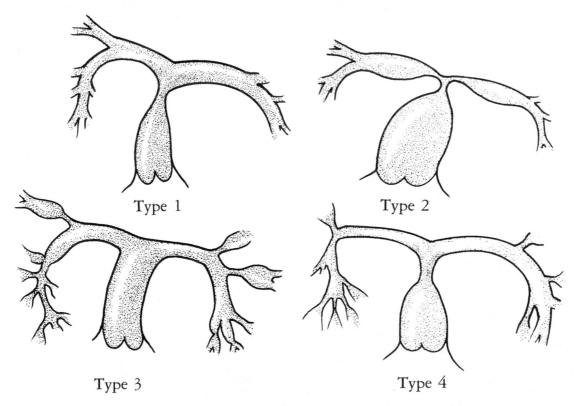

Type 1

Type 2

Type 3

Type 4

Fig. 5-53 Classification of supravalvular pulmonary stenosis. *Type 1* is constriction of the main pulmonary artery. This stenosis can vary from a thin diaphragm to a diffusely hypoplastic artery. *Type 2* is a constriction at the bifurcation of the main pulmonary artery which involves the origins of both the right and left main pulmonary branches. *Type 3* is multiple peripheral stenoses with normal main, right, and left pulmonary arteries. The stenoses usually occur at the origins of peripheral branches and may have poststenotic dilatations. *Type 4* is central and peripheral stenoses. The constrictions are multiple and involve any combination of main, right, and left central arteries with peripheral stenoses. (Modified with permission from Gay BB, Franch RH, Shuford WH et al: The roentgenologic features of single and multiple coarctations of the pulmonary artery and branches, *AJR Am J Roentgenol* 90:599, 1963.)

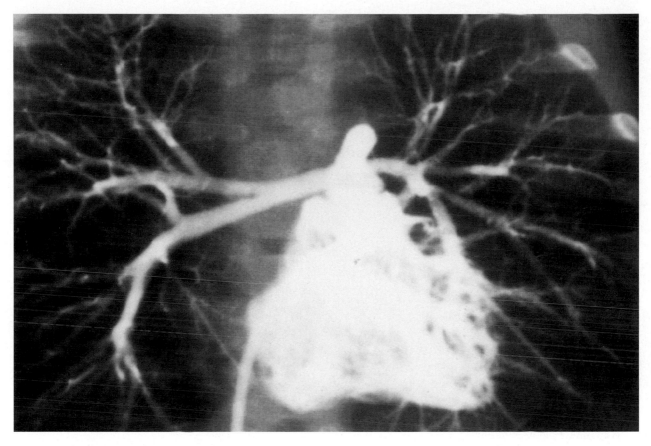

Fig. 5-54   Diffuse hypoplasia of central and peripheral pulmonary arteries.

branches. There may be poststenotic dilatation with variable caliber of the peripheral artery. When evaluating the central variety of pulmonary stenosis at cardiac catheterization, you should use cranial angulation of the beam for the right ventriculogram so that the bifurcation of the main pulmonary artery into the right and left arteries is completely visible. Gay and colleagues have classified the stenoses for surgical therapy according to their location. Type 1 has a single stenosis in the main pulmonary artery. Type 2 occurs at the bifurcation of the main with the right and left pulmonary arteries. Type 3 has only peripheral or branch stenoses. Type 4 is a mixture of the other types (Fig. 5-53).

Diffuse pulmonary artery hypoplasia is a congenital malformation that may occur in isolation or with cardiac anomalies (Fig. 5-54). Centrally located segmental stenoses may be congenital (Fig. 5-55), while peripheral pulmonary arterial stenosis usually are secondary to other diseases (Fig. 5-56). Scarred lung from previous pneumonia, bullous emphysema, recanalized pulmonary emboli, and pulmonary arteritis from Takayasu's disease are common causes.

Acquired supravalvular pulmonary stenosis in the form of pulmonary banding is created intentionally to reduce torrential pulmonary blood flow. The band is correctly

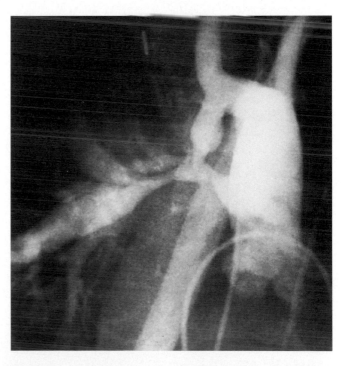

Fig. 5-55   Central pulmonary artery hypoplasia. A Blalock-Taussig shunt (right subclavian artery to right pulmonary artery) is anastomosed to a hypoplastic central pulmonary artery in a patient with pulmonary valve atresia.

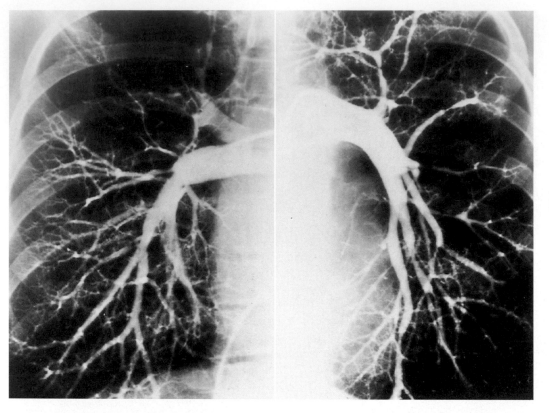

A   **B**

Fig. 5-56   Peripheral pulmonary artery stenosis. Selective injections in the right (**A**) and left (**B**) pulmonary arteries show multiple diffuse stenoses in the smaller parenchymal branches. Several distal branches are occluded.

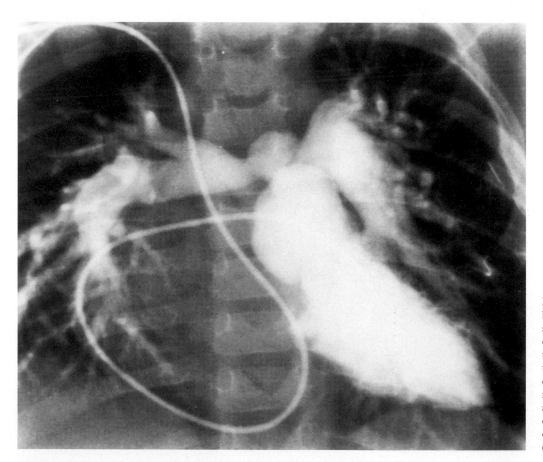

Fig. 5-57   Pulmonary artery bifurcation stenosis. Transposition of the great arteries with congestive heart failure led to the placing of a pulmonary artery band. The band migrated distally, causing stenosis of the main, right, and left pulmonary arteries at the bifurcation. The catheter enters the left ventricle by crossing the atrial septal defect.

positioned above the pulmonary annulus in the main pulmonary artery but may migrate distally causing unwanted branch stenosis (Fig. 5-57). A band placed too close to the pulmonary valve may cause leaflet thickening.

Pulmonary Regurgitation

Pulmonary regurgitation usually is acquired and results from pulmonary arterial hypertension. A congenital cause of pulmonary regurgitation is absence of the pulmonary valve, which is associated with tetralogy of Fallot. This malformation has large pulmonary arteries and a narrow pulmonary annulus creating a stenosis. Conversely, if a patient known to have tetralogy of Fallot paradoxically has large pulmonary arteries, he or she also has pulmonary regurgitation and an absent pulmonary valve.

The general rule that structures on each side of a regurgitant valve dilate is valid in chronic severe pulmonary regurgitation. The right ventricle and the central pulmonary arteries become large.

TRICUSPID VALVE DISEASE

Tricuspid Stenosis

The chest film in tricuspid valve disease is quite variable. The abnormalities in tricuspid stenosis follow the

principle that the chamber behind a severe stenosis is large. Although right atrial enlargement is always seen, the right ventricle and the left heart frequently are also big because tricuspid stenosis is a late sequela of rheumatic mitral stenosis. The superior vena cava and azygos vein are enlarged. In congenital Ebstein anomaly, the film may be strikingly specific with its right atrial and right ventricular enlargement. The right atrium at the junction with the superior vena cava has an unusual rounded appearance (Fig. 5-58). In other types of tricuspid valve disease, the plain film shows nonspecific cardiac enlargement, occasionally with dilatation of the superior and inferior vena cava. In rheumatic heart disease, the features of mitral stenosis predominate: left atrial enlargement and pulmonary artery enlargement. Tricuspid valve calcification rarely may be seen at fluoroscopy. Tricuspid annular calcification has the same causes as mitral annular calcification, namely, dystrophic degeneration from aging and from chronic severe right ventricular hypertension (Fig. 5-59).

Acquired tricuspid stenosis mainly results from rheumatic heart disease, although rare causes are right atrial tumors, the carcinoid syndrome, and pericardial and mediastinal masses external to the heart compressing the tricuspid valve. Rheumatic involvement of the tricuspid valve is invariably associated with enlargement of both the right atrium and right ventricle, thick-

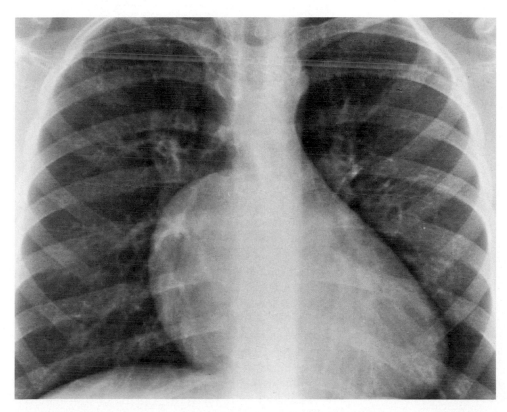

Fig. 5-58 Ebstein anomaly. The round right heart border is a massively enlarged right atrium. A large right ventricle contributes most of the left side and apex of the cardiac silhouette. The pulmonary arteries are slightly enlarged, reflecting the atrial septal defect.

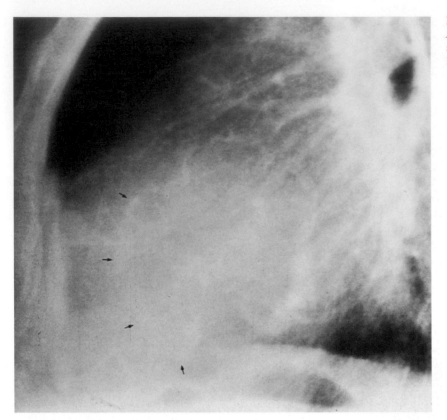

Fig. 5-59 Tricuspid annular calcification. *Arrows* outline the tricuspid annulus. The mitral annulus is also calcified. (Courtesy of Robert E. Dinsmore, M.D.)

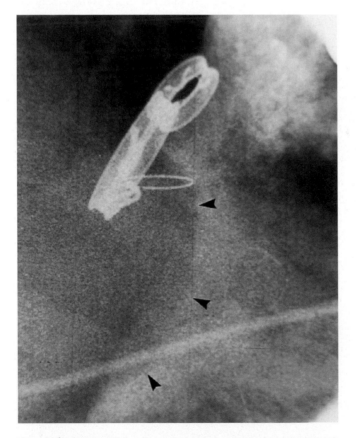

Fig. 5-60 Rheumatic tricuspid stenosis. A right ventriculogram outlines the domed tricuspid valve leaflets *(arrowheads)* in diastole. Bjork-Shiley aortic and mitral valves are present.

Box 5-7   Causes of Tricuspid Stenosis

CONGENITAL

Ebstein anomaly
Isolated tricuspid stenosis

ACQUIRED

Rheumatic heart disease
Carcinoid
Tumors, particularly right atrial myxoma
Endocarditis

ened tricuspid leaflets that have diminished motion, and, occasionally, some nodularity of the chordae. While all these features may indicate rheumatic involvement in the absence of a pressure gradient, doming of the leaflets is consistently found when the stenosis is severe (Fig. 5-60). Unlike stenosis of the semilunar valves, there is rarely a jet of contrast material through a stenotic valve.

Congenital tricuspid stenosis is extremely rare and is associated with severe hypoplasia of the right ventricle.

See Box 5-7 for a summary of the causes of tricuspid stenosis.

Tricuspid Regurgitation

Similar to mitral regurgitation, tricuspid regurgitation occurs when there is an abnormality in one or several parts of the tricuspid apparatus: the annulus, leaflets, chordae, papillary muscles, and right ventricular wall. Dilatation of the right ventricle and the tricuspid annulus secondary to pulmonary artery hypertension from mitral valve disease is the most common cause of acquired regurgitation (Fig. 5-61). When the abnormality causing the right ventricular enlargement is corrected (that is, mitral stenosis), right ventricular size usually returns to normal and the regurgitation ceases.

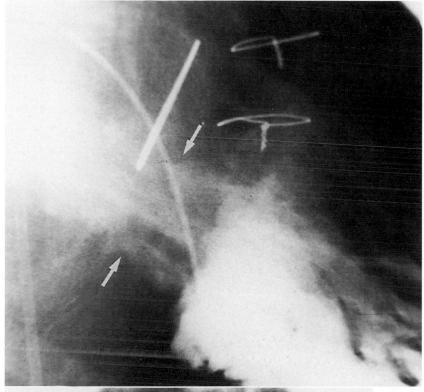

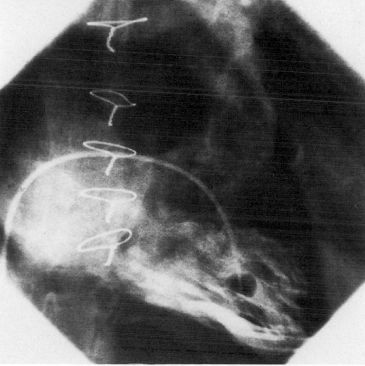

Fig. 5-61 Tricuspid regurgitation. Two patients with tricuspid regurgitation evaluated with right ventriculography. **A,** The jet *(arrows)* of regurgitation is narrower than the tricuspid annulus, suggesting an element of stenosis. **B,** A wide, broad regurgitant stream filled both superior and inferior venae cavae and was grade 3 because the right atrium was more dense than the right ventricle.

The grading of tricuspid regurgitation is similar to that of mitral regurgitation:

Grade 1: Minimal regurgitant jet in systole with rapid clearing

Grade 2: Persistent partial opacification of the entire right atrium

Grade 3: Dense opacification of the right atrium with delayed washout

Grade 4: Right atrium more dense that the right ventricle with filling of the venae cavae

Diseases of the leaflets include rheumatic heart disease, the carcinoid syndrome, infective endocarditis, and trauma. Endocarditis from *Staphylococcus* typically destroys the tricuspid leaflets or causes multiple perforations and small, irregular vegetations on the ventricular side of the leaflets. Infection from *Candida* can produce large fungal tumors that partially obstruct blood flow (Fig. 5-62).

Tricuspid valve prolapse results from redundancy of the leaflets and chordae and occurs in roughly 50% of patients with mitral valve prolapse, with or without Marfan syndrome. The identification of prolapse in the tricuspid valve is identical to that used with the mitral valve. It consists of defining the plane of the tricuspid annulus. Since in systole the normal tricuspid valve leaflets do not extend beyond this plane into the right atrium, when prolapse occurs the tricuspid leaflets move to the right of this plane. These leaflets are large with multiple scallops and may create an eccentric jet, although usually a broad front of the regurgitant stream is visible in the right atrium.

Congenital causes of tricuspid insufficiency involve several parts of the tricuspid apparatus: dysplastic leaflets and chordal attachments without their displacement, Ebstein anomaly with leaflet displacement, or pulmonary atresia with an intact ventricular septum. Right ventricular infarction with ischemia or rupture of the papillary muscles appears as an akinetic or dyskinetic motion of the anterior, diaphragmatic, or septal walls of the right ventricle and is frequently associated with rupture of the interventricular septum.

See Box 5-8 for a summary of the causes of tricuspid regurgitation.

Ebstein Anomaly

Ebstein anomaly of the tricuspid valve is an uncommon malformation that may result in stenosis or regurgi-

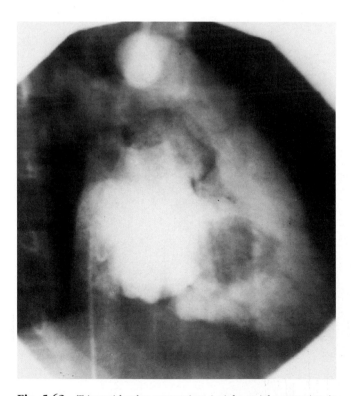

Fig. 5-62   Tricuspid valve vegetation. A right atrial vegetation is outlined as a large circular mass attached to the tricuspid leaflets. A vegetation this large in the setting of endocarditis is typical of *Candida.*

Box 5-8   Causes of Tricuspid Regurgitation

LEAFLET

   Ebstein anomaly
   Carcinoid
   Rheumatic
   Prolapse syndrome
   Endocarditis
   Trauma
   Systemic lupus erythematosus
   Right atrial myxoma
   Cleft leaflet in atrioventricular canal defect
   Tumor deposit
   Dysplastic valve

CHORDAE

   Rupture from trauma, infection, congenital malformation, or cystic medical necrosis

PAPILLARY MUSCLE

   Rupture from ischemia or infarct

ANNULUS

   Right ventricular dilatation from any cause
   Marfan syndrome

RIGHT VENTRICULAR WALL

   Papillary muscle dysfunction from ischemia, infarct, or aneurysm
   Idiopathic hypertrophic subaortic stenosis

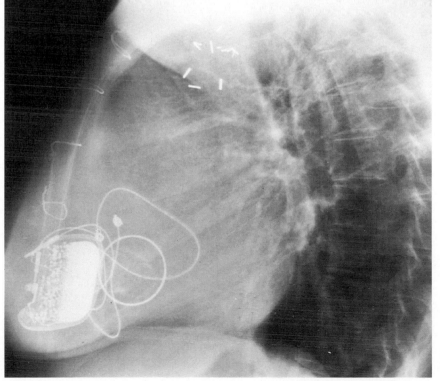

Fig. 5-63 Ebstein anomaly. A Hancock porcine tricuspid valve replacement and a surgically implanted epicardial cardiac pacemaker indicate that this patient had tricuspid stenosis or regurgitation and arrhythmias—complications of Ebstein anomaly. **A,** The right atrium is large because of its projection into the right lung and the distance between the tricuspid valve and the lateral right atrial wall. **B,** The retrosternal space is filled in by the large right ventricle.

tation, or both. In most instances, there is an atrial septal defect or patent foramen ovale. The major anatomic features include displacement of the valve leaflets and their attachments toward the apex of the right ventricle, an "atrialized" portion of the right ventricle between the atrioventricular groove and the leaflet attachment, and dilatation of the right ventricle.

The attachment of the tricuspid leaflets is quite variable; a portion of the septal and posterior cusps usually adheres to the right ventricular wall. The large, redundant anterior leaflet originates several millimeters to several centimeters apically from the atrioventricular groove. Because of this displacement, the chordae tendineae and papillary muscles are also abnormal, ranging from those that are invisible angiographically to a discrete cylindrical muscle mass. The doming of the leaflets has a sail-like appearance during ventricular diastole. In extreme cases, the redundant leaflets may occlude the infundibulum during diastole.

The plain film of the chest in Ebstein anomaly shows a cardiac silhouette that varies from normal to strikingly enlarged. You should suspect this anomaly when you detect right atrial and right ventricular dilatation (Figs. 5-58 and 5-63). The contour of the large right atrium is round and occupies the right cardiac border. It is continuous with the superior vena cava and the right hemidiaphragm in the posteroanterior view. Dilatation

of the right ventricle ordinarily is most visible on a lateral projection. However, if enlargement is massive, the right ventricle will contact the sternum and rotate the entire heart leftward. The result of this motion is that the frontal film will show a convexity in the upper cardiac border which is not the left atrial appendage but rather the right ventricular outflow tract. Further dilatation of the right ventricle can cause it to become the entire left heart border. The size of the pulmonary vessels tends to reflect the amount of blood flowing through them. In those with atrial septal defects and moderate left-to-right shunts, the vascular markings are slightly large; in cyanotic patients with right-to-left flow across the interatrial shunt, the vessels tend to be small because of tricuspid stenosis .

You can make the angiographic diagnosis if the notch of the atrioventricular groove is separate from the displaced leaflet attachments (Figs. 5-64 and 5-65). This "atrialized" portion of the right ventricle is on the right atrial side of the tricuspid leaflets; it beats synchronously with the remainder of the ventricle because this segment contains contractile ventricular muscle. Occasionally, the wall of the atrialized portion of the ventricle may be only a fibrous sac and therefore be akinetic. The dilatation of the right atrium and right ventricle reflects the degree of tricuspid stenosis and regurgitation.

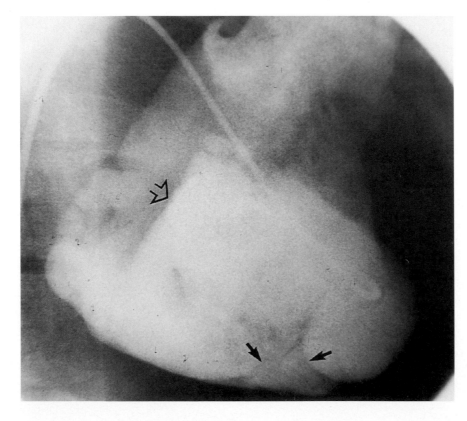

Fig. 5-64 Displaced tricuspid valve leaflets. The *closed arrows* point to the leaflet attachment, which is displaced from the tricuspid annulus *(open arrow)* by 4 cm. Note the large size of the annulus and the poor clearing of contrast media from the right ventricle.

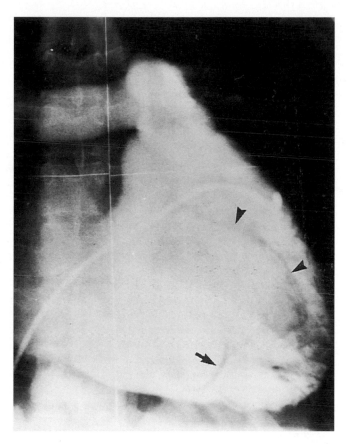

Fig. 5-65 Billowing anterior leaflet in Ebstein anomaly. The anterior leaflet *(arrowheads)* extends into the outflow tract during systole. The posterior leaflet *(arrow)* is apically displaced. The dilated right ventricle forms the entire left border of the cardiac silhouette.

Patients with congenitally corrected transposition and a posteriorly placed right ventricle may have an associated Ebstein anomaly. Tricuspid regurgitation in congenitally corrected transposition should always raise the suspicion of a left-sided Ebstein anomaly; however, the tricuspid leaflet attachment in congenitally corrected transposition without Ebstein anomaly has slight apical displacement so subtle degrees of the leaflet malformation may not be apparent.

Other Imaging Findings

Other imaging modalities nicely show the involvement of the different parts of the tricuspid apparatus Two-dimensional echocardiography is the examination of choice for detecting the stenosis and quantitating the regurgitation with Doppler study. Imaging tumors, vegetations, mediastinal abnormalities, and Ebstein anomaly is easy with MRI, which has the advantage of showing the adjacent pericardium and mediastinum, as well as demonstrating the regurgitant jet on magnetic resonance cineangiography.

SUGGESTED READINGS

Books

Davies MJ: *Pathology of cardiac valves,* Boston, 1980, Butterworth.

Higgins CB: *Essentials of cardiac radiology and imaging,* Philadelphia, 1992, JB Lippincott.

Journals

Anderson RP, Hartmann AF Jr, Aker U, et al: Tricuspid valve prolapse with late systolic tricuspid insufficiency, *Radiology* 107:309, 1973.

Barlow JB, Pocok WA, Promund Obel IW: Mitral valve prolapse: primary, secondary, both or neither? *Am Heart J* 102:140, 1981.

Carey LS, Sellers RD, Shone JD: Radiology findings in the developmental complex of parachute mitral valve, supravalvular ring of left atrium, subaortic stenosis and coarctation of aorta, *Radiology* 82:1, 1964.

Carlsson E, Gross R, Holt RG: The radiological diagnosis of cardiac valvar insufficiencies, *Circulation* 55:921, 1977.

Castaneda-Zuniga WR, Formanek A, Amplatz K: Radiologic diagnosis of different types of pulmonary stenosis, *Cardiovasc Radiol* 1:45, 1978.

Davachi F, Moller JH, Edwards JE: Diseases of the mitral valve in infancy: an anatomic analysis of 55 cases, *Circulation* 43:565, 1971.

Dee PM, Hubbell MM, Rheuban KS, et al: Congenital absence of the pulmonary valve, *Cardiovasc Intervent Radiol* 4:158, 1981.

Desilets DT, Marcano BA, Emmanoulides GC, et al: Severe pulmonary valve stenosis and atresia, *Radiol Clin North Am* 6:367, 1968.

Dinsmore RE, Miller SW: Angiography in acquired valvular heart disease, *Semin Roentgenol* 14:153, 1979.

Fellows KE, Martin EC, Rosenthal A: Angiocardiography of obstructing muscular bands of the right ventricle, *AJR Am J Roentgenol* 128:249, 1977.

Fisher CH, James AE, Humphries JO, et al: Radiographic findings in anomalous muscle bundle of the right ventricle: an analysis of 15 cases, *Radiology* 101:35, 1971.

Freedom RM, Culham JAG, Rowe RD: Angiocardiography of subaortic obstruction in infancy, *AJR Am J Roentgenol* 129:813, 1977.

Gay BB Jr, Franch RH, Shuford WH, et al: The roentgenologic features of single and multiple coarctations of the pulmonary artery and branches, *AJR Am J Roentgenol* 90:599, 1963.

Jeffery RF, Moller JH, Amplatz K: The dysplastic pulmonary valve: a new roentgenographic entity, *AJR Am J Roentgenol* 114:322, 1972.

Katz NM, Buckley MJ, Liberthson RR: Discrete membranous subaortic stenosis. Report of 31 patients, review of the literature, and delineation of management, *Circulation* 56:1034, 1977.

Kelley MJ, Higgins CB, Kirkpatrick SE: Axial left ventriculography in discrete subaortic stenosis, *Radiology* 135:77, 1980.

Lachman AS, Roberts WC: Calcific deposits in stenotic mitral valves. Extent and relation to age, sex, degree of stenosis, cardiac rhythm, previous commissurotomy and left atrial body thrombus from study of 164 operatively-excised valves, *Circulation* 57:808, 1978.

Link KM, Herrera MA, D'Souza VJ, et al: MR imaging of Ebstein anomaly: results in four cases, *AJR Am J Roentgenol* 150:363-367, 1988.

Marin-Garcia J, Tandon R, Lucas RV Jr, et al: Cor triatriatum: study of 20 cases, *Am J Cardiol* 35:59, 1975.

Marks AR, Choomg CY, Sanfilippo AJ, et al: Identification of high-risk and low-risk subgroups of patients with mitral-valve prolapse, *N Engl J Med* 330:1031, 1989.

Miller SW, Dinsmore RE: Aortic root abscess resulting from endocarditis: spectrum of angiographic findings, *Radiology* 153:357, 1984.

Nestico PF, Depace NL, Morganroth J, et al: Mitral annular calcification: clinical, pathophysiology, and echocardiographic review, *Am Heart J* 107:989, 1984

Numan F, Islak C, Berkman T, et al: Behçet disease: pulmonary artery involvement in 15 cases, *Radiology* 192:465, 1994.

Osterberger LE, Goldstein S, Khaka F, et al: Functional mitral stenosis in patients with massive mitral annular calcification, *Circulation* 64:472, 1981.

Pellikka PA, Tajik AJ, Khandheria BK, et al: Carcinoid heart disease. Clinical and echocardiographic spectrum in 74 patients, *Circulation* 87:1188, 1993.

Pflugfelder PW, Landzberg JS, Cassidy MM, et al: Comparison of cine MR imaging with Doppler echocardiography for the evaluation of aortic regurgitation, *AJR Am J Roentgenol* 152:729, 1989.

Pflugfelder PW, Sechtem UP, White RD, et al: Noninvasive evaluation of mitral regurgitation by analysis of left atrial signal loss in cine magnetic resonance, *Am Heart J* 117:1113, 1989.

Ranganthan N, Silver MD, Robinson TI, et al: Idiopathic prolapsed mitral leaflet syndrome. Angiographic-clinical correlations, *Circulation* 54:707, 1976.

Roberts WC: The congenitally bicuspid aortic valve: a study of 85 autopsy cases, *Am J Cardiol* 26:72, 1970.

Roberts WC: Valvular, subvalvular, and supravalvular aortic stenosis. Morphologic features, *Cardiovasc Clin* 5:104, 1973.

Roberts WC: Morphologic features of the normal and abnormal mitral valve, *Am J Cardiol* 51:1005, 1983.

Roberts WC, Morrow AG, McIntosh CL, et al: Congenitally bicuspid aortic valve causing severe, pure aortic regurgitation without superimposed infective endocarditis. Analysis of 13 patients requiring aortic valve replacement, *Am J Cardiol* 47:206, 1981.

Roberts WC, Perloff JK: A clinicopathologic survey of the conditions causing the mitral valve to function abnormally, *Ann Intern Med* 77:939, 1972.

Sechtem U, Pflugfelder PW, Cassidy MM, et al: Mitral or aortic regurgitation: quantitation of regurgitant volumes with cine MR imaging, *Radiology* 167:425, 1988.

Selzer A: Changing aspects of the natural history of valvular aortic stenosis, *N Engl J Med* 317:91, 1987.

Spindola-Franco H, Fish BG, Dachman A, et al: Recognition of bicuspid aortic valve by plain film calcification, *AJR Am J Roentgenol* 139:867, 1982.

Wagner S, Auffermann W, Buser P, et al: Diagnostic accuracy and estimation of the severity of valvular regurgitation from the signal void in cine MR, *Am Heart J* 1178:760, 1989.

Ischemic Heart Disease
  Chest radiograph
    Pulmonary edema
    Heart size
    Aneurysms and ruptures
    Pericardial effusion
  Coronary angiography
    Uses and analysis
    Progression of atherosclerosis
  Extent and location of stenoses
    Common lesion sites
    Left main equivalent disease
  Morphology of coronary atherosclerosis
    Angiographic appearance
    Grading system
    Relationship to coronary syndrome
    Myocardial infarctions
    Other causes of stenosis
  Interpretation of arterial stenoses on angiography
    Determining severity
  Determinants of coronary blood flow
    Normal flow
    Transient variations
    Flow reserve
    Effects of stenosis length and diameter
    Cumulative effects of stenosis
  Coronary collateral vessels
    Significance and development
    Angiographic appearance
  Coronary artery spasm
    Angiographic appearance
    Catheter-induced vs. Prinzmetal syndrome
  Coronary aneurysms
    Causes
  Myocardial bridging
  Coronary dissection
Congenital Anomalies of the Coronary Arteries
  Anomalies of origin

Anomalies of origin and course
    Tetralogy of Fallot
  Anomalies of termination
    Complications
Coronary Bypass Grafting
  Internal mammary artery grafts
  Saphenous vein grafts
    Complications
  Imaging techniques
Left Ventricular Abnormalities in Coronary Disease
  Ventriculogram analysis
    Projection
    Heart rate
    Symmetry
Segmental Wall Motion Abnormalities With and Without Coronary Disease
  Regional wall motion
  Correlation with coronary artery disease
  Factors influencing wall motion
  Left ventricular thrombus
    Calcifications
    Other filling defects
  Left ventricular true and false aneurysm
    Definition and pathologic correlation
    Imaging signs of aneurysm
    False aneurysm
Ventriculography After Aneurysm Resection
Rupture of the Interventricular Septum
  Clinical presentation
  Left ventricular signs
Mitral Regurgitation Resulting from Coronary Artery Disease
  Pathologic causes
  Ventriculographic signs
Suggested Readings

Most coronary artery disease is caused by obstruction in the coronary arteries from atherosclerosis and coronary thrombosis. In the United States nearly 1.5 million people have an acute myocardial infarction annually, a cause of about one fourth of all deaths. Ischemic heart disease consists of those diseases in which blood flow to the myocardium is inadequate to supply normal oxygenation requirements. Signs of coronary artery disease are stable and unstable angina pectoris, acute myocardial infarction, and the complications of inadequate coronary flow, such as arrhythmias, congestive heart failure, ventricular aneurysms, mitral regurgitation, and emboli from left ventricular thrombus. The goals of imaging in patients with coronary artery disease are several: to detect latent arterial obstructions before symptoms appear, to evaluate left ventricular function, to map the location and extent of plaques in the coronary arteries, to evaluate complications like mitral regurgitation and septal rupture, and to judge plaque morphology with an eye to planning medical or surgical relief.

ISCHEMIC HEART DISEASE

Chest Radiograph

The initial plain chest film in patients undergoing acute myocardial infarction is obtained to search for signs of left ventricular failure and to screen for some of the complications of infarction. Nearly half the patients admitted to a coronary care unit have radiologic signs of pulmonary venous hypertension within the first 24 hours after an acute myocardial infarction. Even though many films are taken with portable technique in the supine position, the signs of pulmonary edema have a rather good correlation with the pulmonary capillary wedge pressure. The usual caveat, that low lung volumes can mimic signs of pulmonary edema, is appropriate. Indistinct hilar structures represent early vasculature engorgement and dilatation of the rich mediastinal lymphatics. You will occasionally see dilatation of upper lobe vessels even on supine films before the reticular pattern of interstitial edema develops. The width of the vascular pedicle above and adjacent to the aortic arch is frequently a good indicator of the intravascular volume. Increase in the size of the azygos vein and superior vena cava on serial films suggest the increase in intravascular blood volume and the need for treatment of left ventricular failure.

Pulmonary edema

At times the assessment of pulmonary edema on the chest film does not correlate with the pulmonary capillary wedge pressure. Many variables may be involved including low lung volumes, supine position, layered pleural effusions, and pneumonia. The amount of pulmonary edema seen on the chest film reflects a different hemodynamic parameter than does the pulmonary

artery catheter. The pulmonary capillary wedge pressure is the instantaneous left ventricular end-diastolic pressure. Conversely, the chest film reflects changes in lung water over periods of several hours to a couple of days. If the patient had several episodes of "flash" pulmonary edema during the last several hours, which was subsequently treated and reversed, the lungs still have excess water which has not been carried off by the lymphatic system and other drainage pathways. The therapeutic lag in the chest film findings indicates that the chest film is an average or integral of the lung water status over many hours while the pulmonary artery catheter reflects current left atrial pressure, not the status of the intravascular volume. These facts have important clinical implications because wet lungs have decreased compliance and cause increased breathing effort even when the pulmonary capillary pressure is normal.

Heart size

Initially, most patients undergoing myocardial infarction have a normal heart size. The assessment of an enlarged heart on a supine portable chest film is rather inaccurate and usually not necessary for clinical management. Severe cardiomegaly generally indicates longstanding coronary artery disease with previous infarction or with a major complication (Fig. 6-1).

Aneurysms and ruptures

In addition to chronic left ventricular failure, left ventricular enlargement may also be the result of a true or false aneurysm, chronic mitral regurgitation, or rarely cardiac rupture. Heart enlargement is not a feature of acute mitral regurgitation or rupture of the interventricular septum because the left ventricle needs several hours to several days to dilate enough to be visible on the chest film. The most frequent site of a true left ventricular aneurysm is in the anterolateral and apical wall. Although left ventricular aneurysms may involve any wall segment, aneurysms in the posterolateral wall are frequently false aneurysms. A false left ventricular aneurysm exists when the left ventricle ruptures into a site of previous pericardial adhesions so that the rupture is contained by the pericardium. An increase in size of the left ventricular aneurysm on serial studies is suggestive of a false aneurysm and warrants urgent, definitive evaluation. Calcification of the anterolateral and apical region of the left ventricle usually takes several years after the myocardial infarction that produced the scarring (Fig. 6-2).

Both the papillary muscle rupture and rupture of the interventricular septum produce nearly identical findings on the chest radiograph. Both complications typically have moderate interstitial pulmonary edema with mild enlargement of the pulmonary arteries. There is a mild increase in heart size with signs of enlargement of all four cardiac chambers.

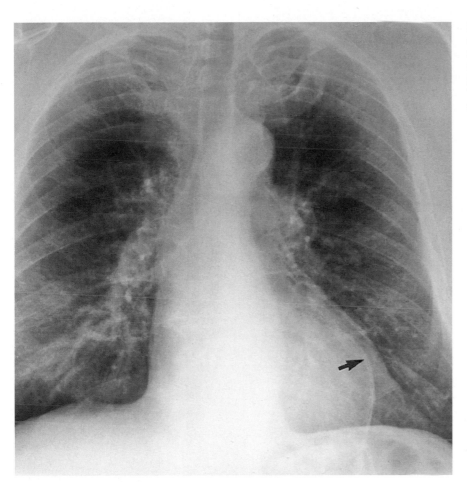

Fig. 6-1 Large left ventricular scar. The arc of calcium *(arrow)* along the anterolateral and apical walls of the left ventricle denotes dystrophic changes in a large scar of several years' duration. The anterolateral wall is thin. There is no outward bulge to indicate an aneurysm.

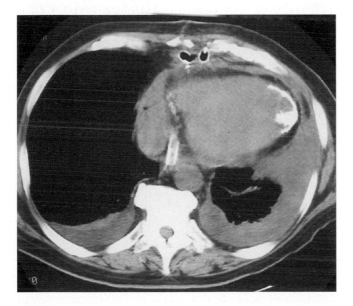

Fig. 6-2 Computed tomography scan of calcified left ventricular apex. The linear calcification at the left ventricular apex is in an old infarct. The polypoid component represents a calcified thrombus. The patient recently had a coronary bypass operation so that anterior mediastinal and pericardial drains, a small pericardial effusion, and bilateral effusions are present.

Pericardial effusion

Pericardial effusion is common after acute myocardial infarction and is seen in about 25% of patients with echocardiography. This small amount of fluid is not visible on chest films but can be inferred if pleural effusions are visible. A large amount of pericardial fluid may result from either hemorrhagic pericarditis, or from cardiac tamponade due to ventricular rupture. Dressler syndrome usually occurs 2 to 10 weeks after infarction, and is manifest on the chest film as pleural effusions, areas of patchy airspace disease, and a large cardiac silhouette.

Coronary Angiography

Uses and analysis

Coronary angiography is used mainly to identify atherosclerotic coronary stenosis and, less often, congenital anomalies and manifestations of other diseases. Each coronary artery is opacified so that its origin, course, and termination are visualized at least in two orthogonal projections. The orthogonal projections are necessary because atherosclerotic stenoses tend to be eccentric; a minor plaque in one projection may appear as a major stenosis in the opposite oblique view (Fig. 6-3). The analysis of a coronary arteriogram for coronary artery disease consists of four tasks. First, the extent and location of stenoses need to be determined. Second, the severity of each stenosis is graded so that a clinical decision can be made regarding both treatment and prognosis. Third, the morphology of the atherosclerotic plaque is graded. Fourth, the size of the vessel distal to the stenosis is evaluated to see if it is a suitable recipient for a bypass graft.

Progression of atherosclerosis

Coronary atherosclerosis begins as lipid deposition in the arterial wall, which appears grossly as a raised, fatty streak. As the lesion progresses, a fibrous cap develops over the endothelial lipid deposit. Disruption of an atherosclerotic plaque results in fissuring and intraluminal thrombosis (Fig. 6-4). The thrombus may lead to intermittent vessel occlusion and unstable angina. Large ulcers at the site of the plaque can cause formation of a fixed thrombus and a chronic occlusion resulting in acute myocardial infarction. Severe stenoses tend to progress to total occlusion about three times more frequently than less severe lesions. Rupture of the coronary vasa vasorum with hemorrhage within the plaque may contribute to plaque disruption (Fig. 6-5).

In patients with unstable angina most coronary stenoses are only of moderate degree. It is the mild to

moderate coronary stenosis that commonly precedes most coronary occlusions in patients with unstable angina. Angiography during acute myocardial infarction usually shows a thrombus in the infarct-related artery. After thrombolysis, many of these patients have an underlying

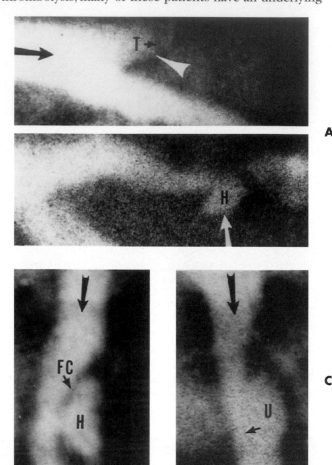

Fig. 6-4 Highly magnified arteriographic images of structurally unstable plaques causing unstable angina or myocardial infarction. **A,** This left anterior descending coronary artery is acutely occluded; 24 hours after intravenous tissue-type plasminogen activator (t-PA), the thrombotic component (*T*) of obstruction is lysed, revealing a pocket of contrast (*H*) protruding beyond the lumen boundaries into presumed plaque and fed through a narrow-necked fissure. This appears to be the arteriographic counterpart of the hemorrhagic pocket (*H*) in Fig. **B. B,** Angiographically visualized plaque hemorrhage. Bleeding into the lipid-rich core of the plaque appears to have formed a hemorrhagic pocket (*H*) that has driven the thin fibrous cap (*FC*) into the lumen, progressively obstructing it. The opposite wall has been remodeled, curving outward to preserve lumen size in the face of the expanding plaque. On cineangiography, contrast enters this pocket from the lumen via small breaks or channels at its upstream shoulder and exits from the middle. **C,** A large ulcer (*U*) is seen after t-PA for unstable angina. This image appears to have been created by full-length erosion or eruption of the fibrous cap, of which only a thin arteriographic vestige remains *(arrow)*. (Reprinted with permission from Brown G, Zhao XQ, Sacco DE, et al: Lipid lowering and plaque regression. New insights into prevention of plaque disruption and clinical events in coronary disease, *Circulation* 87:1781-1791, 1993.)

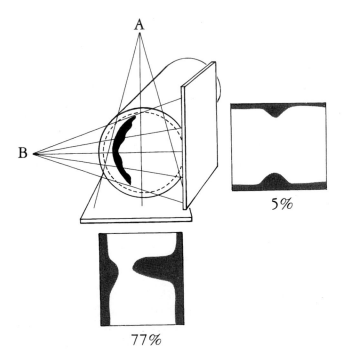

Fig. 6-3 Coronary angiography must be performed in two orthogonal projections because the atherosclerotic lesion is eccentric. In **A** the lumen projects a 77% stenosis, while in **B** only a 5% stenosis is seen.

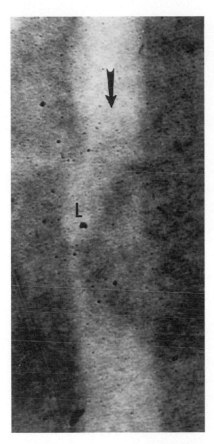 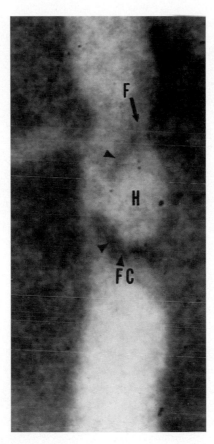 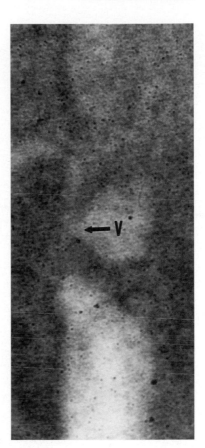

Fig. 6-5 Sequential highly magnified images of the flow of contrast through a right coronary artery plaque disrupted by apparent hemorrhage into its core lipid region. Direction of blood flow is indicated by *large arrow*. Filling and washout of this hemorrhagic intramural pocket (*H*) is delayed relative to flow through the severely narrowed native lumen (*L*). Contrast enters the pocket by the way of an upstream fissure (*F*) and exits via a vent (*V*) at the center of the displaced fibrous cap (*FC*). (Reprinted with permission from Brown G, Zhao XQ, Sacco DE, et al: Lipid lowering and plaque regression: new insights into prevention of plaque disruption and clinical events in coronary disease, *Circulation* 87:1781-1791, 1993.)

lesion with less than 70% stenosis. Those stenoses that later progress usually have eccentric shapes with overhanging edges and are thought to represent plaque disruption. Therefore, the state of the atherosclerotic plaque—whether it is covered with a fibrin cap or has deep fissures which may lead to thrombus—is an important angiographic observation.

Current imaging techniques for ischemic heart disease are used increasingly to differentiate viable from nonviable myocardium in patients with coronary artery disease and left ventricular dysfunction. Acute coronary occlusion generally results in reduced regional myocardial contraction. An acute reduction of blood flow of 80% below a control value in a coronary artery causes akinesis in that segment of the left ventricle, while a 95% reduction causes dyskinesis. Akinesis of a segment of the left ventricle, however, does not reliably distinguish viable myocardium from scar. After reversal of a brief episode of severe ischemia, the abnormal wall segment may return to its normal contractile state, a condition

termed *myocardial stunning. Myocardial hibernation* is a related state in which left ventricular wall motion returns to normal after relief of the ischemia by angioplasty or grafting. These two conditions of reversible left ventricular dysfunction are important to recognize because vigorous treatment of the thrombus or spasm in myocardial stunning and relief of the obstruction in myocardial hibernation may reverse the impaired ventricular performance and potentially salvage the jeopardized myocardium.

Extent and Location of Stenoses

Common lesion sites

Most coronary stenoses occur in the proximal portion of both arteries. The distribution of lesions is rather uniform in the three major arteries. The distribution of coronary stenoses with greater than 50% stenosis is: right coronary artery, 36%; left circumflex artery, 28%; left anterior descending artery, 33%; and left main artery, 3%.

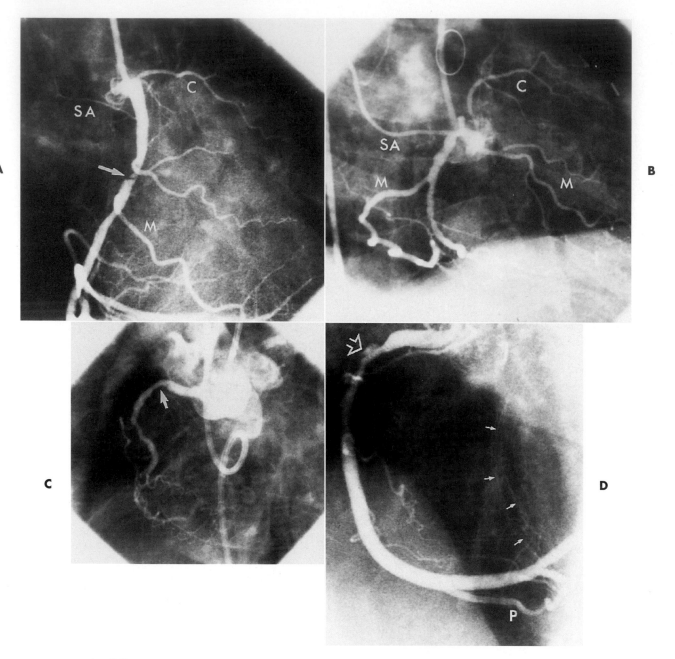

Fig. 6-6 Right coronary stenoses. **A,** In the right anterior oblique view, there is a tapering stenosis ending in an ulcerated plaque *(arrow)* after the second right ventricular marginal branch. **B,** The caudal right anterior oblique view shows diffuse, mildly irregular plaques in the right ventricular marginal branch and distal right coronary artery. **C,** In the left anterior oblique view a nondominant right coronary artery has a proximal 50% stenosis *(arrow)* followed by mild diffuse disease. **D,** A proximal 75% stenosis has a large ulcer *(open arrow)*. Slightly visible collaterals go to septal branches of the left anterior descending artery *(arrows)*. C = conus artery; *SA* = sinoatrial nodal artery; *M* = right ventricular marginal artery; *P* = posterior descending artery.

In the right coronary artery, most severe stenoses develop in its proximal half, although there are occasional severe plaques at the bifurcation of the posterior descending and posterior left ventricular arteries (Fig. 6-6). The right ventricular marginal branch frequently has a severe stenosis at its origin.

The left main coronary artery should not taper. It is usually narrowed either at its ostium or at the bifurcation of the left anterior descending and circumflex arteries. Occasionally, the entire main arterial segment may be uniformly narrowed, but usually one of its ends is more severely involved. Detection of plaques in this segment is

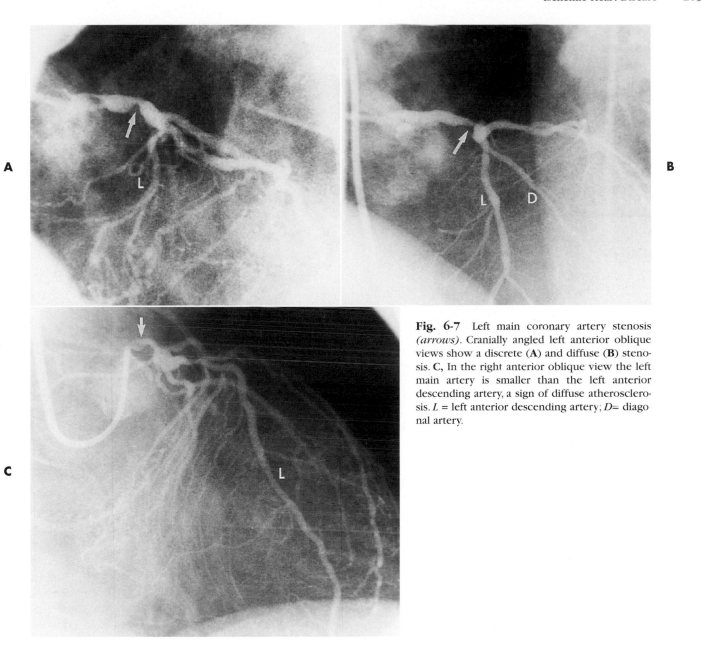

Fig. 6-7 Left main coronary artery stenosis *(arrows)*. Cranially angled left anterior oblique views show a discrete (**A**) and diffuse (**B**) stenosis. **C,** In the right anterior oblique view the left main artery is smaller than the left anterior descending artery, a sign of diffuse atherosclerosis. *L* = left anterior descending artery; *D*= diagonal artery.

particularly important because severe lesions are associated with an increased mortality during cardiac catheterization (Fig. 6-7).

Left main equivalent disease

"Left main equivalent disease" describes the combination of stenoses that would cause a decrease in blood supply similar to that caused by a single stenosis in the left main coronary artery. This concept is applied so that a stenosis at the origin of both the left anterior descending and left circumflex arteries is not a left main equivalent. Either of these stenoses may become more severe but may follow a separate time course. Occlusion of one of these would not result in as large an area of myocardium

becoming ischemic as would a single event in the left main coronary artery. An example of a left main equivalent lesion would be a severe left anterior descending artery stenosis when an occluded right coronary artery is supplied by collaterals from the left anterior descending artery. Here one lesion controls the blood supply to the bulk of the heart. A similar example would be a stenosis in a long left anterior descending artery that extends completely around the apex in place of the usual posterior descending artery. Here also a significant percentage of myocardium is affected by a single stenosis.

Clinically, loss of 40% of the left ventricular myocardium produces cardiogenic shock. A left main or left main equivalent coronary stenosis usually affects this much of

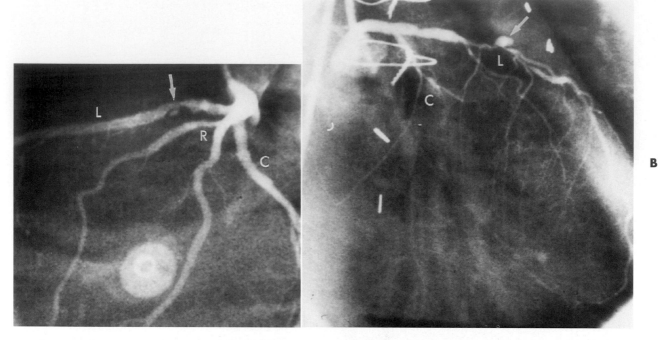

Fig. 6-8   Left anterior descending artery stenoses *(arrows)*. **A,** The lateral projection shows a 50% stenosis associated with a small inferior ulcer in the proximal left anterior descending artery. **B,** A tapering 90% stenosis in the middle segment of the left anterior descending artery has a small superior aneurysm. The left circumflex is occluded after a small first marginal branch. *L* = left anterior descending artery; *R* = ramus medianus; *C* = left circumflex artery.

the myocardium. If collateral vessels supply an adequate perfusion to an occluded vessel, other combinations of coronary stenoses may produce a situation in which one lesion controls the blood supply to a major portion of the left ventricle.

In the left anterior descending artery, stenoses before or after the first large septal branch may have different clinical implications. Patients with chronic stable angina who have a severe stenosis before the first septal branch have a statistically higher mortality when compared with patients who have a stenosis distal to this branch (Fig. 6-8). The first septal branch can supply nearly half of the interventricular septum, a very contractile portion of the ventricle, and is closely related to the conduction system. A stenosis before the first septal branch also frequently involves a large diagonal branch which supplies a portion of the lateral wall. This correlation does not hold in unstable angina pectoris, where there is no association between severe plaques before and after the first septal branch.

Morphology of Coronary Atherosclerosis

Angiographic appearance

The angiographic appearance of coronary atherosclerosis ranges from a single focal plaque to multiple diffuse stenoses with eccentric and ulcerated margins. Isolated stenoses usually are discrete irregularities in the vessel wall, rarely more than 10 mm long. Multiple focal stenoses may be present in series with one another. Diffuse atherosclerosis is occasionally difficult to recognize because no normal-sized vessel is adjacent to the narrowing for comparison.

Atherosclerotic plaques tend to have eccentric and sharp edges which help distinguish them from spasm, which is usually smooth and fusiform. Thrombus within the artery may be distinguished from plaques if contrast medium flows on both sides of the lucency (Fig. 6-9). Occlusive thrombi may be impossible to distinguish from a fibrosed artery, but sharp, slanting edges are more typical of thrombus.

Grading system

Plaque morphology can be analyzed by location, shape, and severity (Box 6-1). Each lesion is resolved into length, calcification, involvement of major branches, presence of adjacent thrombus, tortuosity of the involved segment, and eccentricity of the plaque edges.

Relationship to coronary syndrome

Both clinical and angiographic studies have confirmed that angiographic morphology is correlated with unstable coronary syndromes. Simple plaques with a smooth fibrous covering, smooth borders, and an hour-

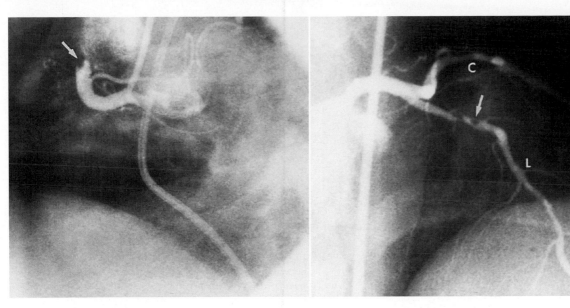

Fig. 6-9 Coronary thrombus *(arrows)*. **A,** In the left anterior oblique view the right coronary artery is occluded by a thrombus. Contrast medium tracks on both sides of the filling defect. **B,** Thrombus has formed on the downstream side of a severe left anterior descending artery stenosis. The angiogram is a cranial right anterior oblique projection. *L* = left anterior descending artery; *C* = left circumflex artery.

glass configuration are associated with stable angina. Complex lesions with plaque rupture, intraplaque hemorrhage, and irregular borders in eccentric stenoses are associated with unstable angina and myocardial infarction (Fig. 6-10).

Myocardial infarctions

Multiple myocardial infarctions result from extensive coronary disease and occur with greater frequency in persons with diabetes. You are more likely to find a decreased ejection fraction in patients with diabetes mellitus, but patients with diabetes and those without do not differ significantly in number and extent of severe stenosis. Type II hyperlipoproteinemia is associated with extensive coronary calcifications and severe involvement of the distal distribution of the coronary arteries (Fig. 6-11). These patients may have an unusual edge in the left sinus of Valsalva at the ostium of the left coronary artery which can make catherization difficult. Patients with type IV hyperlipoproteinemia have a distribution of stenoses similar to that in patients with normal lipid findings.

Other causes of stenosis

There are many causes of coronary stenosis other than atherosclerosis. Frequently, the cause can only be determined by clinical correlation with a systemic disease (Box 6-2). Even then, in the adult age range, it is often impossible to exclude coexisting atherosclerosis (Fig. 6-12). The clinical constellation of chest pain, a positive exercise test, and a normal coronary arteriogram is referred to as syndrome X. The cause of the syndrome is unknown, is not related to large vessel spasm, and may

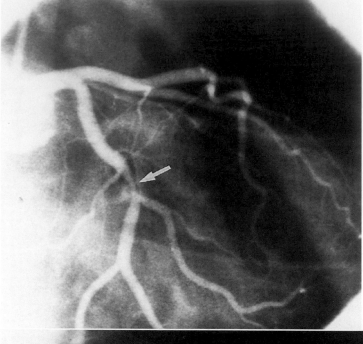

A

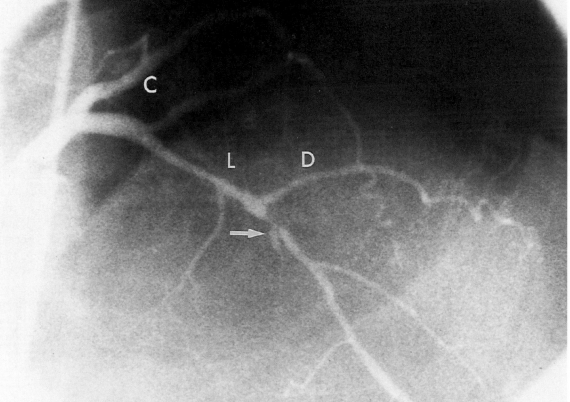

B

Fig. 6-10   Simple and complex stenoses *(arrows)*. **A,** The left circumflex artery has a smooth, tapering symmetric stenosis before the first marginal branch in the caudal right oblique view. **B,** The left anterior descending artery has a complex stenosis after the second diagonal branch, which is eccentric and ulcerated in the cranial right anterior oblique projection. *L* = left anterior descending artery; *C* = left circumflex artery; *D* = diagonal artery.

be related to abnormalities in precapillary vessels that are too small to be seen with coronary angiography. In contrast, myocardial infarction can occur with a normal coronary arteriogram. This event is rare and has been caused by thrombosis with recanalization, coronary spasm, cocaine abuse, viral myocarditis, chest trauma, and carbon monoxide intoxication.

Interpretation of Arterial Stenoses on Angiography

Determining severity

What degree of arterial narrowing constitutes a severe stenosis? Many studies have correlated the degree of stenosis with the ultimate clinical or patho-

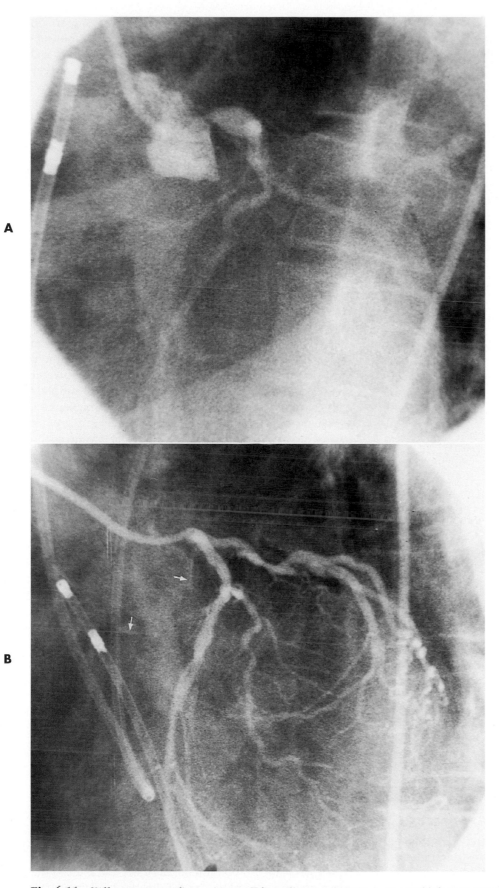

Fig. 6-11   Diffuse coronary disease in type II hyperlipoproteinemia. **A,** An ostial left main stenosis is common. **B,** Slight calcification *(arrows)* in the aortic root is distinctive of this lipid abnormality.

Box 6-2 Examples of Nonatherosclerotic Coronary Disease

CORONARY ANOMALIES

Origin from the pulmonary arteries
Aberrant course between the aorta and the pulmonary artery
Arteriovenous fistula
Intramyocardial bridge

SPASM

Prinzmetal angina
Cocaine abuse
Iatrogenic from catheter or angioplasty

TRAUMA

ARTERITIS

Takayasu disease
Giant cell arteritis
Polyarteritis nodosa
Transplant rejection

EMBOLISM

Thrombus
Tumor
Vegetative or nonthrombotic endocarditis
Cholesterol

INFECTIOUS

Syphilitic stenoses of the coronary ostia
Aortic root abscess
Mucocutaneous lymph node syndrome (Kawasaki disease)

INTIMAL THICKENING

Amyloidosis
Homocysteinuria
Hurler disease

EXTRINSIC COMPRESSION

Cardiac, pericardial, or mediastinal tumor

DISSECTION

Extension of aortic dissection
Spontaneous coronary dissection
Catheter- or angioplasty-induced
Marfan syndrome

COLLAGEN-VASCULAR DISEASE

logic outcome. Severe stenoses correlate well with an impairment in the left ventriculogram. Early clinical studies by Likoff and Proudfit demonstrated a good association between arteriographic evidence of one-, two-, and three-vessel disease with the clinical signs and symptoms of ischemic heart disease. Comparison of arteriograms with postmortem examinations demonstrates a rough correlation with a 50% arterial reduction or 75% area reduction in a coronary artery associated with a transmural myocardial infarct. Because it is easier to measure the greatest percent diameter reduction in a coronary artery from serial views, the diameter and not the area reduction is measured. The severity of the obstructive disease is assessed in each coronary artery segment by comparing the arterial diameter at a point of maximum lumen reduction with a proximal or distal "normal-appearing" artery. A coronary stenosis is graded as the highest percent stenosis seen in all projections.

Because atherosclerotic plaques tend to be eccentric, coronary angiography must be performed in two orthogonal projections so you can identify the maximal arterial narrowing (Fig. 6-13). This system has many limitations. The normal-appearing artery may itself be diffusely diseased. A similar percent stenosis in a smaller distal artery is ascribed the same physiologic consequence, even though flow through a larger proximal arterial segment must be quite different. In a large artery with a greater cross-sectional area, the amount of myocardium supplied by its coronary flow is proportionate to the smaller area supplied by a distal coronary artery. A similar degree of narrowing of a small distal coronary artery produces the same profusion deficit as does the same percent stenosis in a large or proximal artery. The length of a coronary stenosis is important, but is difficult to subjectively evaluate as to the severity of a lesion reducing distal flow. Given these limitations, a 50% or greater stenosis in a patient with ischemic heart disease is defined as a significant stenosis.

Determinants of Coronary Blood Flow

Normal flow

Coronary blood flow in humans is about 60 to 80 ml/min/100 g of myocardium for a cardiac output of 5 L/min. This flow can increase three or four times during vigorous exercise. The hydraulic factors that influence blood flow through a vessel are expressed in Poiseuille's equation

$$Q = \frac{\pi R^4 P}{8 LN}$$

where Q is flow per unit time, R is radius, P is pressure, L is length, and N is viscosity. This equation is strictly valued for nonpulsatile, streamline flow and a uniform viscosity. With some allowance for the transfer of this mathematical principle to a biologic system, the equation helps explain some of the determinants of coronary flow. Under normal conditions, all of the variables in the equation are constant except for the radius of the vessel.

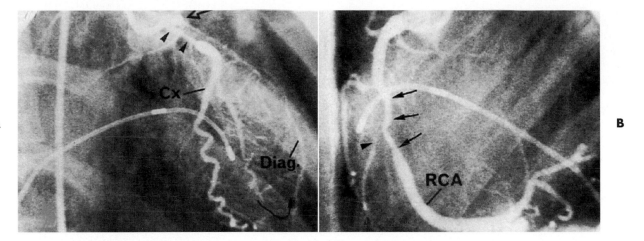

Fig. 6-12   Takayasu's arteritis. **A,** Frontal view of left coronary artery showing complete occlusion of the proximal left anterior descending artery *(open arrow)*, faint collateral flow *(arrow)* to occluded diagonal branch *(Diag)*, and concentric narrowing *(arrowheads)* of the proximal circumflex *(Cx)*. **B,** Lateral view of right coronary artery *(RCA)* showing long, smooth narrowing *(arrows)* of middle segment, involving the origins of the first and second anterior ventricular branches *(arrowhead)*. (From Pasternac A, Lesperance J, Grondin LP, et al: Primary arteritis in Takayasu's disease: a case studied by selective coronary arteriography, *AJR Am J Roentgenol* 128:488, 1977.)

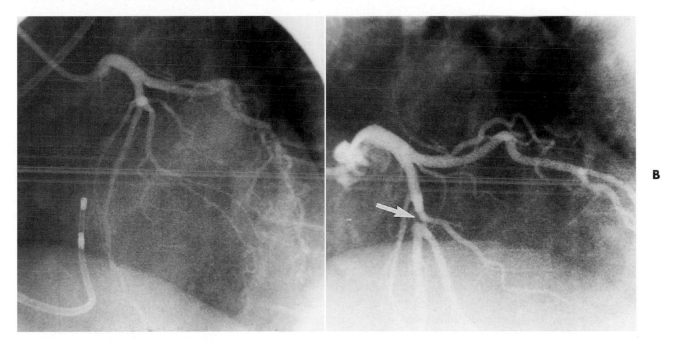

Fig. 6-13   Necessity for multiple projections. The severe stenosis is not visible in the left anterior oblique view **(A)**, but is projected clear of the adjacent diagonal branch in the cranially angled view *(arrow* in **B)**.

However, a number of factors act on the major site of vascular resistance: the precapillary arteriole.

Transient variations

The coronary system autoregulates its blood flow for transient variations in perfusion pressure. Abrupt increases in perfusion pressure (aortic pressure minus right atrial pressure) result in an equivalent increase in coronary blood flow which gradually returns toward the initial value as vascular resistance changes. A similar response occurs when there is a quick decrease in perfusion pressure.

The blood flow through both left and right coronary arteries is influenced by the extravascular resistance supplied by the thick-walled left ventricle. In the left coronary artery, most blood flow is in diastole. In left ventricular hypertrophy, left coronary flow may even reverse. In contrast, right coronary blood flow is more constant and

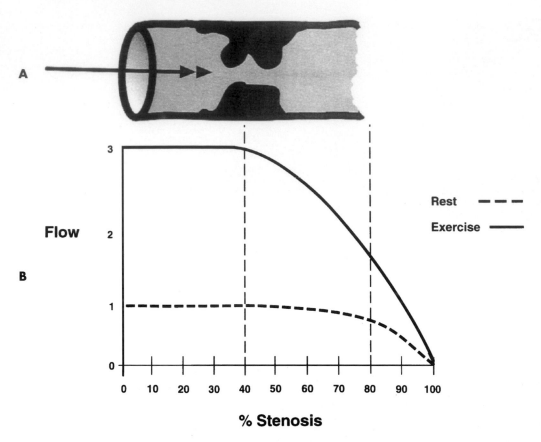

Fig. 6-14   Hemodynamically significant stenosis—a stenosis that reduces flow in the distal artery. **A,** The model is an isolated coronary artery in which a plaque is growing progressively larger. **B,** At rest, when the coronary vasculature is moderately constricted, coronary flow is unchanged until an 80% stenosis is reached because of autoregulation of the vasculature, mainly at the precapillary sphincters. When the experiment is repeated with a vasodilating agent such as exercise, so that the flow is triple the previous resting value, then a 40% stenosis begins to cause a decrease in downstream flow.

occurs rather equally in systole than in diastole. In diseases that increase left ventricular wall tension, resting coronary flow tends to be more phasic. Because left coronary flow occurs mainly during diastole, changes in heart rate can lead to critical alterations in myocardial blood supply. In tachycardia, the diastolic filling period is shortened so blood flow occurs during a shorter time interval. Enhancement of left ventricular contraction, as occurs with aortic stenosis or with sympathetic stimulation, similarly increases the time of the heart in systole and thereby reduces left coronary flow. The opposite effect would occur in a patient on propranolol in whom there is bradycardia and decreased afterload.

Resting coronary blood flow in a normal vascular bed does not decrease until the diameter of the stenosis is at least 80% when compared with the adjacent normal vessel. As a stenosis is gradually increased, the distal vascular bed—mainly at the level of the precapillary arteriole—begins to dilate and therefore reduces the vascular resistance. However, if the vasculature is already maxi-

mally dilated so that autoregulation is no longer present, coronary flow begins to decrease with a stenosis of 30% to 50%. This effect can be seen after pretreatment with a vasodilator but also is thought to occur in the presence of atherosclerosis. In this latter instance, the precapillary sphincters of the distal vascular bed theoretically may slowly dilate from the growth of proximal stenoses.

Flow reserve

Coronary flow reserve is the maximal flow divided by the resting flow. The "50% significant stenosis" then is a rough approximation to this physiologic model. The maximal flow is that which occurs when the coronary vascular bed has undergone maximal vasodilatation. Figure 6-14 shows the relation between coronary blood flow and a focal stenosis in an artery at rest and after maximal vasodilatation.

If a significant stenosis is defined as that which causes coronary blood flow to decrease, a significant stenosis at rest is roughly 80% diameter reduction. However, after maximal vasodilatation, a significant stenosis changes to 40%. The interpretation of these results indicates that stenoses greater than 80% cause a reduction in flow under all circumstances, while stenoses less than 40% are not significant even under conditions where there is maximal vasodilatation. The border zone between 40% and 80% represents the limitation of this method. Unfortunately for clinical decision making, most stenoses fall in this middle zone.

Effects of stenosis length and diameter

The length of the coronary stenosis also determines blood flow although its effect is complex. When the diameter is constricted by less than 50%, stenoses of up to 15 mm in length have little affect on flow during reactive hyperemia. As the diameter of a stenosis is increased to 60%, a 10-mm length results in a reduction in distal flow. Long stenoses in the presence of borderline diameter reduction (40%-60%) may greatly alter coronary hemodynamics during stress. Although Poiseuille's equation suggests that the length of a stenosis would linearly decrease flow, you cannot observe this precisely because there are neural and biochemical factors as well as collateral flow that also regulate blood flow. Moreover, the distal coronary vascular bed may vasodilate in a nonuniform manner from endocardium to epicardium. Since a proximal stenosis reduces coronary pressure, the endocardium becomes anoxic before the epicardium does and has an increased lactate production and a fall in high-energy phosphate mediators. The end result is that vascular resistance distal to a stenosis in an ischemic myocardium varies in a complex way.

Cumulative effects of stenosis

Multiple consecutive stenoses are frequently encountered in clinical practice, and therefore their cumulative effects need to be considered. If a critical stenosis is in series with a mild stenosis, flow is governed by the more severe stenosis. If two critical (i.e., severe enough to reduce blood flow) stenoses are in the same artery, their combined effect is additive.

Coronary Collateral Vessels

Significance and development

Coronary collaterals may develop in the ischemic heart, but their functional significance and mechanism of development are still controversial. True collateral vessels are not seen angiographically in normal hearts. Coronary collateral vessels may be physiologically important and might lessen myocardial ischemia. Cohen compared a group of men who had angiographic evidence of collateral vessels to the left anterior descending artery with another group who did not. Great cardiac vein flow was 55% higher in those with collaterals after

transient balloon occlusion of the left anterior descending artery.

The capacity of collateral vessels to maintain myocardial perfusion varies considerably. Wall segments with abundant collateralization may undergo large infarcts, and conversely totally occluded arteries may be present without a myocardial infarction. The number and size of the collateral vessels correlate poorly with akinetic wall motion and electrocardiographic abnormalities. If a distal segment of an obstructive artery is reconstituted from collaterals, regional left ventricular contraction tends to be less impaired than if the distal segment had such poor collaterals that only minimal flow was visible. Surgeons usually find a larger size to a collateralized artery than is seen angiographically because of flow artifacts and low pressure in the isolated arterial segment.

Angiographic appearance

The angiographic appearance of an epicardial collateral is usually a serpentine, corkscrew artery that goes from the end of an adjacent artery to the end of the occluded artery. Collaterals through the interventricular septum appear differently; they are straight and connect the septal branches from the anterior descending to the posterior descending artery (Fig. 6-15).

There are many pathways in the heart for collateral vessels. Intracoronary collaterals bridge an occluded artery from its proximal to its distal end (Fig. 6-16). This kind may be difficult to distinguish from a recanalized thrombus. Intercoronary collaterals develop between the terminal branches of different arteries (Fig. 6-17). Frequent collateral pathways are from the conus artery of the right coronary artery to the left anterior descending artery (Vieussens ring). Kugel's artery is a collateral which connects the sinoatrial nodal artery to the atrioventricular nodal artery through the interatrial septum. Since the sinoatrial nodal artery can come from either the right coronary or left circumflex artery, and the atrioventricular nodal artery can originate from either a right or left dominant posterior left ventricular artery, there are four pathways that collaterals can take through the atria that can be called Kugel's artery (Fig. 6-18).

Rarely are collaterals visible angiographically in the first few days after myocardial infarction, but they may develop over the following 2 weeks. Several months after a myocardial infarction, most patients develop visible collaterals unless the infarct has organized into a dense scar.

Coronary Artery Spasm

Dynamic forms of coronary obstruction have been recognized for centuries to cause angina and myocardial infarction. In his original description of angina pectoris Heberden wrote that chest pain occasionally occurs with-

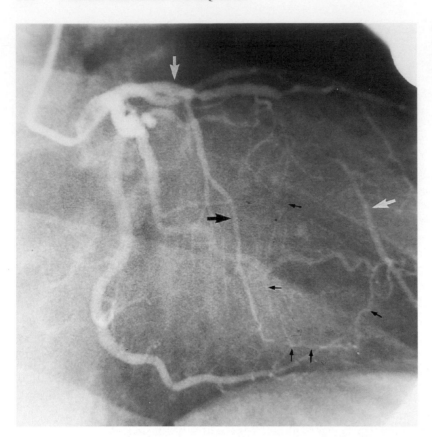

Fig. 6-15   Septal collaterals. The occluded left anterior descending artery *(white arrows)* continues as a diagonal branch. The first septal branch *(large black arrow)* serves as a collateral pathway *(small black arrows)* through other septal branches to the distal anterior descending artery.

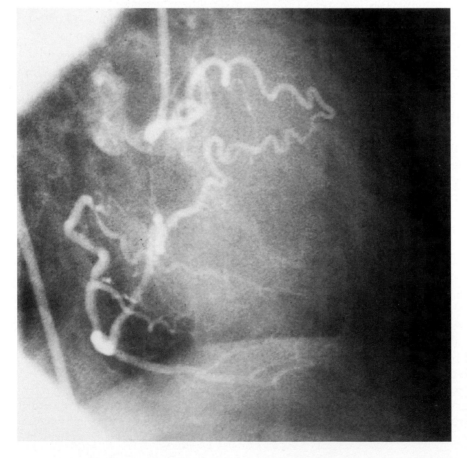

Fig. 6-16   Intracoronary collaterals. The collateral flow around the occlusion in the right coronary artery goes through the conus artery, the collateral vessel in the anterior wall of the right ventricle, and then in a retrograde direction in the marginal branches to the distal right coronary artery.

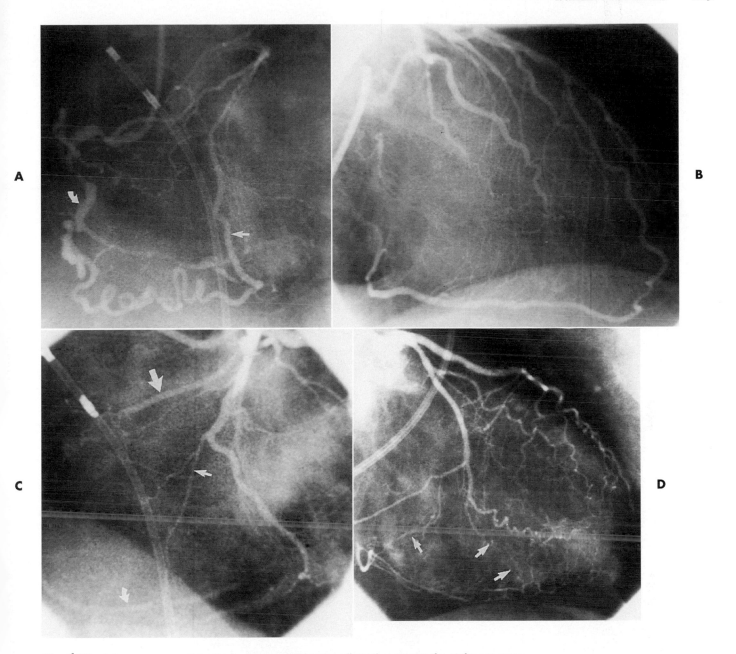

Fig. 6-17   Intercoronary collaterals. **A,** Large, serpentine collateral connects the right coronary artery *(curved arrow)* to the left anterior descending artery *(straight arrow)*. This pathway is called Vieussens' ring. **B,** A collateral vessel as large as the distal left anterior descending artery connects to the posterior descending artery. **C,** A collateral through the crista supraventricularis *(thick arrow)* connects the left anterior descending artery *(thin arrow)* to the distal right coronary artery *(curved arrow)*. **D,** The left circumflex artery serves as collateral supply *(arrows)* to the occluded posterior left ventricular branch of the right coronary artery.

out exertion. In 1910 Osler speculated that spasm of a coronary artery could cause anginal pain. In 1959 Prinzmetal described an unusual syndrome of cardiac pain that occurs almost exclusively at rest, is not precipitated by exertion, and is associated with electrocardiographic ST-segment elevations. Myocardial perfusion scanning and coronary arteriography have shown that spasm may reduce or stop segmental myocardial blood flow.

Angiographic appearance

Coronary spasm is one of a number of causes of myocardial infarction with angiographically normal coronary arteries. The angiographic definition of spasm is a focal stenosis that changes during sequential arterial injections (Fig. 6-19). Occasionally an entire artery will have severe vasoconstriction, but spasm typically is a focal, changeable stenosis. Coronary artery spasm in

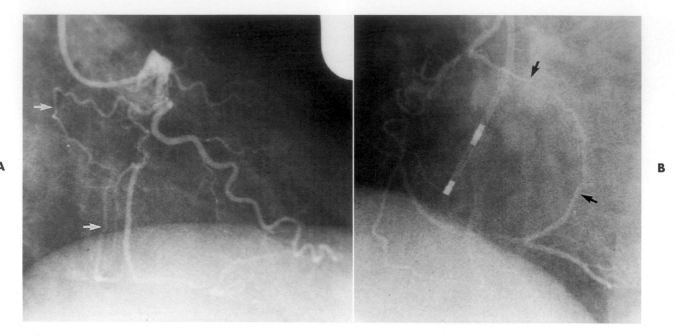

Fig. 6-18 Kugel's artery *(arrows)* connects the proximal right coronary artery to the atrioventricular nodal artery through the atrial septum. The middle segment of the right coronary artery is occluded. **A,** Right anterior oblique view. **B,** Left anterior oblique view.

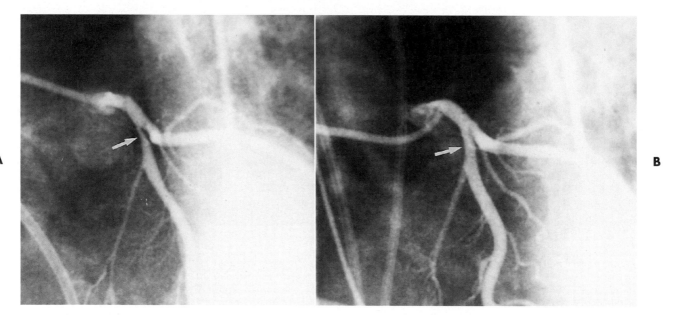

Fig. 6-19 Coronary spasm. **A,** Severe stenosis in the left anterior descending artery *(arrow)* in the cranially angled left oblique view did not change after nitroglycerin administration. **B,** Another study 4 days later shows absence of the previous spasm and a minor fixed stenosis *(arrow)*. This example illustrates that spasm is not always eliminated 5 to 15 minutes after intravenous nitroglycerin.

Prinzmetal variant angina has been seen in the left main, left anterior descending, and circumflex arteries, but spasm in the right coronary artery is more frequent.

Catheter-induced vs. Prinzmetal syndrome

The distinction between catheter-induced spasm and that in Prinzmetal syndrome is difficult, but one caused by a catheter occurs proximally, adjacent to the catheter tip (Fig. 6-20). Catheter-induced spasm usually is seen at the origin of the right coronary artery as a short area with smooth fusiform narrowing. Focal spasm frequently occurs at the site of an atherosclerotic plaque, which may make it difficult to distinguish from fixed disease. Spasm may be slight or it may com-

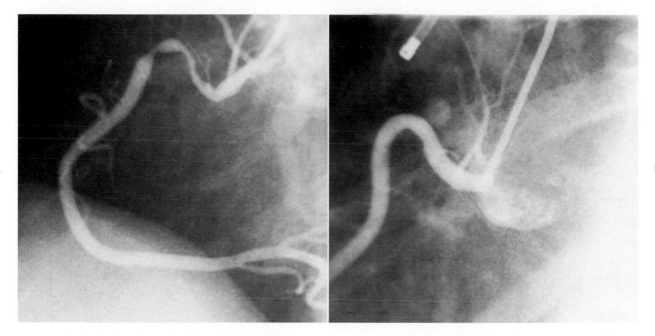

Fig. 6-20   Catheter-induced coronary spasm. Initial injection (**A**) into the right coronary artery produced severe narrowing which was almost completely reversed (**B**) after intracoronary nitroglycerin.

pletely occlude the artery. Because the coronary endothelium has potent factors that can cause spasm as well as thrombus after intimal injury, spasm is frequently seen after percutaneous coronary angioplasty. In this situation, the artery has a sawtooth appearance, which is reversed with nitroglycerin.

Coronary Aneurysms

Coronary artery aneurysms are occasionally discovered during angiographic evaluation of ischemic heart disease and are usually a variant of coronary atherosclerosis (Fig. 6-21). You will frequently find this lesion in the same artery with stenoses and occlusions. Atherosclerosis can produce diffuse ectasia from degeneration of the media and associated elastic elements (Fig. 6-22). In order to distinguish an ectatic artery or poststenotic dilatation from an aneurysm, a useful definition of coronary aneurysm is a dilatation of 50% greater than the preceding normal artery. Most atherosclerotic coronary aneurysms have an adjacent severe stenosis. The saccular aneurysm may overlap and hide the stenosis during angiography so that at least one angiographic projection should profile the neck of the aneurysm.

Causes

Coronary aneurysms are a major manifestation of many systemic diseases. The history of associated cardiac lesions may implicate syphilis, polyarteritis nodosa, trauma, bacterial infections, neoplasm, and a congenital

etiology (Fig. 6-23). Rupture of an atherosclerotic aneurysm is very rare. Rupture is associated with bacterial infected aneurysm, congenital aneurysm of large size, and in arteritis diseases. Diffuse aneurysms have been seen in transplanted hearts that underwent immunologic rejection.

Kawasaki disease is a childhood acute multisystem vasculitis that includes cervical lymphadenopathy, fever, and a rash in the mouth and on the hands and feet. Also called mucocutaneous lymph node syndrome, Kawasaki disease has a myocarditis and pericarditis which may cause congestive heart failure. Aneurysms of the coronary arteries are frequent (Fig. 6-24) and may cause coronary thrombosis, myocardial infarction, and sudden death. About half of the children with coronary aneurysms have angiographically normal-appearing arteries 2 years later. Some aneurysms may be quite large, and rupture is a fatal complication. See Table 6-1 for prognosis of aneurysms in Kawasaki disease.

Table 6-1   Prognosis of aneurysms in kawasaki disease

Size	Prognosis
< 4 mm	Regress to normal size
4-8 mm	Tend to become smaller
> 8 mm	Progress to obstruction or stenosis

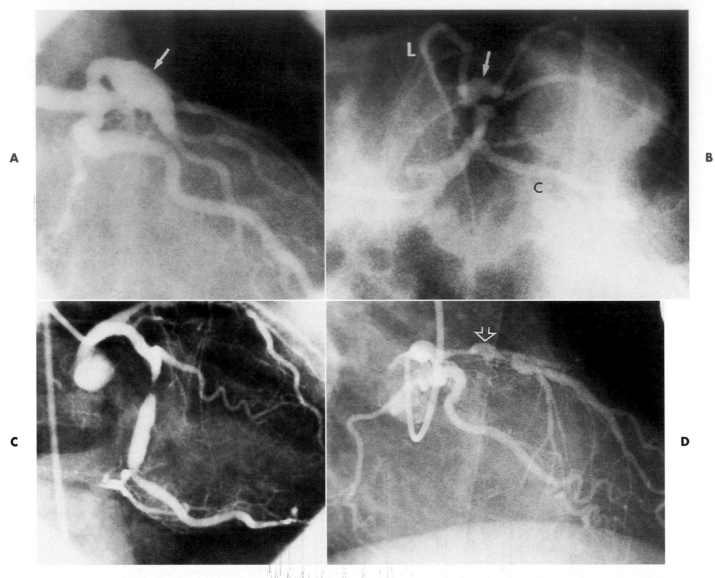

Fig. 6-21 Coronary aneurysms *(arrows)*. **A,** The left anterior descending artery aneurysm is twice the size of the normal artery. **B,** A caudal left anterior oblique projection (spider view) shows an aneurysm in the left anterior descending artery. *L* = left anterior descending artery; *C* = left circumflex artery. **C,** The left circumflex artery in the caudal right anterior oblique view has a fusiform aneurysm after a severe stenosis in a segment that becomes the left posterior descending artery. **D,** Multiple segmental plaques with an intervening normal vessel *(open arrow)* is not to be confused with an aneurysm.

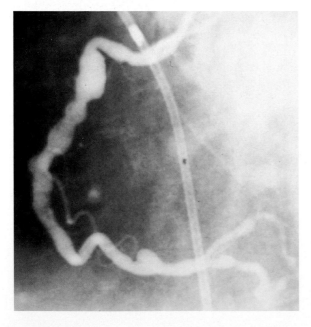

Fig. 6-22 Diffuse ectasia of the right coronary artery with distal saccular aneurysm.

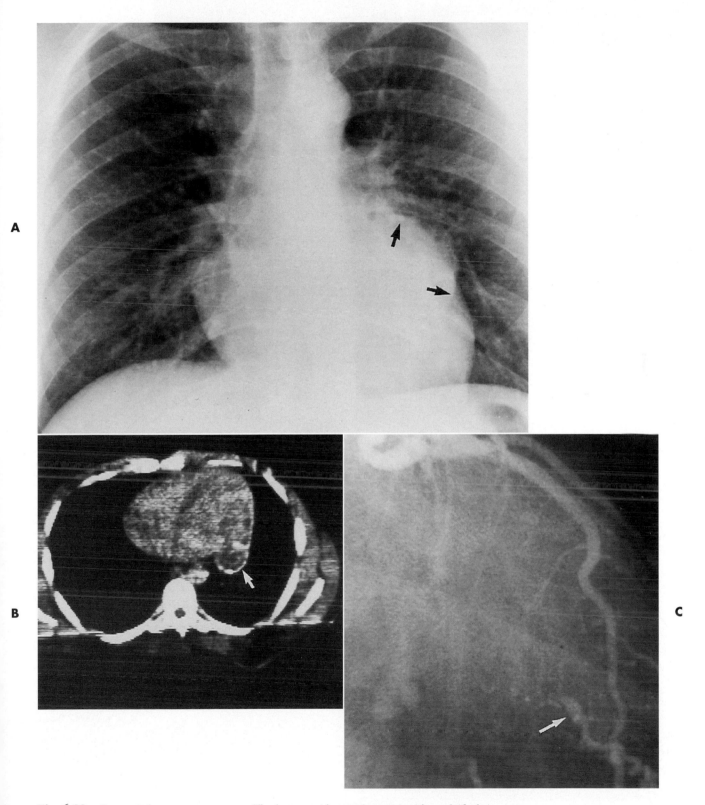

Fig. 6-23   Congenital coronary aneurysm. The large ovoid mass *(arrows)* with a calcified rim was adjacent to the left atrioventricular groove on the chest film (**A**) and computed tomography scan (**B**). **C,** Selective coronary angiography in the right anterior oblique projection shows an occluded left circumflex artery and retrograde filling of a marginal branch *(arrow)* by collaterals.

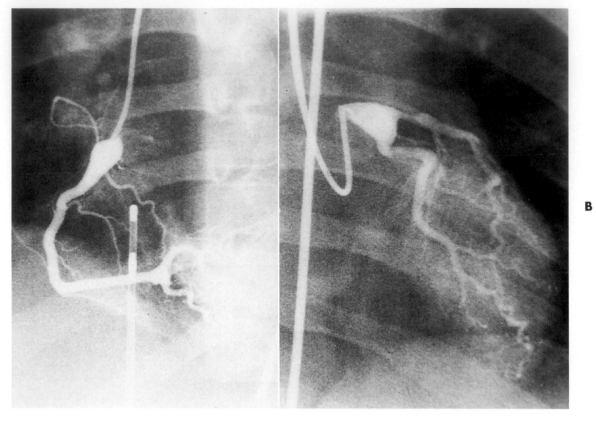

Fig. 6-24   Kawasaki disease. **A,** Coronary aneurysms in the right coronary artery origin. **B,** The left main coronary artery in the same 5-year-old child 2 years after an episode of fever and mucocutaneous signs.

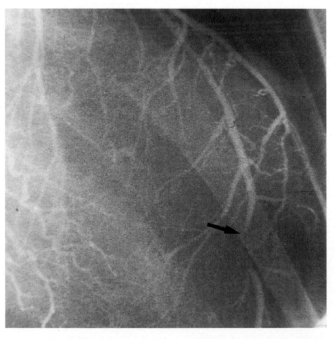

Fig. 6-25   Intramyocardial bridge. The left anterior descending artery *(arrow)* was completely occluded during systole but had a normal caliber at end diastole.

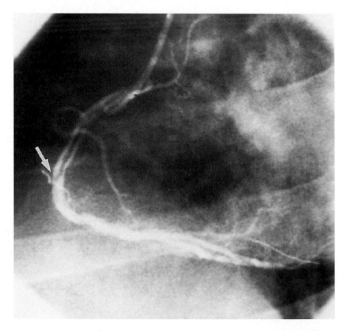

Fig. 6-26   Coronary artery dissection. The right coronary artery has a double-channeled dissection in the proximal and middle segments with moderate reduction in distal flow. The termination of the intimal flap *(arrow)* is at the acute margin.

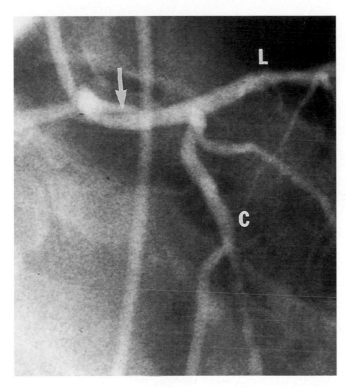

Fig. 6-27 Spontaneous dissection of the left main coronary artery. A small linear filling defect *(arrow)* in the left main coronary artery, seen in the right anterior oblique projection, creates a 50% stenosis but did not appear to reduce distal flow. *L* = left anterior descending artery; *C* = left circumflex artery.

Myocardial Bridging

An intramyocardial bridge is a coronary artery that dips into the myocardium and is completely surrounded by cardiac muscle (Fig. 6-25). This segment of the coronary artery narrows dynamically during systole and returns to its baseline size during diastole. Bridges are seen in about 0.5% to 7.5% of angiographic studies and are usually seen in the left anterior descending artery, although rarely other branches may be affected. Because narrowing takes place during systole and most coronary flow occurs in diastole, mural coronary arteries initially were considered a minor anomaly. However, chest pain and myocardial infarction may occur when the bridge narrows greater than 75% in systole. Because the bridge is usually eccentric, you should obtain views in at least two orthogonal projections.

The septal arteries, which are also intramural, normally show no change in size between systole and diastole. Septal arteries from the left anterior descending artery may occlude during systole in diseases that increase left ventricular wall tension such as aortic stenosis, hypertensive heart disease, and idiopathic hypertrophic subaortic stenosis.

Coronary Dissection

The angiographic appearance of dissection is a linear or spiral lucency within the arterial lumen which represents the intimal flap (Fig. 6-26). The dissection may occlude the distal artery or, as in the aorta, have a false channel with stasis of the contrast medium. Spontaneous dissection occurs in the coronary arteries as it does in most medium-sized arteries (Fig. 6-27). It is seen in pregnancy, Marfan syndrome, and chest trauma. Coronary dissection may occur secondary to an aortic dissection with a retrograde tear. The angiographic catheter may lift a plaque and initiate the downstream tear. After transluminal angioplasty, a short dissection cleft is frequently seen but rarely extends beyond the length of the balloon.

CONGENITAL ANOMALIES OF THE CORONARY ARTERIES

Coronary anomalies can be defined morphologically or hemodynamically. Morphologic variations can arise in the origin, course, or termination of the coronary arteries. These variations may be isolated anomalies or be related to certain forms of congenital heart disease. Coronary anomalies may cause cardiac ischemia. In this group are four major anomalies: (1) coronary fistulas, (2) origin of the left coronary artery from the pulmonary artery, (3) congenital coronary artery stenosis or atresia, and (4) origin of the left coronary artery from the right sinus of Valsalva with the right main coronary artery passing between the right ventricular infundibulum and the aorta. The morphologic classification is used in this discussion.

Anomalies of Origin

Although the usual origin of the left and right coronary arteries is the left and right sinuses of Valsalva respectively, ectopic coronary arteries can arise above the sinuses in the ascending aorta, within the posterior (noncoronary) sinus, low within the sinus adjacent to the leaflet, within the commissure, or in a subvalvular location. The conus artery frequently originates as a separate ostium in the right sinus of Valsalva. There may be no left main artery if the left anterior descending and circumflex arteries arise separately from the left sinus of Valsalva. A common anomaly is the left circumflex artery arising from the right sinus of Valsalva and passing behind the aorta into the left atrioventricular groove (Fig. 6-28). When the left coronary artery originates from the right sinus of Valsalva, it may (1) pass anterior to the right ventricular outflow tract, (2) go between the pulmonary artery and the aorta (Fig. 6-29), or (3) circle posteriorly behind the aorta to get to the left ventricle. Similarly, when the right coronary artery originates from

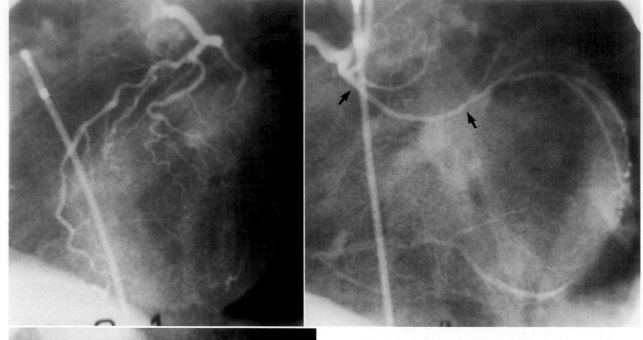

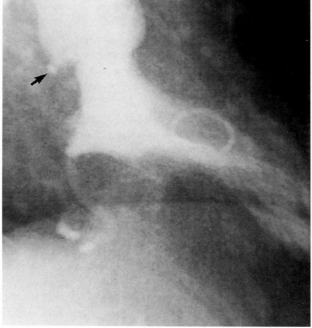

Fig. 6-28   Anomalous left circumflex artery. **A,** Selective injection into the left coronary artery visualized only the left anterior descending artery. **B,** Right coronary artery injection demonstrates a retroaortic left circumflex artery *(arrows).* **C,** A left ventriculogram shows the position of the anomalous circumflex artery *(arrow).* (A small ventricular apical aneurysm secondary to an occluded left anterior descending artery is also present.)

the left sinus of Valsalva by passing between the aorta and the right ventricular infundibulum, it forms an acute angle at its ostium and may be compressed by the two great vessels. Rarely a left coronary artery arises from the right sinus of Valsalva, assumes an intramyocardial course by traversing through the crista supraventricularis, then continues as the left anterior descending and circumflex arteries in their usual locations.

The coronary arteries may have ectopic origins from structures other than the aorta. In this situation, the anomalies include: (1) origin of the left coronary artery from the pulmonary artery, (2) origin of the right coro-

nary artery from the pulmonary artery, (3) origin of both coronary arteries from the pulmonary artery, (4) origin of the conus artery from the pulmonary artery with branching to both right and left circumflex arteries, and (5) origin of the left circumflex artery from the pulmonary artery.

The most common of these is the left coronary origin from the pulmonary artery. This entity, the Bland-White-Garland syndrome, is seen in infants who have a myocardial infarction in the first few months of life. Coronary arteriography shows an empty left sinus of Valsalva. The right coronary artery supplies collaterals to the left coro-

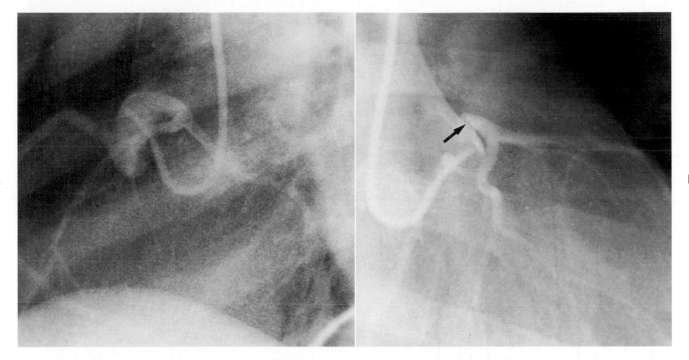

Fig. 6-29   Origin of the left coronary artery from the right sinus of Valsalva. **A,** Injection into the right sinus opacifies both the right and left coronary arteries. **B,** In the right anterior oblique projection, an intimal ridge *(arrow)* is visible as the left coronary artery leaves the right sinus.

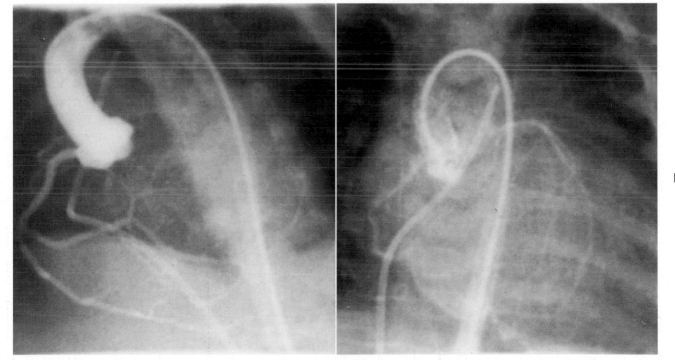

Fig. 6-30   Anomalous origin of the left coronary artery from the pulmonary artery. **A,** Initial aortogram in the cranially angled left oblique projection disclosed absence of the left coronary artery from its usual origin at the left sinus of Valsalva. **B,** The path of coronary filling during cineangiography was right coronary through septal collaterals, to the left anterior descending artery, and then to the pulmonary artery. A catheter in the pulmonary artery helps locate this structure.

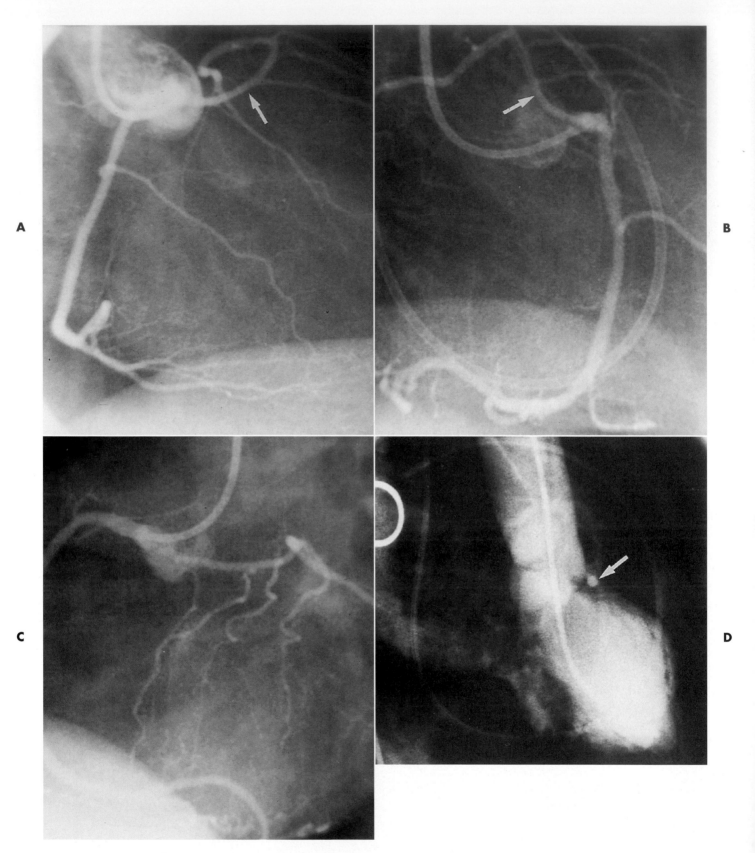

Fig. 6-31 Single right coronary artery with connecting segment to the left anterior descending artery going between the aorta and the right ventricular infundibulum. **A,** Shallow right oblique view shows anterior connecting segment *(arrow)* to the left coronary artery. **B,** Lateral view of artery *(arrow)* between the aorta, which has the angiographic catheter, and the right ventricular outflow tract through which the pulmonary artery catheter passes. **C,** Left oblique view. **D,** Left ventriculogram shows the left coronary artery *(arrow)* to be anterior to the aorta.

nary artery, which fills in a retrograde direction to opacify the pulmonary arteries (Fig. 6-30). The infantile left ventricle may have a segmental wall motion abnormality like that seen in coronary disease in the adult. Left ventricular aneurysms and mitral regurgitation can produce congestive heart failure. Left ventricular aneurysms may completely regress after corrective coronary surgery.

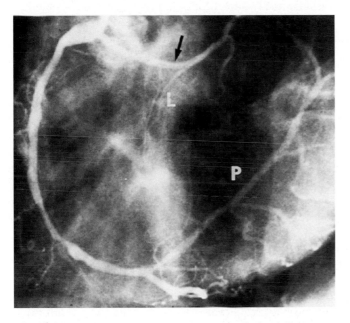

Fig. 6-32 A single right coronary artery. In the left anterior oblique view, the posterolateral branch (*P*) of the distal right coronary continues in the left atrioventricular groove to become the circumflex artery. A bridging artery *(arrow)* from the origin of the right coronary to the vestigial left anterior descending artery (*L*) joins the left circumflex artery to form an arterial ring.

Anomalies of Origin and Course

Major coronary anomalies of location are those that go behind the aorta, between the aorta and the pulmonary artery, or anterior to the right ventricular infundibulum. A prime example of this group is the isolated single coronary artery, which can originate from either the left or right sinus of Valsalva (Fig. 6-31). The most common anomaly is origin of the left circumflex artery from the right coronary artery with a course that goes behind the aorta before supplying the usual circumflex territory. You can usually see this retroaortic course on a right anterior oblique left ventriculogram and it will alert you to the anomaly. Other common variations include the left anterior descending artery coming from the conus artery, and the posterior descending artery continuing around the apex as a long left anterior descending artery (Fig. 6-32).

The anomaly that can cause an angina and sudden death is the aberrant coronary artery which goes between the aorta and the pulmonary artery (Fig. 6-33). These two great arteries expand during systole and may compress the aberrant coronary artery and constrict its flow. This type of anomaly usually has a stenosis at its origin because of an acute angle with the sinus of Valsalva.

Tetralogy of Fallot

A number of types of congenital heart disease have an increased incidence of anomalous coronary arteries, particularly those malformations which alter the positions of the aorta and pulmonary artery. Tetralogy of Fallot, transposition of the great arteries, congenitally corrected transposition, double outlet right ventricle, and single ventricle are several lesions that need proper identifica-

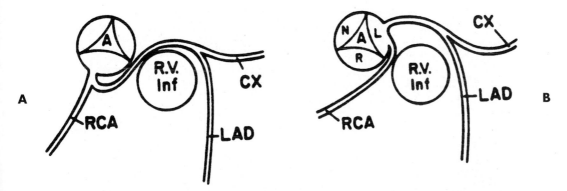

Fig. 6-33 Diagram illustrating the aberrant course taken by the left main coronary artery. **A,** illustrates its beginning at its origin from the right sinus of Valsalva and passing between the aorta (*A*) and the right ventricular infundibulum (*R.V. inf*) to supply the left anterior descending (*LAD*) and the circumflex (*CX*) branches. *RCA* = right coronary artery. **B,** illustrates an aberrant right coronary artery (*RCA*), which arises from the left sinus of Valsalva (*L*) and passes between the aorta (*A*) and the right ventricular infundibulum (*R.V. inf*). *N* denotes noncoronary and *R* right coronary sinus of Valsalva of the aortic valve. (From Case records of the Massachusetts General Hospital. Case 22-1989, *N Engl J Med* 320:1475-1483, 1989, Massachusetts Medical Society. Reprinted by permission of The New England Journal of Medicine.)

tion of artery position for surgical correction. About 5% of patients with tetralogy of Fallot have an anomalous left anterior descending artery originating from the right coronary artery and passing across the anterior right ventricle. This artery lies directly in the path of a surgical ventriculotomy. If transected during the procedure, a major anterior myocardial infarction will result. Other coronary anomalies associated with tetralogy of Fallot are a single left or right coronary artery, fistulas between the coronary arteries and the pulmonary artery, and major aortopulmonary collaterals originating from the descending thoracic aorta. There are similar anomalies in origin and course in the transposition complexes. The coronary arteries in congenitally corrected transposition are reversed in right-to-left mirror image fashion and are a major diagnostic marker for this anomaly.

Anomalies of Termination

Coronary artery fistula is a rare congenital anomaly, but is significant in the differential diagnosis of a continuous murmur. A coronary fistula may occur to any adjacent vascular bed. Fistulas may connect to all four cardiac chambers, the coronary sinus, the right or left superior vena cava, the pulmonary artery, and the systemic arteries (Fig. 6-34). In aortic atresia and pulmonary atresia there are frequently large coronary artery sinuses and fistulas to the ventricles.

Complications

As in other parts of the body, fistulas can be the site of bacterial arteritis, ischemia to distal tissues, and rupture. Complications in the heart are congestive heart failure, infective endocarditis, myocardial infarction, and fistula rupture.

These fistulas are best studied with selective coronary arteriography. Congenital coronary arteriovenous fistulas have a large tortuous artery and vein down to the point of termination (Fig. 6-35). In contrast, acquired fistulas from either trauma (Fig. 6-36) or endocarditis have a normal or slightly dilated artery proximal to the fistula. The arterial bed distal to the fistula may be hypoperfused (a vascular steal), and if long-standing, may have collaterals supplying this lesion. Acute traumatic fistulas initially have normal-sized arteries and veins, but if uncorrected, both of these vessels will dilate. If a fistula opens into the right heart, a left-to-right shunt is present.

CORONARY BYPASS GRAFTING

Aortocoronary grafts are constructed from either the internal mammary arteries or from reversed saphenous veins so that the valves do not impede flow. Rarely, the gastroepiploic artery is brought through the diaphragm as a graft.

Internal Mammary Artery Grafts

The most common procedure is to attach the left internal mammary artery to the proximal left anterior descending artery (Fig. 6-37). Either the right or left internal mammary artery may be used for grafting, but usually not both together, to prevent sternal osteonecrosis. Occasionally these arteries are sequentially grafted to the left anterior descending and to the diagonal artery. The

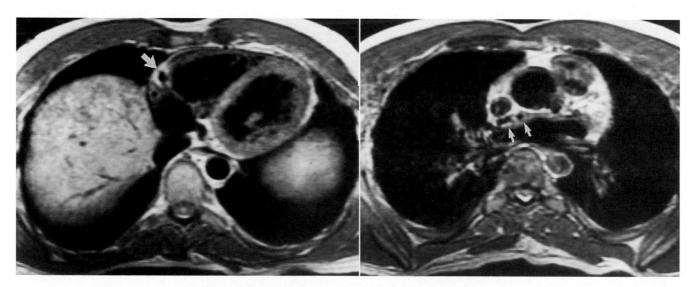

Fig. 6-34 Coronary artery-to-pulmonary artery fistula. **A,** Spin echo MR image shows large right coronary artery *(arrow)*. **B,** A slice at the level of the pulmonary arteries show numerous mediastinal branches *(arrows)* that terminated in the pulmonary artery.

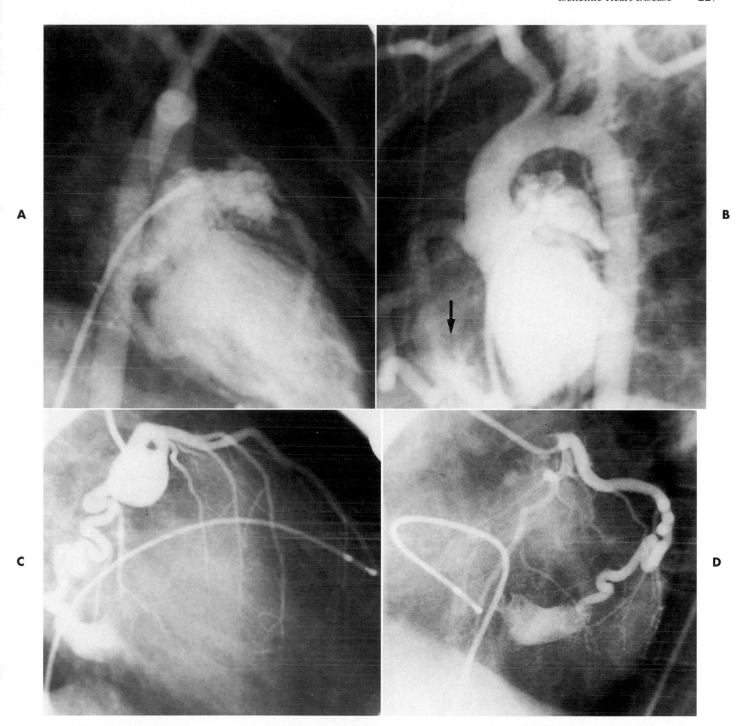

Fig. 6-35   Congenital coronary artery fistulas in two patients. **A** and **B,** Right coronary and left circumflex artery terminate in the right ventricle *(arrow).* **C** and **D,** Left circumflex artery terminates in the coronary sinus.

patency rate of the internal mammary grafts is higher than that of saphenous vein grafts, even though the arterial graft has a slower flow than the venous graft. Unlike the vein graft, the internal mammary arteries do not form intimal hyperplasia, which occurs in all vein grafts during the first year after surgery.

Saphenous Vein Grafts

Saphenous vein grafts have a proximal anastomosis to the ascending aorta several centimeters above the aortic valve (Fig. 6-38). Vein grafts may be constructed so that one or more side-to-side anastomoses are connected with diagonal and marginal arteries that lie in proximity. A side limb can be placed to a saphenous vein graft so that several coronary arteries at a distance from one another may be supplied by a single proximal graft (Fig. 6-39). This type of graft resembles an inverted "Y."

Complications

Complications in venous grafts are usually at the proximal aortic anastomosis or the distal coronary anastomosis. Graft complications in coronary surgery are the same as complications to grafts elsewhere. Occlusion and focal or diffuse stenosis are common, whereas pseudoaneurysm

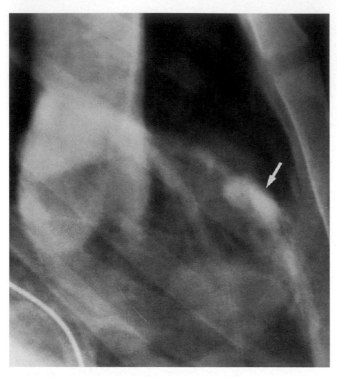

Fig. 6-36 Traumatic fistula from the left anterior descending artery to the right ventricle. Flow through the fistula is small and rapid at the site of the false aneurysm *(arrow)* in the artery.

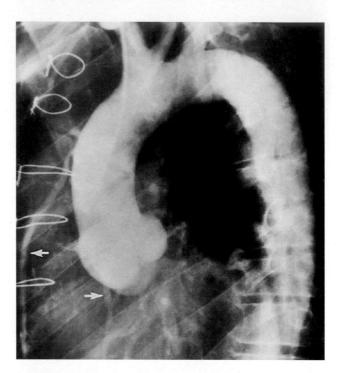

Fig. 6-38 Aortogram to locate graft origins. Patent grafts *(arrows)* are present to the right coronary and left anterior descending arteries.

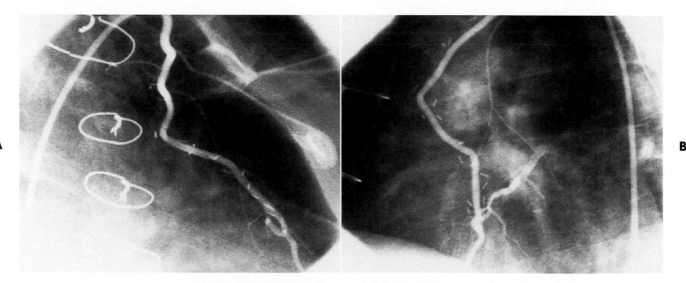

A

B

Fig. 6-37 Internal mammary artery graft to left anterior descending artery. Selective injections into the left internal mammary artery in the **A,** right anterior oblique, and **B,** left anterior oblique projections show an open distal anastomosis. There is both antegrade flow in the left anterior descending artery toward the apex and retrograde flow back through a moderate stenosis.

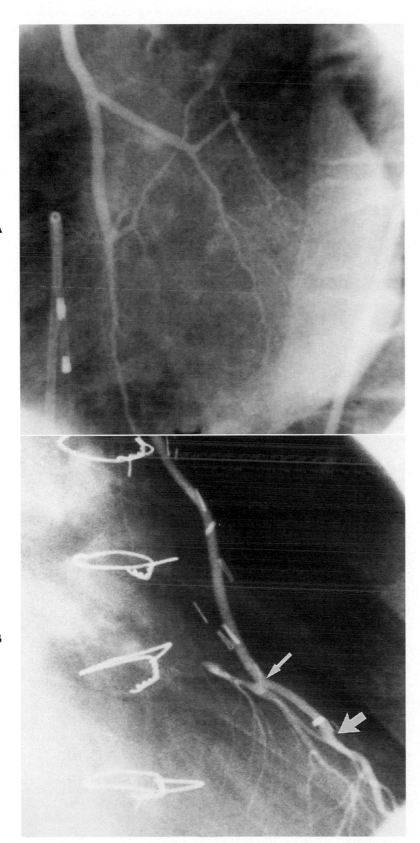

Fig. 6-39 Complex aortocoronary grafts. **A,** Saphenous vein "Y"-graft has one limb to the left anterior descending artery and the other limb to a diagonal branch. **B,** The left internal mammary artery in the right anterior oblique projection has a side-to-side anastomosis *(thin arrow)* to the left anterior descending artery and an end-to-side anastomosis *(thick arrow)* on a diagonal artery.

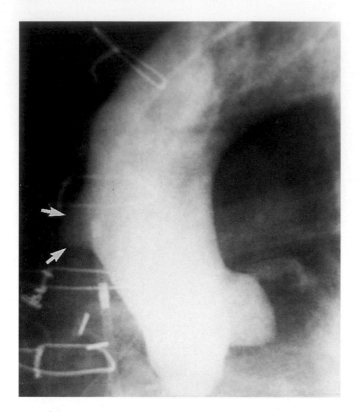

Fig. 6-40 False aneurysm of the aorta. An outpouching in the wall of the aorta *(arrows)* has developed at the site of the graft anastomosis. The graft is occluded.

(Fig. 6-40) at either anastomosis is unusual. Over time, saphenous grafts develop a diffuse stenosis from intimal hyperplasia (Fig. 6-41). Degenerated venous grafts can look like severe atherosclerosis with ragged ulcerated plaques. Unlike coronary artery stenoses, which can be graded by a percent diameter reduction, this method is not accurate when applied to a stenosis in a vein graft because vein grafts are larger than the supplied coronary artery. In a graft four times the size of the native artery a stenosis must have an 80% diameter before it reduces distal flow, but in a graft of the same size as the coronary artery, distal flow would be reduced by about 50% at rest. Because of these difficulties, a thallium exercise test is required to assess the severity of a graft stenosis.

Imaging Techniques

Bypass grafts are usually studied by angiography, although they can be identified with computed tomography, ultrafast computed tomography, and magnetic resonance imaging (MRI). Angiography of bypass grafts is performed by selective injection in the internal mammary artery or in the aortic anastomosis of the vein graft. The flow into the native coronary artery from a graft should occur in both antegrade and retrograde directions (Fig. 6-42). If there is no flow into the proximal coronary artery from the graft, that artery is usually

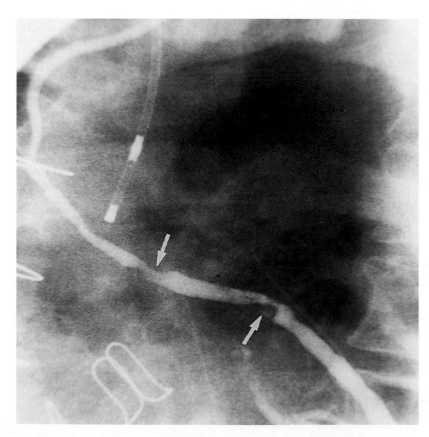

Fig. 6-41 Aortocoronary reversed saphenous vein graft stenoses *(arrows)*. Selective injection into a graft to the left circumflex marginal artery has a moderate stenosis in its middle segment and a severe stenosis distally. These changes are intimal hypertrophy and graft degeneration from development of atherosclerosis in the neointima of the vein. A Carpentier-Edwards valve prosthesis is present.

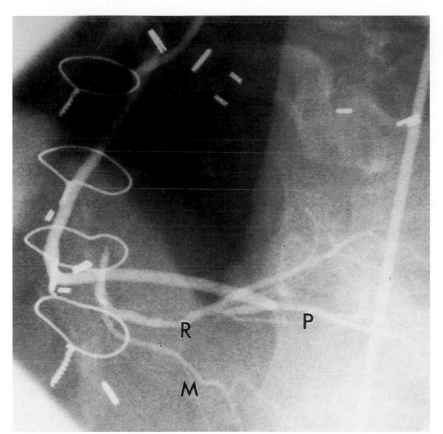

Fig. 6-42 Imaging criteria for a normal aorto-coronary bypass graft. The saphenous vein graft to the posterior descending artery (*P*) has no stenosis in either the aortic anastomosis or the coronary anastomosis. In this left anterior oblique view, there is both antegrade flow in the posterior descending artery and retrograde flow into the distal right coronary artery (*R*). *M* = right ventricular marginal artery.

occluded. Injection into a coronary artery that has a distal graft may show an apparent occlusion in the "watershed" region between the proximal coronary artery and graft insertion. When the coronary artery is stenotic and not occluded before the graft, the graft will fill in a retrograde direction. These complex flow patterns in the graft and the adjacent coronary arteries depend on how much pressure is applied by the angiographer when injecting the graft or artery, and the hemodynamic variables in the arterial system. Collaterals to a grafted artery are not seen when the graft is functioning. Collateral vessels that were present before surgery, unless very large, no longer are visualized, presumably because the collaterals have involuted or because the graft reduces the pressure gradient between the ends of the collateral channels, thereby slowing flow to the collateral.

LEFT VENTRICULAR ABNORMALITIES IN CORONARY DISEASE

The evaluation of segmental and global left ventricular function is a standard part of the imaging evaluation for ischemic heart disease. Ventricular wall motion can be analyzed on tomographic methods such as echocardiography or MRI (Fig. 6-43). Because the angiographic left ventriculogram is a projectional and not a tomo-

graphic image, only those wall segments that are tangential to the x-ray beam can be evaluated. Biplane, rather than single plane, left ventriculograms generally give a more accurate evaluation of segmental wall motion, as well as a better estimate of the ejection fraction.

Ventriculogram Analysis

The ventriculogram is a classic example of "information overload." It contains many structures that are usually moving in different directions at different velocities. Even among experienced observers, one person's dyskinetic wall motion may be another's normal motion. Therefore, it is useful to develop a schema for interpreting the ventriculogram by isolating the components and separately judging their shape and motion. The basis for analyzing the left ventriculogram follows:

Aorta
  1. Is the ascending aorta aneurysmal?
  2. Are the leaflets of the aortic valve thickened? Do they open completely or is there aortic stenosis?

Mitral valve
  1. Are the leaflets domed in diastole (mitral stenosis)?
  2. Is there prolapse in systole?
  3. Are the chordae and papillary muscles thick (mitral stenosis)?

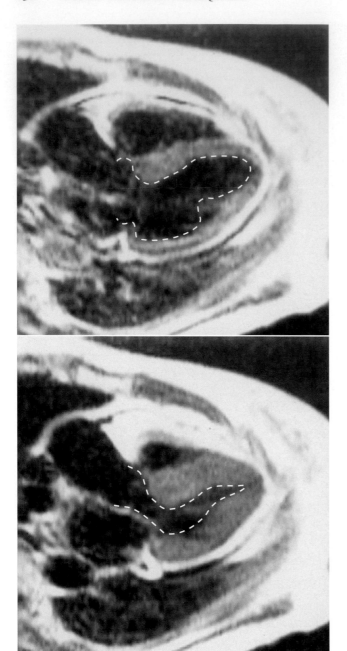

Fig. 6-43 Wall motion analysis by MRI. Spin echo images in diastole (*top*) and systole (*bottom*) were obtained in the long-axis plane perpendicular to the ventricular septum. The *dotted lines* outline the endocardial cavity that was used to calculate the ejection fraction which was 81%. The thickness of the left ventricular muscle has increased in systole to nearly double the diastolic width. The patient had aortic stenosis with left ventricular hypertrophy. (From Miller SW, Brady TJ, Dinsmore RE, et al: Cardiac magnetic resonance imaging: the Massachusetts General Hospital experience, *Radiol Clin North Am* 23:745-764, 1985.)

4. Is the head of the posteromedial papillary muscle halfway between the mitral valve and the left ventricular apex (normal), or is it retracted to lie near the mitral valve (mitral stenosis)?
5. Is there mitral regurgitation?

Left ventricular wall
1. Is there generally symmetric shortening of each segment of the left ventricle between diastole and systole?
2. At end diastole, is the anterolateral wall thicker than 12 mm (hypertrophy)?
3. If a segment is akinetic, is there an adjacent filling defect (thrombus)?

Projection

A few principles of geometry and perception are important to consider, particularly when comparing one examination with another. First, even though most laboratories have a standard examination (30-degree right anterior oblique projection and 60-degree left anterior oblique projection), the same projection of a wall segment is not always the same part of the heart. The actual wall seen is a function of the rotation of the heart in the thorax. For example, the "anterolateral wall" in a patient with right ventricular enlargement that rotates the heart posteriorly may be the anterior segment of the left ventricle. A heart that lies horizontally in the thorax may not project its wall segments exactly as does a heart with a more vertical orientation.

Heart rate

A difference in heart rate may also alter the apparent function. A fast heart rate may incorrectly suggest poor wall motion because there is less filling in diastole. Similarly, a fast heart rate will produce a thicker wall measurement at end diastole because the ventricle is not distended as much as it can be with a longer diastole filling period. For these reasons, the biplane examination is preferred because you can see the septum and posterolateral walls which you cannot see on a single-plane right anterior oblique projection. Cranial angulation in the left anterior oblique view has the advantage of delineating the outflow region of the left ventricle and showing the entire septum and mitral valve without overlap of apical structures.

Symmetry

The normal left ventricle has relatively symmetric synchronous shortening of all segments. However, if the extent of contraction is quantitated, there will be differences in range of motion in normal hearts. The inferior wall on the right anterior oblique projection moves slightly more than does the anterolateral wall. In the left anterior oblique view, the septal excursion may differ slightly from the posterior wall, depending on rotation. The apical tip always moves toward the aortic valve, but in some hearts this excursion may be minimal.

Angiography shows the motion of the endocardium. Fluoroscopy of the heart, particularly in the right anterior oblique view, evaluates the epicardium: the heart-lung border. In the normal person the epicardium in the right anterior oblique view has no motion and should not be mistaken for a myocardial infarct in that region.

SEGMENTAL WALL MOTION ABNORMALITIES WITH AND WITHOUT CORONARY DISEASE

Regional Wall Motion

Regional wall abnormalities are a distinguishing characteristic of coronary artery disease and occur in acute myocardial infarction, myocardial ischemia without infarction, in areas of myocardial scar from a remote infarction, in aneurysms, and in regions of muscle in which there are some viable myocytes interlaced with areas of scar. These changes in wall contraction can occur after only a few minutes of acute coronary occlusion. As ischemia progresses to infarction, first hypokinesis, then akinesis, and then dyskinesis develop. Dyskinesis can represent acute or chronic ischemia as well as an aneurysm or large scar.

Correlation with Coronary Artery Disease

As a general rule, asynergy is noted in areas of previous myocardial infarction and is more common in regions of severely stenosed vessels. However, perfusion, as determined by thallium-201 scintigraphy, correlates more closely with segmental wall motion abnormalities than does coronary anatomy. On the other hand, it is not uncommon to find normal wall motion in a segment of the left ventricle supplied by a severely stenotic coronary artery. These segments tend to have good collaterals and have not had an infarct.

In both acute and chronic myocardial infarction, there are compensatory mechanisms that tend to restore the cardiac output even though a portion of the ventricle is not contracting. These are manifested in a hyperkinetic performance of wall segments that are not involved in the region of ischemia. For example, in anteroseptal infarction, the posterolateral wall may have an excursion twice the normal range.

Factors Influencing Wall Motion

The shape and motion of the interventricular septum is controlled by a number of factors other than the coronary blood supply. The pressure gradient between the right and left ventricle may cause the septum to move abnormally toward the left ventricle in diastole and toward the right ventricle during systole. Such paradoxical motion is seen in right ventricular hypertension from pulmonary stenosis, right ventricular volume overload in atrial septal defects, and rarely after cardiopulmonary

bypass. In addition, patients with both mitral stenosis and mitral valve prolapse may have unusual contraction patterns, particularly in the diaphragmatic wall. Right ventricular volume overload in atrial septal defect or in tricuspid regurgitation is a common example of reversal of the normal left ventricular convexity of the septum. Patients with left bundle branch block and normal coronary arteries occasionally have markedly abnormal segmental wall motion.

Left Ventricular Thrombus

Mural thrombi of the left ventricle occur in the area adjacent to healed myocardial infarcts without aneurysm, in segmental wall aneurysms, and with idiopathic dilated cardiomyopathy with poor wall motion. Left ventricular thrombi do not occur if the wall is contracting normally. The thrombi are usually at the apex, although they may be elsewhere, particularly along the inferior wall and, occasionally, within a false aneurysm. Approximately half of all patients with postinfarction ventricular aneurysm have left ventricular thrombi that are seen at surgery or on necropsy study; however, the angiographic detection of these thrombi is only moderately sensitive and specific. Simpson and colleagues found that roughly 74% of mural thrombi found at surgery are not detected by angiography, and in 10% of patients diagnosed as having thrombi, no thrombi are present at operation.

Calcifications

Left ventricular thrombi may be calcified, particularly when there is calcification of adjacent structures, such as an aneurysm or infarcted papillary muscle. Filling defects that are typical of thrombus may have several appearances (Fig. 6-44). A polypoid shape usually arises in an akinetic apex. This angiographic configuration is a harbinger of systemic embolization. A truncated apex with an adjacent shaggy wall may also indicate thrombus formation (Fig. 6-45). Since the wall of an aneurysm is thin, the presence of a normal or thick wall to the aneurysm indicates a thrombus within the aneurysm.

Other filling defects

Occasionally, other types of filling defects in the ventricle will mimic a thrombus. Large papillary muscles may appear polypoid and can occupy a major portion of the ventricle. Unlike thrombi, they increase in size during systole and are attached to a normally moving wall. Trabeculations and chordae may appear as circular, punctate filling defects. Trabeculations will increase in size during systole and do not show the chaotic, vibrating motion that is associated with thrombi or masses anchored in only one location. Thrombi never occur on a normally moving wall. In idiopathic dilated cardiomy-

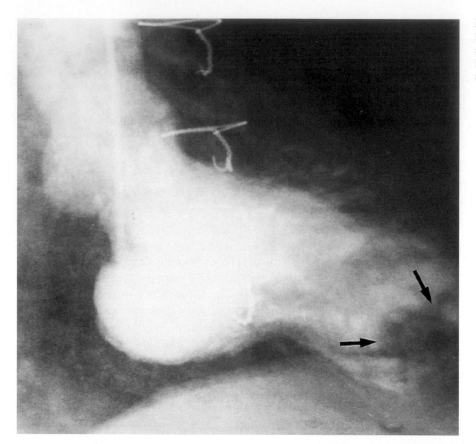

Fig. 6-44 Left ventricular thrombus. The left ventricle in midsystole has a dyskinetic apex and diaphragmatic wall. The thrombus is polypoid (*arrows*) and is attached at the apex.

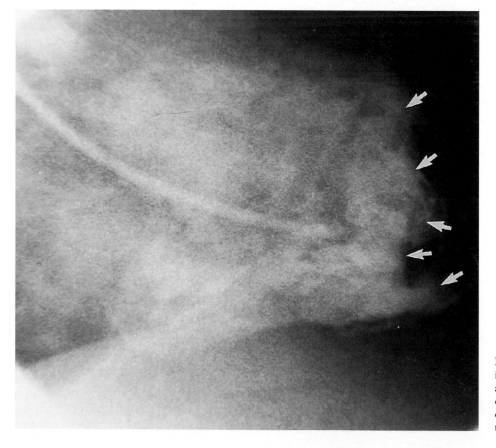

Fig. 6-45 The truncated apex with an irregular contour is a sessile thrombus in a region of akinesis. The catheter is too close to the thrombus and if recognized on the test injection would be repositioned near the mitral valve.

opathy, the apex may be hypokinetic and have an adjacent thrombus. In these patients, there is usually a dilated ventricle and a thinning of the apical wall. In the absence of other indications of left ventricular hypertrophy, a thick apical wall in dilated cardiomyopathy suggests thrombus.

Left Ventricular True and False Aneurysm

Definition and pathologic correlation

Left ventricular aneurysms appear to develop early in the course of myocardial infarction. In more than 50% of patients who develop an aneurysm, it will be present within 24 to 48 hours of the onset of infarction and frequently will still be present 3 months later. In the Coronary Artery Surgery Study (CASS), roughly 8% of patients with coronary artery disease had well-defined left ventricular aneurysms. Although aneurysms can develop with single-artery disease, most left ventricular aneurysms have multivessel coronary disease with severe obstructions. Patients with an anterior aneurysm usually have a greater than 90% stenosis of the proximal left anterior descending artery.

A left ventricular aneurysm is a segment of a left ventricular wall that protrudes from the expected diastolic outline of the ventricular chamber. The wall motion may be either akinetic or dyskinetic. The wall of the aneurysm generally is smooth without the usual trabecular pattern. This definition of a left ventricular aneurysm overlaps with several features of reversible ischemia. During an acute myocardial infarction, the wall segment involved has a dyskinetic motion, which may return to normal if a transmural infarction does not occur.

When the wall thins, a large myocardial scar may develop the appearance of an aneurysm. On imaging studies, a large scar or a small aneurysm may have the same appearance. A functional aneurysm has a normal diastolic contour but a dyskinetic systolic bulge in the region of a large acontractile segment and may contain either reversible ischemic myocardium or scar. In contrast, an anatomic aneurysm has an abnormal protrusion during both systole and diastole because the wall is completely a scar that has stretched (Fig. 6-46).

Imaging signs of aneurysm

Anatomic aneurysms that have been present for more than several months may have a thin rim of calcium outlining their extent. This type of aneurysm may be either akinetic or dyskinetic. The wall of a true aneurysm is quite thin, reflecting that the scar extends from the endocardium through to the pericardium (Fig. 6-47). The aneurysmal segment has a large neck comparable in size to its internal circumference. Within the aneurysm, the wall is usually smooth unless a thrombus is present. The boundaries of the aneurysm are usually discrete and easily discernible. The chest film is not a sensitive test to screen for left ventricular aneurysm. Only one third of angiographically diagnosed aneurysms show contour abnormalities on the chest film. Part of the explanation for this discrepancy is that the septum is not visible on the chest film, and small aneurysms at the apex are obscured by the fat pad. The left ventricle is usually dilated and the remaining wall is hyperkinetic to maintain cardiac output. The uninvolved ventricular wall is frequently hypertrophied, which probably reflects that about one half of patients with aneurysms also have systemic hypertension. Most true aneurysms are in the anterolateral and apical walls (Fig. 6-48) although the inferior (Fig. 6-49) and posterolateral walls occasionally have isolated aneurysms.

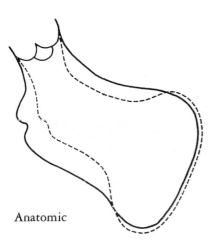

Anatomic

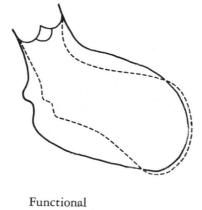

Functional

Fig. 6-46 Types of ventricular aneurysms. The *anatomic aneurysm* has an abnormal bulge during both diastole and systole. The *functional aneurysm* has a normal diastolic contour but, physiologically, has a large acontractile segment. The *solid lines* outline end diastole and the *dotted lines* outline end systole.

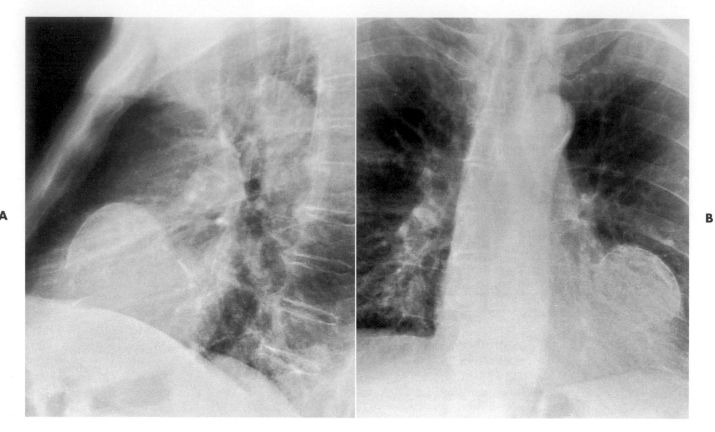

Fig. 6-47 True left aneurysm. **A,** A thin rim of calcium outlines the abnormal left ventricular contour over the anterolateral wall. **B,** On the lateral view, the aneurysm has a broad base and partially projects anteriorly over the right heart.

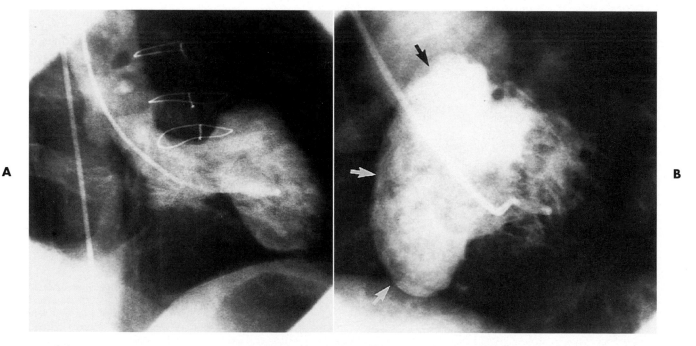

Fig. 6-48 Left ventricular true aneurysm. **A,** A systolic frame shows a large aneurysm with a broad base involving the anterolateral, apical, and diaphragmatic walls. **B,** The left anterior oblique view shows that the aneurysm extends into the septal wall *(arrows)*.

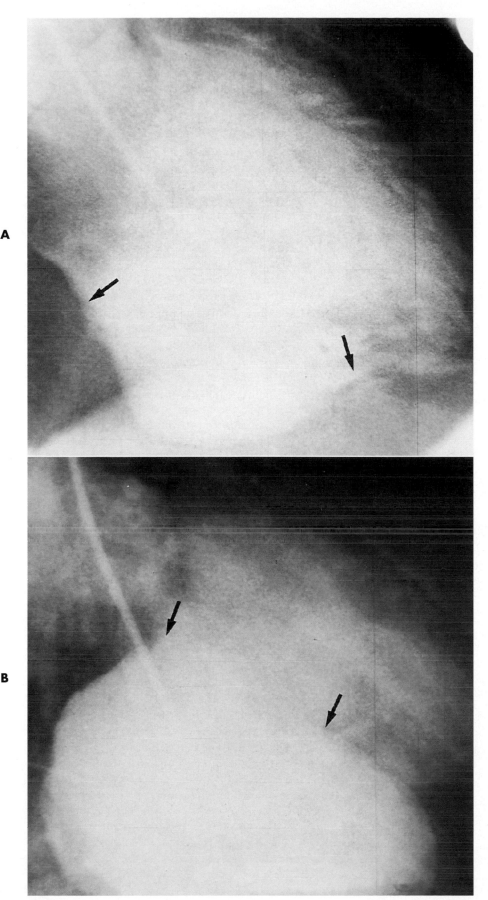

Fig. 6-49 Inferior aneurysms. **A,** The abnormal diastolic contour *(arrows)* extends from the mitral annulus to the diaphragmatic segment and includes the posteromedial papillary muscle. **B,** The saccular aneurysm has a wide neck *(arrows)* which distinguishes it from a false aneurysm, although a false aneurysm may rarely have a neck this large.

False Aneurysm

When the pericardium rather than myocardium composes the wall of the aneurysm, it is a false aneurysm or pseudoaneurysm. The usual cause is a rupture of the left ventricle into the pericardial space after myocardial infarction. Because of adhesions from previous pericarditis, the pericardium locally attaches to the epicardium. This opportunely restrains the ventricular blood from extending into the remaining pericardial space and causing tamponade. Causes that are less common but which have nearly identical appearance include abscess from bacterial endocarditis, surgical ventriculotomy (Fig. 6-50), and penetrating trauma. In contrast to true aneurysms, most false aneurysms resulting from myocardial infarct are on the posterolateral and diaphragmatic sides of the left ventricle (Fig. 6-51).

The left ventriculogram demonstrates a discrete saccular aneurysm whose neck is considerably smaller than the internal circumference of the saccule. Contrast material may not flow into the false aneurysm until late in systole, and it may oscillate into and out of the neck of the

aneurysm without exiting from the left ventricle. Because of the narrow communication with the left ventricular chamber, the opacification of the false aneurysm may persist for many seconds after the injection has ended (Fig. 6-52). The narrow neck of the false aneurysm has also been used as a pathognomonic sign in the scintigraphic assessment in both blood pool scans and MRI (Fig. 6-53).

Frequently the false aneurysm is bigger than the left ventricle and, in fact, may enlarge over serial examinations. This has prognostic significance in that false aneurysms have a high propensity to rupture. Rupture of a true aneurysm is rare, occurring in less than 4% of several necropsy series. In contrast, postmortem series indicate that approximately 45% of false aneurysms rupture.

The coronary arteries in patients with false aneurysms are also severely diseased. However, reflecting the posterior and diaphragmatic location of most false aneurysms, there is frequent occlusion of the right coronary artery, whereas with true aneurysm, occlusion is more common in the left coronary artery.

Cardiac false aneurysm (or changes that look like aneurysms) may result from diseases other than coronary artery disease. Congenital diverticula of the left ventricle may be confused with false aneurysm, but they usually are smaller and occur at the apex. The African cardiomyopathies that have apical aneurysms usually can be distinguished by both their clinical course and the absence of coronary disease. The rare submitral aneurysms found in black Africans are not caused by ischemia. These aneurysms have a narrow neck originating between the mitral annulus and the posteromedial papillary muscle. The large sac lies beneath the left atrium and displaces it superiorly.

VENTRICULOGRAPHY AFTER ANEURYSM RESECTION

Resection of a true aneurysm at the apex leaves a sharply marginated and truncated "new" apex with a vertical orientation. This new apex is akinetic and with its truncation can be confused with a large thrombus. When the resection extends to a wall containing a papillary muscle, mitral valve replacement will be evident. Because rupture of the interventricular septum occurs in association with aneurysm, the reconstructed portion of the septum will be akinetic. Rarely, the pledgets used for suture reinforcement will be visible as a slightly shaggy irregularity. The coronary arteries adjacent to the resection will be abruptly terminated. No large or main coronary arteries are seen adjacent to the ventriculotomy, although there may be a vascular blush.

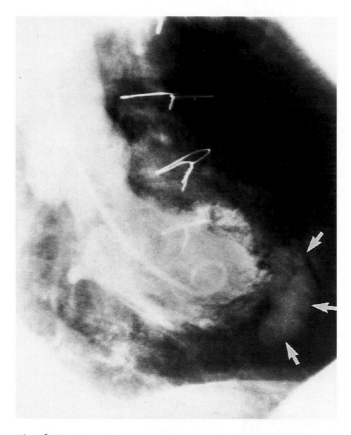

Fig. 6-50   False left ventricular aneurysm after ventriculotomy. The extraluminal collection of contrast *(arrows)* at the apex occurred at the site of a puncture to vent air as the patient came off coronary bypass. The blood is constrained by the adjacent pericardium and mediastinal scarring.

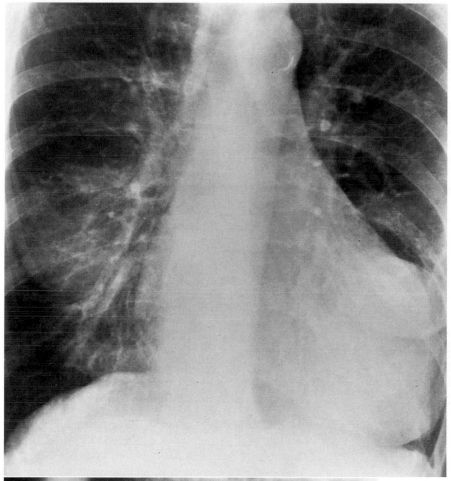

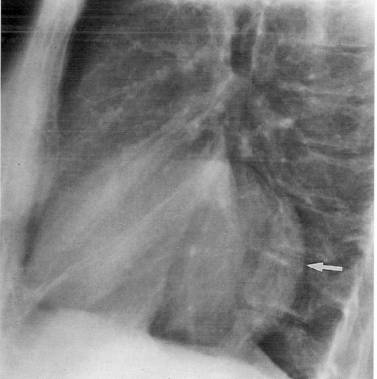

Fig. 6-51 Contour abnormality in left ventricular false aneurysm. The patient had a false aneurysm develop at the site of a true aneurysm. **A,** The anterolateral and apical location is typical of a true aneurysm. **B,** The lateral chest film shows an aneurysm in the posterolateral wall *(arrow),* more typical of a false aneurysm. The chest film cannot distinguish between the types of aneurysms but is more useful for diagnosing their presence and whether they have increased in size.

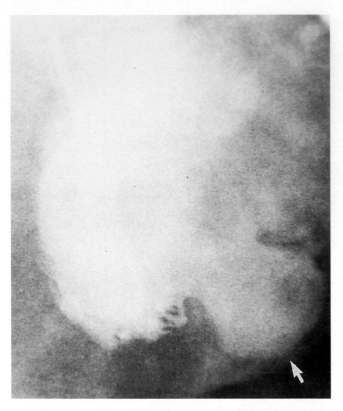

Fig. 6-52 Left ventricular false aneurysm. Left anterior oblique ventriculogram shows a posterolateral aneurysm with a narrow neck. The wall thickness is only 3 mm *(arrow).*

Table 6-2 Chest radiographic abnormalities in rupture of the interventricular septum	
Abnormality	**Percent**
Pulmonary	
Normal	12
Pulmonary venous hypertension	9
Interstitial edema	42
Alveolar edema	36
Pleural effusions	
None	36
Right side	3
Left side	30
Both sides	30
Pulmonary artery enlargement	39
Cardiac enlargement	
Left ventricle	82
Left atrium	6
Right ventricle	3
Right atrium	12

Modified with permission from Miller SW, Dinsmore RE, Greene RE, et al: Coronary, ventricular, and pulmonary abnormalities associated with rupture of the interventricular septum complicating myocardial infarction. *AJR Am J Roentgenol* 131:571, 1978.

RUPTURE OF THE INTERVENTRICULAR SEPTUM

Clinical Presentation

Rupture of the interventricular septum is an uncommon complication of myocardial infarction that occurs in about 1% of those who sustain infarction. If not surgically treated, more than 90% of those with rupture die within 1 year. The appearance of a new systolic murmur within hours to weeks after myocardial infarction, particularly if associated with biventricular failure or cardiogenic shock, suggests ventricular septal defect or ruptured papillary muscle.

Common abnormalities in chest radiographs of patients with a ruptured septum usually show interstitial or alveolar pulmonary edema and left ventricular enlargement (Table 6-2). Enlargement of other chambers is inconstant. Almost half will show pleural effusions, enlargement of the pulmonary arteries, and signs of pulmonary venous hypertension. Occasionally, an unusual configuration of the heart will suggest the presence of an aneurysm in addition to the septal rupture (Fig. 6-54).

Left Ventricular Signs

During left ventriculography, almost all patients have at least one segment with akinesis or dyskinesis. The posterolateral wall is hyperkinetic in some patients, suggesting that the exaggerated motion was partly compensating for the other segments of the ventricle. The septum is always akinetic or dyskinetic.

In the right anterior oblique view, you will see opacification of the pulmonary artery during left ventriculography. This view superimposes the two ventricles. The most inferior wall visible is the diaphragmatic wall of the right ventricle. If the left ventricular diaphragmatic wall is akinetic, the adjacent right ventricular wall behaves similarly. In the left anterior oblique projection, contrast material passes through the rupture to opacify the right ventricle (Fig. 6-55). The margins of the rupture may be difficult to identify but they always are in a region of severe segmental wall motion abnormality. Occasionally, the right ventricular anterior wall will also be akinetic and represent an extension of the diaphragmatic infarct.

After myocardial infarction, ventricular septal defects occur in the muscular septum either posteriorly adjacent to the mitral valve, or anteriorly near the apex. The margins of the rupture are irregular and the flow of contrast media in that region is slow. However, the site of rupture is always in a region of severe segmental wall motion abnormality. Anterolateral and apical akinesis uniformly correspond with an anterior rupture near the apex, whereas posterobasal and diaphragmatic akinesis occur with posterior rupture adjacent to the mitral annulus.

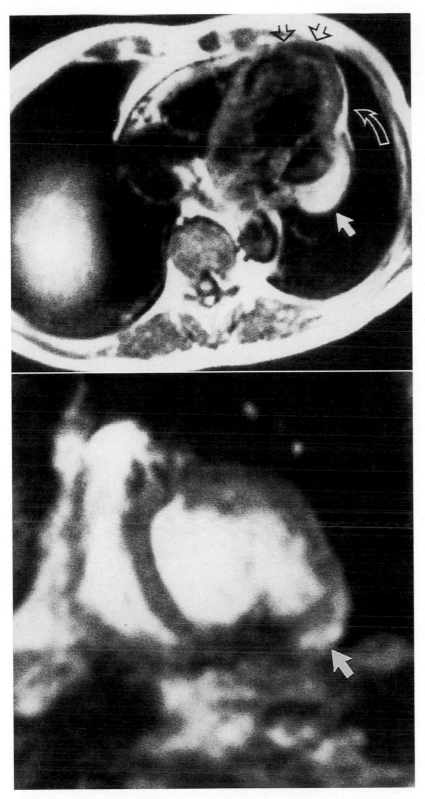

Fig. 6-53 True and false ventricular aneurysm with thrombus in false aneurysm. **A,** Gated MR image demonstrates thinning and low signal intensity of the myocardium in the anteroseptal and apical left ventricle *(open arrows)* representing a true aneurysm. Along the inferoposterior wall is a discrete bulge suggestive of a false aneurysm *(white arrow)*. Adjacent to the pericardium along the anterolateral wall of the left ventricle is a high signal in epicardial fat *(curved arrow)*. The high-signal crescent-shaped region within the false aneurysm lumen represents a combination of thrombus and slow flow. **B,** Gradient echo oblique sagittal view through the left ventricle demonstrates a high signal in the false aneurysm *(arrow)*. The diameter of the mouth of the aneurysm is smaller than the largest diameter of the aneurysm itself, consistent with a false aneurysm. (Reprinted from Kahn J, Fisher MR: MRI of cardiac pseudoaneurysm and other complications of myocardial infarct, *Magn Reson Imaging* 9:159-164, 1991. With permission from Pergamon Press Ltd, Headington Hill Hall, Oxford OX3 OBW, UK.)

The cranial left anterior oblique view elongates the septum and helps to distinguish apical from basal ruptures.

Left ventricular aneurysm, mitral regurgitation, or both are found in roughly three fourths of patients with septal rupture. These exaggerate extensive wall motion abnormalities. The aneurysm may be in the region of the septal rupture or in a separate portion of the ventricle. The mitral regurgitation is the result of a variety of factors, including left ventricular dilatation and papillary muscle dysfunction. Both of these lesions contribute to

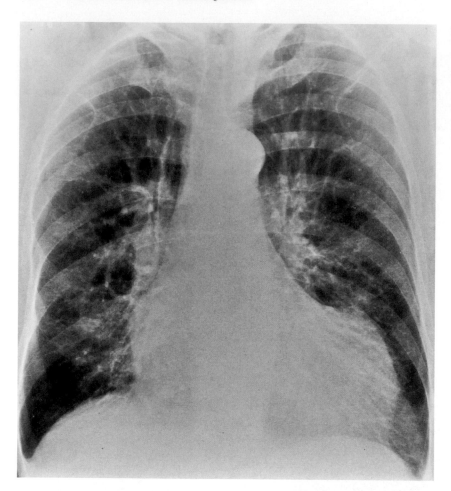

Fig. 6-54 Typical chest film in rupture of interventricular septum. The heart is enlarged with an aneurysm in the anterolateral and apical segments. There is redistribution of blood to the upper lobes and slight interstitial pulmonary edema manifested by Kerley B lines and shaggy bronchovascular walls. The pulmonary vasculature reflects the left ventricular failure and not the left-to-right shunt that is present.

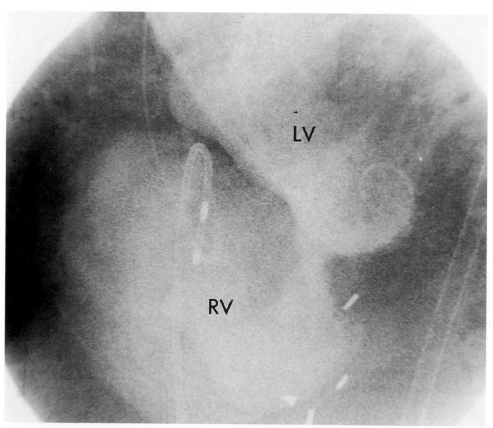

Fig. 6-55 Rupture of the interventricular septum. In a left anterior oblique left ventriculogram, contrast material pours through most of the apical septum of the left ventricle (*LV*) into the dilated right ventricle (*RV*). The right ventricle is large and akinetic with an aneurysm involving most of the anterior wall.

poor left ventricular performance and make catheteriza tion difficult. However, their recognition is essential for proper surgical management.

Extensive coronary artery stenoses are usually present with septal rupture. Severe two- and three-vessel disease is common with rupture of the interventricular septum, yet about 30% with rupture have a significant stenosis in only one coronary artery, either the right coronary or left anterior descending artery. When only one coronary artery is involved, that portion of the artery distal to the occlusion is generally not visualized. This indicates that it is completely occluded or that bridging collateral vessels either have not formed or are not currently functioning. The absence of collaterals and the lack of visualization of the coronary artery distal to a proximal occlusion in a patient with septal rupture is presumably associated with a sizable area of muscle infarction that was present before the septum ruptured. On the other hand, in the absence of a septal rupture or aneurysm, the distal segment of an occluded coronary artery is almost always opacified through collateral vessels. It is possible that edema in the ischemic zone around the infarct compresses existing collateral vessels, and that these small vessels might be visible when the edema regresses.

MITRAL REGURGITATION RESULTING FROM CORONARY ARTERY DISEASE

Pathologic Causes

The mechanism of mitral regurgitation in coronary artery disease appears to be related to the impairment of

the left ventricular wall containing the papillary muscles. This pathologic process has been labeled the papillary muscle dysfunction syndrome, although the papillary muscles and their blood supply are only a partial explanation. The arterioles supplying the papillary muscles are either end-arteries or, at least, are at the termination of a long arterial path. The posteromedial papillary muscle is supplied by left circumflex marginal branches to the posterolateral wall or by branches of the distal right coronary artery; the anterolateral papillary muscle receives blood mainly from diagonal branches of the left anterior descending artery. During systole, the papillary muscles contract and either initiate the action or assist in the support of the mitral apparatus to withstand systolic pressure. Clinically, under situations in which the papillary muscles are ischemic, the adjacent left ventricular wall is also ischemic. Congestive heart failure leading to left ventricular dilatation will change the orientation of the papillary muscles to the mitral leaflets but causes only a trace amount of regurgitation because the muscle around the mitral orifice contracts slightly during systole. Under these circumstances mitral regurgitation of mild to severe degree may result because of incomplete mitral leaflet closure. The spectrum of papillary muscle disorders includes ischemic processes to both the papillary muscle and its adjacent left ventricular free wall. For example, hypokinesis, akinesis, or aneurysm may produce any degree of mitral regurgitation (Fig. 6-56).

Complete rupture of a necrotic papillary muscle is quite rare, and because of its acute severity, usually causes death of the patient. Recent surgical advances have made survival possible for some individuals if this lesion is rec-

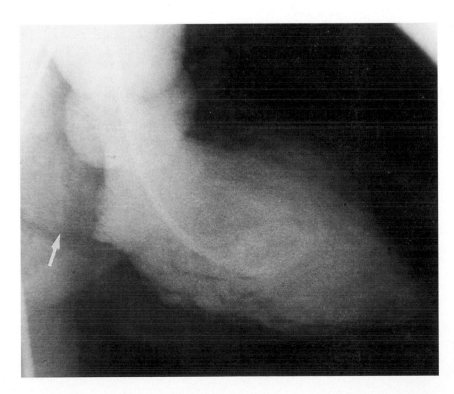

Fig. 6-56 Papillary muscle dysfunction. Mitral regurgitation *(arrow)* has resulted from akinesis of the inferior wall after an infarct.

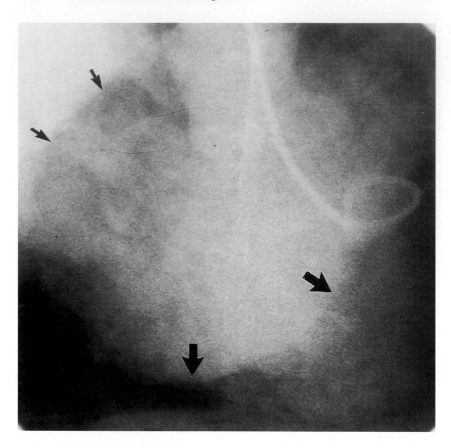

Fig. 6-57 Rupture of a papillary muscle after a myocardial infarct. Right anterior oblique left ventriculogram outlines a large posterobasal aneurysm *(thick arrows)*. The mitral leaflets *(thin arrows)* are visible because there is contrast material in the left atrium from severe regurgitation.

ognized early. The more frequent clinical event is rupture of only one head of the papillary muscle, allowing the attached chordae to partially support both mitral leaflets and to limit somewhat the amount of regurgitation.

Ventriculographic Signs

The left ventriculographic signs of papillary muscle dysfunction include left ventricular enlargement, an akinetic wall that contains a papillary muscle or an adjacent left ventricular aneurysm, calcification in a papillary muscle, and any degree of mitral regurgitation. The papillary muscle may be quite large, swollen with edema associated with myocardial infarction. An erratically moving mitral leaflet with a major portion of its motion in the left atrium indicates a ruptured papillary muscle (Fig. 6-57). In the setting of free mitral regurgitation after myocardial infarction, one or both heads of a papillary muscle must have ruptured, indicating the need for emergent mitral valve replacement.

SUGGESTED READINGS

Books

Marcus ML, Schelbert HR, Skorton DJ, et al: *Cardiac imaging: a companion to Braunwald's heart disease,* Philadelphia, 1991, WB Saunders.

Neufeld HN, Schneeweiss A (eds): *Coronary artery disease in infants and children,* Philadelphia, 1983, Lea & Febiger.

Virmani R, Forman MB (eds): *Nonatherosclerotic ischemic heart disease,* New York, 1989, Raven Press.

Journals

Ambrose JA: Plaque disruption and the acute coronary syndromes of unstable angina and myocardial infarction: if the substrate is similar, why is the clinical presentation different? *J Am Coll Cardiol* 19:1653-1658, 1992.

Ambrose JA, Winters SL, Arora RR, et al: Angiographic evolution of coronary artery morphology in unstable angina, *J Am Coll Cardiol* 7:472-478, 1986.

Baim DS, Kline H, Silverman JF: Bilateral coronary artery–pulmonary artery fistulas. Report of five cases and review of the literature, *Circulation* 65:810-815, 1982

Beckmann CF, Levin DC, Kubicka RA, et al: The effect of sequential arterial stenoses on flow and pressure, *Radiology* 140:655-658, 1981.

Bogaty P, Brecker SJ, White SE, et al: Comparison of coronary angiographic findings in acute and chronic first presentation of ischemic heart disease, *Circulation* 87:1938-1946, 1993.

Bolli R: Myocardial "stunning" in man, *Circulation* 86:1671-1691, 1992.

Brown BG, Gallery CA, Badger RS, et al: Incomplete lysis of thrombus in the moderate underlying atherosclerotic lesion during intracoronary infusion of streptokinase for acute myocardial infarction: quantitative angiographic observations, *Circulation* 73:653-661, 1986.

Brown BG, Zhao ZQ, Sacco DE, et al: Lipid lowering and plaque regression. New insights into prevention of plaque disruption and clinical events in coronary disease, *Circulation* 87:1781-1791, 1993.

Cabins HS, Roberts WC: Left ventricular aneurysm, intra-aneurysmal thrombus and systemic embolus in coronary heart disease, *Chest* 77:586-590,1980.

Cabins HS, Roberts WC: True left ventricular aneurysm and healed myocardial infarction. Clinical and necropsy observations including quantification of degrees of coronary arterial narrowing, *Am J Cardiol* 46:754-763, 1980.

Cipriano PR, Sacks AH, Reitz BA, et al: The effect of stenosis of bypass grafts on coronary blood flow. A mechanical model study, *Circulation* 62:61-66, 1980.

Crouse JR III, Thompson CJ: An evaluation of methods for imaging and quantifying coronary and carotid lumen stenosis and atherosclerosis, *Circulation* 87(suppl 2):II-17–II-33, 1993.

Davies MJ: A macro and mirco view of coronary vascular insult in ischemic heart disease, *Circulation* 82(suppl 2):II-38–II-46), 1990.

Davies SW, Marchant B, Lyons JP, et al: Coronary lesion morphology in acute myocardial infarction: demonstration of early remodeling after streptokinase treatment, *J Am Coll Cardiol* 16:1079-1086, 1990.

Dilsizian V, Bonow RO: Current diagnostic techniques of assessing myocardial viability in patients with hibernating and stunned myocardium, *Circulation* 87:1-20, 1993.

Dulce MC, Duerinckx AJ, Hartiala J, et al: MR imaging of the myocardium using nonionic contrast medium: signal-intensity changes in patients with subacute myocardial infarction, *AJR Am J Roentgenol* 160:963-970, 1993.

Edelman RR, Manning WJ, Pearlman J, et al: Human coronary arteries: projection angiograms reconstructed from breath-hold two-dimensional MR images, *Radiology* 187:719-722, 1993.

Faxon DP, Ryan TJ, Davis KB, et al: Prognostic significance of angiographically documented left ventricular aneurysm from the coronary artery surgery study (CASS), *Am J Cardiol* 50:157-164, 1982.

Feldman RL, Nichols WW, Pepine CJ, et al: Hemodynamic significance of the length of a coronary arterial narrowing, *Am J Cardiol* 41:865-871, 1978.

Fellows KE, Freed MD, Keane JF, et al: Results of routine preoperative coronary angiography in tetralogy of Fallot, *Circulation* 51:561-566, 1975.

Formanek A, Nath P, Zollikoffer C, et al: Selective coronary arteriography in children, *Circulation* 61:84-95, 1980.

Fuster VF, Badimon L, Badimon JJ, et al: The pathogenesis of coronary artery disease and the acute coronary syndrones, *N Engl J Med* 326:242-250, 310-318, 1992.

Gould KL, Kirkeeide RL: Assessment of stenosis severity. In Reiber JIIC and Serruys PW (eds): *State of the art in quantitative coronary arteriography,* Dordrecht, Netherlands, 1986, Martinus Nijhoff, p 209.

Gould KL, Kirkeeide RL, Buchi M: Coronary flow reserve as a physiologic measure of stenosis severity, *J Am Coll Cardiol* 15:459-474, 1990.

Greenberg MA, Fish BG, Spindola-Franco H: Congenital anomalies of the coronary arteries: classification and significance, *Radiol Clin North Am* 27:1127-1146, 1989.

Guidelines for percutaneous transluminal coronary angioplasty. A report of the American College of Cardiology/American Heart Association Task Force on Assessment of Diagnostic and Therapeutic Cardiovascular Procedures (Subcommittee on Percutaneous Transluminal Coronary Angioplasty), *J Am Coll Cardiol* 12:529-545, 1988.

Hamby RI, Wisoff G, Davison ET, et al: Coronary artery disease and left ventricular mural thrombi: Clinical, hemodynamic and angiocardiographic aspects, *Chest* 66:488-494, 1974.

Harding MB, Leither ME, Mark DB, et al: Ergonovine maleate testing during cardiac catheterization: a 10 year perspective in 3,447 patients without significant coronary artery disease or Prinzmetal's variant angina, *J Am Coll Cardiol* 20:107-111, 1992.

Higgins CB, Lipton MJ: Radiography of acute myocardial infarction, *Radiol Clin North Am* 18:359-368, 1980.

Irvin RG: The angiographic prevalence of myocardial bridging in man, *Chest* 81:198-202, 1982.

Kahn K, Fisher MR: MRI of cardiac pseudoaneurysm and other complications of myocardial infarction, *Magn Reson Imaging* 9:159-164, 1991.

Kaski JC, Rosano GMC, Collins P, et al: Cardiac syndrome X. Clinical characteristics and left ventricular function, *J Am Coll Cardiol* 25:807-814.

Kereiakes DJ, Topol EJ, George BS, et al: Myocardial infarction with minimal coronary atherosclerosis in the era of thrombolytic reperfusion, *J Am Coll Cardiol* 17:304-312, 1991.

Kimbiris JB, Iskandrian AS, Segal BL, et al: Anomalous aortic origin of coronary arteries, *Circulation* 58:606-615, 1978.

Kloner RA, Przyklenk K, Patel B: Altered myocardial states: the stunned and hibernating myocardium, *Am J Med* 80(suppl 1A):14, 1986.

Levin DC, Gardiner GA Jr: Complex and simple coronary artery stenoses: a new way to interpret coronary angiograms based on morphologic features of lesions, *Radiology* 164:675-680, 1987.

Li D, Paschal CB, Haacke EM, et al: Coronary arteries: three-dimensional MR imaging with fat saturation and magnetication transfer contrast, *Radiology* 187:401-406, 1993.

Liberthson RR, Dinsmore RE, Bharatic S, et al: Aberrant coronary artery origin from the aorta. Diagnosis and clinical significance, *Circulation* 50:774-779, 1974.

Liberthson RR, Sagar K, Berkoben JP, et al: Congenital coronary arteriovenous fistula. Report of 13 patients, review of the literature and delineation of management, *Circulation* 59:849-854, 1979.

Little WC, Constaninescu M, Appelgate RJ, et al: Can coronary angiography predict the site of a subsequent myocardial infarction in patients with mild-to-moderate coronary artery disease?, *Circulation* 78:1157-1166,1988.

Manning WJ, Li W, Boyle NG, et al: Fat-suppressed breath-hold magnetic resonance coronary angiography, *Circulation* 87:94-104, 1993.

Manning WJ, Li W, Edelman RR: A preliminary report comparing magnetic resonance coronary angiography with conventional angiography, *N Engl J Med* 328:828-832, 1993.

Massie BM, Botvinick EH, Brundage BH, et al: Relationship of regional myocardial perfusion to segmental wall motion. A physiologic basis for understanding the presence and reversibility of asynergy, *Circulation* 58:1154-1163, 1978.

Megnien JKL, Sene V, Jeannin S, et al: Coronary calcification and its relation to extracoronary atherosclerosis in asymptomatic hypercholesterolemic men, *Circulation* 85:1799-1807, 1992.

Meizlish JL, Berger HJ, Plankey M, et al: Functional left ventricular aneurysm formation after acute anterior transmural myocardial infarction, *N Engl J Med* 311:1001-1006, 1984.

Miller SW, Boucher CA: Assessing the adequacy of myocardial perfusion in man: anatomic and functional techniques, *Radiol Clin North Am* 23:589-596, 1985.

Miller SW, Dinsmore RE, Greene RE, et al: Coronary, ventricular, and pulmonary abnormalities associated with rupture of the interventricular septum complicating myocardial infarction, *AJR Am J Roentgenol* 131:571-577, 1978.

Mizuno K, Horiuchi K, Matui H, et al: Role of coronary collateral vessels during transient coronary occlusion during angioplasty assessed by hemodynamic, electrocardiographic and metabolic changes, *J Am Coll Cardiol* 12:624-628, 1988.

Morbidity from coronary heart disease in the United States, NHLBI Data Fact Sheet, Bethesda, MD, June 1990, National Heart, Lung, and Blood Institute.

Ogden JA, Stansel HC Jr: Roentgenographic manifestations of congenital coronary artery disease, *AJR Am J Roentgenol* 113:538-553, 1971.

Pierard LA, Albert A, Henrard L, et al: Incidence and significance of pericardial effusion in acute myocardial infarction as determined by two-dimensional echocardiography, *J Am Coll Cardiol* 8:517-520, 1986.

Proudfit WL, Shirey EK, Sheldon WC, et al: Certain clinical characteristics correlated with extent of obstructive lesions demonstrated by selective cine-coronary arteriography, *Circulation* 38:947-954, 1968.

Reddy K, Gupta M, Hamby RI: Multiple coronary arteriosystemic fistulas, *Am J Cardiol* 33:304-306, 1974.

Schwartz H, Leiboff RH, Bren GB, et al: Temporal evolution of the human coronary collateral circulation after myocardial infarction, *J Am Coll Cardiol* 4:1088-1093, 1984.

Sharifi M, Frohlich TG, Silverman IM: Myocardial infarction with angiographically normal coronary arteries, *Chest* 107:36-40, 1995.

Simpson MT, Oberman A, Kouchoukos NT, et al: Prevalence of mural thrombi and systemic embolization with left ventricular aneurysm. Effect of anticoagulation therapy, *Chest* 77:463-469, 1980.

Stanford W, Thompson BH, Weiss RM: Coronary artery calcification: clinical significance and current methods of detection, *AJR Am J Roentgenol* 161:1139-1146, 1993.

Tunick PA, Slater J, Kronzon I, et al: Discrete atherosclerotic coronary artery aneurysms: a study of 20 patients, *J Am Coll Cardiol* 15:279-282, 1990.

Yacoe ME, Dake MD: Development and resolution of systemic and coronary artery aneurysms in Kawasaki disease, *AJR Am J Roentgenol* 159:708-710, 1992.

CHAPTER 7

Interventional Cardiology

MARGARET A. FERRELL

IGOR F. PALACIOS

Percutaneous Transluminal Coronary Angioplasty
Changes in the arterial wall after angioplasty
Patient selection
Technique
Results of PTCA
Complications of PTCA
Restenosis
Newer Coronary Interventional Devices
Directional coronary atherectomy
Rotablator
Transluminal extraction endarterectomy
Excimer laser
Coronary Stents
Percutaneous Mitral Balloon Valvuloplasty
Patient selection
Patient preparation
Mechanism of PMV
Results
Complications
Long-term follow-up post-PMV
Percutaneous Aortic Valvuloplasty
Technique
Mechanism and results of PAV
Complications of PAV
Coronary Artery Fistulas
Suggested Readings

Interventional cardiology has evolved rapidly since Andreas Gruentzig performed the first coronary angioplasty in 1977. In a relatively brief time, major advances in technology have allowed the expanded application of percutaneous techniques not only to coronary artery disease but also to valvular and congenital heart disease. This chapter reviews current options for the percutaneous treatment of coronary artery disease, including balloon angioplasty, laser ablation, atherectomy devices, and coronary stents. In addition, balloon valvuloplasty for the management of mitral and aortic stenosis and the percutaneous closure of coronary arteriovenous fistulas are addressed.

PERCUTANEOUS TRANSLUMINAL CORONARY ANGIOPLASTY

Balloon percutaneous transluminal coronary angioplasty (PTCA) remains the most common means of percutaneous coronary revascularization. Patient eligibility continues to expand as more sophisticated equipment makes possible the treatment of coronary lesions not previously approachable. Despite increasingly complex coronary anatomy being approached, the immediate success (defined as reduction of a stenosis to less than 50%) of PTCA has continued to increase and is currently in the range of 90%. Unfortunately, severe dissection, abrupt closure, and restenosis continue to limit short-term and long-term success following PTCA.

Changes in the Arterial Wall After Angioplasty

Mechanisms operative in the increased lumen diameter following successful balloon angioplasty include:

1. Fracture and tearing of stenotic plaque
2. Dissection through the intima into the media
3. Dissection of the media and adventitia underlying the plaque
4. Stretching of the normal vessel wall

Patient Selection

The decision to perform angioplasty requires a judgment that takes into consideration the likelihood of success for a given lesion as well as the consequences of procedure failure or complication. Careful patient selection is essential to achieve a high incidence of success with a low incidence of complications. Generally, candidates for PTCA are also candidates for surgical revascularization (coronary artery bypass grafting, CABG), although "compassionate" procedures are carried out in severely ill patients who are not operative candidates.

Details of coronary anatomy are fundamental to the selection of patients for PTCA. Specific angiographic characteristics of the lesions to be dilated are important determinants of PTCA success and complications. An American College of Cardiology/American Heart Association task force subcommittee has issued a lesion-specific classification as a guide for predicting success of PTCA as well as the risk of developing acute vessel closure (Box 7-1). This classification of lesions, based on their angiographic characteristics, is fundamental to selecting the method of revascularization for any given lesion; that is, balloon angioplasty vs. laser vs. directional atherectomy, and so forth.

Technique

PTCA is generally carried out from the femoral artery, although the brachial approach is an alternative source of arterial access. You should select a guiding catheter according to the vessel to be dilated and obtain initial angiograms of the target vessels as references for wire passage and to enable evaluation of progress during the procedure. Guidewire selection considers the nature of the stenosis and the mechanical features of the available wires. Wires vary in size (.010, .014, .016, and .018 in.), flexibility, visibility, steerability, and trackability (the ability to advance a dilating catheter over a wire). Once you have selected a wire, you shape a gentle curve onto the tip of the wire and advance it through the guiding catheter across the lesion into the distal vessel. You then advance the balloon dilatation catheter to the level of the lesion for inflation.

Balloon dilatation catheters vary in diameter, length, catheter stiffness, and balloon material (compliance). There are two general types of catheters: over-the-wire and on-the-wire devices (Fig. 7-1). In the over-the-wire systems, the balloon catheter has a central wire lumen along its entire length which increases trackability and allows the exchange of balloon catheters while maintaining wire position, a feature that may be of importance if a lesion has been difficult to negotiate with the wire. A variation of this system is the monorail or rapid exchange device where only the distal portion of the balloon catheter has a central wire lumen and the remainder of the wire is side by side with the catheter shaft. In some ways this is easier to handle, but the lack of a central wire along the entire length of the catheter decreases pushability and may be insufficient for difficult lesions.

Another over-the-wire style of catheter is the perfusion catheter. These catheters have a central perfusion

---

Box 7-1   Classification of Coronary Artery Lesions for Angioplasty: Lesion-Specific Characteristics

TYPE A LESIONS (MINIMALLY COMPLEX)

Discrete (length <10 mm)
Concentric
Readily accessible
Nonangulated segment (<45 degrees)
Smooth contour
Little or no calcification
Less than totally occlusive
Not ostial in location
No major side branch involvement
Absence of thrombus

TYPE B LESIONS (MODERATELY COMPLEX)*

Tubular (length 10–20 mm)
Eccentric
Moderate tortuosity of proximal segment
Moderately angulated segment (>45 degrees, <90 degrees)
Irregular contour
Moderate or heavy calcification
Total occlusions less than 3 months old
Ostial in location
Bifurcation lesions requiring double guidewires
Some thrombus present

TYPE C LESIONS (SEVERELY COMPLEX)

Diffuse (length >2cm)
Excessive tortuosity of proximal segment
Extremely angulated segments (>90 degrees)
Total occlusions less than 3 months old or bridging collaterals
Inability to protect major side branches
Degenerated vein grafts with friable lesions

From Ryan TJ, Bauman WB, Kennedy JW, et al: Guidelines for percutaneous transluminal coronary angioplasty. A report of the American College of Cardiology/American Heart Association Task Force on Assessment of Diagnostic and Therapeutic Cardiovascular Procedures (Committee on Percutaneous Transluminal Coronary Angioplasty), *J Am Coll Cardiol* 22:2033-2054, 1993.

*Although the risk of abrupt vessel closure may be moderately high with type B lesions, the likelihood of a major complication may be low in certain instances such as in the dilatation of total occlusions less than 3 months old or when abundant collateral channels supply the distal vessel.

---

lumen with proximal entry ports and distal perfusion ports on either side of the balloon which allow for passive distal coronary perfusion during balloon inflation. This feature is useful in patients who are unable to tolerate balloon inflation owing to severe chest pain or hemodynamic compromise. In addition, these catheters allow prolonged balloon inflation in the event of coronary dissection or abrupt vessel closure and can be left in place while the patient is transferred for bypass surgery.

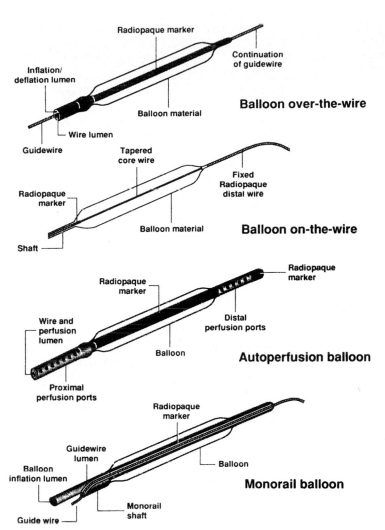

Fig. 7 1 Balloon angioplasty catheter designs. (From Freed M, Grines C (eds): *The manual of interventional cardiology,* Birmingham, MI, 1992, Physician's Press.

The on-the-wire balloon catheters have a segment of wire fixed to the distal balloon top and the entire apparatus is steered as one unit through the stenosis. Although of lower profile than the over-the-wire systems, one disadvantage is the need to remove the entire system and recross the lesion in order to change balloon catheters.

You should choose the balloon size by the diameter of the normal adjacent arterial segment. Undersizing a lesion results in residual stenosis at the dilatation site and oversizing increases the risk of coronary dissection. Frequently, the guiding catheter diameter is used as a reference in a given angiogram and the target vessel diameter is determined by comparison: 7F guide = 2.3 mm outer diameter; 8F = 2.6 mm; 9F = 3.0 mm; 11F = 3.6 mm. Following adequate dilatation, perform repeat angiography in orthogonal views to assess the acute results of the procedure.

Results of PTCA

As mentioned earlier, the immediate success rate of PTCA approaches 90% (residual stenosis <50% with no major complications) (see Table 7-1). The National Heart, Lung, and Blood Institute (NHLBI) sponsored the original PTCA registry from 1979 to 1982 and found the most common reasons for failure to be the inability to cross the lesion with the dilating catheter, failure to reach the lesion because of vessel tortuosity, and inability to adequately dilate the lesion despite crossing with both the wire and the catheter.

There have been no clinical features found to accurately predict success. Immediate outcome is independent of sex, prior myocardial infarct, rest angina, history of smoking, or diabetes.

Angiographic features found to correlate directly with poor outcome are as follows:

Severity of initial stenosis
Presence of calcium
Presence of intraluminal thrombus
Location of lesion in right coronary artery

Angiographic variables that have not been found to correlate with acute success are:

Table 7-1 Coronary artery lesion characteristics and angioplasty success

Variable	Success (%)	P Value
Artery location		
Left main	100	.037
LAD	89.3	
LCx	91.7	
RCA	83.7	
Bypass graft	96.3	
Stenosis site		
Proximal	88.5	NS
Mid	86.7	
Distal	91.1	
Prior PTCA (same site)		
Yes	95.8	
No	88.2	
Stenosis (%)		
60-74	95.7	< .001
75-89	90.2	
90-99	84.2	
100	69.3	
Translesional gradient (mm Hg)		
≤ 39	95.0	NS
40-49	95.2	
50-59	96.0	
60-69	96.3	
≥ 70	98.1	
Artery size (diameter in mm)		
≤1.9	94.7	NS
2.0-2.4	88.2	
2.5-2.9	88.8	
3.0-3.4	88.5	
3.5-3.9	88.1	
≥ 4	92.1	
Stenosis length (mm)		
1-9	90.1	NS
10-19	93.1	
≥ 20	81.8	
Eccentric morphology		
Yes	89.2	NS
No	88.6	
Calcification		
Yes	81.7	.007
No	89.7	
Thrombus		
Yes	82.0	.029
No	89.6	

Modified from Savage MP, et al: Clinical and angiographic determinants of primary coronary angioplasty success, *J Am Coll Cardiol* 17:22-28, 1991. Reprinted with permission from the American College of Cardiology.

LAD, left anterior descending artery; LCx, left circumflex artery; RCA, right coronary artery; PTCA, percutaneous transluminal coronary angioplasty.

Lesion eccentricity
Proximal vs. distal location in vessel
Vessel size
Stenosis length
Translesional pressure gradient

Traditionally, patients with multivessel coronary artery disease unresponsive to medical therapy have been considered candidates for surgical revascularization. However, depending on lesion location and morphology, multivessel PTCA can be over 95% successful in relieving ischemia.

Contraindications to PTCA in patients with multivessel disease are:

* Left main stenosis equivalent
* Complicated lesions that supply a large amount of viable myocardium
* Left main disease with no patent bypass grafts to either the left anterior descending or circumflex artery
* Presence of critical lesions in two major vessels, one of which is technically unsuitable for PTCA

Complications of PTCA

Earlier data found that roughly 20% of cases had complications. More recent data suggest that it is now less than 10% and that less than 5% of patients require emergency surgery.

A higher incidence of complications is found in

* Women
* Lesions with stenosis greater than 90%
* Right coronary lesions
* Unstable angina patients
* Patients more than 60 years old

Since plaque fracture and intimal tearing are part of the mechanism of successful balloon angioplasty, a significant number of procedures have angiographic evidence of dissection. Consequently, coronary dissection should be considered a complication of PTCA only when it is associated with luminal obstruction. The frequency of dissection appears to increase with increasing lesion complexity. The clinical outcome relates to the morphology of the tear. The majority of dissections not resulting in luminal narrowing heal within 3 months with almost no angiographic signs of a previous stenosis.

Risk factors for acute closure and ischemic complications in the presence of dissection are:

* History of unstable angina
* Chronic total occlusion
* Residual stenosis greater than 30%
* Dissection length greater than 15 mm
* Transient occlusion in laboratory

The NHLBI classification of coronary dissection is shown in Table 7-2. The incidence of cardiac events is increased in types C through F.

Management of PTCA-induced coronary dissection is influenced by the location of the lesion, presence of

Table 7-2 Coronary artery dissection: NHLBI classification

Dissection type	Description	Angiographic appearance
A	Minor radiolucencies within the coronary lumen during contrast injection with minimal or no persistence after dye clearance.	
B	Parallel tracts or double lumen separated by a radiolucent area during contrast injection with minimal or no persistence after dye clearance.	
C	Extraluminal cap with persistence of contrast after dye clearance from the coronary lumen.	
D	Spinal luminal filling defects.	
E[†]	New persistent filling defects.	
F[†]	Those non-A–E types that lead to impaired flow or total occlusion.	

Reproduced with permission from Freed M, and Grines C (eds): *The manual of interventional cardiology,* Birmingham, MI, 1992, Physician's Press.

[†]May represent thrombus

thrombus or calcium, and the residual stenosis. For small dissections without significant obstruction, no specific measures are necessary. Dissections accompanied by impaired coronary flow or significant narrowing of the residual lumen are frequently managed with prolonged low-pressure inflation, often with an autoperfusion catheter. Newer interventional devices such as the atherectomy catheter for excision of local intimal flaps and coronary stents can successfully manage local dissections and are discussed later.

The "no-reflow" phenomenon following PTCA is where coronary flow is severely reduced following PTCA despite the absence of angiographic evidence of severe stenosis, thrombus, occlusive dissection, or embolization. Possible explanations of this unusual phenomenon include embolization of the distal capillaries, which cannot be detected by angiography; spasm of the microcirculation; small-vessel edema; and endothelial cell injury. Initially, when you observe the no-reflow phenomenon you should obtain orthogonal views to ensure that an occlusive dissection is not present at the site.

Management strategies include intracoronary nitroglycerin, intracoronary verapamil, intracoronary thrombolysis, and the placement of an intraaortic balloon pump in order to increase coronary flow.

Restenosis

Despite the ability to treat increasingly complex coronary lesions, the accelerated response of the arterial wall to PTCA injury continues to limit the long-term success rate. Angiographic evidence of restenosis occurs in 30% to 40% of patients.

Defining restenosis remains controversial and there are several definitions (Box 7-2). Pathologically, restenosis is primarily a fibroproliferative response to balloon injury and involves smooth muscle cell migration and proliferation as well as connective tissue synthesis. Experimental evidence suggests that vascular injury, local thrombin generation, platelet-derived mitogens, and shear stress influence the smooth muscle response which ultimately leads to recurrent plaque formation

Box 7-2 Commonly Employed Definitions of Restenosis

1. An increase of ≥30% from the immediate postangioplasty stenosis to the follow-up stenosis (NHLBI-1)

2. An initial stenosis <50% after angioplasty, increasing to ≥70% at follow-up angiography (NHLBI-2)

3. An increase in stenosis at follow-up angiography to within 10% of the predilation stenosis (NHLBI-3)

4. A loss of ≥50% of the gain achieved by angioplasty (NHLBI-4)

5. A postangioplasty stenosis of <50% increasing to > 50% at follow-up angiography

6. A decrease in the lesion minimal luminal diameter of > 0.72 mm from the immediate postangioplasty stenosis to the follow-up stenosis

From Holmes DR, Schwartz RS, Webster MWI: Coronary restenosis: what have we learned from angiography? *J Am Coll Cardiol* 17:14B-22B, 1991. Reprinted with permission from The Amercan College of Cardiology.

NHLBI = National Heart, Lung, and Blood Institute definition.

and accelerated atherosclerosis. In addition, elastic recoil and vascular remodeling of the vessel wall play a role in early loss of lumen diameter following angioplasty. As new technology is applied to more complicated patient subsets, the restenosis rate is likely to increase and randomized trials of patients with complicated coronary anatomy are required to compare different technologies and their rates of restenosis. Currently, angiographic predictors of restenosis after PTCA include the presence of intraluminal thrombus at the angioplasty site, residual stenosis, PTCA of total occlusions, long lesions, and specific lesion locations. A higher rate of restenosis is noted in the proximal left anterior descending artery, in saphenous vein bypass grafts, in ostial lesions, and in lesions occurring on a bend. Despite numerous investigations of drug regimens aimed at preventing restenosis, a significant impact has not been made. Ongoing studies include thromboxane inhibitors, angiotensin-converting enzyme (ACE) inhibitors, serotonin antagonists, low-molecular-weight heparin, and HMG CoA (3-hydroxy-3-methylglutaryl coenzyme A) reductase inhibitors.

NEWER CORONARY INTERVENTIONAL DEVICES

Attempts to improve on the acute and long-term results of balloon angioplasty have led to the development of new coronary intervention technologies including atherectomy, mechanical ablative devices, lasers, and stents. Each has strengths and shortcomings and as their appropriate applications are defined, these devices will be useful in approaching specific problematic lesions (Table 7-3).

Directional Coronary Atherectomy

Directional coronary atherectomy (DCA, a registered trademark of Simpson Coronary AtheroCath, Devices for Vascular Intervention, Redwood City, CA) employs a small rigid cylinder with a 10-mm-long cutting window mounted at the end of a catheter which can be inserted over a standard guidewire. Because of the directional nature of the plaque excision and the rigid cylinder in which the blade is housed, the device is best suited for eccentric lesions in straight arterial segments and less well suited for tortuous vessels or calcified segments which are nonpliable.

To use the device, you fluoroscopically position the cutting window against the atheromatous plaque and inflate a balloon on the side of the catheter opposite the window to stabilize the device against the plaque. You then advance the 2000-rpm rotating blade along the cylinder, excise the plaque, and push it into the nose cone of the device. After deflating the balloon, you can reposition the cutting window according to the morphology of the lesion and then perform further cuts.

The DCA acute success rate is between 80% and 90%, depending on the lesion, and the acute closure rate is less than 4%. Despite excellent acute angiographic results, the restenosis rate ranges between 36% and 50%. Most are associated with saphenous vein grafts, longer lesions (>10 mm), restenosis lesions, and smaller vessels (<3 mm). Consequently, the favorable impact of atherectomy on long-term outcome is likely to be apparent in shorter lesions located in large vessels (Fig. 7-2). The risk of coronary dissection with DCA is less than with PTCA (37% vs. 11%), but the risk of perforation is higher (0.8% vs. 0.3%). The risk of abrupt vessel closure is about the same (4.2%). Another successful application of DCA is "rescue atherectomy," the use of atherectomy catheter following failed balloon angioplasty due to dissection or thrombosis at the site (Fig. 7-3).

Rotablator

In percutaneous coronary rotational ablation using the Rotablator (a registered trademark of Heart Technology, Seattle), a small burr studded with diamond microchips is mounted on a shaft that tracks along a guidewire. The burr rotates at 140,000 to 190,000 rpm. This emulsifies the atheromatous plaque into small particles (5-10 μm) which pass through the coronary microcirculation into the reticuloendothelial system. Because of the limited size of the burrs (1.0-2.5 mm), patients frequently require adjunctive PTCA. The primary success rate in complex lesions is 90% to 95%, and non-Q-wave

Table 7-3   Comparison of newer interventional devices

Clinical	DCA	TEC	Rotablation	ELCA
Success (%)	85–96	90–98	85–95	85–99
Average	90	95	90	95
Diameter stenosis (%) without adjunct PTCA	5–20	30–40	35–45	45–50
Adjunct PTCA required (%)	Uncommon	32–85 (60)	30–40	40–78 (60)
Unfavorable lesions	Calcified, dissected diffuse, old SVG, complex, inexperienced op	Eccentric	NA	Ostial, chr occl, dissection
Complications (%)				
Overall	2.3–18 (5)*	2–5	3–5	5
Acute closure	1.0–3.7	1–3	6–10	2.7–7.0 (5)
Dissection	4.5	1.4	3–8	2–14 (10)
Spasm	2.5	NA	3–4	2–8
Thrombosis	NA	0.5	NA	2–6
AMI	4.8		6	2–3
Q wave	0–1.5 (1)	0.5	0.9	
Non Q wave	1.3–8.0 (5)		2.5–20 (5)	
Em CABG	1.5–6.8 (3)	5.0–7.5 (3.5)	1–2	2.0–3.5
Embolization	1.0–6.9 (2)	1.4	10–20	1–2
Perforation	1–3 (1)	1–2	Rare	1.0–7.7 (1)
Death	0–0.6 (0.2)	1.5–2.0	Rare	0.3
Vascular repair	1.6–3.0 (2)	NA	NA	NA
Restenosis (%)	30–50	40–45	30–50	30–60
Risk factors	>1 cm length, <3 mm diam, SVG, resten, subintimal resect, diffuse	NA	SVG, os, prox LAD	SVG, chr occl post ELCA > 30%

Reproduced with permission from Lau KW, Sigwart U: Novel coronary interventional devices: an update, *Am Heart J* 123:497-506, 1992.

NA, not available; *SVG,* saphenous vein grafts; *op,* operator; *prox,* proximal; *diam,* diameter; *resten,* restenosis; *resect,* resection; *os,* ostial; *chr occl,* chronic occlusion; *DCA,* directional coronary atherectomy; *TEC,* transluminal extraction–endarterectomy catheter; *ELCA,* excimer laser coronary angioplasty; *AMI,* acute myocardial infarction; *Em,* emergency; *CABG,* coronary artery bypass grafting; *LAD,* left anterior descending artery; *PTCA,* percutaneous transluminal coronary angioplasty.

*Numbers in parentheses are averages.

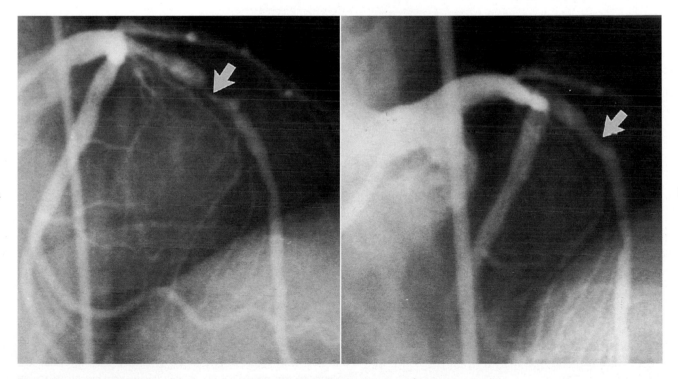

A

B

Fig. 7-2   Directional atherectomy. **A,** The initial angiogram demonstrates an eccentric severe stenosis *(arrow)* in the proximal left anterior descending artery. **B,** Following directional atherectomy, the stenosis is no longer apparent and full lumen diameter is restored.

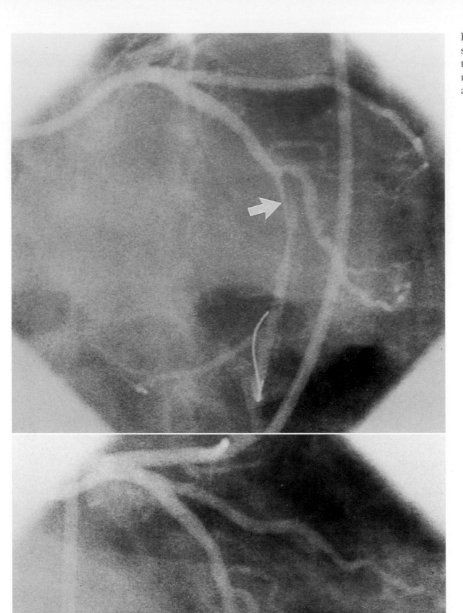

Fig. 7-3 Rescue atherectomy. **A,** A large dissection *(arrow)* compromises the lumen of the circumflex artery. **B,** Following atherectomy, the dissection is no longer present and the area has a smooth contour.

A

B

infarction occurs in between 1% and 6% and may represent distal embolization. The Rotablator appears to be most useful for lesions which are (1) calcified, (2) ostial, (3) diffuse over a long segment, and (4) cannot be dilated by the balloon technique despite high balloon inflation pressures (Fig. 7-4).

Transluminal Extraction Endarterectomy

The transluminal extraction endarterectomy catheter (TEC, a registered trademark of Interventional Technologies, Inc., San Diego) is an over-the-wire mechanical device for simultaneous excision and aspiration of

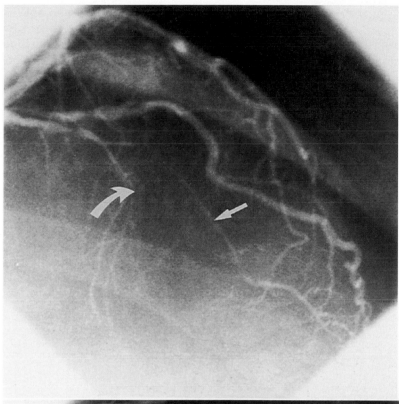

A

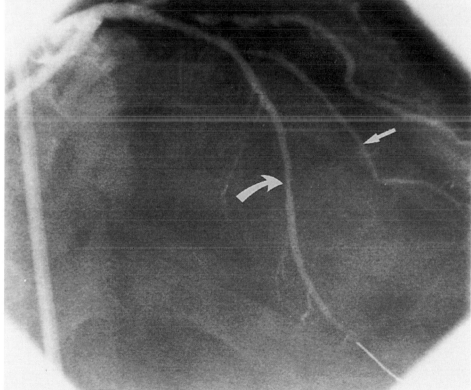

B

Fig. 7-4 Rotablator treatment of a totally occluded left anterior descending artery. **A,** The initial angiogram demonstrates proximal stenosis followed by complete occlusion *(curved arrow)* of the left anterior descending artery. The second diagonal artery *(straight arrow)* has decreased flow. **B,** Following wire passage, this region was treated with two Rotablator catheters of incremental size as well as adjunct balloon angioplasty. The result is restoration of flow in the left anterior descending artery. Flow in the diagonal branch is restored.

atheromatous plaque. Two blades mounted in a conical configuration rotate at 750 rpm and excise debris which is aspirated through a central channel.

The primary success rate exceeds 90% in both native coronaries and saphenous vein grafts. As with the Rotablator, adjunctive PTCA is often necessary. Major complications occur at a rate similar to PTCA and preliminary data suggest that the TEC device may be useful for thrombus-containing lesions, degenerated vein grafts, and ostial disease.

Excimer Laser

Among the various lasers for coronary application, the most experience has been with excimer laser coronary angioplasty (ELCA). These multifiber catheters emit pulsed energy in the ultraviolet spectrum (308 nm) and ablate only when the catheter tip is in direct contact with the atheromatous plaque. A variety of sizes of over-the-wire catheters are available, 1.3, 1.6, 2.0, and 2.2 mm. The pulses ablate approximately 50 μm of tissue per pulse with minimal thermal effects. Since the catheters ablate a channel approximating the catheter diameter, patients usually require adjunctive PTCA. There is a 90% preliminary success rate and ELCA appears promising in lesions traditionally difficult for balloon angioplasty (ostial lesions, saphenous vein grafts > 3 years old, and lesions > 10 mm). See Box 7-3 for lesions that are appropriate and inappropriate for ELCA. Encouraging initial results suggest that excimer laser angioplasty should be rigorously compared with balloon angioplasty in these clinical settings. In

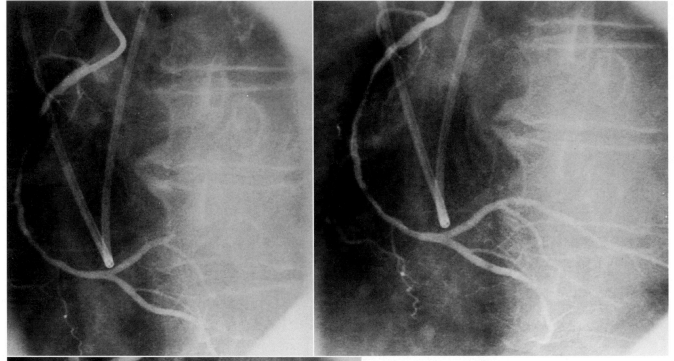

A

B

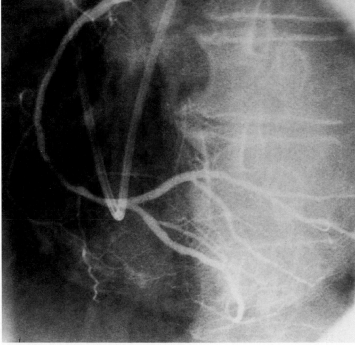

C

Fig. 7-5 Excimer laser angioplasty. **A,** The initial angiogram demonstrates a long severely diseased segment with calcification in the proximal and mid right coronary artery. **B,** Following the passage of a 1.3-mm excimer laser catheter, there is improved lumen diameter over the segment. **C,** Adjunct balloon angioplasty results in restoration of lumen diameter.

a recently developed directional laser catheter, the laser fibers are eccentrically located to one side of the catheter which facilitates the ablation of eccentric plaque. Clinical results with this catheter are awaited (Fig. 7-5).

Coronary Stents

Endovascular stents are used to lower the incidence of abrupt closure and to decrease late restenosis.

Box 7-3 Excimer Laser Angioplasty and Lesion Appropriateness

DESIRABLE LESIONS

Diffuse lesions
Ostial lesions
Total occlusion which can be crossed with a guidewire

LESIONS TO AVOID

Bifurcation lesions
Lesions in tortuous vessels
Eccentric lesions (unless using a directional laser catheter)

Currently, four different stent designs have been successfully implanted in the coronary circulation: the self-expanding Wallstent, and three balloon-expandable stents, the Palmaz-Schatz stent, the Gianturco-Roubin stent, and the Wiktor stent (a registered trademark of Medtronic, Inc., Minneapolis). In the United States, the most experience has been gained with the balloon-expandable stainless steel Palmaz-Schatz stent. To use a stent, you should predilate the lesion with a conventional angioplasty balloon. This allows the advancement of the delivery catheter over the .014 to 0.18-in. guidewire. You then crimp the stent onto a delivery balloon (if using a system in which the stent is not premounted) and deploy it at the stenosis site by balloon inflation. These stents can almost always be placed successfully. In early studies the vascular complication rate was high and included pseudoaneurysms, arteriovenous fistulas, and retroperitoneal hemorrhages.

Diabetes, small lumen diameter, and stenting of the left anterior descending artery are associated with higher rates of restenosis. In saphenous vein grafts, the restenosis rate is 22% for primary stent placement and 28% for a graft that had a previous angioplasty (Fig. 7-6).

Rigorous anticoagulation regimens have traditionally been required before, during, and following stent placement. This has limited patient eligibility for these devices.

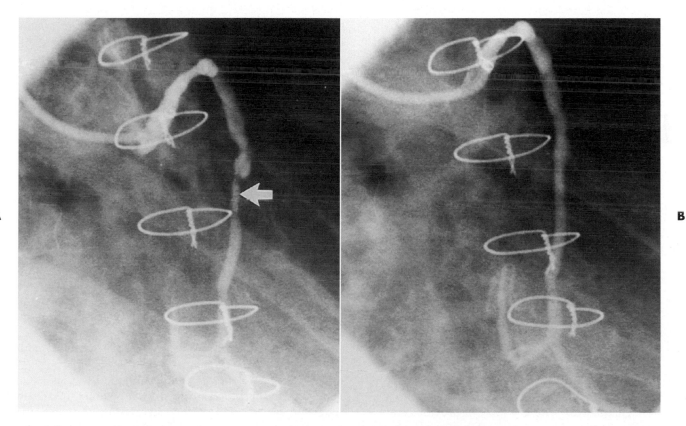

A   **B**

Fig. 7-6   Palmaz-Schatz stent in a saphenous vein graft. **A,** The initial angiogram demonstrates a severe stenosis in the midportion of a vein graft to the right coronary artery *(arrow)*. **B,** Following placement of a 4.0-mm diameter, 15-mm-long stent, the region of the stenosis is widely patent.

Although regimens may vary, the current trend is toward a less aggressive anti-coagulation approach in hopes of decreasing bleeding complications without compromising the success rate.

Coronary stents have been successfully deployed in the setting of PTCA failure due to significant recoil and dissection. Stenting would expected to be less effective in the setting of PTCA failure due to thrombus accumulation at the site because the stent itself is a thrombogenic device. Initial data suggest an increased risk of subacute thrombosis when angiographic evidence of thrombus is present at the time of stent deployment. Therefore, although emergency stenting may be useful in certain patients, there appears to be an increased risk of subacute thrombosis and these patients require careful anticoagulation and follow-up.

PERCUTANEOUS MITRAL BALLOON VALVULOPLASTY

Since its introduction in 1985 by Inoue, percutaneous mitral balloon valvuloplasty (PMV) has become an efficacious nonsurgical technique for the treatment of patients with symptomatic mitral stenosis. There are several techniques for PMV, most of which require transseptal left heart catheterization and use an antegrade approach to the mitral valve. You can accomplish antegrade PMV by using a single or a double balloon technique. For retrograde PMV, however, you need two balloon-dilating catheters which you will advance from the right and left femoral arteries over guidewires that have been snared from the descending aorta. These guidewires have been previously advanced across the septum from the femoral vein into the left atrium, the left ventricle, and the ascending aorta.

Patient Selection

Selection of patients should be based on symptoms, physical examination, and two-dimensional and Doppler echocardiographic findings. The criteria required for patients to be considered for PMV include:

1. Symptomatic mitral stenosis
2. No recent embolic events
3. Less than grade 2/4 mitral regurgitation by contrast ventriculography
4. No evidence of left atrial thrombus by two-dimensional echocardiography

You should perform transesophageal echocardiography whenever the transthoracic echocardiogram is inconclusive and in all patients with a history of previous embolic events. Patients with previous embolic events should be anticoagulated with warfarin with a therapeutic pro-

thrombin time for at least 3 months before PMV. Patients with left atrial thrombus should be excluded.

Patient Preparation

Antibiotics should be started before the procedure: dicloxacillin 500 mg orally every 6 hours for four doses.

All patients should undergo right and transseptal left heart catheterization. It is best to catheterize the right heart from the right internal jugular vein and the left heart from the right femoral vein using a transseptal sheath and a transseptal needle. Following the transseptal catheterization, administer 100 units/kg of heparin. Patients over 40 years old should also undergo coronary angiography.

Both before and after PMV, you should perform hemodynamic measurements, cardiac output, cine left ventriculography, and an oxygen saturation run to evaluate the presence of a left-to-right shunt following the procedure. After transseptal catheterization, advance a 7F flow-directed balloon catheter through the Mullin's sheath, into the left atrium, and across the mitral valve into the left ventricle. Then maneuver the catheter across the aortic valve into the descending aorta and insert a .038-in. exchange length wire through the catheter while removing the sheath and catheter, and leaving the wire behind in the descending aorta. Advance a 5-mm balloon-dilating catheter to the atrial septum and dilate the septum. You then place a second guidewire in the descending aorta using a double lumen catheter and remove the double lumen catheter leaving behind the two guidewires. If a second guidewire cannot be positioned in the aorta, a .038-in. Amplatz wire with a curved tip can be placed in the left ventricular apex as the second wire. In patients with prosthetic aortic valves, both wires can be apical wires, using care to inflate the balloons separately during the procedure and avoiding forward motion of the balloons during inflation to prevent left ventricular perforation by the balloon catheters.

Once the wires are in position, choose balloon catheters according to the patient's body surface area, and advance them over the guidewires and across the mitral valve. You should take care to ensure that the proximal portions of the balloons are beyond the atrial septum to decrease the likelihood of a left-to-right shunt after the procedure. You can then inflate the balloons until the indentations produced by the stenotic mitral valve are no longer visible. Generally, you will need one to three inflations. Figure 7-7 demonstrates the initial "waist" of the balloons at the level of the stenotic mitral valve as they are inflated.

The single-balloon technique also entails transseptal puncture. In this procedure, you advance an Inoue balloon catheter into the left atrium and position it across the mitral valve in a partially inflated position. This is performed without the aid of a wire. Once across the valve, fur-

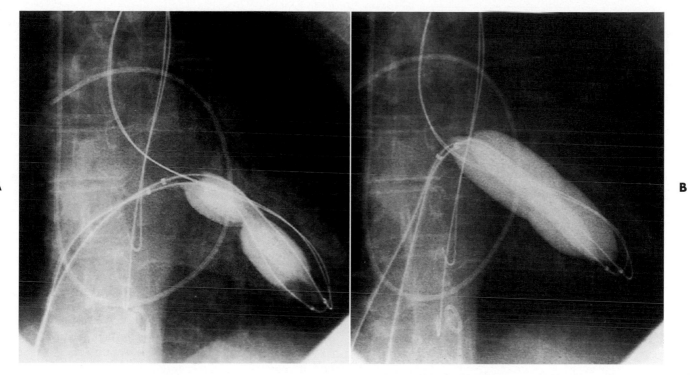

Fig. 7-7   Percutaneous mitral valvuloplasty using the two-balloon technique. **A,** Two wires cross the atrial septum, pass through the mitral valve, and enter the descending aorta. Initially, the balloons are partially inflated with a waist at the level of the stenotic mitral valve. **B,** Full inflation of both balloons resolved the mitral valve stenosis.

ther inflate the balloon which preferentially inflates only the distal portion. Then pull back the apparatus toward the left atrium until the ventricular portion of the balloon is snug against the valve, and fully inflate the balloon.

Mechanism of PMV

The mechanism of successful PMV involves splitting of the fused commissures of the valve toward the mitral annulus, resulting in commissural widening. In addition, patients with calcific mitral stenosis may have increased valve flexibility due to fracture of the calcified deposits in the valve leaflets. Undesirable mechanical effects include tears of the mitral leaflet and chordae, left ventricular perforation, atrial septum tears, and ruptures of the chordae, mitral annulus, or papillary muscles.

Results

In most series, successful PMV increases mitral valve area from less than 1.0 cm² to greater than 2.0 cm² with an associated increase in cardiac output and a decrease in the transvalvular gradient. An important predictor of the immediate and long-term results of PMV is the Massachusetts General Hospital morphologic echocardiographic score (see Chapter 2). This scores leaflet rigidity, leaflet thickening, valvular calcification, and sub-

---

Box 7-4   PMV Procedural Outcome

DIRECTLY RELATED

Selection of appropriate balloon

INVERSELY RELATED

Valvular calcification (by fluoroscopy)
Atrial fibrillation
Previous surgical commissurotomy
Age
Presence and severity of mitral regurgitation prior to procedure

---

valvular disease from 0 to 4 and then the four categories are summed. A higher score represents a heavily calcified, thickened, immobile valve with extensive thickening and calcification of the subvalvular apparatus. Among the four components, the best predictors of a suboptimal result from PMV are poor leaflet mobility with leaflet thickening and subvalvular disease.

The increase in mitral valve area observed after PMV is inversely related to the valve score by this system and the best outcome is obtained in patients with a score of less than 8.

See Box 7-4 for PMV procedural outcome.

Complications

Mortality and morbidity with PMV are low and similar to surgical commissurotomy. In the series of 432 patients from Massachusetts General Hospital there was a 0.7% mortality and no death has been recorded in the last 300 cases. The incidence of thromboembolic episodes and stroke was 1.1%. Severe mitral regurgitation occurred in 2.0% of patients, transient heart block in 0.4% of patients, and pericardial tamponade in 1.3% of patients. Tamponade occurred from ventricular perforation in two patients and from transseptal puncture in the other four patients. PMV was associated with 16% incidence of left-to-right shunt immediately after the procedure and the pulmonary-to-systemic flow ratio was greater than 2:1 in nine patients. Follow-up of patients after PMV with left-to-right shunts demonstrated that the defect closed spontaneously in 59% and was small and well tolerated in the remainder. In recent comparisons between the single Inoue balloon technique and the double balloon technique there are no significant differences in the acute success rate or the complication rate.

Long-Term Follow-Up Post-PMV

Over 90% of post-PMV patients survive past 4 years. Those patients with a higher echocardiographic score, a calcified mitral valve under fluoroscopy, and a smaller adjusted balloon diameter used during PMV had a higher mortality.

Eighty-seven percent of the patients were free of mitral valve replacement at 4-year follow-up and 83% were New York Heart Association class 1 or 2 at follow-up. Predictors of mitral valve replacement were post-PMV mitral regurgitation, larger residual mitral valve gradient post PMV, atrial fibrillation, and a history of previous surgical commissurotomy. Patients with echocardiographic scores of less than 8 had a significantly greater survival and freedom from events (death, mitral valve replacement, and New York Heart Association class 3 or 4) than those patients with echocardiographic scores greater than 8. Patients with scores of less than 8 had a 99% 4-year survival as opposed to a 75% 4-year survival in patients with scores greater than 8. The symptoms of mitral stenosis severe enough to require another PMV or mitral valve replacement recurred in 18%.

PERCUTANEOUS AORTIC VALVULOPLASTY

Percutaneous aortic balloon valvuloplasty (PAV) is a palliative treatment for patients with calcific aortic stenosis. Since the first report from France in 1986, more than 2000 patients have undergone PAV. This technique has been used in patients with severe aortic stenosis who are at high risk for aortic valve replacement, including those who are very elderly, have major related medical conditions, and those who have depression of left ventricular function.

Technique

The technique of PAV is not complex. A balloon is passed either retrograde (via the femoral or brachial arteries) or antegrade (transseptal) through the aortic valve. The retrograde approach is more frequently used. In the retrograde approach, after crossing the valve and determining resting hemodynamics, you then advance a .038-in. Amplatz wire through the retrograde catheter and place it in the left ventricular apex. The catheter is then removed, but the wire remains coiled in the left ventricular apex. You then advance a dilating balloon catheter over the guidewire, place it across the valve, and inflate.

The antegrade technique is performed by entering the left atrium via transseptal puncture using a modified Brockenbrough needle and a Mullin's sheath. You pass a balloon wedge catheter through the Mullin's sheath, into the left ventricle, and then antegrade through the stenotic aortic valve. You then pass a soft .038-in. wire through the catheter into the ascending and descending aorta and remove the Mullin's sheath. A 6- or 8-mm balloon-dilating catheter is then used to dilate the atrial septum and the aortic valve. After removing this catheter, you advance the appropriate dilating balloon (15-23 mm).

Multiple balloon inflations are usually needed to relieve the stenosis. Inflations as long as 1.0 to 1.5 minutes are usually tolerated well. Some patients experience a marked fall in blood pressure with balloon inflation so that inflations must be limited to 15 to 20 seconds. When severe hypotension occurs during balloon inflation and no movement of the inflated balloon is seen under fluoroscopy, it is likely that the balloon is large enough to fill the aortic annulus. Under these circumstances, larger or multiple balloons may increase the risk of rupture of the aortic annulus, aortic leaflets, or left ventricular outflow tract. A significant increase in aortic regurgitation and annulus tears occurs when PAV is performed with an effective ratio of balloon dilating area to aortic annulus area greater than 1.1. You should choose the size of the dilating balloon catheter by careful measurement of the aortic annulus by echocardiography or aortography so that it will produce hypotension with full balloon inflation. When a single-balloon PAV gives suboptimal results, you can use the double balloon technique taking care not to injure the annulus, valve, or outflow tract.

Mechanism and Results of PAV

Results following PAV relate to the underlying valve disorder. The increase in the aortic valve area is inversely related to the New York Heart Association functional class and to the severity of stenosis before PAV. Fresh postmortem studies of patients with degenerative calcific aortic stenosis in whom commissural fusion is minimal show that fracture of calcium deposits in the aortic leaflets increases the aortic valve area. In patients with commissural fusion (such as rheumatic aortic stenosis and in some patients with noncalcific bicuspid valve stenosis), PAV produces commissural splitting with or without cuspal cracking. In addition, PAV produces stretching of the aortic wall at nonfused commissural sites. Stretching is transient and is responsible for the cases of early restenosis seen in some patients. Although opening of the fused commissures is probably the most effective mechanism of PAV, commissure fusion seldom occurs in elderly patients with calcific aortic stenosis.

PAV results in a decrease in aortic gradient and a modest increase in aortic valve area in the majority of patients with degenerative calcific stenosis. Generally, the mean systolic gradient decreases by one half, the cardiac output increases minimally, and the aortic valve area approximately doubles. Failure of PAV (no increase in valve area) occurs in only 3% of patients.

Complications of PAV

Mortality with PAV is low and in-hospital mortality (approximately 5%) is primarily influenced by the presence of other major medical problems. Vascular complications requiring surgery occur in 9% to 15% of patients and have decreased with the introduction of lower-profile balloons. There is less than a 2% incidence of thromboembolic events and stroke, and even less occurrence of transient heart block (0.5%). No change in aortic regurgitation occurs in most patients, but severe regurgitation can occur, particularly in those patients dilated with a balloon/annulus ratio of greater than 1.1. Pericardial tamponade, rupture of the aortic annulus, and damage to the leaflets occur in less than 1% of patients.

Although PAV results in immediate hemodynamic and symptomatic improvement in most patients, the long-term results show that restenosis occurs in half of these patients 6 to 12 months after PAV. Four major identifiers associated with increased 30-day mortality are (1) systolic pressure less than 100 mm Hg with functional class IV congestive heart failure, (2) blood urea nitrogen (BUN) greater than 30 mg/dl, (3) use of antiarrhythmic drugs, and (4) cardiac output less than 3 L/min. At 30 days post procedure there is roughly a 10% mortality due to cardiovascular-related causes. A natural history study of PAV candidates who had no intervention revealed that PAV provides modest increase in actuarial survival at 1 year but no increases at $2^1/_2$ years. In a recent series of patients undergoing PAV, only 3 of 46 patients survived longer than 2 years. Thus, it seems reasonable to recommend PAV only for those patients (1) who are not surgical candidates, (2) who require major noncardiac surgery and are found to have critical aortic stenosis, and (3) as a bridge to aortic valve replacement in patients with cardiogenic shock due to critical aortic stenosis.

CORONARY ARTERY FISTULAS

Coronary artery fistulas represent direct connections between the coronary arteries and one of the cardiac chambers or vessels around the heart. They usually occur in isolation and rarely cause symptoms before the age of 20 years. Although embolization procedures have been used in the management of congenital heart disease as well as for closure of arteriovenous fistulas elsewhere in the body, only recently have these techniques been applied to the management of coronary artery fistulas. Complications and symptoms arise later in life and include dyspnea on exertion, cardiac failure, myocardial ischemia, infective endocarditis, atrial fibrillation, and rupture. Traditionally, surgical ligation has been the treatment.

Several percutaneous embolization techniques have now been applied to coronary fistula closure, including detachable balloons, umbrellas, and coils. The choice of the device is somewhat arbitrary in many patients and familiarity with all three techniques will likely increase the success rate in a given patient. Coils can be delivered through a very small catheter, whereas umbrellas require a large arterial sheath (between 7F and 11F, depending on the umbrella size). Since numerous coils are frequently delivered, they may not be ideally suited to vessels that are short or have side branches near the region where the coils will be deployed and umbrellas may be more effective in these settings.

Potential complications from percutaneous closure of coronary fistulas include embolization or migration of the device, infection, elevation of myocardial enzymes, and arrhythmias during the procedure. Long-term follow-up of patients managed with percutaneous techniques is not yet available.

SUGGESTED READINGS

Books

Grossman W, Baim DS: *Cardiac catheterization, angiography and intervention,* ed 4, Philadelphia, 1991, Lea & Febiger.
Topol EJ: *Textbook of interventional cardiology,* ed 2, Philadelphia, 1994, WB Saunders.

Journals

Anderson HV, Cox WR, Roubin GS: Mortality of acute closure following coronary angioplasty (abstract), *J Am Coll Cardiol* 9:20A, 1987.

Bell MR, Reeder GS, Garratt KN, et al: Predictors of major ischemic complications after coronary dissection following angioplasty, Am J Cardiol 7(16):1402-1407, 1993.

Bernard Y, Etievent J, Mourand JL: Long-term results of percutaneous aortic valvuloplasty compared with aortic valve replacement in patients more than 75 years old, J Am Coll Cardiol 20:796-801, 1992.

Bittle JA, Sanborn TA: Excimer–laser-facilitated coronary angioplasty. Relative risk analysis of acute and follow-up results in 200 patients, Circulation 86:71-80, 1992.

Block PC, Tuzcu EM, Palacios IF: Percutaneous mitral balloon valvotomy, Cardiol Clin 9:271-287, 1991.

Bourassa MG, Lesperance J, Eastwood C: Clinical, physiologic, anatomic and procedural factors predictive of restenosis after percutaneous transluminate coronary angioplasty, J Am Coll Cardiol 18:368-376, 1991.

Carrozza JP, Kuntz RE, Levine MJ: Angiographic and clinical outcome of intracoronary stenting: immediate and long-term results from a large single-center experience, J Am Coll Cardiol 20:328-337, 1992.

Cohen DJ, Kuntz RE, Gordon SPF: Predictors of long-term outcome after percutaneous balloon mitral valvuloplasty, N Engl J Med 327:1329-1335, 1992.

Davidson CJ, Harrison K, Pieper KS: Determinants of one-year outcome from balloon aortic valvuloplasty, Am J Cardiol 68:75-80, 1991.

Dean LS: Complications and mortality of percutaneous balloon mitral commissurotomy. A report from the National Heart, Lung, and Blood Institute Balloon Valvuloplasty Registry, Circulation 85:2014-2024, 1992.

Detre KM, Holmes DR Jr, Holubkov RMS, and coinvestigators of the National Heart, Lung and Blood Institute's Percutaneous Transluminal Coronary Angioplasty Registry, Circulation 82:739-750, 1990.

Fisch C: Guidelines for percutaneous transluminal coronary angioplasty. A report of the American College of Cardiology/American Heart Association Task Force on assessment of diagnostic and therapeutic cardiovascular procedures (Subcommittee on Percutaneous Transluminal Coronary Angioplasty), J Am Coll Cardiol 12:529-545, 1988.

Fishman RF, Kuntz RE, Carrozza JP Jr: Long-term results of directional coronary atherectomy: predictors of restenosis, J Am Coll Cardiol 20:1101-1110, 1992.

Freed M, Grines C (eds): The manual of interventional cardiology, Birmingham, MI, 1992, Physician's Press.

Herrmann HC, Buchbinder M, Clemen MW: Emergent use of balloon-expandable coronary artery stenting for failed percutaneous transluminal coronary angioplasty, Circulation 86:812-819, 1992.

Hinohara T, Rowe MH, Robertson GC: Effect of lesion characteristics on outcome of directional coronary atherectomy, J Am Coll Cardiol 17:1112-1120, 1991.

Hinohara T, Robertson GC, Selmon MR: Restenosis after directional coronary atherectomy, J Am Coll Cardiol 20:623-632, 1992.

Hofling B, Gonschior P, Simpson L: Efficacy of directional coronary atherectomy in cases unsuitable for percutaneous transluminal coronary angioplasty (PTCA) and after unsuccessful PTCA, Am Heart J 124:341, 1992.

Holmes DR, Schwartz RS, Webster MWI: Coronary restenosis:

what have we learned from angiography?, J Am Coll Cardiol 17:14B-22B, 1991.

Hostetler MD, Dunn MI: Percutaneous balloon aortic valvuloplasty: Dr. Bailey revisited, J Am Coll Cardiol 20:802-803, 1992.

Ip JH, Fuster V, Israel D: The role of platelets, thrombin, and hyperplastia in restenosis after coronary angioplasty, J Am Coll Cardiol 17:77B-88B, 1991.

Isom OW, Rosengart TK: Percutaneous aortic valvuloplasty: off the bandwagon, again, J Am Coll Cardiol 20:804-805, 1992.

Kahn JK, Rutherford BD, McConahay DR: Results of primary angioplasty for acute myocardial infarction in patients with multivessel coronary artery disease, J Am Coll Cardiol 16:1089-96, 1990.

Lau KW, Sigwart U: Novel coronary interventional devices: an update, Am Heart J 123:497-506, 1992.

Lee L, Erbel R, Brown TM: Multicenter registry of angioplasty therapy of cardiogenic shock: initial and long-term survival, J Am Coll Cardiol 17:599-603, 1991.

Liberthson RR, Sagar K, Berkoben JP: Congenital coronary arteriovenous fistula. Report of 13 patients, review of the literature and delineation of management, Circulation 59:849, 1979.

Lincoff AM, Popma JJ: Abrupt vessel closure complicating coronary angioplasty: clinical, angiographic and therapeutic profile, J Am Coll Cardiol 19:926-935, 1992.

Litvack F, et al: Percutaneous excimer laser coronary angioplasty, Am J Cardiol 66:1027-1032, 1990.

MacIsaac AI, Bass TA, Buchbinder M, et al: High speed rotational atherectomy: outcome in calcified and noncalcified coronary artery lesions, J Am Coll Cardiol 26:731-736, 1995.

NHLBI Balloon Valvuloplasty registry participants: Percutaneous balloon aortic valvuloplasty. Acute and 30-day follow-up results in 674 patients from the NHLBI balloon valvuloplasty registry, Circulation 84:2383-2397, 1991.

O'Keefe JH Jr, Rutherford BD, McConahay DR: Multivessel coronary angioplasty from 1980 to 1989: procedural results and long-term outcome, J Am Coll Cardiol 16:1097-1102, 1990.

Perry SB, Keane JF, Bain DS, et al: Transcatheter closure of coronary artery fistulas, J Am Coll Cardiol 20:205-209, 1992.

Reidy JF, Anjos RT, Qureshi SA: Transcatheter embolization in the treatment of coronary artery fistulas, J Am Coll Cardiol 18:187-192, 1991.

Ryan TJ, Bauman WB, Kennedy JW, et al: Guidelines for percutaneous transluminal coronary angioplasty. A report of the American College of Cardiology/American Heart Association Task Force on Assessment of Diagnostic and Therapeutic Cardiovascular Procedures (Committee on Percutaneous Transluminal Coronary Angioplasty), J Am Coll Cardiol 22:2033-2054, 1993.

Safian RD, Niazi KA, Strzelecki M, et al: Detailed angiographic analysis of high-speed mechanical rotational atherectomy in human coronary arteries, Circulation 88:961-968, 1993.

Sanborn TA, Torre SR, Sharma SK: Percutaneous coronary excimer laser-assisted balloon angioplasty: initial clinical and quantitative angiographic results in 50 patients, J Am Coll Cardiol 17:94-99, 1991.

Sanborn TA, Bittle JA, Hershman RA, et al: Percutaneous coronary excimer laser-assisted angioplasty: initial multicenter experience in 141 patients, *J Am Coll Cardiol* 17:169B-173B, 1991.

Santoian EC, King SB III: Intravascular stents, intimal proliferation and restenosis, *J Am Coll Cardiol* 19:877-879, 1992.

Savage MP, Goldberg S, Hirshfeld JN: Clinical and angiographic determinants of primary coronary angioplasty success, *J Am Coll Cardiol* 17:22-28, 1991.

Schatz RA, Baim DS, Leon M: Clinical experience with the Palmaz-Schatz coronary stent. Initial results of a multicenter study, *Circulation* 83:148-161, 1991.

Schatz RA, Goldberg S, Leon M: Clinical experience with the Palmaz-Schatz coronary stent, *J Am Coll Cardiol* 17:155B-159B, 1991.

Sigwart U, Urban P, Golf S: Emergency stenting for acute occlusion after coronary balloon angioplasty, *Circulation* 78:1121-1127, 1988.

Tuzcu EM, Block PC, Palacios IF: Comparison of early versus late experience with percutaneous mitral balloon valvuloplasty, *J Am Coll Cardiol* 17:1121-1124, 1991.

Warner M, Chami Y, Johnson D, et al: Directional coronary atherectomy for failed angioplasty due to occlusive coronary dissection, *Cathet Cardiovasc Diagn* 24:28-31, 1991.

Pericardial and Myocardial Diseases

Pericardial Diseases

Anatomy

Parietal and serous pericardium, lateral attachments, sinuses, and recesses

Normal appearance on chest radiography, CT, and MRI

Pericardial effusion

Normal pressure–volume relations, cardiac tamponade, and congestive heart failure

Appearance of effusion on CT and MR

Pericardial effusion syndromes

Infection, collagen diseases, metabolic diseases, and tumors

Myocardial infarction

Dressler syndrome

Postpericardiotomy syndrome

Radiation pericarditis

Cardiac tamponade

Constrictive pericarditis

Calcifications

Comparison with restrictive cardiomyopathy

Congenital absence of the pericardium

Location of defects

Radiologic signs

Pericardial masses

Myocardial Diseases

Cardiac masses

Primary tumors, vegetations, thrombi, and cardiomyopathies

Normal variants

Tumors and cysts

Metastatic tumors

Primary tumors

In children (rhabdomyoma, fibroma)

In adults (myxoma, papillary fibroelastoma)

Malignant cardiac tumors

Imaging abnormalities

Vegetations

Thrombus

Cardiac lesions in AIDS

Cardiomyopathies

Classifications

Dilated cardiomyopathy

Restrictive cardiomyopathy

Hypertrophic cardiomyopathy

Imaging abnormalities in cardiomyopathies

Distinguishing features of the cardiomyopathies

Suggested Readings

PERICARDIAL DISEASES

Anatomy

Parietal and serous pericardium, lateral attachments, sinuses, and recesses

Like the pleura and peritoneum, the normal pericardium may not be seen along its entire course, but it becomes more visible when diseased and thickened. The inner serous layer of the pericardium is the epicardium—the glistening membrane attached to the surface of the heart. The adventitia of the great vessels blend with the serous pericardium to become the parietal pericardium—the fibrous sac that creates the pericardial cavity. The parietal pericardium attaches anteriorly to the superior pericardiosternal ligament, inferiorly to the central tendon of the diaphragm, and posteriorly to the esophagus and descending aorta (Fig. 8-1). The transverse sinus of the pericardium is posterior to the heart behind the ascending aorta and pulmonary arteries, and it extends from the superior vena cava on the right side to the strip of pericardium above and behind the left pulmonary veins. The oblique sinus separates the posterior wall of the left atrium from the posterior pericardium over the esophagus; it is bounded by the inferior vena cava inferiorly, the pulmonary veins laterally, and the strip of pericardium between the right and left superior pulmonary veins superiorly. The superior pericardial recess connects the upper level of the

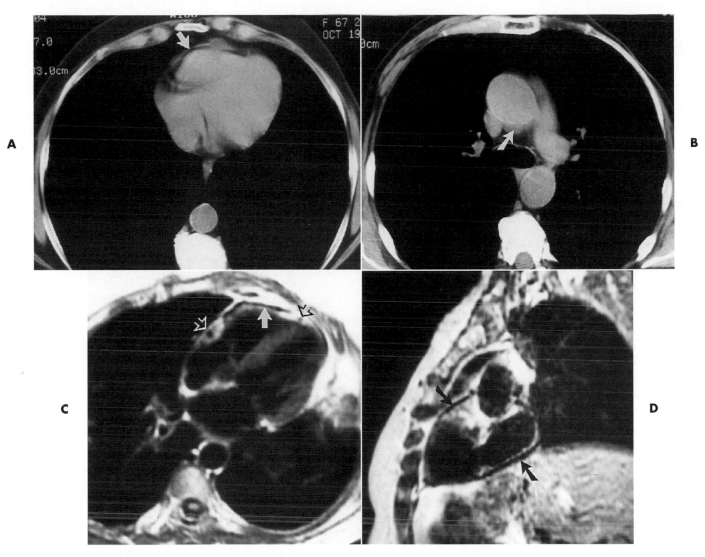

Fig. 8-1   Normal pericardium. **A,** CT appearance of normal pericardium *(arrow)* medial to a metastasis. The low density tissue on both sides of the pericardium is epicardial and pericardial fat. **B,** Superior recess *(arrow)* of the transverse sinus. **C,** MRI of pericardium *(arrow)* in four-chamber view. Note the right coronary and left anterior descending arteries *(open arrows).* **D,** Recesses *(arrows)* over the right ventricle and the diaphragm leading into the oblique sinus.

transverse sinus between the ascending aorta and the main and right pulmonary arteries; on computed tomography (CT) and magnetic resonance imaging (MRI) scans, this recess can mimic an aortic dissection, a thickened aortic wall from aortitis, or enlarged lymph nodes.

Normal Appearance on Chest Radiography, CT, and MRI

Of great aid in imaging the pericardium is the fat that covers the outside of the parietal pericardium and the fat over the surface of the heart, particularly in the atrioventricular grooves. The visibility of the parietal pericardium is increased because it is sandwiched between these two fatty layers. However, in extremely lean patients the pericardium may not be visible. You can occasionally see the pericardium on the lateral chest film as a white band between the lucencies of the pericardial and epicardial fat (Fig. 8-2). On CT and MR images the normal thickness of the pericardium behind the sternum is about 2 mm and may approach 4 mm near the diaphragm. The thickness of the normal pericardium is made up of the width of the fibrous sac and the normal 25 to 50 ml of fluid in the pericardial space.

Laterally the pericardium is usually not visible on CT and MRI scans because of motion blurring and pixel misregistration. On MR images chemical shift artifacts blur the pericardium in the frequency encoding direction, and

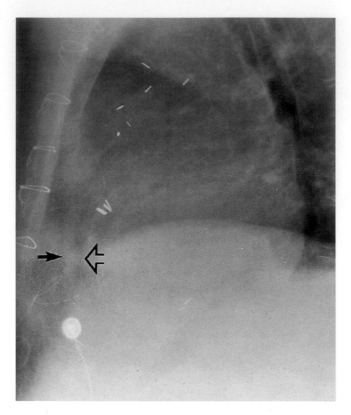

Fig. 8-2 Pericardial fluid. Lucencies outline fat on the epicardium *(open arrow)* and outside the pericardium *(solid arrow)*, denoting pericardial fluid or thickening. The "double lucency sign" denotes an abnormality if it exceeds 4 mm in width.

motion artifacts degrade the resolution in the phase encoding direction. The motion of the pericardial fluid during cardiac contraction appears as an increased signal on MR sequences that are sensitive to motion, such as gradient-echo sequences and phase reconstructed images.

Pericardial Effusion

Normal pressure–volume relations, cardiac tamponade, and congestive heart failure

The normal pericardial space in the adult can be distended with 150 to 250 ml of fluid acutely before cardiac tamponade results. Cardiac tamponade is a low cardiac output caused by excess fluid in the pericardial space that compresses the heart. In congestive heart failure when pulmonary edema and pleural effusions are visible, the amount of fluid in the pericardial space also increases. The effusions (less than 1 cm in width) seen in congestive heart failure rarely cause hemodynamic consequences.

In tamponade the cardiac size on the chest radiograph is slightly to markedly increased. The heart has a "water bottle" appearance in which both its sides are rounded and displaced laterally (Fig. 8-3). The differential diagnosis is global cardiomegaly or a huge anterior mediastinal tumor.

Appearance of Effusion on CT and MR

The appearance of a pericardial effusion on CT and MR images depends on the type of fluid. When blood is in the pericardial cavity the Hounsfield numbers on a CT scan are mildly increased to roughly 40 units. Pericardial effusions typically have a low signal intensity on CT images in the range of 10 to 20 hounsfield units. In MR images the T1 and T2 values depend on the type of hemoglobin (for example, oxyhemoglobin, deoxyhemoglobin, or methoxyhemoglobin), the age of the hematoma, the ingress of oxygenated blood, and the clearance of the hematoma by the pericardial lymphatic system. Spin-echo MR scans show a low signal intensity pericardial effusion, partly from the low protein content but also from the fluid motion, which causes phase dispersion (Fig. 8-4).

Pericardial Effusion Syndromes

Infection, collagen diseases, metabolic diseases, and tumors

The most common cause of pericardial effusion is myocardial infarction with left ventricular failure. An increase in either right or left heart pressure may also cause a pericardial effusion. Many infectious and metabolic diseases, tumors, radiation, drug reactions, and collagen disorders such as systemic lupus erythematosus and scleroderma typically cause small pericardial effusions. Uremic pericarditis occurs in about 50% of the patients with chronic renal failure and is an indication for dialysis. Most effusions do not lead to cardiac tamponade.

Common diseases that form pericardial effusions are listed in Box 8-1. Infectious agents that cause pericarditis with resultant effusions are usually coxsackievirus group B and echovirus type 8. Tuberculous pericarditis is uncommon except in patients with acquired immunodeficiency syndrome (AIDS). Although many bacterial, viral, or fungal agents can cause pericarditis, the most common organisms are *Staphylococcus*, *Hemophilus influenza*, and *Neisseria meningitidis*. In addition to a hematogenous source, pericardial infections result from extension from a myocardial abscess related to infective endocarditis, and from mediastinal abscesses caused by fistulas from carcinoma of the lung and esophagus. Loculated pericardial fluid can represent hematoma (Fig. 8-5), abscess, lymphocele, or compartmentalization by fibrous adhesions from previous pericarditis. Loculated pericardial effusions can appear similar to pericardial cysts.

Myocardial infarction

Dressler syndrome   About 5% of patients have pericardial effusions after myocardial infarction. Dressler syndrome is the development of pericardial and pleural effusions 2 to 10 weeks after a myocardial infarction (Fig. 8-6). These effusions may be hemorrhagic and can

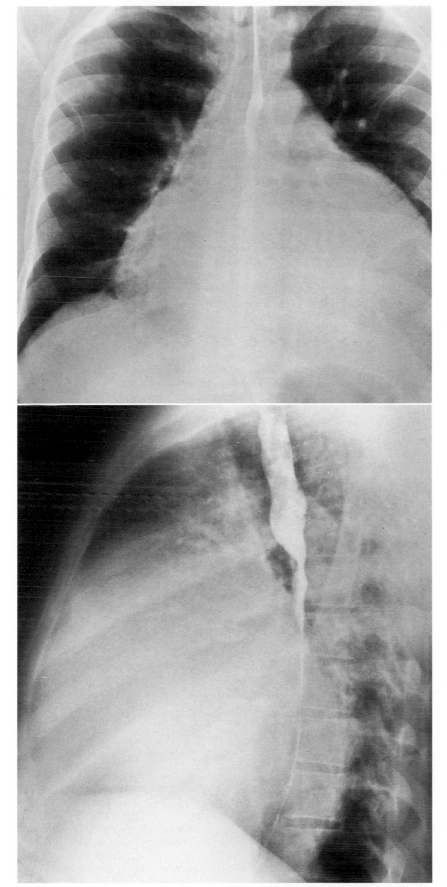

Fig. 8-3 Recurrent chronic pericarditis. **A,** The large heart shadow represents several liters of pericardial fluid surrounding a normal sized heart. **B,** Barium in the esophagus is not displaced posteriorly indicating that the left atrium has a normal size. Given the overall size of the mediastinum, it is not possible for the heart itself to be this large without left atrial enlargement, so the leading diagnosis must be pericardial effusion.

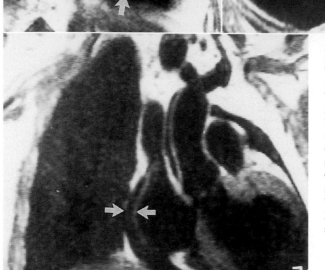

A

B

C

Fig. 8-4 MRI of pericardial effusion with spin-echo pulse sequences. **A,** Pericardial effusion is the region with signal void *(arrows)* around the left ventricle, which is covered by a layer of fat. The pericardial space extends superiorly into the aortic-pulmonary window and beneath the main pulmonary artery. **B,** An axial view shows the pericardial fluid *(arrows)* layering anteriorly around the ascending aorta. The mediastinum has lipomatosis. **C,** The pericardial space extends laterally to the right atrium *(arrows)*. The effusion in the space between the aorta and the superior vena cava outlines the pericardium extending into the top of the aortic arch.

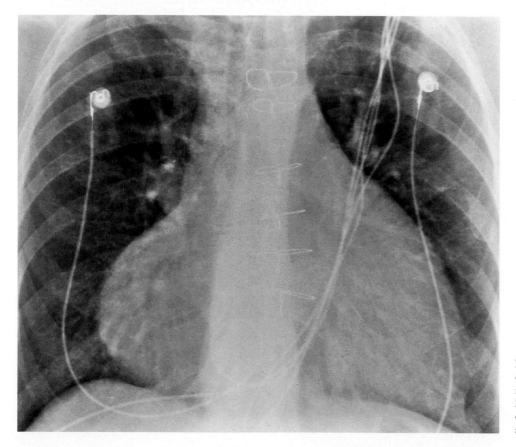

Fig. 8-5 Loculated pericardial effusion. The large, rounded, right mediastinal border is a loculated hematoma over the right atrium that occurred several days after coronary artery bypass surgery.

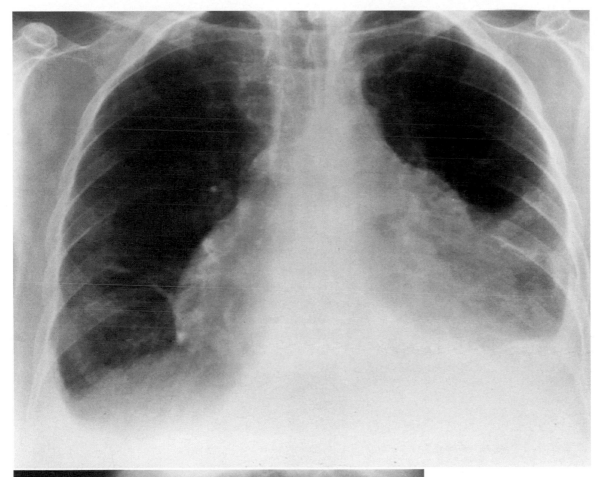

A,

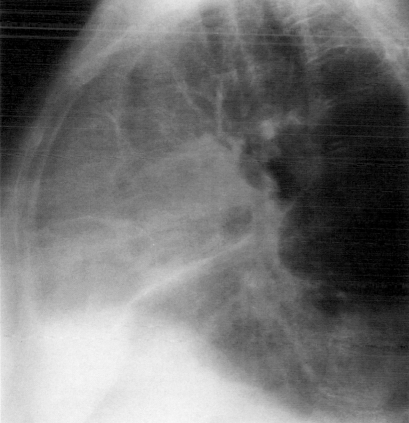

B,

Fig. 8-6 Dressler syndrome. **A,** A large, pericardial effusion and bilateral pleural effusions developed 6 weeks after myocardial infarct. Note the unusual rounding of the pericardium over the left atrial appendage. **B,** The lateral film shows a dense anterior mediastinum, reflecting the tense upward bowing of the pericardium. (Reprinted with permission from Miller SW: Imaging pericardial disease, *Radiol Clin North Am,* 27:1113-1125, 1989.)

result in cardiac tamponade, particularly if the patients have been given anticoagulant medication.

Postpericardiotomy syndrome Patients with postpericardiotomy syndrome develop fever, pericarditis, and pleuritis more than 1 week after the pericardium has been incised. Pericardial effusions alone are quite common after cardiac surgery, therefore the diagnosis requires pleural effusions and typical pericardial chest pain. Like Dressler syndrome, the etiology is presumably on an autoimmune basis.

Radiation pericarditis Radiation pericarditis is a complication of radiation therapy used for breast carcinoma, Hodgkin disease, and nonHodgkin lymphoma. This complication occurs with a delay of at least several months after radiotherapy in patients who have received a mediastinal dose of more than 40 GY. An effusion from recurrent tumor can be difficult to distinguish from one caused by radiation.

Box 8-1 Common Causes of Pericardial Effusions

SEROUS

Congestive heart failure
Hypoalbuminemia
Radiation
Collagen disease
    Systemic lupus erythematosus
    Rheumatoid arthritis
    Scleroderma
Myxedema
Drug reaction
    Procainamide
    Hydralazine

BLOODY

Acute myocardial infarct
Trauma, including cardiac surgery
Chronic renal disorder
Anticoagulants
Neoplasm

PURULENT

Bacterial
    Staphylococcus
    Streptococcus
    Pneumococcus
    Neisseria
Viral
    Coxsackievirus
    Human immunodeficiency virus (HIV)
    Echovirus
Tuberculosis
Fungal and parasitic

Cardiac tamponade

Enlargement of the cardiac silhouette on the chest radiograph usually is not apparent until 250 ml of fluid is in the pericardial space. Diagnostic mimics of large pericardial effusions include four-chamber cardiac enlargement and a large anterior mediastinal tumor in front of the heart. In recurrent pericarditis, pericardial fluid may accumulate slowly so that several liters may be present without tamponade occurring.

In cardiac tamponade the fluid within the pericardial space compresses the heart and decreases the return of blood to the right side of the heart, leading to decreased cardiac output. Although tamponade is usually caused by a bloody or serous effusion, air in the pericardial space can also create a tension pneumopericardium, especially in children who are on assisted ventilation. Penetrating chest trauma and fistulas from the adjacent bronchus, esophagus, or stomach also may introduce air into the pericardium.

The heart size may be normal in cardiac tamponade if the accumulation is rapid as in heart laceration or rup-

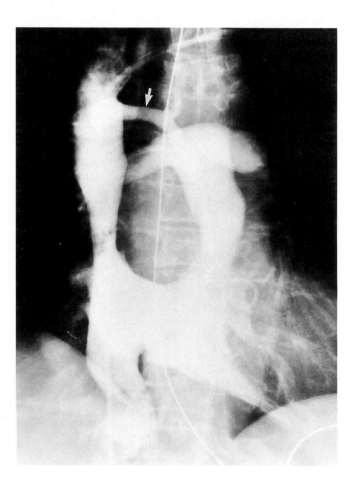

Fig. 8-7 Cardiac tamponade. Superior vena cavagram demonstrates a lateral concavity of the superior vena cava. The lateral wall of the right atrium is straight and the septal wall of the right ventricle is concave. Reflux into the azygos vein *(arrow)* and inferior vena cava reflects high filling pressures.

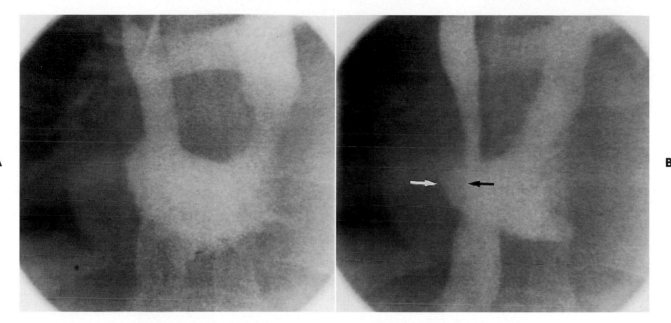

Fig. 8-8   Dynamic change in the shape of the superior vena cava during atrial diastole **(A)** and atrial systole **(B)** in cardiac tamponade. The anterolateral wall of the right atrium remains convex *(white arrow)*, whereas the posterior wall segment is concave *(black arrow)*. Note the markedly increased distance between the right lung and the right atrial cavity. (From Miller SW, Feldman L, Palacios I et al. Compression of the superior vena cava and right atrium in cardiac tamponade, *Am J Cardiol* 50:1287, 1982. Reprinted with permission from *American Journal of Cardiology.*)

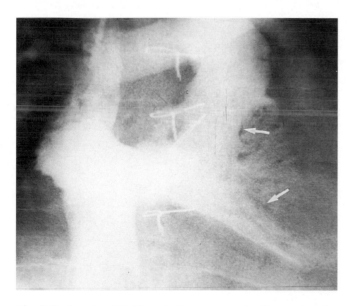

Fig. 8-9   Loculated fluid producing tamponade after aortic valve surgery. Anterior mediastinal hematoma has compressed the right ventricle *(arrows).*

ture. A typical chest film in cardiac tamponade has a wide cardiac silhouette with little abnormality in the lungs. Pulmonary edema is rarely seen in cardiac tamponade unless another disease, such as left ventricular failure from myocardial infarction, is also present.

The angiographic signs of cardiac tamponade indicate the location of fluid and its degree of cardiac compres-

sion. If there is an abnormal amount of pericardial fluid but no abnormality in the intracardiac pressures or cardiac output, the angiogram will show only the increased separation of the cardiac chambers from the adjacent interface. When tamponade is present both the inferior and superior venae cavae dilate to variable degrees. Sometimes the azygos vein is dilated. Retrograde passage of contrast material into the azygos vein is common in severe tamponade and indicates the hemodynamic resistance to cardiac inflow (Fig. 8-7). The superior vena cava normally changes shape between systole and diastole, but this motion is augmented in tamponade (Fig. 8-8). With echocardiography the right atrial border straightens and becomes concave. The thin-walled right ventricle may also be compressed and concave, but this sign should not be mistaken for septal hypertrophy or anterior loculated effusions (Fig. 8-9).

Constrictive Pericarditis

Constrictive pericarditis is a thickening of the pericardium that restricts diastolic filling of the heart. It may occur after pericarditis from any etiology but is more frequently ascribed to viral or tuberculous pericarditis, uremia with pericardial effusion, and after cardiac surgery presumably from blood left in the pericardium. Dense fibrous tissue covers the outer surface of the heart and obliterates the pericardial space. Later the thickened pericardium may calcify. Effusive-constrictive pericarditis

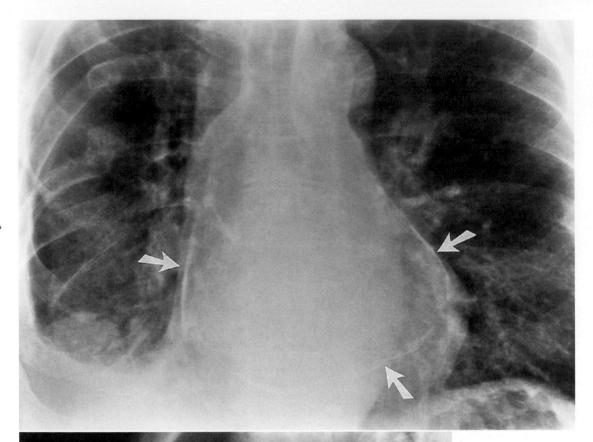

A

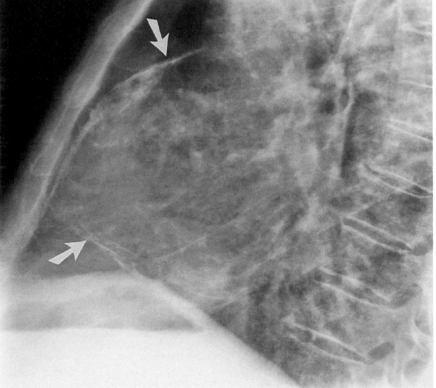

B

Fig. 8-10 Pericardial calcification. "Eggshell calcification" outlines the heart border *(arrows)* over both ventricles and the right atrium.

is a disease in which hemodynamic signs of constriction remain after a pericardial effusion has been aspirated.

Calcifications

On the chest radiograph the pericardium is calcified in about 50% of patients with constrictive pericarditis.

The calcium may be quite thin and linear and appear as "eggshell calcification" around the margins of the heart (Fig. 8-10). The etiology of this type of calcification is speculative, but it is seen mainly after viral and uremic pericarditis. A second type of pericardial calcification is a shaggy, thick, and amorphous deposition, which histor-

A

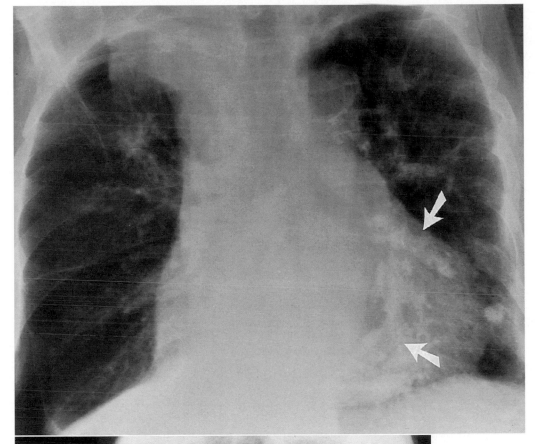

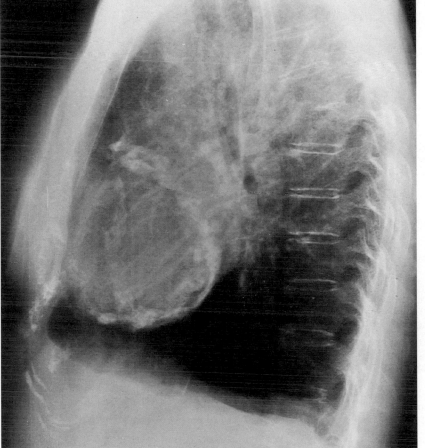

B

Fig. 8-11 Constrictive pericarditis. Clumps of calcium developed mainly in the atrioventricular grooves in a patient with tuberculosis.

ically was rather specific for tuberculosis (Fig. 8-11). The calcium is particularly obvious in regions of the heart where normal fat is found, namely in the atrioventricular grooves. Calcium in the atrioventricular region may indent the heart focally, producing "extrinsic" tricuspid and mitral stenoses. However, a calcified pericardium does not necessarily imply that constriction exists.

Comparison with restrictive cardiomyopathy

Constrictive pericarditis may be impossible to distinguish from restrictive cardiomyopathy based on hemodynamic tracings alone (Table 8-1). Although MRI and echocardiography may show an abnormally thick pericardium, CT is the best imaging procedure to use in searching for a calcified pericardium (Fig. 8-12). The pericardium in a restrictive cardiomyopathy does not

calcify. The presence (but not the absence) of pericardial calcium is strong evidence that a constrictive and not restrictive physiology is present. Patients with constrictive pericarditis usually have a pericardial thickness greater than 5 mm. MRI frequently shows no pericardial space and a thick rind of fat around the heart (Fig. 8-13). Because of the restriction to right ventricular filling, the right atrium, venae cavae, and hepatic veins are dilated. A pitfall in examining calcific pericarditis with MRI is that the calcified pericardium has a signal void (Fig. 8-14). Coronary arteriography shows that the coronary arteries do not reach the heart-lung interface as they should because they are epicardial vessels (Fig. 8-15). The left ventriculogram in constriction shows an abnormal diastolic relaxation. The normal diastolic motion is a rapid expansion in early diastole followed by a slower

Table 8-1	Radiologic features differentiating constrictive pericarditis from restrictive (nondilated) cardiomyopathy	
Feature	**Constrictive pericarditis**	**Restrictive cardiomyopathy**
Cardiothoracic ratio	<0.50*	>0.50
Pericardial calcification	Present	Absent
Motion of medial right atrial wall and crista supraventricularis	Normal	Restricted
Coronary artery location in relation to mediastinal silhouette	Separated†	Adjacent
Right atrial border	Straight or concave	Convex
Right atrial wall thickness	Increased	Normal or increased
Coronary artery motion	Decreased	Normal

*In effusive-constrictive pericarditis the ratio is usually greater than 0.50.

†Also separated when pericardial fluid is present.

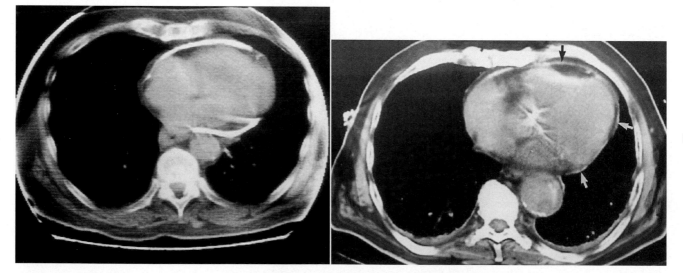

A   **B**

Fig. 8-12 Constrictive pericarditis. **A,** A band of calcium in the anterior pericardium extends from the right atrioventricular groove to near the left phrenic nerve. The posterior calcium is in the left atrioventricular groove. **B,** In another patient, the arrows point to a thin rim of calcified pericardium. (Courtesy of Robert M. Steiner, MD.)

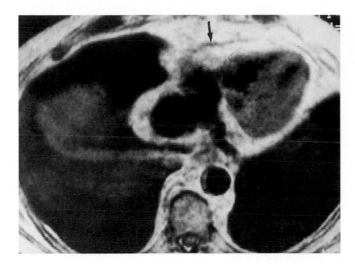

Fig. 8-13 MRI of constrictive pericarditis. A thick rind of fat around the heart is the only marker of an obliterated pericardial space. Anteriorly, abundant pericardial and epicardial fat is on each side of the pericardium *(arrow)*. The abundant fat is not specific for constrictive pericarditis, nor is the normal width of the pericardium evidence that pericardial constriction does not exist.

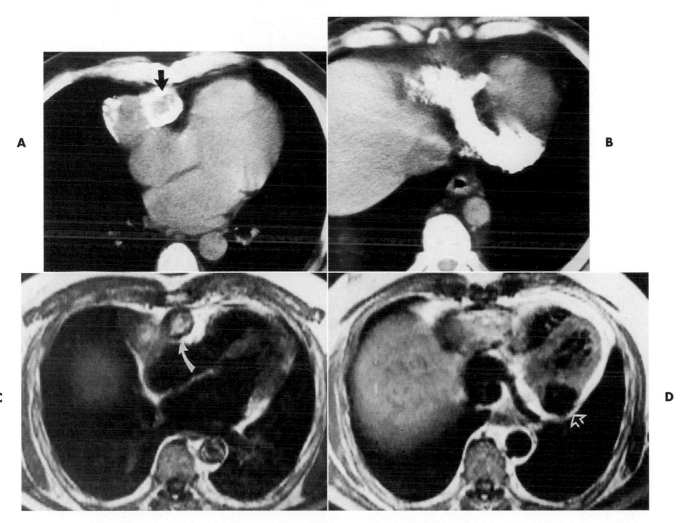

Fig. 8-14 Tuberculous pericarditis. **A** and **B,** CT images show dense calcification in the left atrioventricular groove. A tubercular abscess *(arrow)* with a rim of calcium is in the right atrioventricular groove. **C** and **D,** MR images obtained with spin-echo pulse sequences and cardiac gating show inhomogenous signal intensities in the abscess *(arrow)* and a rim of signal void representing the calcification in the left atrioventricular groove *(open arrow)*. The heart is covered by a 5- to 10-mm layer of fat. The calcium in the left atrioventricular groove has no signal. (Reprinted with permission from Miller SW: Imaging pericardial disease, *Radiol Clin North Am,* 27:1113-1125, 1989.)

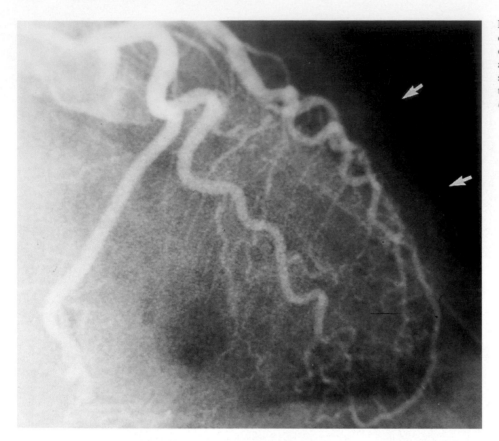

Fig. 8-15 Coronary angiography in constrictive pericarditis. The thick pericardium in a patient with rheumatoid arthritis is delineated by the thick space between the coronary arteries on the epicardium and the lung border *(arrows)*.

rate of volume increase at the end of diastole before the atrial contraction. In constriction, however, the last half of diastole has no volume change on the ventriculogram, analogous to the "dip and plateau" contour on the hemodynamic pressure tracings.

Congenital Absence of the Pericardium

Location of defects

Congenital absence of the pericardium may involve all or part of the parietal pericardium. Most defects are partial and involve a defect over the left atrial appendage and adjacent pulmonary artery (Fig. 8-16). Defects in the diaphragmatic part of the pericardium and partial defects over the right atrium and superior vena cava are much less common, and total absence is extremely rare. About 20% of patients with pericardial defects have associated heart and mediastinal abnormalities, including atrial septal defect, patent ductus arteriosus, tetralogy of Fallot, bronchogenic cysts, and pulmonary sequestration. Patients with partial pericardial defects are at risk for having part of the heart herniate through the defect, which could cause local strangulation of that part of the heart. In partial absence over the left side, the left atrial appendage may be strangulated.

Radiologic signs

Most of these defects can be identified on the plain chest film (Fig. 8-17). Defects on the left side of the medi-

astinum rotate the heart in that direction producing levocardia. The radiologic signs of absent pericardium include (1) a prominent notch between the aorta and the pulmonary artery, which is filled with interposed lung; (2) lung between the heart and the diaphragm; (3) continuity of the pericardial space with the pleural cavity on CT scans; and (4) lung between the right atrium and the right ventricular outflow tract.

Pericardial Masses

Focal masses in the pericardium may originate in the heart, in the pericardium, or in adjacent structures. Pericardial metastases are found in half of those patients dying from breast or lung carcinoma. Primary pericardial masses are usually cysts or lipomas. Cysts in pericardial teratomas contain all three germ layers, whereas intrapericardial bronchogenic cysts contain two germ layers. Seventy percent of cysts occur in the right cardiophrenic angle; the rest occur in the left cardiophrenic angle and in the anterior mediastinum. Not all pericardial masses are tumors. Bronchogenic cysts develop in the neonate and are quite rare. Herniation of abdominal contents into the pericardium can occur through a partial absence of the diaphragm. Purulent pericarditis can progress to a pericardial abscess. Tomographic images show a locally thickened pericardium or an intrapericardial mass displacing adjacent cardiac structures. MRI shows increased signal on T2-

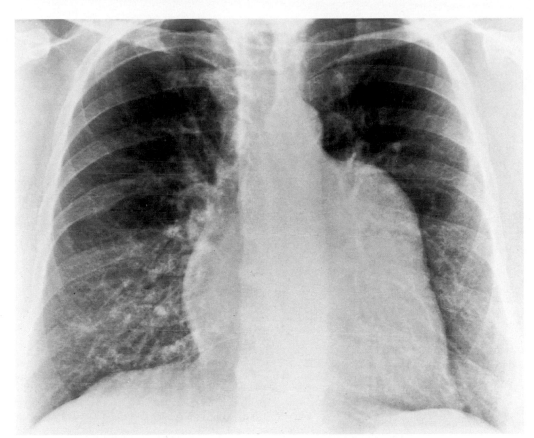

Fig. 8-16 Partial absence of the pericardium. The unusual shape of the left mediastinal contour about the heart does not readily conform to either the pulmonary artery segment or the left atrial appendage. The concave aortic-pulmonary window helps to exclude valvular pulmonary stenosis and right ventricular enlargement from pulmonary artery hypertension.

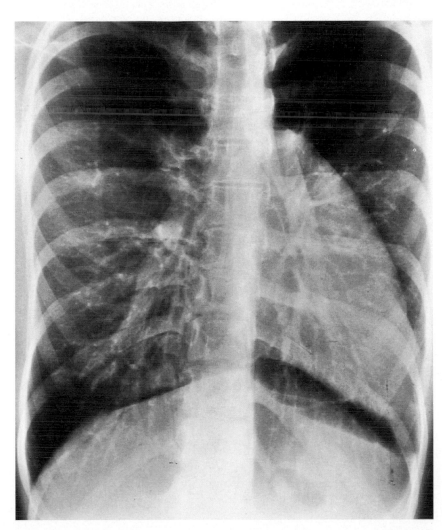

Fig. 8-17 Absence of the pericardium. The lucency beneath the heart is interposition of lung between the heart and the diaphragm. The left border is unusually convex, and the mediastinum is shifted to the left. The aortic-pulmonary window has an acute angle with lung in the left side of the mediastinum usually occupied by the pericardium. Shunt vasculature is also present from an atrial septal defect.

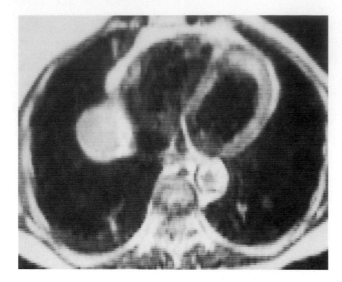

Fig. 8-18 Pericardial cyst. The spherical mass in the right atrio-ventricular groove on a T2-weighted image has a higher signal intensity than the myocardium. On T1-weighted images the fluid in the cyst is slightly less than myocardium. (Reprinted with permission from Miller SW: Imaging pericardial disease, *Radiol Clin North Am,* 27:1113-1125, 1989.)

weighted scans of both cysts and abscesses, but cysts tend to be spherical, whereas abscesses have spiculated borders reflecting the inflammatory process (Fig. 8-18).

MYOCARDIAL DISEASES

Cardiac Masses

Primary tumors, vegetations, thrombi, and cardiomyopathies

Myocardial diseases are abnormalities of the cardiac muscle. Cardiac tumors, thrombi, and vegetations are typical myocardial masses. Echocardiography and MRI are the best methods for imaging these masses, whereas angiography and CT scanning are more useful for imaging masses in the mediastinum, which impinge on the heart or great arteries. Cardiomyopathies are usually diffuse myocardial diseases, but they may also have isolated focal components or a patchy, inhomogeneous distribution. The functional aspects—ventricular volumes, ejection fraction, filling pressures, and wall thickness—must be combined with the anatomic characteristics to correctly diagnose the cardiomyopathies. Because of the importance of the hemodynamic parameters, you should correlate the imaging studies with pressure measurements at catheterization or with Doppler studies.

Normal variants

Not all cardiac masses are tumors. Extracardiac masses may indent the heart, particularly the low pressure right and left atria, and produce a concavity that may be mistaken for a primary cardiac tumor. An example is an

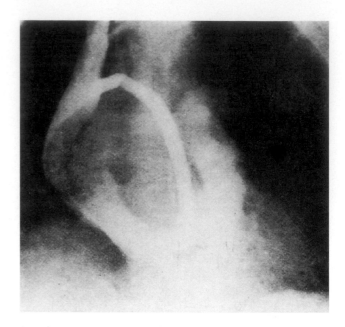

Fig. 8-19 Pseudotumor of the right atrium. Superior vena caval injection shows a large filling defect in the right atrium. The right ventricle was displaced to the left, and the right atrium was distorted to the right side. At operation a saccular aortic aneurysm was found to occupy the space between the superior vena cava and the left and right atria. Note the filling of the azygos vein. (Reprinted with permission from Wollenweber J, Giuliani ER, Harrison CE et al: Pseudotumors of the right heart, *Arch Intern Med* 121:169, copyright 1968, American Medical Association.)

aneurysm in the aortic root that deforms the right atrium and compresses the superior vena cava and adjacent pulmonary artery (Fig. 8-19). The eustachian valve of the inferior vena cava may be large and mobile and misinterpreted as a vegetation; however, its flaplike appearance adjacent to the inferior vena cava should distinguish it from a pathologic right atrial mass. A tumor in the mediastinum can extrinsically displace the superior vena cava and the pulmonary artery (Fig. 8-20). Rarely, the mitral and tricuspid valves may have a large amount of redundant tissue, which appears as a mobile mass on the valve. Atrioventricular canal defects also have an unusual amount of valve tissue, which is rarely large enough to prolapse into the right ventricular outflow region and cause pulmonary stenosis. Large trabeculations in the right ventricle usually are not confused with a tumor, but occasionally a large moderator band has the appearance of a mass if it extends to the apex. The moderator band can be distinguished from a thrombus because the band enlarges as it contracts during systole and is on a moving wall. Linear filling defects in the left ventricle are also common, are unrelated to the mitral valve, and are false tendons that traverse the lower third of the left ventricular cavity.

Tumors and cysts

Although quite uncommon, tumors and cysts of the heart are easily recognized by using the wide variety of

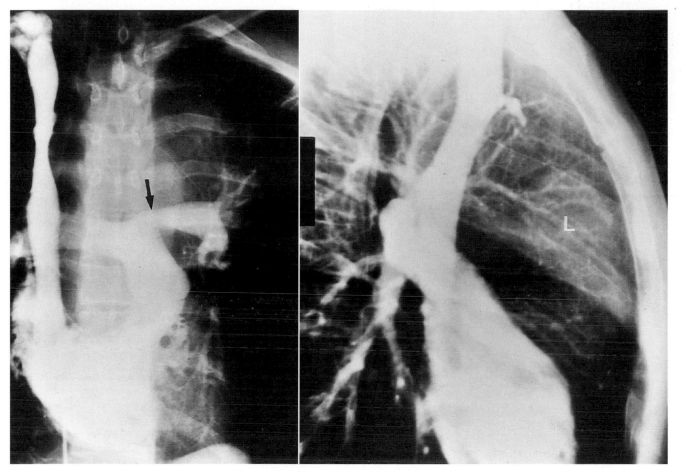

Fig. 8-20   Extrinsic displacement of the heart and great vessels by tumor. Large anterior mediastinal lymphoma *(L)* has displaced the superior vena cava posteriorly. The mass effect of the tumor has created a stenosis at the origin of the left pulmonary artery *(arrow)* and in the superior vena cava near the azygos region.

imaging techniques available. In addition to diagnosis, the imaging procedures help define the extent of the lesion and determine its effect on cardiac function. If surgical resection is a possibility, the involvement of adjacent structures such as the coronary arteries is critical information for planning. If a pericardial cyst is enlarging, CT-guided fine needle aspiration is diagnostic and frequently curative.

Metastatic tumors

Metastatic tumors to the heart and pericardium are 20 to 40 times more frequent than primary heart tumors (Fig. 8-21). Melanoma, leukemia, and malignant lymphoma (Fig. 8-22) are the tumors that more frequently metastasize to the heart. Because of their adjacent location, lung and breast tumors frequently go to the pericardium during the terminal stage of the disease. However, almost any malignant tumor, except those arising from the central nervous system, may metastasize to the heart and pericardium. Tumors that metastasize to

the lungs via the blood stream may extend into the heart along a pulmonary vein (Fig. 8-23). Seeding of the endocardium (Fig. 8-24) can be difficult to distinguish from an embolus because many patients with cancer have a hypercoagulable state. A nodular deformity of a heart chamber is strong evidence that the mass is a tumor.

Primary Tumors

In children (rhabdomyoma, fibroma)

Primary tumors of the heart are rare. In children, rhabdomyomas constitute 40% of all cardiac tumors; fibromas (Fig. 8-25), myxomas, and teratomas occur less frequently. Rhabdomyoma is found in patients with tuberous sclerosis. These tumors are frequently multiple and most occur in the ventricular septum. Metastatic Wilms tumor (Fig. 8-26) frequently is identified as a filling defect in the inferior vena cava extending into the heart. (See Table 8-2 for tumors and cysts of the heart and pericardium.)

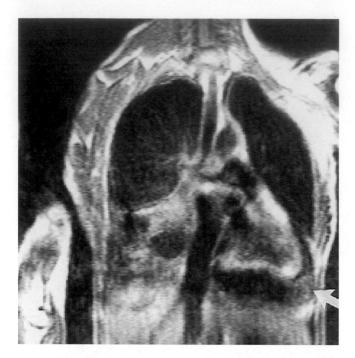

Fig. 8-21 Pericardial metastasis. A bronchogenic carcinoma in the right hilum has produced collapse of the right-middle and lower lobes. The inferior vena cava is displaced toward the left. A large pericardial effusion surrounds the heart and a pericardial metastasis *(arrow)*. (Reprinted with permission from Miller SW, Brady TJ, Dinsmore RE et al: Cardiac magnetic resonance imaging: the Massachusetts General Hospital experience, *Radiol Clin North Am* 23:745-764, 1985.)

In adults (myxoma, papillary fibroelastoma)

In adults, myxomas constitute 25% of benign cardiac tumors. Angiosarcomas, rhabdomyosarcomas, mesotheliomas, and fibrosarcomas are the most common primary malignant cardiac tumors. Although cardiac neoplasms do not metastasize or invade locally, many of these tumors act in a malignant manner by causing arrhythmias, obstruction, and embolism.

Myxoma is the most common primary benign heart tumor. Most myxomas arise in the atria with the left atrium involved four times as often as the right atrium. Most atrial myxomas arise from the interatrial septum. A "dumbbell" myxoma is one that has grown through the fossa ovalis and extends into both the right and left atria. Some patients may have a syndrome of multiple myxomas that appear throughout life and require multiple surgical resections.

Most myxomas are polypoid and are quite changeable during the cardiac cycle. Many have fronds that may move erratically as the tumor prolapses through a valve (Fig. 8-27). About 10% of left atrial myxomas have a calcified stock, which may be seen fluoroscopically. The appearance of myxomas in the ventricles is similar. These ventricular myxomas can be distinguished from vegetations in that they do not arise from the valve leaflets. On spin-echo sequences myxomas have the same signal

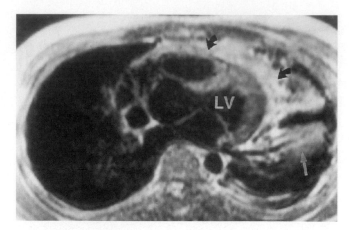

Fig. 8-22 Non-Hodgkin lymphoma involving the pericardium. The tumor *(black arrows)* diffusely involves the anterior mediastinum and part of the left lung *(white arrow)*. The black line that represents the pericardium on spin-echo images is absent over the right ventricle and left ventricle *(LV)*.

Table 8-2   Tumors and cysts of the heart and pericardium

Type	Percent
BENIGN	
Myxoma	24
Lipoma	8
Papillary fibroelastoma	8
Rhabdomyoma	7
Fibroma	3
Hemangioma	3
Teratoma	3
Mesothelioma of the AV node	2
Granular cell tumor	1
Neurofibroma	1
Lymphangioma	<1
SUBTOTAL	60%
Pericardial cyst	15
Bronchogenic cyst	1
SUBTOTAL	16%
MALIGNANT	
Angiosarcoma	7
Rhabdomyosarcoma	5
Mesothelioma	4
Fibrosarcoma	3
Malignant lymphoma	1
Extraskeletal osteosarcoma	1
Neurogenic sarcoma	1
Malignant teratoma	1
Thymoma	1
Leiomyosarcoma	<1
Liposarcoma	<1
Synovial sarcoma	<1
SUBTOTAL	24%

Modified with permission from McAllister HA, Fenoglia JJ: *Tumors of the cardiovascular system.* In Hartmann WH, Cowan WR (editors): *Atlas of tumor pathology* (Fasc.15, 2nd series), Washington, DC, 1978, Armed Forces Institute of Pathology.

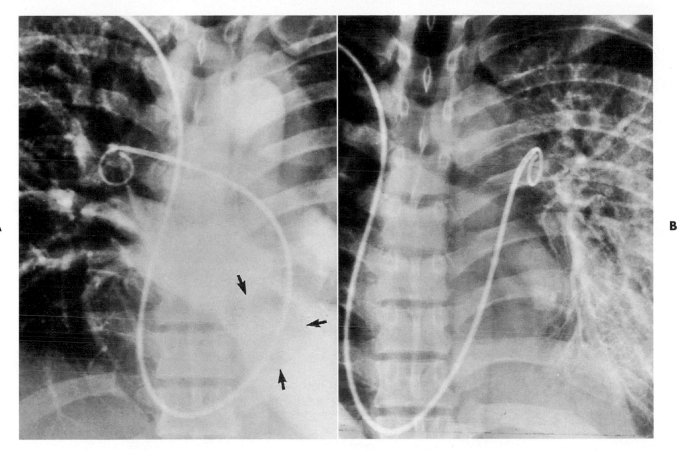

Fig. 8-23 Metastatic tumor to the heart and the mediastinum. Unilateral left pulmonary edema developed in a man with known extremity osteosarcoma. **A,** A filling defect *(arrows)* in the left atrium is adjacent to the left pulmonary veins and mitral valve. The mediastinum is wide from metastases. **B,** Selective left pulmonary artery injection does not opacify the pulmonary veins, indicating tumor encasement.

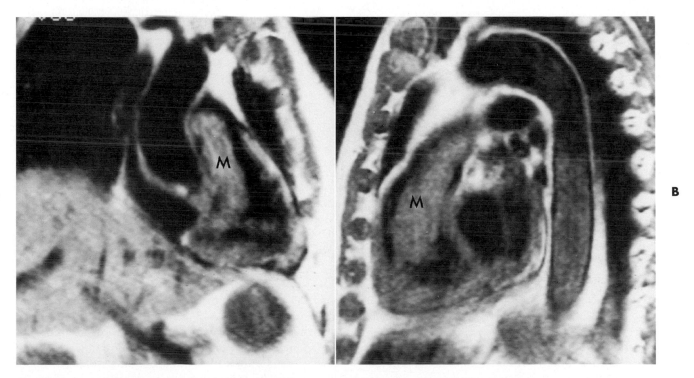

Fig. 8-24 Metastatic fibrosarcoma to the right ventricle. The mass *(M)* extends from the region of the tricuspid annulus through the right ventricular outflow region into the main pulmonary artery. At surgery the mass was found to be mostly a thrombus on top of a small tumor.

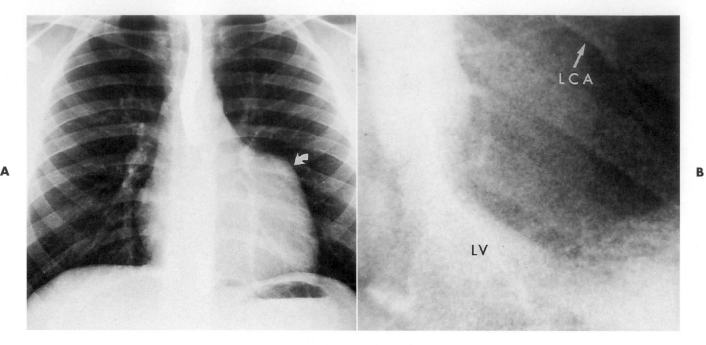

Fig. 8-25   Intracardiac fibroma. **A,** Chest film shows the mass *(arrow)* at the junction of the left atrium and the left ventricle. **B,** The anterobasal left ventricle *(LV)* is displaced inferiorly and the left coronary artery *(LCA)* is pushed superiorly, indicating an intracardiac mass.

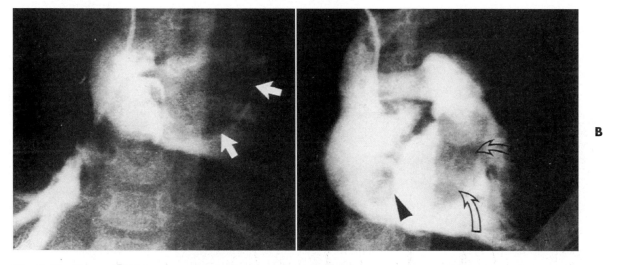

Fig. 8-26   Metastatic Wilms tumor. **A,** Injection at the level of the inferior vena cava and the right atrium shows reflux into the hepatic vein but no reflux into the vena cava proper. The right atrium is filled with contrast, and a lucent tumor mass is in the right ventricle *(white arrows)*. **B,** Injection in the right atrium shows a lucent tumor mass in the right atrium *(arrowhead)* and in the right ventricle *(curved arrows)* extending into the outflow tract. (Reprinted with permission from Slovis TL, Cushing B, Reilly BJ et al: Wilm's tumor to the heart: clinical and radiologic evaluation, *AJR Am J Roentgenol* 131:263, 1978.)

intensity as adjacent myocardium on both T1-weighted and T2-weighted images (Fig. 8-28). This distinguishes them from lipomas, which are much brighter, and from cysts, which enhance with T2 weighting.

Papillary fibroelastomas are small tumors (1 cm or less), that are difficult to see angiographically but are encountered on other imaging modalities as polypoid tumors attached to one of the four heart valves. Lipomas are benign tumors that have a spherical shape and a sharp demarcation with adjacent ventricular myocardium.

Lipomatous hypertrophy of the interatrial septum (LHIS) is a common tumor in the right atrium (Fig. 8-29). Best studied by MRI, it consists of large masses of fatty tissue in the interatrial septum with occasional extension

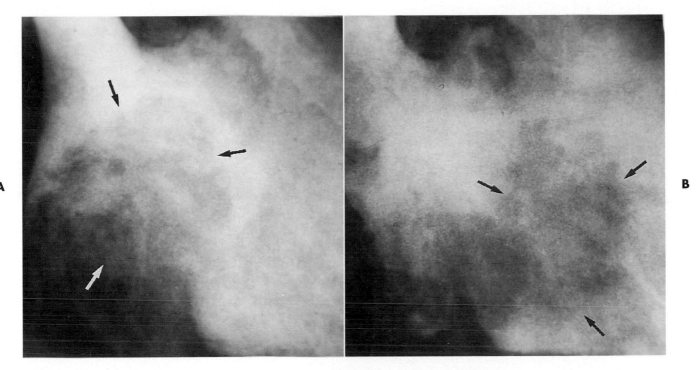

Fig. 8-27   Right atrial myxoma. **A,** After a superior vena caval injection, contrast material outlines a mass in the right atrium. **B,** During ventricular filling, the mass prolapses into the right ventricle.

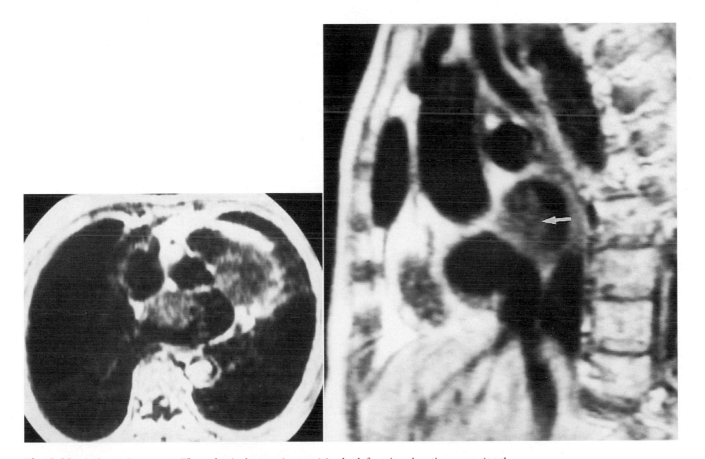

Fig. 8-28   Left atrial myxoma. The spherical mass *(arrows)* in the left atrium has the same signal characteristics as the mediastinum and the heart, and it is attached to the interatrial septum.

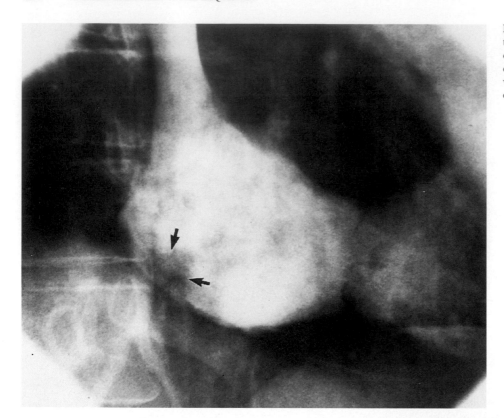

Fig. 8-29 Lipomatous hypertrophy of the interatrial septum. A superior vena caval injection shows a small filling defect *(arrows)* in the right atrium, which is a fatty deposit near the entrance to the inferior vena cava.

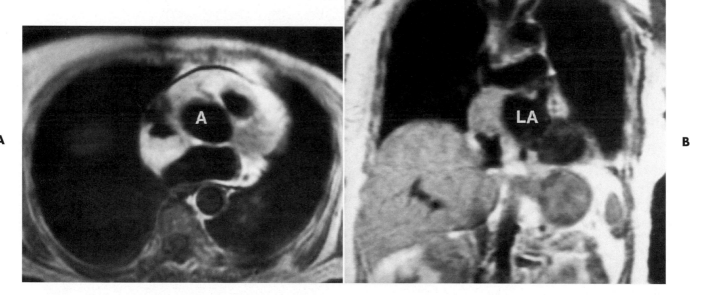

A

B

Fig. 8-30 MRI of lipomatous hypertrophy of the interatrial septum. **A,** The high signal intensity fat in the right atrium is adjacent to the interatrial septum and produces a concavity into the left atrium. *A* = aorta. **B,** The coronal plane image with fat suppression shows a mass occupying the upper half of the right atrium at the junction with the superior vena cava. There are extensions of this tumor into the right atrial appendage and medially adjacent to the tricuspid valve. *LA* = left atrium.

into the left and right atria (Fig. 8-30). These masses are benign and not associated with body obesity, but they can produce supraventricular arrhythmias. The MRI examination is used to map the extent of the fat, to document any caval obstruction, and to verify the tissue with fat suppression sequences.

Malignant cardiac tumors

Malignant cardiac tumors have a similar appearance regardless of their histologic diagnoses. Angiosarcoma typically involves the right side of the heart and is an irregular infiltrating mass that diffusely involves many structures (Fig. 8-31). The venae cavae may be partially

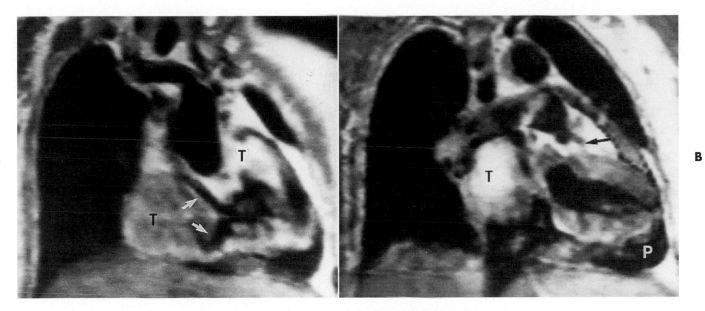

Fig. 8-31 Spin-echo sequences of angiosarcoma. **A,** An irregularly lobulated mass *(T)* in the right atrium and superior vena cava partially occludes *(arrows)* systemic inflow into the right ventricle. The tumor extends around the aortic root and between the aorta and pulmonary artery. **B,** A more posterior slice shows the tumor in the interatrial septum and nearly occluding *(arrow)* the right ventricular outflow tract. A moderate pericardial effusion *(P)* is lobulated around the apex.

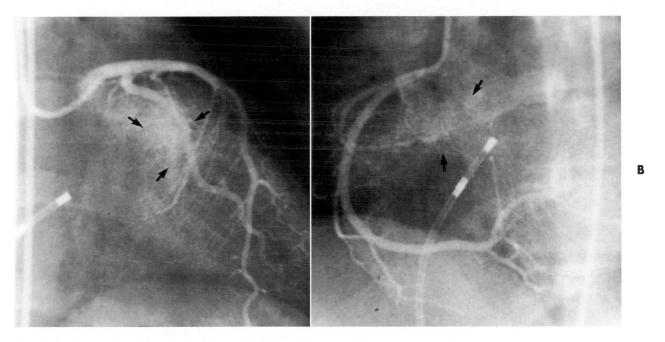

Fig. 8-32 Vascular blush from hemangioma. The intramural extent of the tumor is visualized as an intense blush *(arrows)* of contrast media, which cleared slowly and faintly, drained to the adjacent ventricle. **A,** Tumor in the anterior wall of the right ventricle is fed by marginal branches of the right coronary artery. **B,** Contrast pooling in the interventricular septum comes mainly from a large septal artery.

obstructed, the right atrial cavity narrowed, the right ventricle distorted, and the pulmonary outflow region narrowed. Coronary angiography frequently demonstrates patent arteries, but extrinsic stenosis and obstruction are well known. You can occasionally see a neovascular blush as well as a tangle of tumor vascularity (Fig. 8-32), but that is more common with myxo-

mas. Tumor emboli from left atrial myxoma may obstruct the coronary arteries and cause a myocardial infarction.

Imaging abnormalities

Box 8-2 lists the variety of imaging abnormalities that may be seen with cardiac tumors.

Box 8-2   Imaging Signs of Cardiac Tumor

Extrinsic displacement of the heart and great vessels
Compression or occlusion of venae cavae, pulmonary arteries, or veins
Pericardial fluid or thickening
Intracavity filling defects
Decreased wall motion
Angiographic tumor stain and neovascularity
Focal MRI change in T1 and T2 values
Asymmetric pulmonary edema from pulmonary vein occlusion

Vegetations

Vegetations on heart valves have characteristic imaging features that may be present with or without the classic clinical triad of fever, heart murmur, and positive blood cultures. Nodularity and calcification of valve leaflets are seen in noninfected bicuspid aortic valves and in mitral valves with rheumatic stenosis. However, larger pedunculated masses attached to the valve leaflets are characteristic of vegetations. These masses may prolapse through the valve and occasionally embolize. Aortic root abscess is another complication of infective endocarditis and appears as irregular cavities adjacent to the sinuses of Valsalva. Rarely an aortic root abscess forms a fistula to an adjacent heart chamber, pericardium, or pulmonary artery. In addition to the pericarditis of systemic lupus erythematosis, the cardiac valves and myocardium in this disease are affected in more than half of patients in the terminal stage. Nonbacterial thrombotic endocarditis (Libman-Sacks endocarditis) has vegetations that are considerably smaller than those in bacterial endocarditis and frequently occur beneath the cusps. In contrast, the vegetations in infective endocarditis frequently occur on the line of closure of the leaflets.

Thrombus

Whether a cardiac mass is a tumor or a thrombus can frequently be decided by the clinical situation. Thrombi are common in the left ventricle after a myocardial infarction or in the presence of a known ventricular aneurysm. In patients with atrial fibrillation, particularly when they have rheumatic heart disease, left atrial thrombi are common (Fig. 8-33), whereas myxoma is quite rare. Conversely, peripheral embolization in a patient with no overt sign of heart disease is commonly the first sign of a left atrial myxoma. Thrombi can develop in any part of the heart, but the etiology of the thrombus may be unique to a particular chamber (Box 8-3).

Some imaging characteristics are quite reliable in distinguishing tumor from thrombus. Thrombi occur on car-

---

Box 8-3   Cardiac Thrombus by Location

LEFT ATRIUM

Mitral valve disease
Atrial fibrillation
Tumor from pulmonary veins

RIGHT ATRIUM

Embolic
    Thromboembolism
Tumor
        Renal cell carcinoma
        Hepatocellular carcinoma
Foreign body

LEFT VENTRICLE

Cardiomyopathy
Myocardial infarction with scar or aneurysm
Vegetation from endocarditis on mitral valve

RIGHT VENTRICLE

Trauma
Cardiomyopathy
Myocardial infarction with scar or aneurysm
Vegetation from endocarditis on tricuspid valve

---

diac walls that are akinetic. A focal mass on a moving atrial or ventricular wall is not a thrombus but more likely is an anomalous muscle bundle in the right ventricle, a multiheaded papillary muscle in the left ventricle, an imaging artifact caused by slowly flowing blood, or a tumor. Thrombi can have many shapes in the four cardiac chambers. A shaggy linear density next to a Swan-Ganz catheter is a typical appearance of a foreign body thrombus. In the left ventricle after myocardial infarction, a thrombus in the apex may appear to truncate the ventricle making the apex appear thick, whereas in an infarct the wall should be thin. Polypoid thrombi are easily recognized in any heart chamber. When the thrombus is layered smoothly along a wall it may not be identified. A clue to the presence of a layered thrombus in the left ventricle is a smooth wall rather than the normally fine trabeculations.

Cardiac Lesions in AIDS

Myocarditis is a common autopsy finding in patients who have died from AIDS, with nearly half having disease in the heart or pericardium. Even though these patients have multiple infections, an agent is rarely identified in the heart. The histopathologic picture is a focal lymphocytic myocarditis. Many infectious agents occasionally are cultured, such as *Mycobacterium avium-intracellulare, Toxoplasma* (Fig. 8-34), *Cryptococcus, Cytomegalovirus,* and human immunodeficiency virus

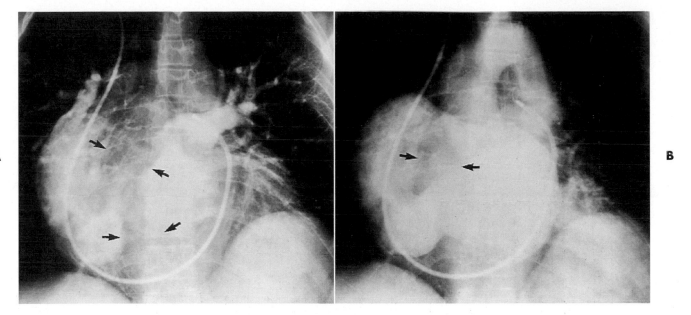

Fig. 8-33   Left atrial thrombus. Several irregular filling defects *(arrows)* are present in the large left atrium on the early **(A)** and late **(B)** phases of a pulmonary angiogram. At surgery for mitral stenosis, 110 g of thrombus were removed. (Courtesy of Robert E. Dinsmore, M.D.)

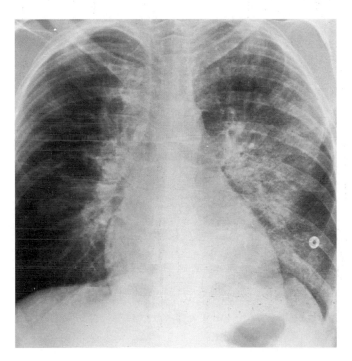

Fig. 8-34   Toxoplasma myocarditis in a patient with AIDS. Although the heart size is normal, 200 ml of pericardial fluid was present at autopsy. Bronchopneumonia is seen in both lungs.

(HIV). Kaposi sarcoma, which is histologically difficult to distinguish from angiosarcoma, and lymphoma are the major pericardial and heart tumors (Fig. 8-35). The pericardium frequently has fibrinous pericarditis from uremia or infection and may have a moderate effusion. Vegetations of both infective and nonbacterial endo-

carditis have been found on all four heart valves. Congestive heart failure with pulmonary edema from left ventricular failure may have a similar clinical presentation as a dilated cardiomyopathy. The right ventricle may be dilated from pulmonary artery hypertension secondary to pulmonary infection or emboli.

Cardiomyopathies

Cardiomyopathies are heart muscle diseases in which congenital, pericardial, valvular, and coronary causes have been excluded by appropriate clinical, hemodynamic, or imaging methods. Primary cardiomyopathies have an unknown etiology whereas secondary cardiomyopathies have an etiologic diagnosis and therefore are potentially reversible with appropriate therapy. Alcoholic, Adriamycin (doxorubicin), and ischemic cardiomyopathies are examples of known causes and produce similar clinical signs, such as ventricular failure, but may require different therapy.

Classifications

The WHO/ISFC Task Force classifies primary cardiomyopathies as (1) dilated cardiomyopathy, (2) hypertrophic cardiomyopathy; and (3) restrictive cardiomyopathy. Although many patients fit easily into one of these groups, many have features that overlap several categories. Arrhythmogenic right ventricular dysplasia, an increasingly common diagnosis, is one such cardiomyopathy that cannot easily be classified into one of the three major groups.

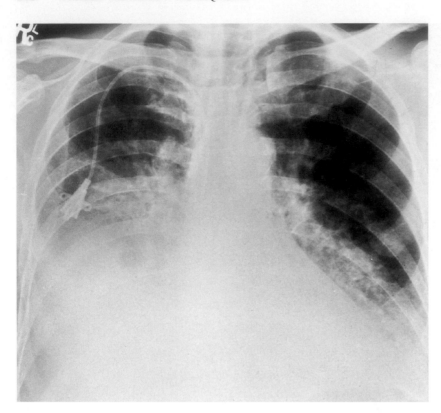

Fig. 8-35 Lymphocytic myocarditis in the immunodeficiency syndrome appearing like a dilated cardiomyopathy. Large bilateral pleural effusions partially mask a dilated heart with a small pericardial effusion.

Dilated cardiomyopathy

Dilated cardiomyopathy causes dilatation of both right and left ventricles. Typically the left ventricle is enlarged with global hypokinesis, whereas the right ventricle is less dilated and typically has a less severe contraction abnormality. Mild mitral and tricuspid regurgitation are common because of the ventricular dilatation. Patients with this condition have decreased ejection fractions with reduced stroke volumes and may have decreased cardiac output. Systolic function is depressed, but diastolic function is nearly normal. As the left ventricle dilates to a moderate degree, segmental wall motion abnormalities may appear. For example, the apex may be akinetic. Mural thrombi are frequently found in the apex and have a laminated appearance. Because global wall motion is not unique to this abnormality, cardiac imaging not only measures the left ventricular ejection fraction but also helps exclude other types of heart disease. The chest film generally shows cardiomegaly and pulmonary venous hypertension with little or no pulmonary edema (Fig. 8-36). The paradox of a huge heart and clear lungs is a diagnostic clue that a dilated cardiomyopathy may be present. Global reduction in left ventricular wall motion may also be seen in acute viral myocarditis; in eosinophilic myocarditis; and as atypical presentations in other types of cardiomyopathies such as those with infective etiologies (Chagas disease), granulomatous heart disease (sarcoid), and infiltrative heart disease (amyloid). Peripartum cardiomyopathy (Fig. 8-37) also has global hypokinesis of both ventricles and occurs dur-

ing the last trimester of pregnancy or during the first several months post partum. Known causes of dilated cardiomyopathy are listed in Box 8-4.

Arrhythmogenic right ventricular dysplasia is a rare cardiomyopathy associated with arrhythmias and sudden death in young individuals and is similar to Uhl anomaly, which is a congenital defect of the right ventricular myocardium from birth, causing right heart failure in infancy. The right ventricular anterior wall is replaced by fatty fibrous tissue. Cine right ventricular angiography shows regional akinesis or aneurysms with global right ventricular dilatation and tricuspid regurgitation. MRI is performed with a surface coil to maximize resolution of the anterior heart (Fig. 8-38). The free wall of the right ventricle has no visible myocardium in systole or diastole and has mainly fat on a fibrous thin wall between the cavity and the pericardium. Fat-suppressed images may help in resolving the residual wall, which is about a pixel wide.

Restrictive cardiomyopathy

Restrictive cardiomyopathy, the least common type, has features that overlap other types of cardiomyopathy. In this condition the heart has normal ventricular size and contractility but a diastolic relaxation abnormality. In this disease's earliest form, hearts are neither dilated nor hypertrophied, but as the disease progresses, a combination of both enlargement and a thick left ventricular wall (at times ≥ 1.5 cm) may develop. Because of the stiff right and left ventricles, the right and left atria dilate in response to filling the ventricles under increased dias-

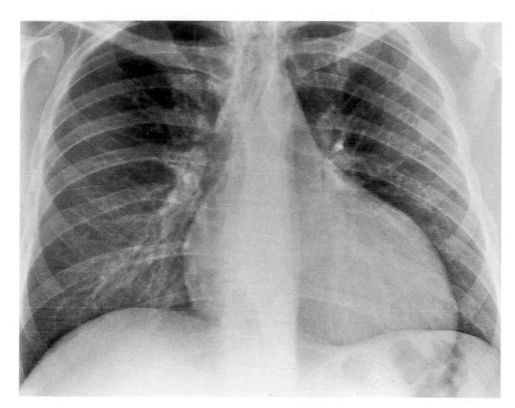

Fig. 8-36 Dilated cardiomyopathy. The heart has enlargement of all four chambers. The azygos vein and superior vena cava are slightly dilated reflecting high central venous pressure.

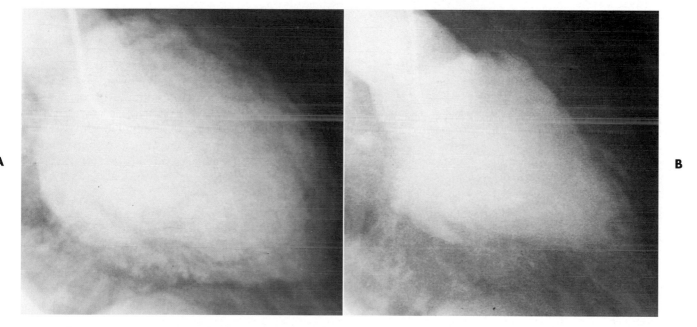

A   **B**

Fig. 8-37 Peripartum cardiomyopathy. End-diastolic (**A**) and end-systolic (**B**) frames from a left ventriculogram show large volumes with a correspondingly decreased ejection fraction and slight mitral regurgitation.

tolic pressures. Flow into the ventricles typically is rapid in early diastole followed by a plateau with little filling in late diastole. Dilated venae cavae, large atria, and small ventricles also are present in constrictive pericarditis. Indeed it may be impossible to distinguish these two entities by their hemodynamic features only. The pres-

ence of a thickened and calcified pericardium is relatively specific for constrictive pericarditis and is best imaged by CT scanning. However, about 50% of patients with constrictive pericarditis do not have a calcified pericardium, and some patients with restrictive cardiomyopathy may have slight thickening of the pericardium.

Box 8-4   Known Causes of Dilated Cardiomyopathy

Idiopathic
Myocarditis
Coronary artery disease
Human immunodeficiency virus (HIV)
Peripartum cardiomyopathy
Alcohol
Principal pharmacologic agents
    Doxorubicin, bleomycin, antiretroviral agents
    Many classes of drugs including antibiotics,
       anticonvulsants, diuretics, and antiinflammatory
       agents (many of these may cause restrictive
       cardiomyopathy)
Cobalt
Phenothiazines
Carbon monoxide
Lead
Cocaine
Mercury
Connective tissue diseases
    Scleroderma, systemic lupus erythematosus,
       dermatomyositis
    Sarcoidosis
Endocrine disorders
    Hypothyroidism, acromegaly, thyrotoxicosis, Cushing
       disease, pheochromocytoma, diabetes mellitus
Infections
    Viral (coxsackievirus, cytomegalovirus, human
       immunodeficiency virus [HIV])
    Rickettsial
    Bacterial (diphtheria)
    Mycobacterial
    Fungal
    Parasitic (toxoplasmosis, trichinosis, Chagas disease)
Neuromuscular causes
    Duchenne muscular dystrophy
    Facioscapulohumeral muscular dystrophy
    Erb limb-girdle dystrophy
    Myotonic dystrophy
    Friedreich ataxia

Modified with permission from Dec GW, Fuster V: Idiopathic dilated cardiomyopathy, *N Engl J Med,* 331:1564-1575, 1994; and Kasper EK, Agema WRP, Hutchins GM et al: The causes of dilated cardiomyopathy: a clinicopathologic review of 673 consecutive patients, *J Am Coll Cardiol* 23:586-590, 1994.

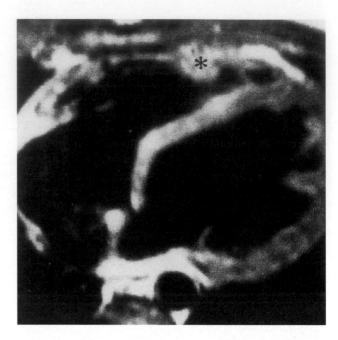

Fig. 8-38 Arrhythmogenic right ventricular disease. Cardiac gated spin-echo image shows regional wall thinning at the anterior free wall of the right ventricle with increased signal intensity in adjacent circumscribed region *(asterisk)* and in most of the interventricular septum, corresponding to fatty replacement. (Reprinted with permission from Auffermann W, Wichter T, Breithardt G et al: Arrhythmogenic right ventricular disease: MR imaging vs. angiography, *AJR Am J Roentgenol* 161:549-555, 1993.)

Because of these difficulties, multiple imaging modalities along with a myocardial biopsy are frequently necessary to distinguish these two entities (Fig. 8-39). Constrictive pericarditis may be cured by surgical stripping of the pericardium, whereas operation on a patient with restrictive cardiomyopathy carries an increased anesthetic risk, making accurate preoperative diagnosis essential.

Restrictive cardiomyopathies are associated with extracellular infiltration of protein; granulomas; and cellular or fibrous infiltration such as amyloidosis, sarcoidosis, radiation fibrosis, carcinoid, and eosinophilic endomyocardial fibrosis. Patients with hemochromatosis and the glycogen storage diseases, inborn errors of metabolism, develop restrictive cardiomyopathies because of an intracellular accumulation of excessive iron or lipids (Box 8-5).

Hypertrophic cardiomyopathy

Hypertrophic cardiomyopathy is characterized by disproportionate hypertrophy of the left ventricle and occasionally of the right ventricle. The disease is distinctive and needs to be separated from secondary and acquired hypertensive heart disease (Box 8-6). Initially this disease was called idiopathic hypertrophic subaortic stenosis or hypertrophic obstructive cardiomyopathy. Subsequently it became clear that subaortic obstruction was only one feature of cardiac hypertrophy. Now hypertrophic cardiomyopathy is typically subdivided into those patients with left ventricular outflow obstruction and those without. Mild nonobstructive hypertrophy of the left ventricle is common in many conditions that cause an increased afterload of the left ventricle, such as hypertension, aortic stenosis, and coarctation. The hypertrophy in these diseases usually is concentric and uniform.

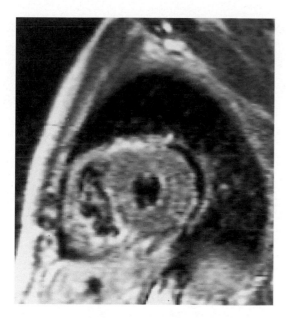

Fig. 8-39 Amyloid heart disease. A short-axis image using a spin-echo sequence (TE = 60 msec) delineated the concentric thick walls of both right and left ventricles. There is a slight inhomogeneous appearance to the myocardium. A small pericardial effusion is layered posteriorly. (Reprinted with permission from Miller SW, Brady TJ, Dinsmore RE et al: Cardiac magnetic resonance imaging: the Massachusetts General Hospital experience, *Radiol Clin North Am* 23:745-764, 1985.)

Hypertrophic cardiomyopathy has an unusual amount of wall thickening in relation to the left ventricular pressure. The disease is genetically transmitted as an autosomal dominant trait with variable penetrance. Histology shows myocardial fibers of varying size and in disarray, that is the fibers are not aligned with each other as in the normal heart. The hypertrophy may be concentric or localized to the apex, the free wall of the left ventricle, or to a segment of the interventricular septum. This spectrum of segmental hypertrophy has lead to the mnemonics ASH (asymmetric septal hypertrophy) and DUST (disproportionate upper septal thickening). Occasionally the right ventricular infundibulum may be stenotic. The hallmark of obstructive hypertrophic cardiomyopathy is a dynamic subvalvular aortic stenosis. In diastole the left ventricular outflow tract is open or slightly stenotic because of upper septal hypertrophy. But in systole an increasing stenosis develops as the anterior leaflet of the mitral valve moves into the outflow region. This abnormal motion of the mitral valve increases throughout systole and frequently causes the valve to touch the ventricular septum, creating an occlusion of the outflow from the left ventricle. The systolic anterior motion (SAM) of the mitral valve is variable. Physiologic maneuvers that decrease the size of the left ventricle or increase its contractility worsen the aortic stenosis, whereas those maneuvers that increase its size or decrease its contractility lessen or abolish the pressure gradient.

Box 8-5 Restrictive Cardiomyopathy

Amyloidosis
Sarcoidosis
Hemochromatosis
Infiltrative diseases
    Glycogen storage disease
    Fabry disease
Löffler endocarditis
Metastases to the heart
Radiation

Box 8-6 Hypertrophic Cardiomyopathy

GENETIC HYPERTROPHIC CARDIOMYOPATHY (HCM)

Obstructive HCM
    Subaortic stenosis
    Midventricular stenosis
Nonobstructive HCM
    Symmetric hypertrophy
    Asymmetric hypertrophy
        Septal hypertrophy
        Apical hypertrophy
        Midventricular hypertrophy

ACQUIRED OR SECONDARY HCM

Essential hypertension
Renal parenchymal and renovascular diseases
Adrenal diseases
Endocrine diseases including pheochromocytoma
Left ventricular outflow obstruction
    Aortic stenosis
    Coarctation
    Takayasu disease
Chronic high output states such as arteriovenous fistulas

Although ASH and SAM are characteristic of obstructive cardiomyopathy, neither is specific. ASH can be seen in children under 2 years in whom the heart retains its neonatal structure with the wall thickness of both ventricles being nearly equal. Pulmonary stenosis may cause right ventricular hypertrophy, which causes the septum to be more than 1.3 times the thickness of the left ventricular free wall, the criterion for asymmetric septal thickening. A posterior myocardial infarction thins the posterior wall, whereas the septum retains its normal thickness. Occasionally the septum is segmentally thicker for unknown reasons in hypertensive heart disease and in valvular aortic stenosis. In the same way SAM is not entirely specific for hypertrophic cardiomyopathy. In transposition of the great arteries the anterior leaflet of the mitral valve may move abnormally in one third of newborns with this malformation. In this instance the SAM is a dynamic subpulmonary stenosis as the pulmonary artery is connected to the left ventricle.

Imaging abnormalities in cardiomyopathies

The abnormalities that can be seen by imaging techniques are listed in Box 8-7. On the chest film the heart size is usually normal, but it can have severe biventricular enlargement from hypertrophy (Fig. 8-40). Left atrial enlargement and pulmonary edema occur when the left ventricle is too stiff to allow normal diastolic filling. Tomographic imaging is required to assess the location and amount of hypertrophy (Fig. 8-41). Echocardiography and occasionally angiography show the abnormal mitral valve motion (Fig. 8-42). Several types of contraction abnormalities are frequently seen in the left ventricle. Lack of base-to-apex shortening, which appears as apical akinesis, is a sign of the muscle-bound heart and not an area of scar from coronary disease. Cavity obliteration usually occurs at the apex at end-systole (Fig. 8-43), although it may occur only in the middle segment of the ventricle or rarely in the outflow

---

Box 8-7   Imaging Signs of Hypertrophic Cardiomyopathy with Obstruction (Idiopathic Hypertrophic Subaortic Stenosis)

Mitral regurgitation
Systolic anterior motion (SAM) of the anterior leaflet of the mitral valve
Hyperkinetic ventricular free wall
Hypokinetic septum
Ventricular hypertrophy
    Asymmetric septal hypertrophy (ASH)
    Concentric hypertrophy after long-term severe outflow gradient
Early systolic closure of the aortic valve
Thickening of the aortic leaflets
Phasic coronary flow
Right ventricular outflow narrowing
Left atrial enlargement
Mitral annular calcification
Septal artery compression during systole

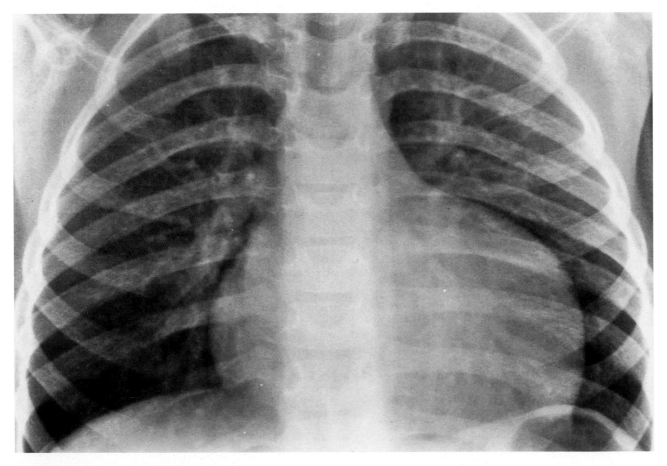

Fig. 8-40   Hypertrophic cardiomyopathy. The left heart border is uplifted and laterally displaced indicating both right and left ventricular enlargement.

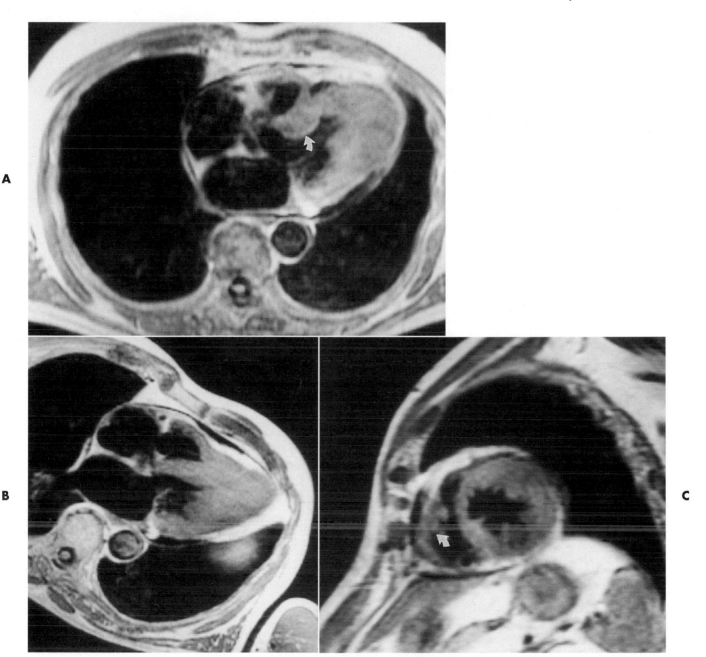

Fig. 8-41 Hypertrophic cardiomyopathy. **A,** An axial spin-echo image shows a thick apex measuring 30 mm (normal ≤ 12 mm) and a lobular upper septal hypertrophy *(arrow)*. **B,** The four-chamber view at end-diastole (there is white blood in the descending aorta) shows severe apical hypertrophy of both right and left ventricles. **C,** A short-axis view demonstrates the moderate hypertrophy in the right ventricular free wall *(arrow)*. The lateral wall of the left ventricle is asymmetrically thicker than the septum.

region. The left ventricle may have an unusual shape because of the segmental hypertrophy (Fig. 8-44). The papillary muscles may touch at end-systole, producing obliteration of the cavity at the midventricular level (Fig. 8-45). Cranially angled left anterior oblique (LAO) left ventriculography may define the left ventricular outflow region and the mitral valve. The best projection results from angling the image intensifier cranially

about 30 degrees in a 60-degree LAO projection. This view allows the entire left ventricular septum to project onto the film and the anterior mitral leaflet to be tangential to the x-ray beam.

Mitral regurgitation in obstructive hypertrophic cardiomyopathy is directly related to the degree of SAM of the anterior leaflet (Fig. 8-46). The amount of mitral regurgitation is usually mild and alleviated with medical

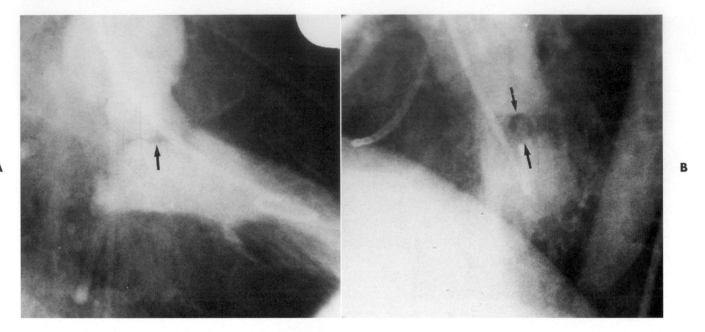

Fig. 8-42 Systolic anterior motion of the anterior leaflet of the mitral valve. **A,** In the RAO view the thick horizontal lucency *(arrow)* below the aortic valve is the mitral leaflet curving anteriorly to touch the septum. **B,** In the LAO view the thick mitral leaflet is 1 cm below the aortic valve and almost touches the septum.

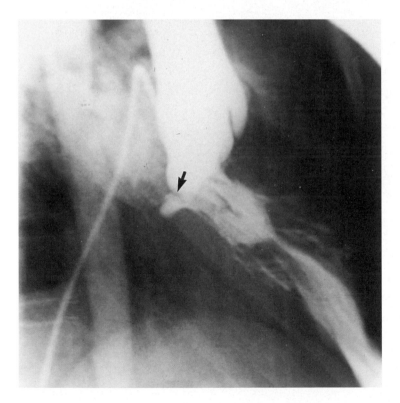

Fig. 8-43 Hypertrophic cardiomyopathy. A left ventriculogram via the transseptal route demonstrates lack of apical contractions with no base-to-apex shortening. The large papillary muscles touch at end-systole, producing obliteration of the cavity at the midventricular level. One of the aortic leaflets is thickened. Systolic motion of the anterior leaflet of the mitral valve *(arrow)* has resulted in mild mitral regurgitation.

therapy. However, a small number of patients have such severe mitral regurgitation that septal myotomy or mitral valve replacement is necessary.

Other angiographic signs of hypertrophic cardiomyopathy include abnormalities in the aortic valve and in the coronary arteries. Frequently the aortic leaflets are mildly thickened and flutter during systole. In echocardiography part of this motion is identified to represent early systolic closure of the aortic valve. The left coronary artery may show phasic flow, particularly in the sep-

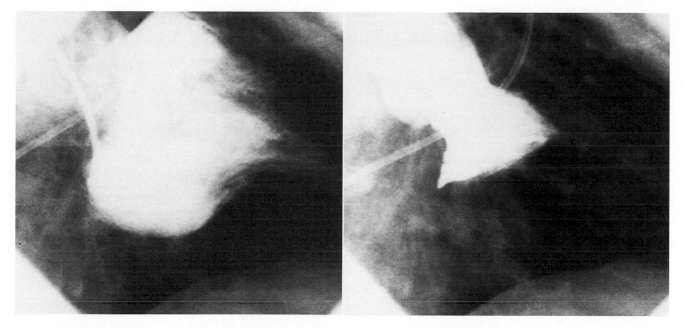

Fig. 8-44 Left ventricular apical obliteration in hypertrophic cardiomyopathy. **A,** End-diastolic RAO frame shows a spadelike left ventricle with huge anterolateral and posteromedial papillary muscles. **B,** At end-systole most of the left ventricular cavity is obliterated.

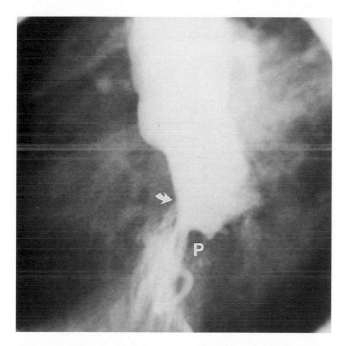

Fig. 8-45 Midventricular hypertrophy. The LAO ventriculogram shows the medial notch *(arrow)* of the septal hypertrophy, which almost touches the posteromedial papillary muscle *(P)*.

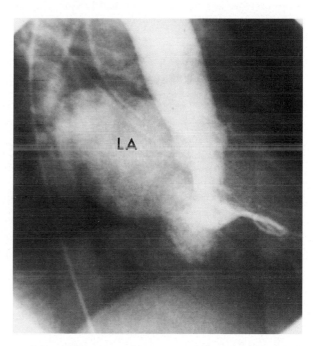

Fig. 8-46 Mitral regurgitation in hypertrophic cardiomyopathy. A systolic frame in the RAO projections shows apical cavity obliteration. Severe mitral regurgitation opacifies the left atrium *(LA)*.

tal branches, that reflects the high wall pressure. The angiographic contrast material may even reverse direction during systole. If the complication of bacterial endocarditis occurs on the damaged aortic or mitral valve leaflets, imaging may show vegetations, regurgitation, or myocardial abscesses.

Distinguishing features of the cardiomyopathies

The diagnostic evaluation of the cardiomyopathies frequently requires cardiac imaging, hemodynamic pressure measurements, and occasionally an endomyocardial biopsy. Table 8-3 lists imaging features that distinguish the three types of cardiomyopathies.

Table 8-3   Left ventricular abnormalities in the cardiomyopathies

	Dilated	Restrictive	Hypertrophic
LV cavity size	Increased	Normal to increased	Normal to decreased
Free wall thickness	Slightly increased, normal, or decreased	Slightly to moderately increased	Septal to free wall ratio > 1.3
Mitral regurgitation	Mild to moderate	Variable	Without obstruction: none to mild With obstruction: mild to severe
Wall motion	Global hypokinesis	Normal to decreased	Hyperkinetic
Mural thrombi	Frequently	Occasionally	None
Systolic function	Decreased	Normal	Normal to increased
Diastolic function	Normal	Decreased	Normal to decreased
Ejection fraction	Decreased	Normal to decreased	Normal to increased
Cardiac output	Decreased	Normal to decreased	Decreased, normal, or increased

SUGGESTED READINGS

Books

McAllister HA, Fenoglia JJ: *Tumors of the cardiovascular system.* In Hartman WH, Cowan WR (editors): *Atlas of tumor pathology* (Fasc. 15, 2nd series), Washington, DC, 1978, Armed Forces Institute of Pathology.

Shabetai R: *The pericardium,* New York, 1981, Grune & Stratton.

Spodick DH: *Pericardial diseases. Cardiovascular clinics,* Vol 7, No 3, Philadelphia, 1976, FA Davis,

Journals

Abrams HL, Adams DF, Grant HA: The radiology of tumors of the heart, *Radiol Clin North Am* 9:299, 1971.

Auffermann W, Wichter T, Breithardt G et al: Arrhythmogenic right ventricular disease: MR imaging vs angiography, *AJR Am J Roentgenol* 161:549-555, 1993.

Black CM, Hedges LK, Javitt MC: The superior pericardial sinus: normal appearance on gradient-echo MR images, *AJR Am J Roentgenol* 160:749-751, 1993.

Brandenburg RO, Chazov E, Cherian G et al: Report of the WHO/ISFC Task Force on definition and classification of cardiomyopathies, *Circulation* 64:437A, 1981.

Buckley BH, Hutchins GM: Atrial myxomas: a fifty-year review, *Am Heart J* 97:639, 1979.

Cammarosano C, Lewis W: Cardiac lesions in acquired immune deficiency syndrome (AIDS), *J Am Coll Cardiol* 5:703-706, 1985.

Choe YH, Im J, Park JH et al: The anatomy of the pericardial space: a study in cadavers and patients, *AJR Am J Roentgenol* 149:693, 1987.

Cyrlak D, Cohen AJ, Dana ER: Esophagopericardial fistula: causes and radiographic features, *AJR Am J Roentgenol* 141:177-179, 1983.

Dec GW, Fuster V: Idiopathic dilated cardiomyopathy, *N Engl J Med* 331:1564-1575, 1994.

Feigen DS, Fenoglio JJ, McAllister HA et al: Pericardial cysts. A radiologic-pathologic correlation and review, *Radiology* 125:15, 1977.

Gale ME, Kiwak MG, Gale DR: Pericardial fluid distribution: CT analysis, *Radiology* 162:171, 1987.

Glazer GM, Gross BH, Orringer MB et al: Computed tomography of pericardial masses: further observations and comparisons with echocardiography, *J Comput Assist Tomogr* 8:895, 1984.

Gomes AS, Lois JF, Child JS et al: Cardiac tumors and thrombus: evaluation with MR imaging, *AJR Am J Roentgenol* 149:895-899, 1987.

Green CE, Elliot LP, Coghlan HC: Improved cineangiographic evaluation of hypertrophic cardiomyopathy by caudocranial left anterior oblique view, *Am Heart J* 102:1015, 1981.

Hamada S, Takamiya M, Ohe T et al: Arrhythmogenic right ventricular dysplasia: evaluation with electron-beam CT, *Radiology* 187:723-727, 1993.

Hancock EW: Subacute effusive-constrictive pericarditis, *Circulation* 43:183, 1971.

Im JG, Rosen A, Webb WR et al: MR imaging of the transverse sinus of the pericardium, *AJR Am J Roentgenol* 150:79, 1988.

Isner JM, Carter BL, Bankoff MS et al: Differentiation of constrictive pericarditis from restrictive cardiomyopathy by computed tomographic imaging, *Am Heart J* 105:1019, 1983.

Kaminsky ME, Rodan BA, Osborne DR et al: Post-pericardotomy syndrome, *AJR Am J Roentgenol* 138:503, 1982.

Kaplan KR, Rifkin MD: MR diagnosis of lipomatous infiltration of the interatrial septum, *AJR Am J Roentgenol* 153:495-496, 1989.

Kasper EK, Agema WRP, Hutchins GM et al: The causes of dilated cardiomyopathy: a clinicopathologic review of 673 consecutive patients, *J Am Coll Cardiol* 23:586-590, 1994.

Kaul S, Fishbein MC, Siegal RJ: Cardiac manifestations of acquired immune deficiency syndrome: a 1991 update, *Am Heart J* 122:535-544, 1991.

Keren A, Popp RL: Assignment of patients into the classification of cardiomyopathies, *Circulation* 86:1622-1633, 1992.

Ledford DK: Immunologic aspects of cardiovascular disease, *JAMA* 268:2923-2929, 1992.

Levy-Ravetch M, Auh YH, Rubenstein WA et al: CT of the pericardial recesses, *AJR Am J Roentgenol* 144:707, 1985.

Lund JT, Ehman RL, Julsrud PR et al: Cardiac masses: assessment by MR imaging, *AJR Am J Roentgenol* 152:469-473, 1989.

Maron BJ, Epstein SE: Hypertrophic cardiomyopathy. Recent observations regarding the specificity of three hallmarks of the disease: asymmetric septal hypertrophy, septal disorganization and systolic anterior motion of the anterior mitral leaflet, *Am J Cardiol* 45:141, 1980.

Masui T, Finck S, Higgins CB: Constrictive pericarditis and restrictive cardiomyopathy: evaluation with MR imaging, *Radiology* 182:369-373, 1992.

McMurdo KK, Webb WR, von Schulthess GK et al: Magnetic resonance imaging of the superior pericardial recesses, *AJR Am J Roentgenol* 145:985, 1985.

Miller SW: Imaging pericardial disease, *Radiol Clin North Am* 27:1113-1125, 1989.

Moncada R, Baker M, Salinas M et al: Diagnostic role of computed tomography in pericardial heart disease: congenital defect, thickening, neoplasms, and effusions, *Am Heart J* 103:263, 1982.

Park JH, Kim YM, Chung JW et al: MR imaging of hypertrophic cardiomyopathy, *Radiology* 185:441-446, 1992.

Protopapas Z, Westcott J: Left pulmonic recess of the pericardium: findings at CT and MR imaging, *Radiology* 196:85-88, 1995.

Pugatch RD, Braver JH, Robbins AH et al: CT diagnosis of pericardial cysts, *AJR Am J Roentgenol* 131:515, 1978.

Reynen K: Cardiac myxomas, *N Engl J Med* 333:1610-1617, 1995.

Sagrista-Sauleda J, Permanyer-Miralda G, Soler-Soler J: Tuberculosis pericarditis: ten-year experience with a prospective protocol for diagnosis and treatment, *J Am Coll Cardiol* 11:724, 1988.

Schiavonne WA, O'Donnell JK: Congenital absence of the left portion of parietal pericardium demonstrated by nuclear magnetic resonance imaging, *Am J Cardiol* 55:1439, 1985.

Sechtem U, Edwards JE: Irradiation-induced pericarditis, *Chest* 75:560, 1979.

Sechtem U, Tscholakoff D, Higgins CB: MRI of the normal pericardium, *AJR Am J Roentgenol* 147:239, 1986.

Sharma OP, Maheshwari A, Thaker K: Myocardial sarcoidosis, *Chest* 103:253-258, 1993.

Shirani J, Roberts WC: Clinical, electrocardiographic and morphologic features of massive fatty deposits ("lipomatous hypertrophy") in the atrial septum, *J Am Coll Cardiol* 22:225-238, 1993.

Soulen RL, Stark DD, Higgins CB: Magnetic resonance imaging of constrictive pericardial disease, *Am J Cardiol* 55:480, 1985.

Takasugi JE, Godwin JD: Surgical defects of the pericardium: radiographic findings, *AJR Am J Roentgenol* 152:951, 1989.

Tyberg TI, Goodyer AVN, Hurst VW III et al: Left ventricular filling in differentiating restrictive amyloid cardiomyopathy and constrictive pericarditis, *Am J Cardiol* 47:791, 1981.

CHAPTER 9

Congenital Heart Disease

Segmental Analysis of Cardiac Malformations
Cardiac axis and visceral situs
Atrial morphology
Ventricular morphology
Atrioventricular connections
Relations of the great arteries
Ventriculoarterial connections
Associated malformations
Malpositions and Abnormal Connections
Cardiac connections and positions
Left and right atria
Ventricular looping
Dextrocardia
Levocardia
Mesocardia
Heterotaxy and the syndromes of asplenia and polysplenia
Atrioventricular discordance
Congenitally corrected transposition of the great vessels
(Levotransposition of the great arteries)
Angiographic anatomy
Coronary artery patterns
Isolated ventricular inversion
Straddling atrioventricular valves
Ventriculoarterial discordance
Complete dextrotransposition of the great arteries
Angiographic anatomy and technique
Surgical procedures
Partial transposition of the great arteries
Double-outlet right ventricle
Double-outlet left ventricle
Anomalies of aortopulmonary septation
Truncus arteriosus
Chest film abnormalities
Imaging features
Hemitruncus arteriosus
Aortopulmonary septation
Anatomically corrected malposition of the great arteries

Abnormal connections of the pulmonary veins
Total anomalous pulmonary venous connection
Chest film findings
Partial anomalous pulmonary venous connection
Cardiotyping
Septal Defects, Hypoplasias, and Atresias
Atrial septal defects
Patent foramen ovale
Ostium secundum and primum defects
Sinus venosus defects
Less common defects
Chest film features
Imaging techniques and features
Atrioventricular septal defects
Complete atrioventricular canal defects
Partial or incomplete atrioventricular canal defects
Segmental analysis
Chest film abnormalities
Angiographic features
MRI features
Ventricular septal defects
Classifications
Chest film findings
Imaging features
Patent ductus arteriosus
Characteristics
Complications
Infant chest film abnormalities
Adult chest film abnormalities
Angiographic examination
Single ventricle
Definition
Chest film features
Angiographic examination
Tricuspid atresia
Characteristics
Anatomy

        Chest film abnormalities

        Angiographic findings

    Pulmonary atresia with intact ventricular septum

        Classification

        Anatomic features

        Chest film abnormalities

        Angiographic examination

    Tetralogy of Fallot

        Characteristics

        Anatomy

        Chest film abnormalities

        Angiographic examination

        Severe pulmonary lesions

        Postoperative evaluation

    Hypoplastic left heart syndrome

        Characteristics

        Chest film abnormalities

        Angiographic examination

Differential Diagnosis in Congenital Heart Disease

    Pattern recognition and triangulation approach

    Segmental analysis

    By pulmonary pattern

    By age

    By prevalence

Suggested Readings

SEGMENTAL ANALYSIS OF CARDIAC MALFORMATIONS

Complex malformations, particularly those associated with malposition, are diagnostically very challenging and call for precise and complete morphologic description. You can classify most malformations in a logical manner if you sequentially diagnose the position and connections of the atria, the ventricles, and the great arteries.

The steps for the segmental diagnostic approach to cardiac malformations are:

1. Atrial segment: Use abdominal and thoracic situs to determine the position of the right and left atria. Identify the atria—distinguished by their appendages and caval connections.
2. Ventricular segment: Determine the cardiac axis—is the apex on the right or left side? Define the ventricular type—which is the right and which is the left ventricle?
3. Determine atrioventricular connections: concordant—right atrium to right ventricle, left atrium to left ventricle; discordant—right atrium to left ventricle, left atrium to right ventricle.
4. Aortic position: Classify anteroposterior and lateral aortic positions in relation to the pulmonary artery.

5. Great artery connections: Determine the connection of each ventricle with the aorta and pulmonary artery.
6. Identify associated malformations: septal defects; inlet or outlet obstruction; regurgitant valves; vena cava, pulmonary, aortic anomalies.

Cardiac Axis and Visceral Situs

The situs is determined by chest and abdominal radiographs. Situs solitus and situs inversus are recognized by the asymmetry of the tracheobronchial tree and by the positions of the abdominal organs. Symmetrically lobed lungs, midline liver, gastrointestinal malrotations, asplenia, and polysplenia denote the heterotaxy syndrome (Fig. 9-1), which can also be recognized by isomerism of the atria. *Isomerism* means both atria have features of the right atrium or of the left atrium. The *visceral-atrial rule* is that the right and left atria develop on the same side as the thoracic and abdominal viscera do. In situs solitus, the right atrium is on the right side of the mediastinum and the left atrium is on the left side. In situs inversus, the morphologic right atrium is on the left side and the left atrium lies on the right side. In situs ambiguous, right and left sides cannot be determined because the lungs and abdomen are symmetric. For example, in asplenia there are two right (trilobed) lungs and both atria are morphologically right atria. In polysplenia there are two (bilobed) left lungs and both atria are morphologic left atria.

In most persons, the major portion of the heart lies slightly to the left of midline. The cardiac apex denotes the location of the heart within the thorax. Dextrocardia (Fig. 9-2), levocardia (Fig. 9-3), and mesocardia then indicate the possible positions of the heart. Using this terminology, a *cardiac malposition* is any heart that does not have a leftward cardiac axis in situs solitus. A malposition includes dextrocardia in situs solitus and levocardia in situs inversus (Fig. 9-4), as well as dextrocardia in situs inversus. All of these positions represent deviation from normal embryologic development without necessarily implying any hemodynamic or morphologic derangement. In primary dextrocardia, the main defect is in the heart. There are two types of *primary dextrocardia:* (1) dextroversion wherein the heart is rotated or pivoted so that its apex lies on the right side with the atria as a fulcrum, and (2) mirror image dextrocardia. In *secondary dextrocardia,* the heart is normal, but the mediastinum is shifted to the right owing to extracardiac abnormalities that involve the lungs, pleura, or skeleton (see Box 9-1). Examples of the latter include pneumothorax, congenital herniation of the gastrointestinal tract into the thorax, and thoracolumbar scoliosis (Fig. 9-5).

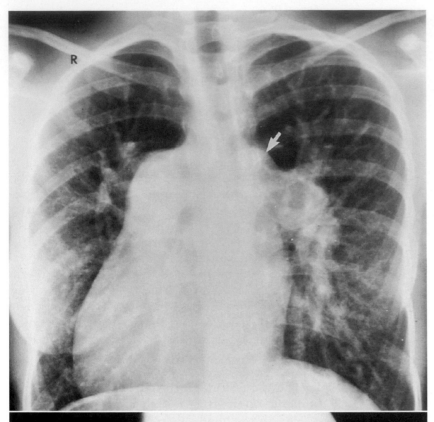

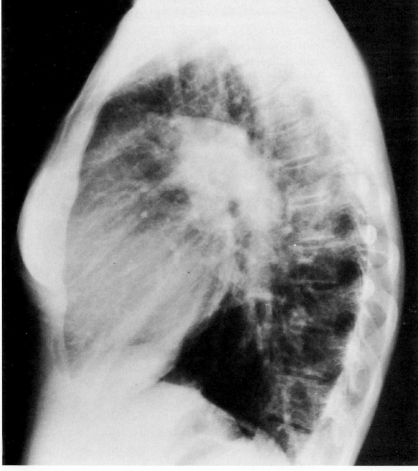

Fig. 9-1 Polysplenia in the heterotaxy syndrome. In the frontal view (**A**), the stomach is on the right side, as is the lowest leaf of the diaphragm. Both mainstem bronchi are below their adjacent pulmonary arteries. The aortic arch is not visible. The azygos vein (*arrow*) is large because of the absence of the intrahepatic portion of the inferior vena cava (azygos continuation). In the lateral view (**B**) both right and left pulmonary arteries project above and posterior to the trachea, which is a sign of bilateral left lungs. An atrial septal defect with pulmonary arterial hypertension has produced the large pulmonary arteries.

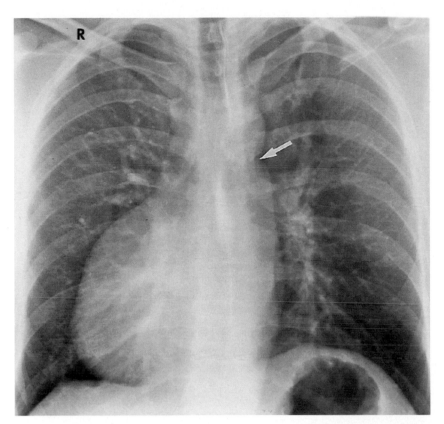

Fig. 9-2 Dextrocardia. The cardiac apex lies on the right side, while the abdominal and tracheobronchial structures are on their normal sides. Slight rib notching and an indentation in the descending aortic shadow *(arrow)* denote coarctation of the aorta. A ventricular septal defect is reflected in the large pulmonary arteries.

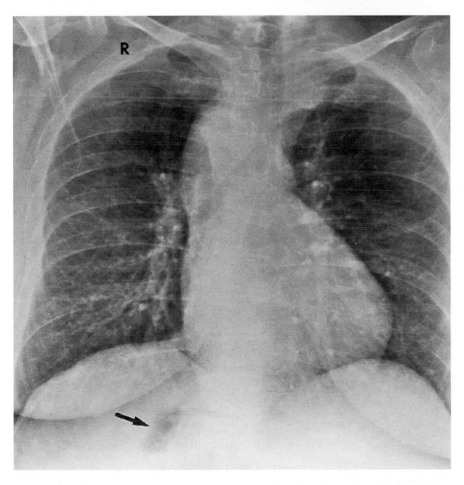

Fig. 9-3 Levocardia. The right-sided stomach bubble *(arrow)* and the asymmetric mainstem bronchi with the left-sided epiarterial bronchus are diagnostic of situs inversus. Therefore, the left cardiac apex, which represents levocardia, is discordant with the body situs. Tetralogy of Fallot is present with a right aortic arch.

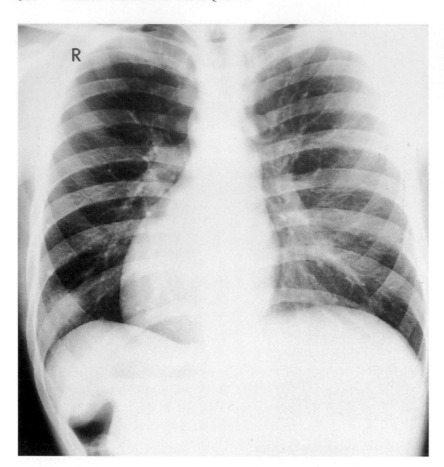

Fig. 9-4 Situs inversus. The right and left sides of the abdomen and thorax are reversed in a mirror-image fashion. The spleen, stomach bubble, and lowest leaf of the diaphragm are on the right side of the abdomen. The left-sided lung has an epiarterial bronchus, indicating a morphologic right lung.

Box 9-1   Types of Dextrocardia

PRIMARY DEXTROCARDIA

Dextroversion. The left ventricle is to the *left* of the right ventricle, as it is in the normal heart.
Mirror-image dextrocardia. The left ventricle is to the *right* of the right ventricle.

SECONDARY DEXTROCARDIA

Skeletal causes
  Scoliosis
  Sternal or rib deformity
Lung causes
  Pneumonectomy
  Collapse
  Pneumothorax
  Unilateral airtrapping
Pleural causes
  Herniation of the gut into the left thorax

Atrial Morphology

With rare exceptions, the morphology of the atria corresponds closely with the situs of the tracheobronchial tree and the abdominal viscera. Of the various criteria for distinguishing between right and left atria, the most reliable are the shape of the atrial appendage and the connection to the inferior vena cava. The right atrial appendage is broad and pyramidal, while the left atrial appendage is thin with a narrow neck. The inferior vena cava almost always connects with the right atrium. This is true even in the "absence" of the inferior vena cava and azygos continuation. In this entity, there is no intrahepatic portion of the cava, but the hepatic veins connect to the subdiaphragmatic portion of the inferior vena cava which joins the right atrium. The superior vena cava is a poor landmark of atrial morphology because bilateral cavae may be present or the right superior vena cava may be absent, and there may be a connection of either the right or left superior vena cava into either atrium or into the coronary sinus. As an example, in situs inversus totalis, the morphologic right atrium is on the left side and the morphologic left atrium lies on the right side of the body, while the right-sided lung has two lobes and the left-sided lung has three lobes. When thoracic isomerism exists in the heterotaxy syndrome, bilateral morphologic right atria are seen in the asplenia syndrome and bilateral left atria in polysplenia.

Ventricular Morphology

When the right and left ventricles are normal, identification of the two ventricles is relatively simple (see Table

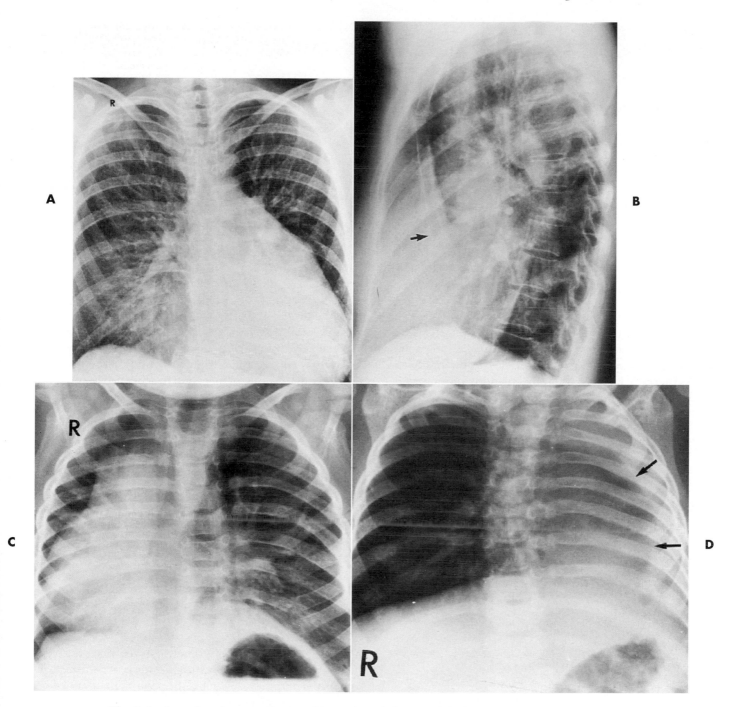

Fig. 9-5   Secondary dextrocardia caused by positional changes of the heart and mediastinum. **A** and **B,** Levoposition caused by severe pectus excavatum *(arrow)*. **C,** Hypoplasia of the right lung producing dextroposition. **D,** Agenesis of the left lung. The *arrows* show the extent to which the right lung has herniated across the anterior mediastinum to lie in the left hemithorax.

9-1). The normal right ventricle has coarse, trabeculated walls when compared with the smooth-walled left ventricle. The right ventricle has a contractile muscle called the conus or infundibulum between the tricuspid and pulmonary valves, while the left ventricle has mitral-aortic continuity with no intervening muscle. The right ventricle has trabeculations and papillary muscles on its septum, whereas in the left ventricle these structures are not pre-

sent on the septum. A bicuspid (mitral) atrioventricular valve is a part of the left ventricle, while a tricuspid atrioventricular valve is part of the right ventricle, although either of these valves may have a cleft or be absent.

When some of the structures used to identify the ventricles are congenitally absent or malformed, the identification of the two ventricles becomes confusing. To clarify this situation, identify the three anatomic segments in

Table 9-1 Normal ventricles	
Right ventricle	**Left ventricle**
Coarse, trabeculated walls	Smooth walls
Contractile muscle (conus, infundibulum) between tricuspid and pulmonary valves	Mitral-aortic continuity with no intervening muscle
Trabeculations and papillary muscles on septum	Septum free from trabeculations and papillary muscles
Tricuspid atrioventricular valve	Bicuspid (mitral) atrioventricular valve
Complex triangular shape	Spheroidal shape

the normal ventricle: (1) the inlet or *inflow tract,* (2) the *trabecular part,* and (3) the outlet or *outflow tract.* The inlet segment in the right ventricle is smooth and adjacent to the tricuspid valve; in the left ventricle it is between the papillary muscles and the mitral valve. The trabecular segment constitutes the body of the ventricle distal to the insertion of the papillary muscles. This trabeculated segment is a key feature in the angiographic distinction between the two ventricles. In the right ventricle, there are large, coarse trabeculations, prominent in both systole and diastole. In the left ventricle, the wall is smooth in diastole but has fine trabeculations during systole. The ventricular outlet portion of the right ventricle is a tubular muscular structure, the conus, which separates the inlet and outlet valves. In the left ventricle, the outlet is smooth and has a deficiency of muscle between the inlet and outlet valves.

When one or more of these three ventricular segments is absent, the heart may be called a single ventricle. Similar terminology for hearts that lack at least one of the three ventricular segments are as follows:

Single ventricle
Univentricular heart
Common ventricle
Double-inlet left ventricle
Double-inlet right ventricle
Undifferentiated ventricle

There is general agreement that an inflow tract must be present for a chamber to be considered a ventricle. The trabecular portion determines if the chamber is of the right or left ventricular type. In these instances, the single ventricle consists of one large chamber that receives both atrioventricular valves. (Note that this definition excludes mitral or tricuspid atresia.) If only the trabecular and outflow segments are present, this structure is called an outlet chamber. Examples of such hearts are the univentricular heart of the left ventricular type, with or without a rudimentary outflow chamber. Difficulties arise in this classification scheme when part of an inlet or outlet valve overrides the septum. In this situation, rather than make an arbitrary decision, a description of

the amount of overriding is appropriate. In general, when either the inlet or outlet valve is associated with more than 50% of a ventricle, it is considered to be a part of that ventricle. Examples of this condition include straddling tricuspid valves and a double-outlet right ventricle.

Inversion of a chamber occurs when a structure that normally lies on the right side is situated on the left side, or vice versa. In the asymmetric body, situs inversus totalis is an example of inversion in which all body structures are isomers to those in situs solitus. In describing the relation of the ventricles to one another, it may be difficult to distinguish true inversion from a cardiac rotation due to an extrinsic abnormality. Locate the ventricular septum as seen through the mitral and tricuspid valves. In the normal, noninverted right ventricle, the septum is on the left side as viewed through the tricuspid valve. In the normal left ventricle, the septum is on the right side as viewed through the mitral valve.

Atrioventricular Connections

The atrioventricular connections are called concordant when the right atrium connects to the right ventricle and the left atrium connects to the left ventricle. When the right atrium connects to the left ventricle and the left atrium connects to the right ventricle, the ventricles are discordant in relation to the atria. In the heterotaxy syndrome, in which either two right atria or two left atria may exist, the atrioventricular connection is ambiguous. This schema is less clear when either atresia of one of the atrioventricular valves exists or when one of the atrioventricular valves straddles the interventricular septum. When there is a double-inlet or a straddling atrioventricular valve, the tensor apparatus (the attachments of the chordae tendineae) may connect to either side of the interventricular septum.

Relations of the Great Arteries

The position of the aorta is described relative to the pulmonary artery in both the anteroposterior and lateral

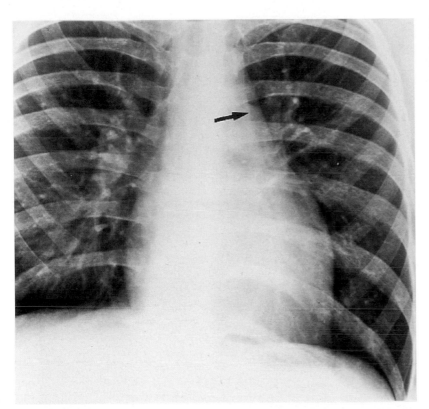

Fig. 9-6 Congenitally corrected transposition of the great arteries. The abnormal leftward course of the ascending aorta is visible as a mediastinal line *(arrow)* as it becomes the aortic arch.

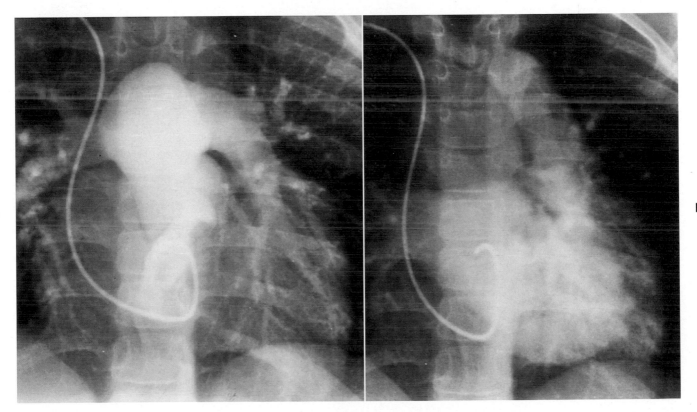

A   B

Fig. 9-7 Levomalposition of the aorta. **A,** A left ventriculogram in congenitally corrected transposition of the great arteries shows the pulmonary artery to the right of the aorta. **B,** On the levophase, the right ventricle connects to the aorta, which is on the left side of the pulmonary artery. The left aortic arch forms the border of the left side of the mediastinum.

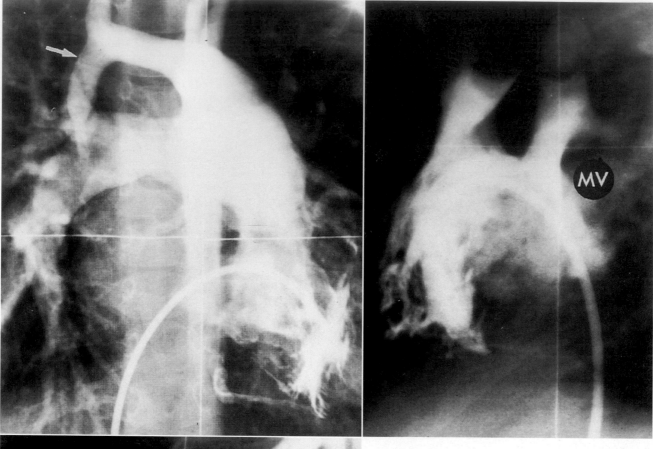

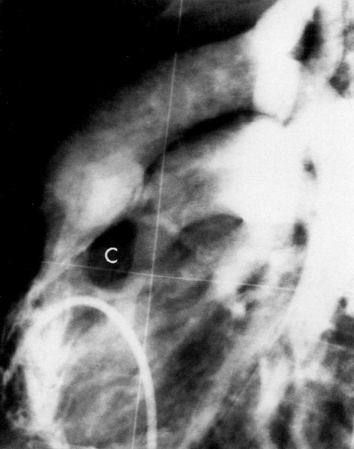

Fig. 9-8   Transposition of the great arteries with levo-malposition of the aorta. **A,** Both the pulmonary artery and aorta fill from a right ventricular injection. The left aortic arch is the convexity in the left superior mediastinum. The right subclavian artery-to-right pulmonary artery graft (Blalock-Taussig shunt) is patent *(arrow)*. Early **(B)** and late **(C)** frames in a lateral projection show a large ventricular septal defect. The mitral valve *(MV)* below the conus to the pulmonary artery is shown in diastole. The crista supraventricularis *(C)* is the lucency between the bilateral conus. The aortic valve is anterior to the pulmonary valve and at the same height. Note the bilateral conus in **B.** (Courtesy of Kenneth E. Fellows, M.D.)

planes (Fig. 9-6). In the normal heart, the aorta is to the right of and posterior to the pulmonary artery. An anterior aorta to the right of the pulmonary artery is common in transposition of the great arteries. An aorta to the left of and anterior to the pulmonary artery is typical in, but not diagnostic of, corrected transposition. Then there is a characteristic leftward convexity of the aorta (Fig. 9-7).

Ventriculoarterial Connections

The pulmonary valve is part of the pulmonary artery (not part of the right ventricle) and the aortic valve is part of the aorta. When the pulmonary artery or the aorta is related to, or overrides more than 50% of, a particular ventricle, it is defined as being connected to that ventricle. This association is particularly strong when there is a continuity between an atrioventricular valve and the semilunar valve. Concordant connections exist when the left ventricle is connected to the aorta and the right ventricle to the pulmonary artery. Discordant connections result when the left ventricle is connected to the pulmonary artery and the right ventricle to the aorta. This latter connection is also called *transposition.* When both great arteries arise predominantly from one ventricle, there is a double-outlet right ventricle or double-outlet left ventricle. The final type of arterial connection is a single-outlet heart of which there are three varieties: (1) only the aorta may be connected to the heart when there is pulmonary valve atresia; (2) only a pulmonary artery may be connected to the heart when there is aortic valve atresia; and (3) where there is a persistent truncus arteriosus in which the pulmonary arteries, aorta, and coronary arteries all arise above the truncal valve in the ascending aorta.

The ventricular outflow tracts may be one of four distinct types:

1. Bilateral conus
2. Subaortic conus
3. Subpulmonary conus
4. Bilaterally deficient conus

Certain types of conus are associated with particular malformations:

- Normally related great arteries have a subpulmonary conus.
- Transposition of the great arteries has a subaortic conus with mitral-pulmonary continuity.
- Double-outlet right ventricle typically has a bilateral conus (Fig. 9-8).
- Double-outlet left ventricle has a bilaterally deficient conus.

Associated Malformations

These defects may actually dominate the clinical presentation. Septal defects may be in the atrial septum, the interventricular septum, or peripherally between the aorta and pulmonary arteries. An example of the latter is patent ductus arteriosus and aortic-pulmonary window. Stenoses, atresias, hypoplasia, and regurgitation may exist at the atrioventricular or arterial valves or in relation to the inflow and outflow regions of these valves. Finally, there are anomalies in the connection of the systemic veins (particularly with a left superior vena cava) and in the connections of the pulmonary veins. Abnormal pulmonary and systemic venous connections are particularly prevalent in the asplenia and polysplenia syndromes. In asplenia, there are bilateral right atria so that the pulmonary veins connect either to the superior vena cava or the portal system. In polysplenia with two left atria, the pulmonary veins may connect to either or both atria.

MALPOSITIONS AND ABNORMAL CONNECTIONS

Cardiac Connections and Positions

You can unequivocally describe most cardiac malpositions using the basic concepts of segmental analysis of the atria, the ventricles, and the great vessels and their associated relations, connections, and associated malformations.

Left and right atria

Although there are exceptions, the position of the morphologic right and left atria is directly determined by the symmetry of the thoracic and abdominal contents. The right atrium lies on the side that contains the trilobed lung and the liver, while the left atrium connects to the thorax on the side of the bilobed lung and the spleen. These relationships are very precise when there are no caval anomalies. The symmetric determination of the atrial position and morphology is ambiguous in bilateral right or left lungs and in asplenia or polysplenia.

Ventricular looping

The next step is identification of the two ventricles as either *d*-loop or *l*-loop. These terms refer to the embryologic looping of the straight tube of the heart. A *d*-loop brings the cardiac apex initially to the right with the morphologic right ventricle anterior to the left ventricle; the normal heart has a *d*-loop. Final looping of the heart tube places the apex to the left with the left ventricle lying on the left-hand side of the interventricular septum as viewed through the tricuspid valve. A helpful but not infallible method of localizing the ventricles is the "loop rule": the position of the aorta with respect to the pulmonary artery corresponds to a particular ventricular looping. Without regard to anteroposterior positions, when the aorta is located to the right of the pulmonary artery, a ventricular *d*-loop is probable. When the aorta is to the left of the pulmonary artery, a ventricular *l*-loop is probable. The coronary arteries are also helpful for locating the position of the ventricles. The right coronary artery marks the atrioventricular sulcus of the right ventricle, and the anterior descending artery marks the interventricular sulcus. When there is an *l*-loop heart, the right coronary artery is to the left of the anterior descending artery.

Dextrocardia

Dextrocardia signifies that the apex of the heart is directed toward the right. Primary dextrocardia exists because of an embryologic abnormality. This type of dextrocardia can exist with any type of situs position (Fig. 9-9). When dextrocardia exists with situs inversus, the atrial and ventricular relations have a mirror image to their positions in the usual situs solitus. When the dextrocardia exists in situs solitus, the term *isolated dextrocardia* is frequently applied. It is clear then that dextrocardia can occur in situs solitus, inversus, and ambiguous. Many associated cardiac anomalies exist in primary dextrocardia. Frequent conditions include ventricular septal defect, transposition of the great arteries, corrected transposition of the great arteries, double-outlet right ventricle, and juxtaposition of the atrial appendages.

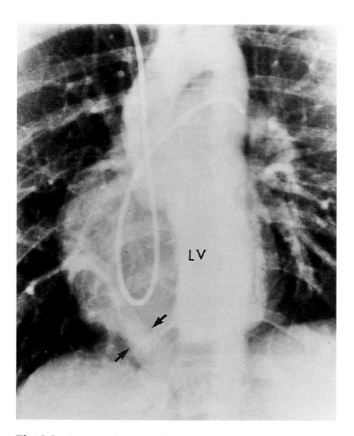

Fig. 9-9 Primary dextrocardia (dextroversion). The levophase of a pulmonary angiogram outlines a smooth-walled left ventricle *(LV)*, which is the anterior ventricle because the heart is rotated to the right. An anomalous right inferior pulmonary vein *(arrows)* connects to the inferior vena cava (scimitar syndrome).

The goal of echocardiography, magnetic resonance imaging (MRI), and angiography is to define the position and location of each chamber of the heart and their connections and relations with one another and with the great arteries. In those malpositioned hearts in which the location of the interventricular septum is not known before angiography, posteroanterior and lateral projections serve as initial guidelines. Frequently, the projections can be reversed for a malposition; that is, those structures that are normally best seen in the left anterior oblique projection in the normal heart would be studied in the right anterior oblique projection in dextrocardia. As a rule, the dextrocardia itself does not cause clinical problems, but rather the associated malformations mandate medical or surgical alleviation.

Levocardia

Strictly speaking, *levocardia* means that the cardiac apex is left-sided. Isolated levocardias are those hearts that are left-sided when situs inversus is present. This anomaly occurs in less than 1% of all of congenital cardiac malformation patients compared with a 2% incidence of dextrocardia in patients with congenital heart disease. With levocardia, the position of the thoracic and abdominal organs ranges from partial to complete situs inversus and also to heterotaxy (Fig. 9-10). Severe malformations are always associated with levocardia and frequently include ventricular septal defect, complete atrioventricular canal defects, and pulmonary stenosis or atresia. Isolated levocardia may be suspected on the chest film with a right-sided stomach bubble and left-sided liver shadow and a left cardiac apex. In contrast, in extrinsic levocardia the heart is intrinsically normal but the mediastinum is shifted from skeletal or pulmonary abnormalities (Fig. 9-11).

Mesocardia

Mesocardia is a variant of dextrocardia and levocardia. In this condition, the heart lies in the midline without a distinct apex pointing to either side. These patients may have situs solitus, inversus, or ambiguous of the atria and have similar associated defects.

Heterotaxy and the syndromes of asplenia and polysplenia

Heterotaxy is the abnormal arrangement of organs that differ from that in situs solitus or situs inversus. In these patients the thoracic and abdominal contents have a degree of symmetry, unlike those in situs solitus or inversus where right- and left-sided organs exist together. In the thorax, both lungs may be trilobed with bilateral epiarterial bronchi, or both lungs may be bilobed with bilateral hypoarterial bronchi. In the abdomen, the asymmetry is also frequently lost. The liver may be midline. The attachment of the mesentery, which usually

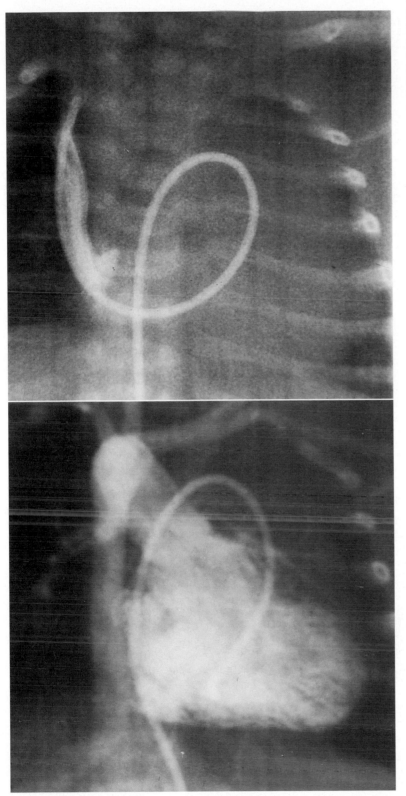

Fig. 9-10 Levocardia with polysplenia. **A,** The catheter in the inferior vena cava has a high, left-sided loop indicating hemiazygos continuation before it enters the right superior vena cava. **B,** Posteroanterior view shows a single ventricle with a subaortic conus. The right aortic arch supplied a patent ductus arteriosus. The ventricle had pulmonary atresia and a complete atrioventricular canal.

runs from the left upper quadrant to the right lower quadrant, may have a midline attachment. The spleen may be absent (asplenia), bilobed with multiple accessory spleens, or multiple small spleens (Fig. 9-12) may be found throughout the mesentery (polysplenia). Situs ambiguous exists when either the right and left sides of the lungs, heart, and abdomen are similar, or where a right-left relationship is difficult to identify. (See Boxes 9-2 and 9-3 for summaries of the characteristics of asplenia and polysplenia.)

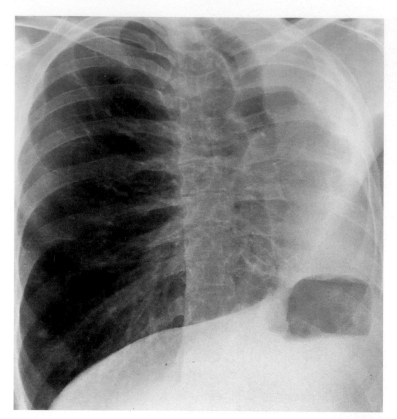

Fig. 9-11 Secondary levocardia. Because of a left pneumonectomy, the heart has moved with the mediastinum into the extreme left side of the thorax. The huge right lung now crosses the midline to fill much of the left hemithorax. The heart is invisible because of the oblique interface the right lung makes with the shifted mediastinum.

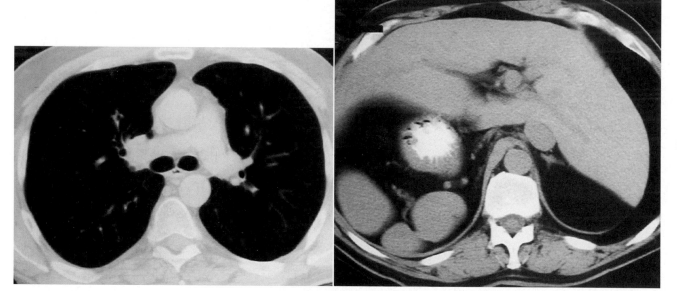

A **B**

Fig. 9-12 Heterotaxia. **A,** The mainstem bronchi are below the pulmonary arteries bilaterally. **B,** The abdominal situs is inverted with multiple small spleens occupying the right side of the abdomen. The liver is midline and occupies nearly equal space in the right and left sides of the abdomen.

Splenic anomalies with malpositions and malformations in multiple organ systems have been recognized since 1826 when Martin and later Ivemark described the absence of the spleen in cyanotic congenital heart disease. Complex cardiac malformations are typical when the type of thoracic and abdominal situs abnormality is uncertain or has features of both situs solitus and situs inversus (Table 9-2).

Segmental analysis of the defects in hearts associated with asplenia begins with the atria and the atrial septum.

Table 9-2 Cardiovascular abnormalities in asplenia and polysplenia*

Abnormality	Asplenia (%)	Polysplenia (%)
Superior vena cava		
Bilateral	53	33
Right	34	33
Left	10	33
Uncertain	3	—
Inferior vena cava		
Right-sided	60	—
Left-sided	28	—
Uncertain	12	—
Azygos continuation	—	84
Anomalous pulmonary veins	84	50
Total anomalous connection	72	—
Partial anomalous connection	12	—
Cardiac apex		
Left	56	58
Right	41	42
Uncertain	3	—
Aortic arch		
Left	56	33
Right	38	67
Unknown	6	—
Great vessels		
Normally related	19	84
Transposition of great arteries	72	8
Double-outlet right ventricle	9	8
Pulmonary valve		
Normal	22	58
Stenosis	34	33
Atresia	44	9
Patent ductus arteriosus	56	50
Absent coronary sinus	83	42
Single ventricle	44	8
Ventricular septal defects	90†	67

*Modified from Rose V, Izukawa T, and Moes CAF: Syndromes of asplenia and polysplenia: a review of cardiac and non-cardiac malformations in 60 cases with special reference to diagnosis and prognosis, *Br Heart J* 37:840, 1975.

†Eighty-four percent of the ventricular septal defects in asplenia were of the atrioventricular canal type.

On the chest film, the external contours of the heart frequently do not conform to the expected heart chambers (Fig. 9-13). Almost all of these hearts show a common atrioventricular valve frequently associated with separate, large atrial septal defects in the primum and secundum location. The size and location of these atrial defects are such that the malformation is called a common atrium. The ventricles also almost invariably have major malformations. About one fourth of the ventricles are inverted (as seen in corrected transposition) and half of the hearts have a univentricular chamber with a rudimentary outflow tract. Anomalies of the great vessels, including transposition of the great arteries and double-outlet right ventricle, have an incidence of 3% to 30%. Angiographically, the posteroanterior and lateral projections are best to allow identification of their right-left relationships. Anomalies in the ventricular septum and semilunar valve stenosis are common so that filming is also done with the x-ray beam parallel to the interventricular septum with cranial angulation. Since two thirds of persons with asplenia have anomalous systemic venous or pulmonary venous connections, or both, these malformations frequently complicate catheterization.

The features of the heart in polysplenia are quite variable and, in fact, there occasionally is no cardiac malformation. With a femoral vein approach, you can recognize azygos continuation by the course of the catheter around the azygos arch (Fig. 9-14). You should not make the diagnosis of tricuspid atresia if the catheter tip fails to pass leftward through the heart above the diaphragm but instead should continue advancing the catheter superiorly until it goes around the azygos arch.

Atrioventricular Discordance

In the schema of segmental cardiac analysis, after recognition of the atria and ventricles, the next step is to determine whether the connections between them are either concordant or discordant. Atrioventricular discordance means that the right atrium is connected to the left ventricle and the left atrium is connected to the right ventricle. Implicit in this definition is the presence of two atria, two atrioventricular valves, and two ventricles. This diagnosis is not appropriate when atrial

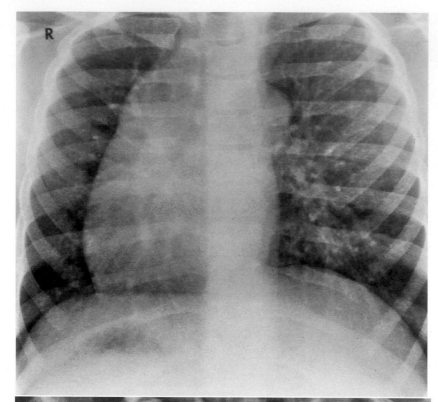

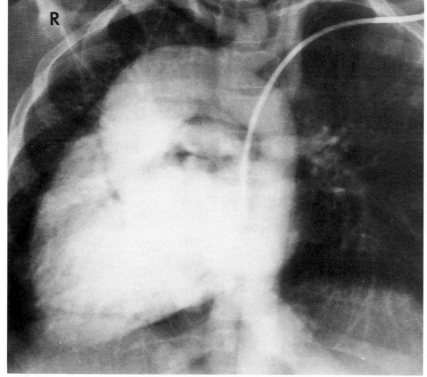

Fig. 9-13 Heterotaxia syndrome with dextrocardia. **A,** The stomach bubble is on the right, as is the cardiac apex. The unusual shape of the heart suggests a complex cardiac malformation. The lungs have shunt vascularity. **B,** The angiogram shows that the right side of the heart is the right ventricle, which connects to the pulmonary artery. The aorta fills simultaneously through a ventricular septal defect and forms the broad curve in the right anterior mediastinum. Comparing with the chest film, the small convexity above the left hilum is an azygos continuation, which is not opacified on this angiogram.

identification is indeterminate in situs ambiguous or when there is a single common atrioventricular valve. Similarly, distinct right and left ventricles are necessary for this definition, although a ventricular septal defect may exist. Atrioventricular discordance may be present in either situs solitus or situs inversus and may be accompanied by ventriculoarterial concordance or discordance. Discordance of both the atrioventricular and the ventriculoarterial segments is called congenitally corrected transposition of the great arteries. Atrio-

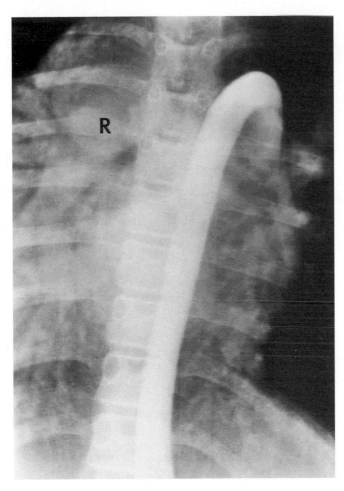

Fig. 9-14 Hemiazygos continuation in a patient with polysplenia and dextrocardia. An injection into the left femoral vein opacified the hemiazygos vein adjacent to the costovertebral sulcus before it emptied into a left superior vena cava.

ventricular discordance with concordance of the ventricles and great arteries, a rare malformation, is called ventricular inversion.

Congenitally corrected transposition of the great vessels (levotransposition of the great arteries)

In 1875 Rokitansky reported a form of transposition in which blood passed in normal serial fashion through the pulmonary and systemic circuits. The right atrium was connected to the left ventricle, which was connected to the pulmonary artery. On the oxygenated side of the lungs, the left atrium was connected to the right ventricle, which was connected to the aorta. The atrioventricular valves always correspond with their ventricles, even when there is atrioventricular discordance. That is, the mitral valve is a left ventricular structure, and the tricuspid valve is a right ventricular structure. In congenitally corrected transposition of the great vessels, the aorta lies to the left of and anterior to the pulmonary

artery, while the pulmonary valve lies to the right and posterior. The aortic valve is usually somewhat anterior to the pulmonary valve, although the two great vessels may be exactly lateral to each other. The ascending aorta frequently has an unusual course, passing in a direction toward the left shoulder so that occasionally a distinctive contour in the left side of the mediastinum is visible on the chest film.

If there are no other defects, this malformation causes no hemodynamic problems and may go undetected during a normal life span. Unfortunately, associated malformations are the rule, and their site and severity determine the clinical course. Ventricular septal defects are frequent (Fig. 9-15) and may be large enough to cause pulmonary arterial hypertension. These defects are usually in the membranous septum adjacent to the pulmonary valve; muscular defects and supracristal defects are less common. Generally, the left-sided atrioventricular valve (i.e., the valve between the left atrium and the right ventricle) is displaced slightly into the ventricle in a manner resembling Ebstein anomaly. If the displacement is more than a few millimeters (because the tricuspid valve is usually displaced to the apex by that amount), the diagnosis of Ebstein anomaly is quite likely. Pulmonary stenosis is frequently associated with ventricular septal defect and may be caused by a malformed valve, a subpulmonary membrane, by aneurysms of the membranous ventricular septum, or, rarely, by accessory tissue in the atrioventricular valve or a muscular bar in the subpulmonary region.

Angiographic anatomy and technique Cardiac catheterization for congenitally corrected transposition may induce frequent disturbances in conduction and rhythm, including atrioventricular block and dissociation. However, in the well-equipped laboratory with current pharmacologic and electrical methods of counteracting these arrhythmias, the catheterization procedure itself should cause a minimum of extra morbidity.

Angiography begins with the conventional posteroanterior and lateral projections. These establish the atrioventricular connections, the morphology of the ventricles, and the position of the aorta and pulmonary artery. As you discover associated malformations, you will frequently need additional injections in specialized views, particularly in cases of dextrocardia. The position of the venous and arterial catheters frequently give the first clue to a corrected transposition (Fig. 9-16). In situs solitus and levocardia, the venous catheter passes through the heart in the midline to reach the pulmonary arteries. On the lateral view, the catheter in the pulmonary artery is posterior to its usual location, which is where the aorta should be in normal hearts. The retrograde arterial catheter has a distinctive curve in the ascending aorta as its course becomes convex medially and to the left before entering the heart. On the lateral view, the aortic

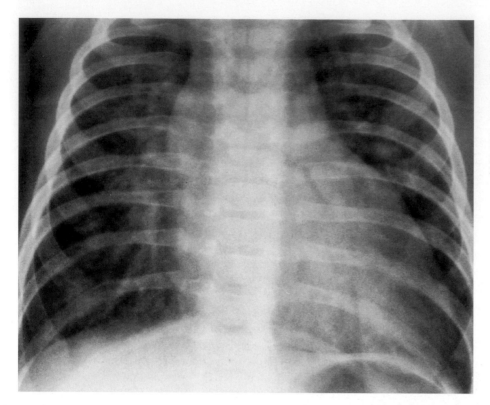

Fig. 9-15 Congenitally corrected transposition of the great arteries with ventricular septal defect. The leftward course of the ascending aorta is not apparent on the chest film. The leftward cardiac apex represents the right ventricle, which is enlarged because of the ventricular septal defect. The main pulmonary artery is not part of the mediastinal interface with the lung because it is central; the hilar and peripheral pulmonary arteries are large from the left-to-right shunt.

catheter is anterior and superior to the venous catheter. The venous and arterial catheters indicate the fundamental relationship between the aorta and the pulmonary artery in corrected transposition with situs solitus and levocardia; the pulmonary artery lies to the right and posterior, while the aorta is anterior and to the left.

In corrected transposition with situs solitus and levocardia, angiography initially consists of right and left ventriculography in the posteroanterior and lateral projections. In the posteroanterior projection, the ventricles lie nearly side by side with the interventricular septum, seen on end. The left ventricle lies slightly inferior to the right ventricle and has a triangular shape with the mitral valve lying medially and to the right. The mitral valve of the left ventricle connects to the right atrium and lies in continuity with the pulmonary valve. The left ventricular outflow region is short and vertically oriented, with the anterior leaflet of the mitral valve on the medial side and the membranous portion of the interventricular septum forming the superior and lateral wall.

In the lateral view, the left ventricle appears to "stand on its apex" with a conical shape whose apex is in the diaphragmatic-sternal angle. The anterior wall of the left ventricle extends superiorly into a distinctive pouch that is characteristic of inverted ventricles, namely the anteriorly placed left ventricle (Fig. 9-17). This recess is separate from both the mitral and pulmonary valves and is the most anterior and superior structure of either ventri-

cle. The outflow portion of the left ventricle in the lateral projection is posterior and connects to a pulmonary artery which is beside or posterior to the aorta. The posterior wall of the left ventricle beneath the pulmonary valve is the membranous septum, and the anterior wall forms a neck above the blind recess and below the pulmonary valve.

In the frontal view, the right ventricle is to the left of and slightly superior to the left ventricle (Fig. 9-18). In this position, the right ventricle has an oval to triangular shape and the usual coarse trabeculations. The tricuspid annulus is in the posteroanterior plane separated from the aortic valve by the muscular infundibulum. This morphologic right ventricle connects with the left atrium. The crista supraventricularis in this projection is the medial wall of the infundibulum above the tricuspid valve. In the lateral projection, the crista is the posterior wall of the infundibulum and separates the tricuspid from the aortic valve.

The aortic valve appears higher than the pulmonary valve and is the border-forming structure in the left side of the upper half of the mediastinum. Unlike in the normal heart, the main pulmonary artery does not form any interface with the lung on the frontal chest film.

Different ventricular patterns and shapes occur in situs inversus and in other rare malformations. Since the aortic arch may lie on either the left or right side, the distinctive mediastinal contour of aorta (which is frequent-

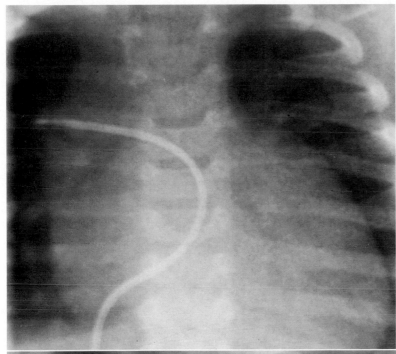

A

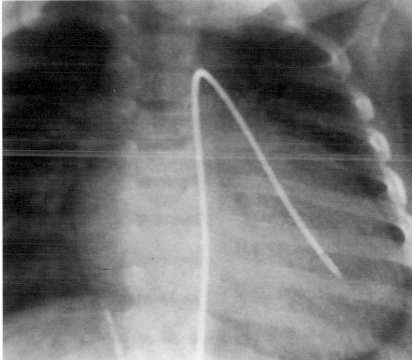

B

Fig. 9-16   Catheter positions in congenitally corrected transposition of the great arteries. **A,** The catheter in the inferior vena cava passes through the right atrium and left ventricle to end in the pulmonary artery. **B,** The retrograde aortic catheter ends in the right ventricle. The ascending aorta lies to the left of the pulmonary valve.

ly not present in situs solitus with classic corrected transposition) may not be visible on the standard chest films.

Since about one third of patients with corrected transposition have tricuspid regurgitation (i.e., from the right ventricle connected to the left atrium), you should perform a right ventriculogram during catheterization. The apically displaced tricuspid leaflets of Ebstein anomaly are usually the cause of the regurgitation, but there are occasionally other leaflet abnormalities. The injection is best made in the frontal projection so that the tricuspid annulus is tangential to the x-ray beam. When there is severe regurgitation in infants, the details of the leaflets and the origin of their insertion are frequently difficult to identify. If technical factors such as arrhythmia and

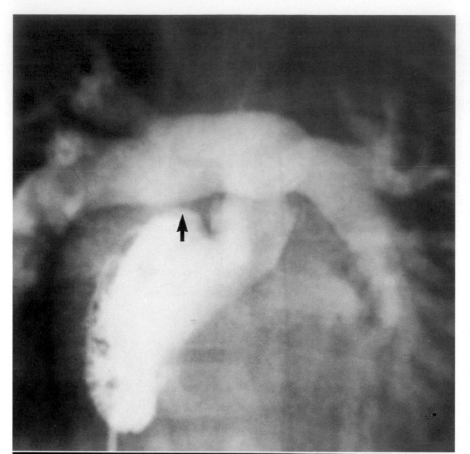

A

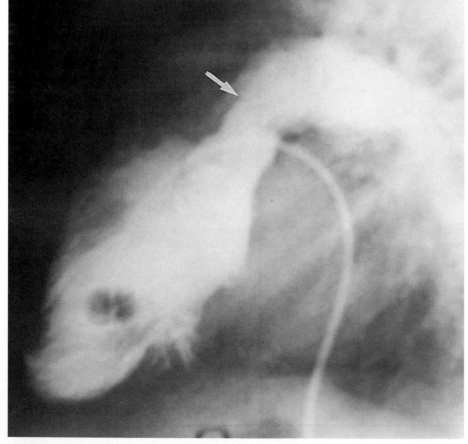

B

Fig. 9-17 Angiography of the left ventricle in congenitally corrected transposition of the great arteries. **A,** The septum runs obliquely, inferiorly on the right, and then superiorly on the left side. The distinctive recess *(arrow)* is typical of an inverted ventricle. **B,** The lateral view shows the pulmonary valve *(arrow)* posterior to the aortic valve.

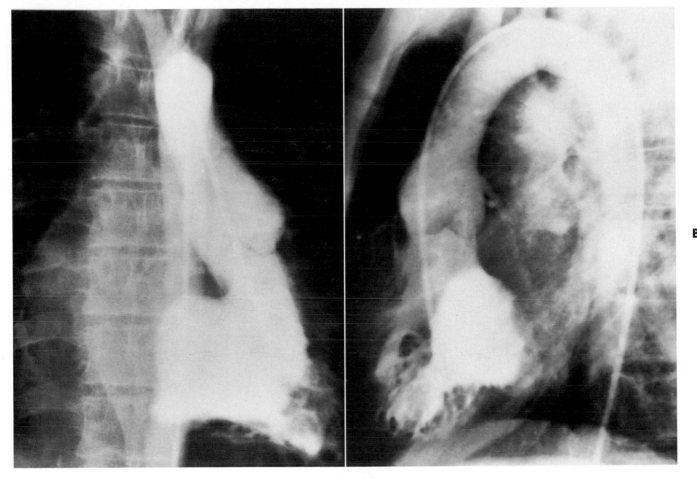

Fig. 9-18 Angiography of the right ventricle in congenitally corrected transposition of the great arteries. **A,** The subaortic conus of the right ventricle connects to the leftward ascending aorta, the border forming structure of the left side of the mediastinum **B,** The aortic valve is anterior to the heart and lies in a horizontal plane.

catheter position can be excluded, you should presume that severe regurgitation into the left atrium is associated with a "left-sided" Ebstein anomaly (Fig. 9-19). The tricuspid annulus is adjacent to the right coronary artery, which may be opacified during the ventriculogram.

Coronary artery patterns The coronary anatomy in congenitally corrected transposition of the great vessels is unique to inverted ventricles. Therefore, the diagnosis of atrioventricular discordance can be made by coronary arteriography. The position of the catheter in the ascending aorta relative to the mediastinal contour demonstrates that the aortic valve lies to the left of the pulmonary artery. The right coronary artery supplies the morphologic right ventricle, and the left coronary artery provides an anterior descending branch in the interventricular sulcus and a variable circumflex branch over the morphologic left ventricle (Fig. 9-20). In congenitally corrected transposition of the great arteries, the right coronary artery passes to the left and

inferior in the atrioventricular groove between the left atrium and right ventricle. Distally, this artery branches into the atrioventricular nodal branch, the posterior descending artery, and a variable set of branches to the inferior portion of the left ventricle (Fig. 9-21). The marginal branches over the right ventricular epicardial surface tend to be large with numerous branches. In contrast, the left coronary artery lies anterior and to the right of the right coronary artery. The left main coronary artery continues mainly as the anterior descending branch which has numerous septal and diagonal branches. The circumflex artery in the atrioventricular groove between the right atrium and left ventricle tends to be vestigial. The position of the coronary arteries within the thorax may be different because of dextrocardia or other relative rotations, but the coronary distribution corresponds uniquely to the respective ventricle. When confusing ventricular morphology does not allow identification of the right or left ventri-

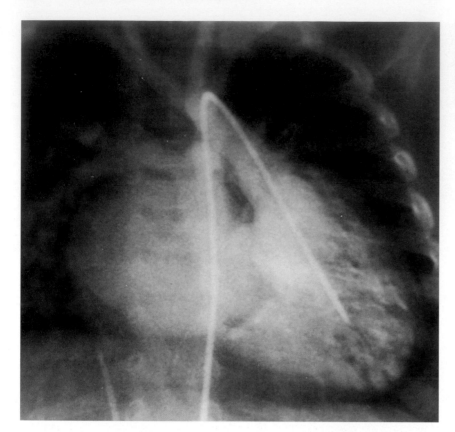

Fig. 9-19 Ebstein anomaly in congenitally corrected transposition of the great arteries. Injection into the right ventricle has resulted in severe regurgitation into the left atrium. In contrast to isolated Ebstein anomaly, the tricuspid leaflets are poorly seen, and have little apical displacement. A ventricular septal defect has allowed opacification of the pulmonary arteries.

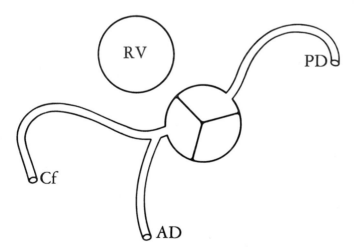

Fig. 9-20 Coronary arteries in corrected transposition of the great arteries. The aortic valve is anterior and to the left of the right ventricular infundibulum *(RV)*. The posterior descending artery *(PD)* originates posteriorly and follows the atrioventricular groove between the left atrium and right ventricle. The circumflex artery *(Cf)* lies in the atrioventricular groove between the right atrium and left ventricle, while the anterior descending artery *(AD)* follows the interventricular sulcus. With situs solitus, the coronary arteries appear to be the mirror image of those in the normal heart.

cle, visualization of the coronary arteries permits accurate identification of the ventricles.

Isolated ventricular inversion Atrioventricular discordance with ventriculoarterial concordance is termed *isolated ventricular inversion.* The segmental connections for the venous side of the heart are right atrium to left ventricle to aorta, and for the systemic side the left atrium to right ventricle to pulmonary artery. As originally reported by the Van Praaghs (1966), the pulmonary artery arises anteriorly and to the left of the aorta (Fig. 9-22). A large subaortic ventricular septal defect is adjacent to the septal leaf of the tricuspid valve. The aorta may also originate anterior to the pulmonary artery. The position of the atrioventricular and ventriculoarterial connections that constitute the diagnosis are best visualized with biplane ventriculograms in the frontal and lateral projections.

Straddling atrioventricular valves Malposition of the atrioventricular valves completely or partially across a ventricular septal defect represents a mixed form of atrioventricular connection. The tensor apparatus of the mitral and tricuspid valves is complex and includes the annulus, leaflets, chordae, and papillary muscles. With a straddling atrioventricular valve, the leaflets connect

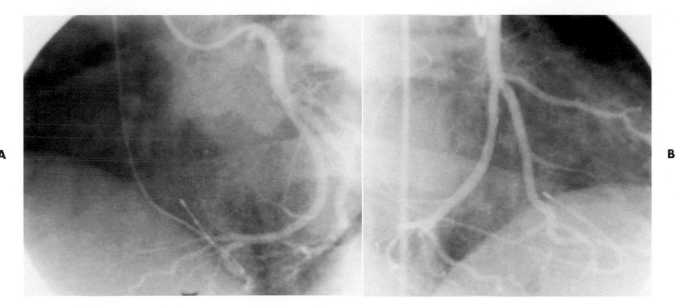

Fig. 9-21   Right coronary artery in situs solitus and congenitally corrected transposition of the great arteries is inverted from its location in the normal heart in the left **(A)** and right **(B)** anterior oblique projections.

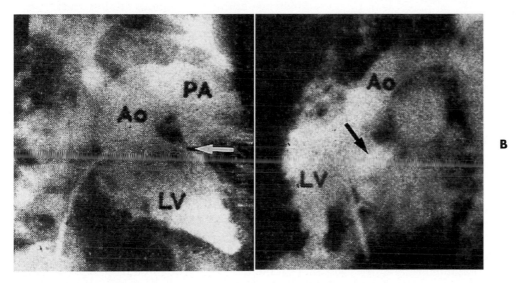

Fig. 9-22   Ventricular inversion. Anteroposterior **(A)** and lateral **(B)** angiograms show the aorta *(Ao)* arising from the anterior left ventricle *(LV)* and the pulmonary artery *(PA)* from the posterior right ventricle. A high ventricular septal defect *(arrows)* is present below the aortic valve, along with a lower muscular defect. The abdominal viscera and atria are located normally, as indicated by the position of the catheter in the inferior vena cava. (From Van Praagh R, Van Praagh S: Isolated ventricular inversion: a consideration of the morphogenesis, definition and diagnosis of nontransposed and transposed great arteries, *Am J Cardiol* 17:395, 1966.)

across the ventricular septum through a septal defect. Peripherally, the chordae or the papillary attachments may cross the septal defect to attach in the contralateral ventricle. Most of these valves represent a type of complete atrioventricular canal defect. An overriding atrioventricular valve has its annulus on both sides of a septal defect. An atrioventricular valve then may be straddling, overriding, or both.

Ventriculoarterial Discordance

The next stage in the segmental analysis concerns the connections and relations of the great arteries with respect to the ventricles. There are a number of ventriculoarterial malformations, most of which are a transposition of the great arteries or one of its variants. A complete description of a ventriculoarterial defect involves three aspects:

1. The anteroposterior relationship of the aorta and pulmonary artery
2. The connection of the aorta and the pulmonary artery to the right and left ventricles
3. The presence of a conus beneath the aortic and pulmonary valves

If a conus is present, there is contractile tissue between the atrioventricular and semilunar valves.

The most common variety of ventriculoarterial discordance is transposition of the great arteries. In this sense, "transposition" means that the two great arteries are abnormally placed with respect to the interventricular septum: the aorta connects to the right ventricle and the pulmonary artery to the left ventricle. As an illustration, complete dextrotransposition of the great arteries exists when the aorta is anterior and to the right and connected to the right ventricle, while the pulmonary artery is posterior and to the left and connected to the left ventricle. The term *partial transposition* applies to variations that do not meet the strict criteria of complete transposition, and includes double-outlet right ventricle and double-outlet left ventricle.

Complete dextrotransposition of the great arteries

In 1797 Baillie described the heart of an infant in which the aorta connected to the right ventricle and the pulmonary artery to the left ventricle. The term *transposition of the aorta and pulmonary artery* is ascribed to Farre in 1814. Since that time there has been controversy about whether it should be defined by the abnormal anteroposterior position of the great arteries, or by the abnormal connections to the ventricles. Transposition of the great arteries is a ventriculoarterial abnormality in which the aorta originates above the right ventricle and the pulmonary artery originates over the left ventricle.

Complete transposition of the great arteries after tetralogy of Fallot is the second most common cause of cyanosis from heart disease in infancy. In this malformation, the systemic and pulmonary circulations connect in parallel, in contrast to the serial connection in the normal infant. The blood flow through the lungs returns to the left atrium and to the left ventricle only to pass again through the lungs; in a similar fashion, the systemic venous and arterial circulations form a closed loop. For life to be sustained, mixing must occur between these two circuits. Therefore, one of the objectives of imaging is to determine the location and amount of these intracardiac or extracardiac shunts. The foramen ovale is almost always patent but is too small for adequate mixing. Occasionally, a secundum atrial septal defect will allow a large shunt to provide adequate mixing of oxygenated blood at this level. Ventricular septal defects occur in about one third of babies with transposition

and, when present, may result in congestive heart failure from the large blood flow. Extracardiac shunts may occur, as in patent ductus arteriosus or with bronchopulmonary connections to the pulmonary vascular bed. The ductus arteriosus remains patent in one fourth to one half of infants who do not receive prostaglandin E_1 and allows blood to flow from the pulmonary artery to the aorta if the pulmonary vascular resistance is high, and from the aorta to the pulmonary artery when the high fetal pulmonary artery pressures fall below the systemic blood pressure.

Besides the ventricular septal defect, the other major associated malformation is obstruction to blood entering the pulmonary arteries. About one fourth of those with transposition of the great arteries have some form of pulmonary stenosis. The site of obstruction usually is in the subpulmonary region and consists of a variety of causes:

- Anomalous attachment of the mitral valve
- Accessory endocardial tissue
- Subpulmonary membrane
- Subpulmonary fibromuscular tunnel
- Aneurysm of the membranous outflow tract

Valvular pulmonary stenosis also occurs from a unicuspid or bicuspid valve. Dynamic pulmonary stenosis is common in those patients with an intact ventricular septum and is caused by systolic anterior motion of the mitral valves, like that in idiopathic hypertrophic subaortic stenosis.

The typical chest radiograph in the first few days of life of a child with transposition of the great arteries shows mild cardiomegaly, a narrow superior mediastinum, and increased size of the pulmonary vessels that is consistent with a left-to-right shunt. All of these signs are variable and, in fact, the chest radiograph may appear normal. The size of the pulmonary vessels depends on the amount of blood carried by them: if the degree of mixing between the pulmonary and systemic circuits is small or if there is some type of pulmonary stenosis, the pulmonary vessels will be small; if there are large intracardiac or extracardiac shunts, the pulmonary vessels are large (Fig. 9-23).

Angiographic anatomy   When complete transposition of the great arteries is suspected, angiography consists of right and left ventriculography and aortography. In the standard posteroanterior and lateral projections, the right ventricle demonstrates the typical coarsely trabeculated body and cylindrical infundibulum which connects to the aortic valve and aorta. A catheter passed through the right atrium and right ventricle and around the aortic arch has a distinctive shape (Fig. 9-24). The right ventriculogram demonstrates that the aorta is medial and anterior to the pulmonary artery (Fig. 9-25). In contrast to the normal heart, the plane of the aortic valve is parallel to the long axis of the body. The subaortic

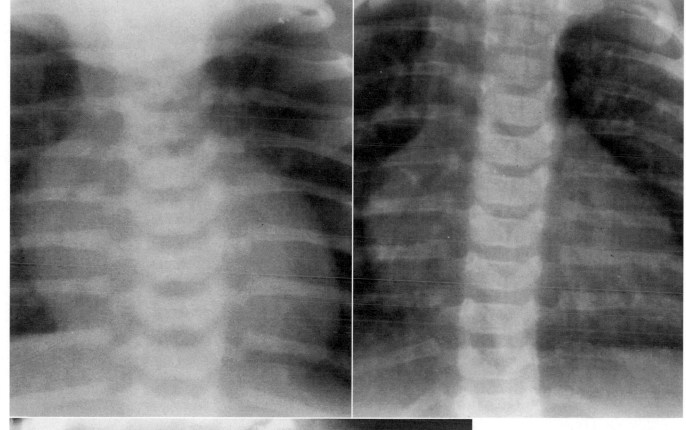

A

B

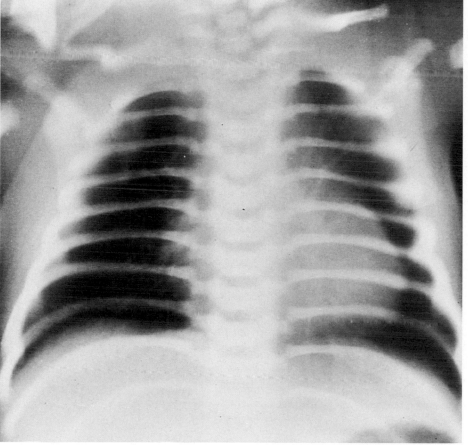

C

Fig. 9-23 Chest film abnormalities in transposition of the great arteries. **A,** The common presentation is a slightly enlarged heart and large pulmonary arteries which suggests increased pulmonary blood flow The mediastinum is narrow with an unusual appearance because of the absence of the thymic shadow. **B,** A less typical radiograph shows cardiomegaly and huge, indistinct pulmonary vessels indicating severe intracardiac shunting from the ventricular septal defect. **C,** The rare occurrence of pulmonary atresia with transposition of the great arteries is reflected in the tiny hilar vessels. In these three patients **(A, B,** and **C),** the circulation to the lungs was reliably indicated by the size of the hilar pulmonary vessels.

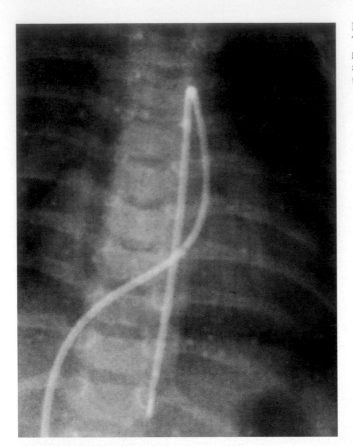

Fig. 9-24 Catheter position in transposition of the great arteries. The catheter passes through the right atrium and right ventricle and goes around the aortic arch. A similar catheter configuration is seen in a normal heart with a patent ductus arteriosus, but does not pass through the aortic arch.

A

B

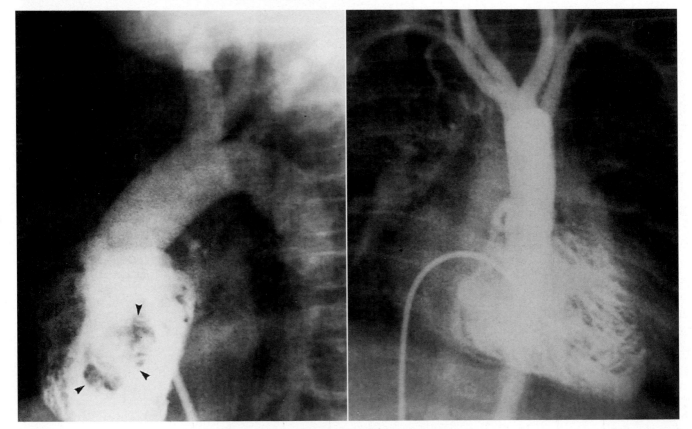

Fig. 9-25 The right ventriculogram in transposition of the great arteries. **A,** In the lateral view the tricuspid valve *(arrowheads)* is separated from the aortic valve by the contractile outflow tract. The aortic valve is anterior to its usual location in the normal heart. The posterior aspect of the valve tilts inferiorly (the "untucked" aorta). **B,** In the frontal view the midline aorta originates from the right ventricle medial to the pulmonary artery segment.

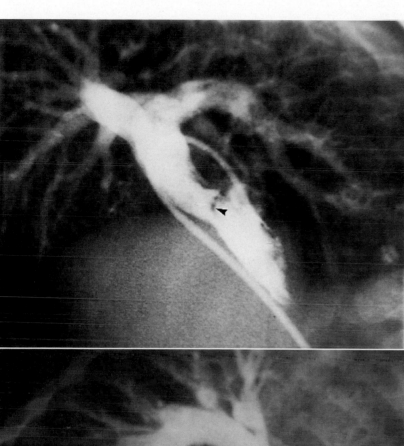

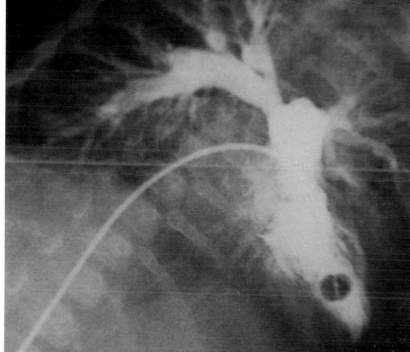

Fig. 9-26 The left ventriculogram in transposition of the great arteries. **A,** The long-axis oblique projection places the ventricular septum and the outflow region in the plane of the film. In this systolic frame, the left ventricle is connected to the pulmonary arteries. The pulmonic valve lies posterior and to the left of the aorta. A subpulmonary stenosis *(arrowhead)* extends from the region of the mitral valve. **B,** The complementary right anterior oblique view shows a mild stenosis at the origin of the right pulmonary artery.

conus elevates the position of the aortic valve superior to the pulmonary valve and creates the "untucked" aorta.

In complete transposition, left ventriculography locates a posterior left ventricle, which connects directly to the pulmonary valve and main pulmonary artery (Fig. 9-26). There is no subpulmonary conus; i.e., the mitral valve lies adjacent to the pulmonary valve. The interventricular septum usually lies parallel to the anterior chest wall. In hearts with normal pulmonary artery pressures, the interventricular septum may appear concave to the left ventricle, reflecting the systemic pressures in the right ventricle. In the cranial left anterior oblique projection, ventricular septal defects are visible with streaming of contrast material into the right ventricle.

Development of left ventricular outflow tract obstruction with or without ventricular septal defects is best evaluated with oblique cranially angled views. The upper aspect of the ventricular septum may protrude dynamically into the subpulmonary region during systole. If the mitral leaflets are drawn toward the septum during sys-

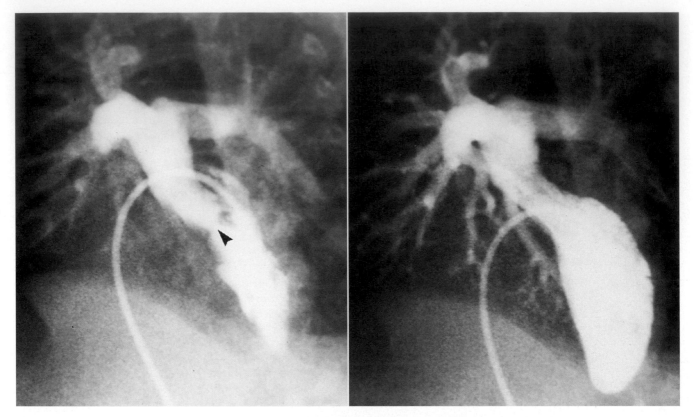

Fig. 9-27   Dynamic subpulmonary stenosis in transposition of the great arteries. In systole **(A)**, a subpulmonic lucency *(arrowhead)* extends from the septum to the mitral valve. In diastole **(B)**, no obstruction is apparent. This obstruction was the anterior leaflet of the mitral valve which moved anteriorly during systole.

tole, similar to the same motion seen in idiopathic hypertrophic subaortic stenosis, subpulmonary obstruction develops with an increase in the left ventricular afterload (Fig. 9-27). A fixed form of subpulmonary stenosis is the fibromuscular ridge or membrane visible as an irregular, radiolucent line on the interventricular septum. This ridge may be more visible during systole when the subpulmonary region is contracted.

Aortography, particularly in the left anterior oblique or lateral projections, completes the examination by identifying the height and posteroanterior location of the aortic valve and the inclination of the plane of the annulus. Associated malformations, such as coarctation, other aortic arch anomalies, and patent ductus arteriosus, are frequently detected in this way when they are not recognized by the hemodynamic measurements (Fig. 9-28).

Surgical procedures   There are several interventional and surgical procedures to correct the cyanosis in dextrotransposition of the great arteries. The atrial septum can be enlarged by balloon angioplasty or by surgical excision of the interatrial septum (Blalock-Hanlon procedure). The caval and pulmonary venous circulations can be reversed by a Senning or Mustard proce-

dure. In the Senning repair, the right atrial wall and interatrial septum are sewn to redirect the caval blood into the left ventricle and the pulmonary venous blood into the right ventricle. The Mustard operation also transposes the path of blood in the atria but uses pericardial tissue rather than the atrial wall. In the arterial switch (Jatene) operation, the ascending aorta and pulmonary arteries are divided above the sinus of Valsalva and the coronary arteries are excised from the aorta. The coronary arteries are replanted in the new aortic root, which is connected to the left ventricle. The pulmonary artery bifurcation is brought anterior and anastomosed to the right ventricular sinuses.

Partial Transposition of the Great Arteries

Double-outlet right ventricle

Double-outlet right ventricle is a congenital cardiac defect in which both great arteries originate exclusively from the morphologic right ventricle. The only outlet for the left ventricle is through the ventricular septal defect, which is usually large but may be restrictive. The malformation occurs in two varieties, depending on the location of the ventricular septal defect in relation to the

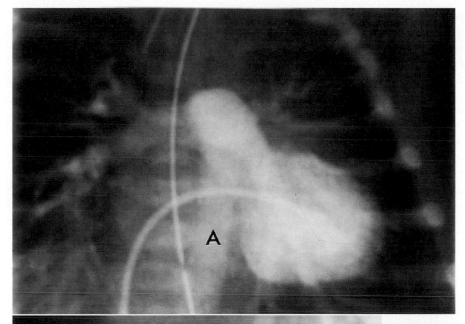

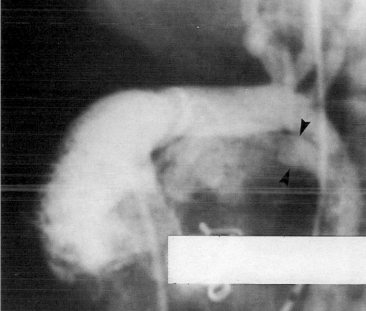

Fig. 9-28   Patent ductus arteriosus associated with transposition of the great arteries. Left ventricular **(A)** and right ventricular **(B)** injections visualize the left ventricle connecting to the pulmonary artery and the right ventricle to the aorta *(A)*. The descending aorta, but not the aortic arch, fills during the left ventriculogram. The ductus *(arrowheads)* originates after the left subclavian artery.

aorta and pulmonary artery. In the more common type, the ventricular septal defect is adjacent to the aorta with the pulmonary outflow situated on the far side of the right ventricle. In the less common type, the Taussig-Bing heart, the ventricular septal defect is adjacent to the pulmonary outflow, while the aorta resides on the far side of the right ventricle. The aorta is usually to the right of the pulmonary artery, either slightly to the front or directly to the side, but it may arise in front of the pulmonary artery. Although there are rare exceptions, bilateral conus is a major criterion for distinguishing double-outlet right ventricle from tetralogy of Fallot or complete transposition of the great arteries. Bilateral conus is recognizable

by muscle between each atrioventricular valve and the semilunar valves. These features place the aortic and pulmonary valves on approximately the same level in the transverse plane.

In addition to the ventriculoarterial malformation and the requisite ventricular septal defect, there are usually a large number of associated anomalies. Subpulmonary stenosis is frequent, occasionally in conjunction with a bicuspid or absent pulmonary valve. Partial or complete atrioventricular canal defects form a spectrum of abnormally formed leaflets. Subaortic stenosis is recognizable by hypoplasia or hyperkinesis of the aortic conus. Extracardiac anomalies abound and include anomalous pulmonary venous connection, bilateral superior vena cava, patent ductus arteriosus, coarctation and interruption of the aortic arch, and the heterotaxy syndrome.

The angiographic evaluation of double-outlet right ventricle necessitates biplane right and left ventriculograms. Simultaneous opacification of both great arteries after a ventriculogram is a typical feature of this malformation, but one artery may fill before the other when premature ventricular contractions occur or when there is subpulmonary or subaortic stenosis.

If double-outlet right ventricle is suspected, angiography in the posteroanterior and lateral views identifies the position of the aorta and pulmonary artery. The angled oblique views, particularly the left ventriculogram, show the abnormalities in the atrioventricular valves and the location and size of the ventricular septal defect. The plane of the ventricular septum is in the normal left anterior oblique projection in those hearts in situs solitus and *d*-loop ventricles. If there are inverted ventricles, the typical ventricular septum is sagittal and therefore aligned on the posteroanterior view.

There are many angiographic features characteristic of double-outlet right ventricle in situs solitus (Fig. 9-29). In the frontal view, the heavily trabeculated right ventricle partially overlies the posterior left ventricle. Both semilunar valves have the same height and are separated from the rest of the heart by a bilateral conus. The central lucency between the aortic and pulmonary outflow tracts is the crista supraventricularis. On the lateral view, there is discontinuity between the atrioventricular valves and the semilunar valves. Behind the great arteries and the mitral valve there is a notch that represents the ven-

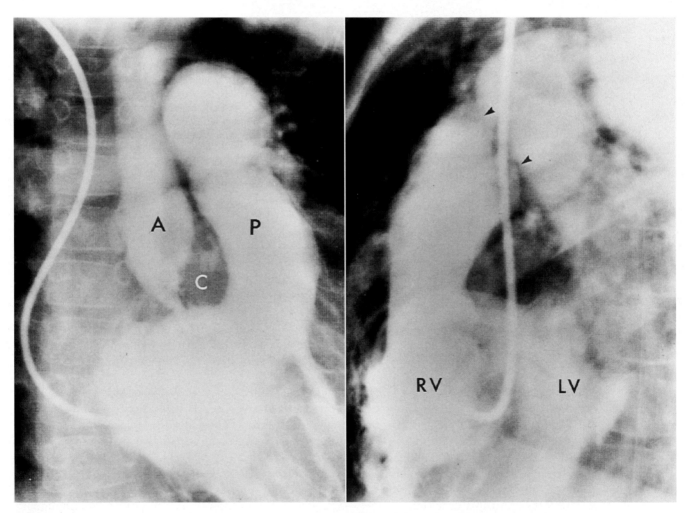

Fig. 9-29 Angiographic features of double-outlet right ventricle. **A,** In the frontal projection, the aorta originates adjacent to the ventricular septal defect. Severe subaortic stenosis narrows the outflow tract to a few millimeters. The crista supraventricularis *(C)* is common to both the subaortic and subpulmonary conus. *A* = aorta; *P* = pulmonary artery. **B,** In the lateral view, the left ventricle *(LV)* is opacified through a large ventricular septal defect. The aorta is not visualized, as it lies beside and is obscured by the large pulmonary artery. A loose pulmonary band *(arrowheads)* is present. *RV* = right ventricle.

triculoinfundibular recess. The conus under both great arteries generally overlaps completely so that unless one artery fills before the other, the relation of the conus to the ventricle may be difficult to recognize. In the uncommon Taussig-Bing type of double-outlet right ventricle (Fig. 9-30), the pulmonary artery is adjacent to the ventricular septal defect.

Pulmonary stenosis (Fig. 9-31), both the subvalvular and valvular varieties, exists in about one half of patients with double-outlet right ventricle. Conversely, subaortic stenosis occurs in about 20% of patients with this defect. Since the semilunar valves tend to lie on a transaxial

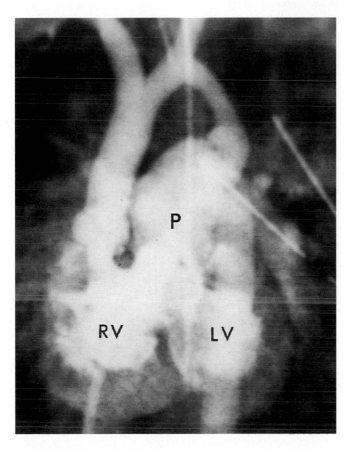

Fig. 9-30   Taussig-Bing malformation. In this double-outlet right ventricle *(RV)*, a small bilateral conus is present with moderate subaortic stenosis. The pulmonary artery *(P)* originates above the ventricular septal defect. An aortic coarctation is associated with mild hypoplasia of the arch. The large ventricular septal defect is the only outlet of the left ventricle *(LV)*.

plane, nonangled films in the frontal plane project the annulus of both the aortic and pulmonary valves in tangent. An injection in the outflow tract or directly beneath the crista supraventricularis may aid in making these outflow obstructions visible. (See Table 9-3 for differential diagnosis of double-outlet right ventricle.)

Double-outlet left ventricle

Double-outlet left ventricle is a rare type of partial transposition. In its complete form, both the aorta and pulmonary artery connect above the left ventricle. This malformation has one great artery and half of the other great artery arising above the left ventricle. Since this classification involves only the ventriculoarterial relations, it is not surprising that double-outlet left ventricle comprises a heterogeneous group of malformations that are associated with multiple anomalies and malpositions of the atrioventricular segments. Anomalies associated with double-outlet left ventricle are:

• Stenosis or atresia of any of the four cardiac valves
• Preductal coarctation
• Patent ductus arteriosus
• Ebstein anomaly
• Situs inversus

Most hearts with this malformation have a bilaterally absent conus, although there may be a subpulmonary or subaortic conus.

The purpose of imaging in double-outlet left ventricle is to identify the associated anomalies as well as to locate the position of the great arteries. Since the only outlet for the right ventricle is through the ventricular septal defect, a right ventricular injection alone may allow misinterpretation of this defect for another form of transposition or even for tetralogy of Fallot. To recognize double-outlet left ventricle you must be able to visualize both great arteries over the left ventricle, or one artery over the ventricular septal defect and the other over the left ventricle (Fig. 9-32). With this definition there is usually, but not always, continuity between the mitral valve and either the aortic or pulmonary valves. For example, in complete transposition of the great arteries with a ventricular septal defect, the pulmonary and mitral valves are adjacent and the aorta may override the ventricular septal defect; if the aorta is malpositioned so that more than 50% of its annulus corresponds to the left ventricle,

Table 9-3 Differential diagnosis of double-outlet right ventricle		
Findings in Double-Outlet Right Ventricle	**Alternative Findings**	**Alternative Diagnosis**
Bilateral conus	Pulmonary mitral continuity	Transposition of great arteries
	Aortic-mitral continuity	Tetralogy of Fallot

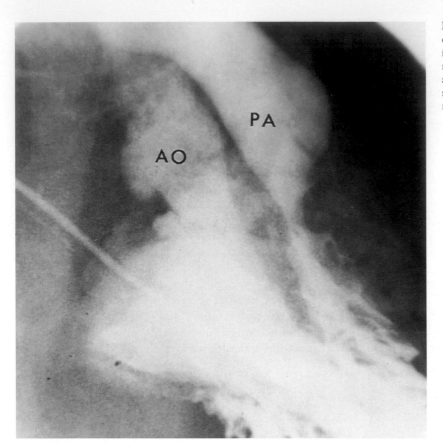

Fig. 9-31 Subpulmonary stenosis associated with double-outlet right ventricle. A right ventricular injection opacifies both the aorta *(AO)* and the pulmonary artery *(PA)*. On other views, the aorta was adjacent to the ventricular septal defect. There is severe bulboventricular malalignment with the pulmonary valve sharply angled toward the ventricle.

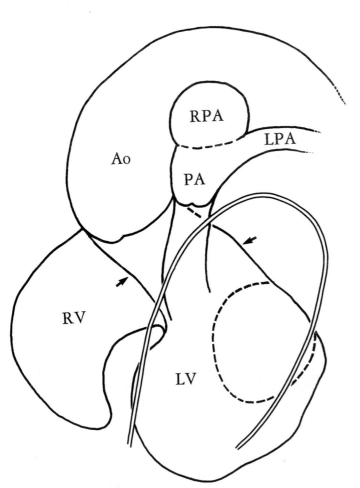

Fig. 9-32 Double-outlet left ventricle. The aortic valve projects equally over both ventricles above a large ventricular septal defect *(arrows)*. There is hypoplasia of the pulmonary valve, subpulmonic infundibulum, and main pulmonary artery. *RV* = right ventricle; *LV* = left ventricle; *Ao* = aorta; *RPA* = right pulmonary artery; *LPA* = left pulmonary artery; *PA* = main pulmonary artery.

then there is double-outlet left ventricle rather than complete transposition.

Anomalies of Aortopulmonary Septation

Truncus arteriosus

Truncus arteriosus is a congenital malformation in which only one great artery arises from the base of the heart and gives origin to the systemic, pulmonary, and coronary arteries proximal to the aortic arch. Buchanan first described this in 1864 from an autopsy specimen. In 1949 Collett and Edwards described five types of truncus arteriosus based on the connections of the pulmonary artery and the aorta (Fig. 9-33):

Type 1: Truncus divides into an ascending aorta and a main pulmonary artery, which then divides to supply both lungs

Type 2: Separate origin of the right and left pulmonary arteries from the posterior wall of the truncus

Type 3: Origin of the pulmonary arteries from the right and left sides of the truncus

Type 4: No pulmonary arteries originate from the ascending aorta, and the pulmonary supply comes from either a patent ductus arteriosus or bronchial arteries from the descending aorta. It is now known that type 4 truncus is an incorrect classification because it is a tetralogy of Fallot with pulmonary valve atresia.

Type 5: Aortopulmonary septal defect

This classification assumed that all hearts with this defect have a ventricular septal defect and only one semilunar valve. Truncus arteriosus can be differentiated from aortic or pulmonary valve atresia because a nubbin of the atrctic valve is usually found in the latter.

A later classification by Van Praagh et al. in 1965 relies on the absence of either the primitive fourth or sixth aortic arches. They classify four types of truncus:

Type A1: A separate main pulmonary artery (identical to Collett-Edwards type 1)

Type A2: Absent main pulmonary artery with separate origin of both pulmonary arteries from the common trunk (identical to Collett-Edwards types 2 and 3)

Type A3: Absence of one pulmonary artery with this lung being supplied by collateral vessels

Type A4: Interruption, hypoplasia, or coarctation of the aortic isthmus associated with a large patent ductus arteriosus

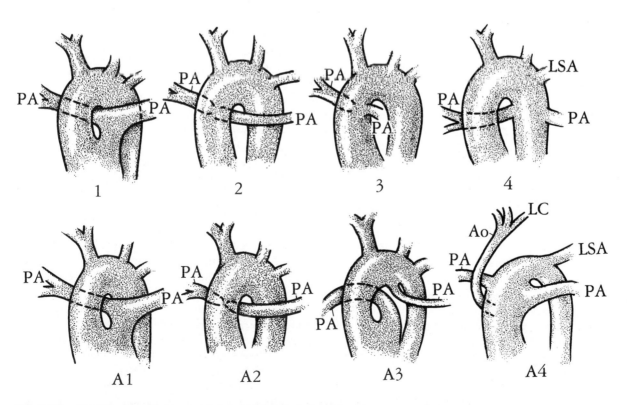

Fig. 9-33   Classification of truncus arteriosus. *Top row:* Collett-Edwards types 1 to 4. *Bottom row:* Van Praagh types A1 to A4. *PA* = pulmonary artery; *LSA* = left subclavian artery; *LC* = left carotid artery; *Ao* = aorta.

Types A1, A2, and A3 then represent agenesis of the sixth embryonic aortic arch which normally becomes the proximal main pulmonary artery, and type A4 results from agenesis of the fourth embryonic aortic arch. This latter classification has the advantage of recognizing the high incidence of aortic arch interruptions with truncus arteriosus.

The truncus usually is centered over a ventricular septal defect but may originate predominately from either ventricle. The mitral valve is in fibrous continuity with the truncal valve. The tricuspid valve may be adjacent to the truncal valve or a septal band may intervene. There is no subtruncal conus. The truncal (semilunar) leaflets are tricuspid in about 70% of patients but may have from two to five cusps. The truncal valve can be either stenotic or regurgitant with prolapse of one or more cusps. The pulmonary arteries, originating either as a main artery or separately supplying each lung, may also be stenotic at their origins.

Aortic arch anomalies with truncus arteriosus are common, with a right arch present in 20% to 40% and an interrupted arch in 20%. The arch interruptions, Van Praagh type A4, are associated with a large patent ductus arteriosus, which may be mistaken for the aortic arch; the patent ductus arteriosus supplies most of the thorax and inferior part of the body and usually the left subclavian artery. Because the ductus arteriosus contains contractile tissue, patients with type A4 truncus arteriosus may physiologically have no blood supply to most of the thorax and abdomen when the ductus contracts and closes.

The coronary circulation is quite variable in its origin. There is frequently an ectopic high origin of one or both coronary arteries. There is a single coronary artery in 13%, usually arising from the posterior cusp. The left coronary artery tends to arise from a more posterior level than in normal hearts.

Chest film abnormalities The chest film usually shows substantial cardiac enlargement (Fig. 9-34) and an engorged pulmonary vasculature. Both ventricles are enlarged because of the central shunting across the ventricular septal defect. In the neonate, the thymic shadow hides the pulmonary arteries and aortic arch, but in older children there may be a concave pulmonary artery segment. The shape of this segment reflects not only the absence of the right ventricular origin of the pulmonary artery but also the posterior position of the pulmonary arteries behind the truncus and ascending aorta. Also, in type A2, the left pulmonary artery originates above the right pulmonary artery. In some patients, the pulmonary arteries may appear to be elevated away from the cardiac silhouette. The size of the peripheral pulmonary arteries reflects the amount of blood flowing through them; they are generally large except when there is pulmonary artery stenosis.

Imaging features In addition to establishing the diagnosis of truncus arteriosus, it is essential to image the pulmonary arteries to see if there is stenosis. Left ventriculography shows truncal-mitral continuity, and right ventriculography shows the relation of the tricuspid valve to the truncal valve (Fig. 9-35). To establish the degree of truncal regurgitation and the presence of arch interruption, it is usually necessary to perform aortography (Fig. 9-36).

The truncal valve lies posterior in the usual location of an aortic valve. The plane of the truncal annulus tips anteriorly, similar to that in complete transposition of the great arteries; this helps to differentiate truncus arteriosus from aortopulmonary septation and from tetralogy of Fallot with pulmonary atresia.

In contrast to normal hearts or those with tetralogy of Fallot, the pulmonary arteries in truncus arteriosus originate from the posterior aspect of the aorta. Truncus types A1 and A2 may be difficult to distinguish when the main pulmonary artery is short. Steep cranially angled views may be helpful. Selective angiography of each pulmonary artery may visualize their origins by backward reflux. Angiography in type A3 shows only one pulmonary artery arising from the truncus; the other lung is supplied by collaterals from the descending aorta. If the left pulmonary artery is not visible following ventricular or truncal injections, you should perform aortography with the catheter at the aortic isthmus to search for the left pulmonary artery. You may recognize type A4 truncus on a ventriculogram as a small ascending aorta that comes from the right anterolateral aspect of the pulmonary artery. It may be difficult to identify whether the catheter has passed around the aortic arch or through a patent ductus arteriosus.

MRI can provide a valuable adjunct to angiography and echocardiography by noninvasively locating the mediastinal pulmonary arteries (Fig. 9-37). Spin echo images are obtained in the coronal and axial planes for the origins of the pulmonary arteries. Small arteries near the lung border are better identified with flow sequences like cine gradient-recalled techniques or phase reconstruction.

Hemitruncus arteriosus

In hemitruncus one of the pulmonary arteries originates from the aorta and the other from the right ventricle. There are separate aortic and pulmonary valves which distinguish hemitruncus from truncus type A3. The lung connected to the aorta is subject to the systemic pressure and has aneurysmal hilar branches and serpentine peripheral vessels. The lung supplied by the right ventricle has normal vasculature. The aortic arch tends to be large and may displace the trachea away from the side of the arch. It is right-sided in 20% to 30%. When the thymus does not obscure the mediastinum, the right boundary is the edge of the large ascending aorta.

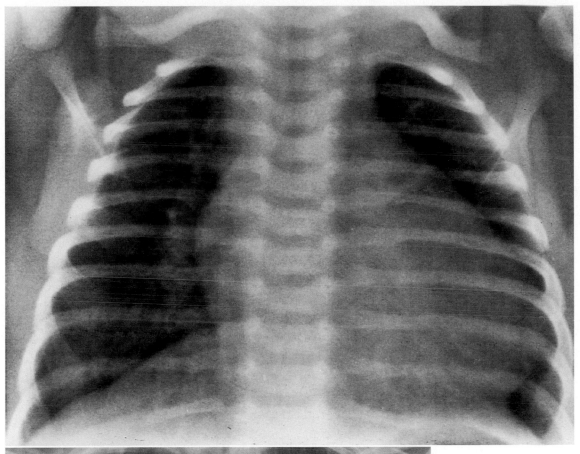

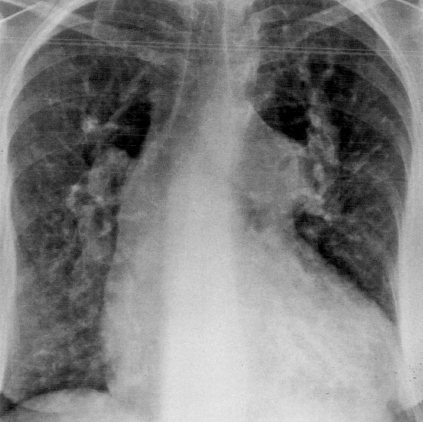

Fig. 9-34   Chest film in truncus arteriosus. **A,** In the infant, the large central shunting is reflected by the huge heart and the bilateral large pulmonary hilar vessels. **B,** In the unusual person who survives to adulthood, the pulmonary vasculature is large and tortuous from pulmonary arterial hypertension.

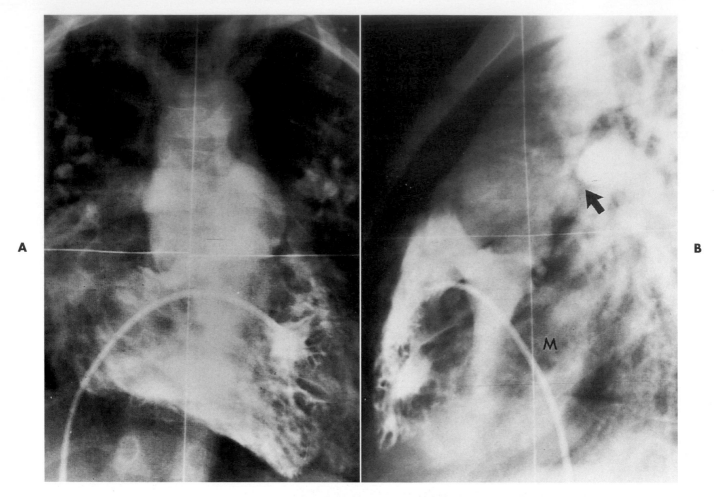

Fig. 9-35 Angiography of truncus arteriosus. The right ventriculogram in the frontal **(A)** and lateral **(B)** projection shows the large truncal valve straddling the ventricular septal defect. The mitral valve *(M)* in diastole shows continuity with the truncal valve. Note that the angle of the truncal valve is untucked and angled anteriorly. The *arrow* points to a pulmonary artery band. (Courtesy of Kenneth E. Fellows, M.D.)

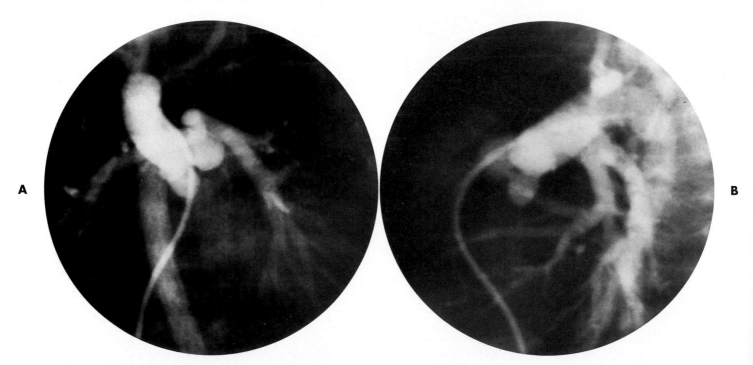

Fig. 9-36 Truncus arteriosus. **A,** The right anterior oblique truncal arteriogram shows the right aortic arch with mirror-image branching. **B,** The lateral view shows a tricuspid truncal valve without regurgitation. The pulmonary arteries originate posteriorly from the truncus.

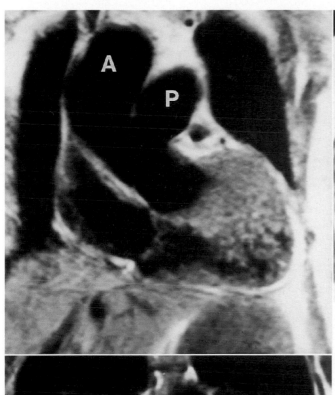

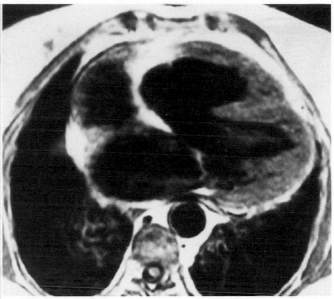

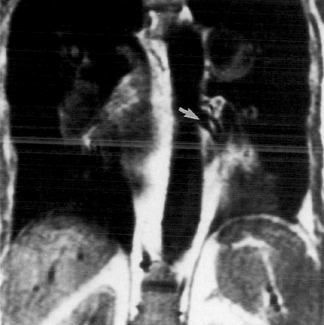

Fig. 9-37 MRI of truncus arteriosus. **A,** The coronal slice shows the large heart with the trunk originating as the single great artery from the heart. *A* = aorta; *P* = pulmonary artery. **B,** The axial slice shows the four heart chambers and the large ventricular septal defect. **C,** The descending thoracic aorta has several aortopulmonary arteries *(arrow)* supplying the left lower lobe.

Large patent ductus arteriosus, tetralogy of Fallot with pulmonary atresia, and aortopulmonary septation are the other major cardiac anomalies to be differentiated from truncus arteriosus. If two semilunar valves are identified, the diagnosis is not truncus. To make this distinction it may take injections in both right and left ventricles, particularly since a ventricular septal defect is also present in all of these malformations. A blind infundibular chamber in the right ventricle is typical of tetralogy of Fallot with pulmonary atresia. During right ventriculography in the lateral projection, this chamber is seen as an outpouching anterior to the aorta; this chamber is not present in truncus arteriosus.

Aortopulmonary septation

Separate aortic and pulmonary valves and a defect between the ascending aorta and the main or right pulmonary artery are characteristic of aortopulmonary septation (Fig. 9-38). This rare malformation is also called aortopulmonary septal defect and aortic pulmonary window. The defect is usually in the left lateral wall of the ascending aorta and connects with the right lateral wall of the pulmonary trunk. The defect can extend from the annulus of the two semilunar valves to involve the ascending aorta to varying degrees. About half have aortic arch interruption or a preductile coarctation.

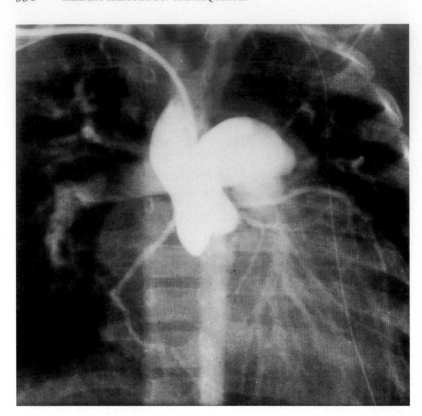

Fig. 9-38 Aortopulmonary septation. Injection into the ascending aorta simultaneously opacifies both the aortic and pulmonary valves. The descending aorta is opacified before the aortic arch, indicating a patent ductus arteriosus.

Anatomically corrected malposition of the great arteries

In this malformation, the left ventricle ejects into the aorta and the right ventricle into the pulmonary artery. However, the great arteries are abnormally related to one another. In situs solitus, the aorta is to the left of the pulmonary artery. The ventriculoarterial connections are normal, but their relations are malpositioned (Fig. 9-39). The levotransposed aorta is characteristic of corrected transposition of the great arteries, and if the loop rule applies, indicates ventricular inversion and *l*-looping of the ventricles. Levotransposed aorta rarely occurs in other types of malformations, including those that defy the loop rule and have noninverted ventricles.

Abnormal Connections of the Pulmonary Veins

Anomalous connection of all or part of the pulmonary veins into the systemic venous circuit has been known since 1739 in its partial form and in its total form since 1798. These variations in pulmonary venous connections are uncommon, occurring in 0.4% of autopsy specimens. The hemodynamic consequence of anomalous pulmonary venous connection depends on the number and location of the abnormally connected veins, the existence and size of an accompanying atrial septal defect, and the resultant degree of pulmonary vascular obstruction. The first angiographic documentation of partial anomalous pulmonary venous return is credited to Dotter and colleagues, who in 1949 injected a large bolus of contrast material into a peripheral vein in two patients who had anomalous pulmonary veins in the right lung that drained into the inferior vena cava.

Total anomalous pulmonary venous connection

All pulmonary veins may connect anomalously in three ways: (1) in a supracardiac manner to a vena cava; (2) to the heart, in particular to the right atrium or coronary sinus; and (3) to a vein below the diaphragm. The most common anomaly is connection of all pulmonary veins to a systemic vein in the thorax. The one or two veins draining each lung merge to form a common confluence behind the left atrium but without connecting to it. The outflow of this common vein may go into the left innominate vein, the right superior vena cava, or to the azygos or hemiazygos system of veins. When the connection is to a vein on the left side of the mediastinum, this vascular structure could be either a left superior vena cava or an anomalous vertical vein. Most vertical veins in the supracardiac type of total anomalous pulmonary venous drainage do not connect to the coronary sinus, hemiazygos, or left atrium, as a left superior vena cava would. Therefore it is actually an anomalous vein between the common pulmonary vein and the left innominate vein. This anomalous vertical vein may pass posterior to the pulmonary artery or may pass between the left mainstem bronchus and the left pulmonary

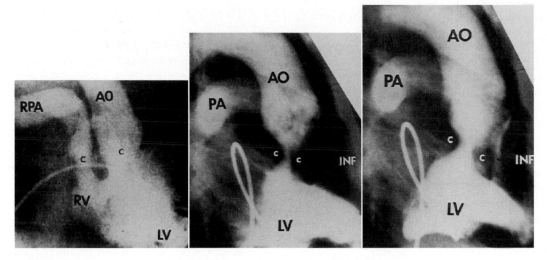

Fig. 9-39 Anatomically corrected levomalposition of the great arteries. *Left:* Frame from a selective left ventricular cineangiocardiogram in the anteroposterior projection. The venous catheter is in the left-sided, morphologic left ventricle *(LV)*. Contrast material opacifies a large chamber, a morphologic left ventricle, and a hypoplastic right ventricular outlet chamber *(RV)*. The right pulmonary artery *(RPA)* is seen. The left pulmonary artery is probably absent. The aorta *(AO)* originates above the morphologic left ventricle and is to the left of the pulmonary artery. Bilateral conal myocardium *(c)* is evident. *Middle* and *right:* Selected radiographs from the left ventricular biplane angiogram in the lateral projection. The semilunar valves are at the same level and appear side by side in this projection. The pulmonary artery *(PA)* originates above the right ventricular outlet chamber and is slightly anterior. The aortic valve is clearly separated from the mitral valve by subaortic conal myocardium *(c)*, which is quite dynamic. The right ventricular infundibulum *(INF)* is very narrow and becomes even narrower with systole *(right)*. Bilateral conal myocardium is thus present. (From Freedom RM, Harrington DP: Anatomically corrected malposition of the great arteries. Report of 2 cases, one with congenital asplenia: frequent association with juxtaposition of atrial appendages, *Br Heart J* 36:207, 1974.)

artery. In the latter instance, an obstruction to flow may occur by compression of these adjacent structures onto the anomalous vein.

In the intracardiac type of total anomalous pulmonary venous connection, the common pulmonary vein connects directly to the right atrium or coronary sinus, either as one vessel or with separate connections of two or more of the pulmonary veins. The intracardiac type of anomaly is frequently accompanied by polysplenia or asplenia with the associated bilateral superior vena cava and azygos continuation. The pulmonary veins may also attach to the coronary sinus, in which case this structure is considerably enlarged.

The infracardiac type of anomalous pulmonary connection always demonstrates pulmonary vascular obstruction. In this type, a venous channel from the common pulmonary vein passes inferiorly through the diaphragm at the esophageal hiatus to connect with the portal vein or its tributaries or the ductus venosus. In the extreme form, which represents atresia of the common pulmonary vein, all egress from the common pulmonary vein is absent except into minute venous channels adjacent to the esophagus.

The physiology of this malformation then is determined by the amount of mixing of oxygenated blood, the amount of blood that reaches the left ventricle and systemic circulation, and the degree of pulmonary vascular obstruction. Most of these patients have either an atrial septal defect or patent foramen ovale, which serves as the conduit to the systemic circulation. The blood flow is bidirectional at the right atrium, passing either into the left atrium or into the right ventricle and pulmonary artery. Increased pulmonary blood flow occurs in the supracardiac and cardiac level anomalies. Decreased pulmonary blood flow can, of course, occur from an Eisenmenger reaction with an increase in the precapillary vascular resistance. In the infracardiac type, the pulmonary venous return is obstructed mainly by the portal circulation. The physiologic consequences are signs of pulmonary venous hypertension and pulmonary edema.

Chest film findings The findings on the chest film depend on the same variables that control the blood flow to the heart and lungs. When there is no pulmonary venous obstruction, typically in the supracardiac and intracardiac types, the chest film generally demonstrates cardiomegaly and large pulmonary vessels. The right atrial and ventricular contours appear prominent, and there is no evidence of left atrial enlargement, even on the barium esophagogram. The right superior vena cava is dilated when it is part of the circuit that receives pulmonary venous drainage. The only sign pathognomonic of the supracardiac variety that is seen on the chest film is the "snowman" configuration (Fig. 9-40). The anomalous left vertical vein forms the convex left superior mediastinal border as it joins the dilated left innominate vein. The enlarged right superior vena cava protrudes into the right lung, completing the head of the snowman.

In those cases that are obstructive, the chest film is quite different (Fig. 9-41). Generally, the heart is of normal size without prominence of any chamber. The striking abnormality occurs in the lungs which show evidence of pulmonary edema. An interstitial pattern is invariably present in the infracardiac type. Interstitial and alveolar pulmonary edema and, occasionally, Kerley B lines are frequently mistaken for noncardiac causes of pulmonary consolidation, such as neonatal pneumonia, aspiration, respiratory distress syndrome, and transient tachypnea of the newborn.

The angiographic technique for identifying the course and location of the anomalous veins begins with pulmonary arteriography. In the supracardiac variety with the anomalous left vertical vein, the vein itself may be injected directly. In the newborn, this structure may be fragile so that indirect opacification from a more peripheral site is desirable. A main pulmonary artery angiogram in the posteroanterior projection demonstrates the pulmonary veins on the levophase (Fig. 9-42). In the lateral view, the confluence of veins appears behind the usual position of the left atrium before it ascends into the anomalous vertical vein to join the left innominate vein. If other cardiac defects are discovered, additional injections will clarify their morphology.

In the intracardiac type, the location of the anomalous connection may be difficult to identify because of overlapping cardiac chambers. Pulmonary angiography with late filming for the levophase structures shows opacification of the coronary sinus or right atrium before the left atrium (Fig. 9-43).

The infracardiac variety is distinctive and has considerably reduced blood flow (Fig. 9-44). For this reason, the levophase of the pulmonary angiogram should extend for 10 to 12 seconds until you can see the long venous

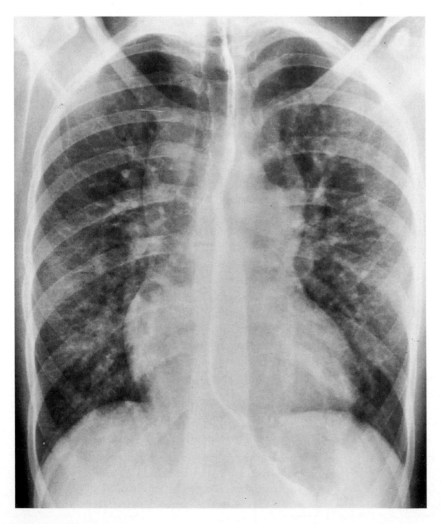

Fig. 9-40   Chest film in supracardiac type of total anomalous pulmonary venous connection. The pulmonary vessels are large, consistent with increased pulmonary blood flow. The abnormal mediastinum (the "snowman") is caused by the dilated right superior vena cava on the right side and by the anomalous vertical vein draining both lungs on the left side.

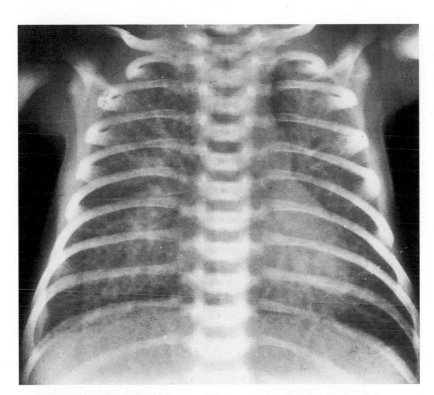

Fig. 9-41 Chest film in total anomalous pulmonary venous connection to the portal vein. The small heart size reflects the diminished inflow to the left side of the heart through an atrial septal defect. Pulmonary edema and a small heart are sentinel features of the infracardiac type of total anomalous pulmonary venous connection.

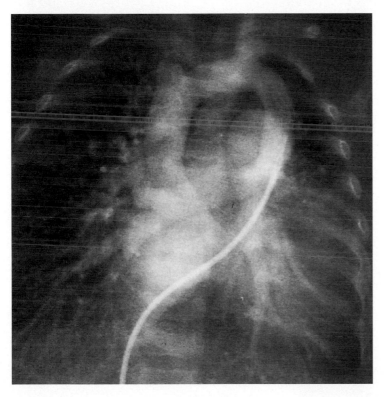

Fig. 9-42 Total anomalous venous connection to vertical vein. Levophase of pulmonary angiogram in the anteroposterior projection shows all pulmonary veins connecting behind the left atrium to form an anomalous vertical vein. This structure forms the left mediastinal border and joins the left innominate vein. The right superior vena cava is dilated and occupies the right side of the mediastinum.

channel extending below the diaphragm to enter the portal vein.

Partial anomalous pulmonary venous connection

Partial anomalous pulmonary venous connection is present when one or more, but not all, of the pulmonary veins connect to a systemic vein (Fig. 9-45). The veins of the right lung have 2 to 10 times the number of anomalous connections as do those from the left lung. When an anomalous vein exists, it usually connects to the nearest adjacent systemic vein or to the right atrium (Fig. 9-46). For example, the right superior pulmonary vein usually

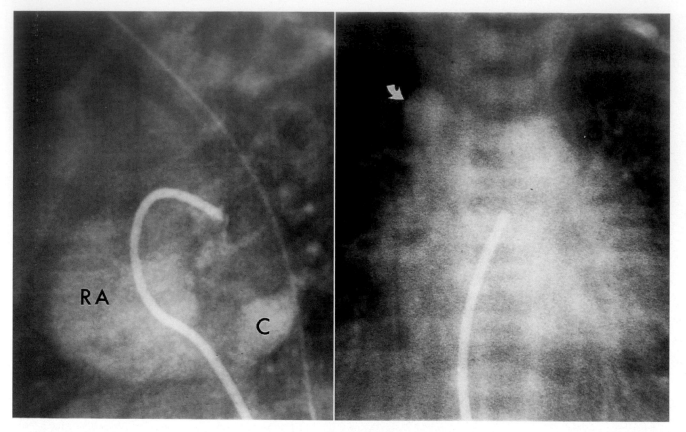

Fig. 9-43   Unusual type of total anomalous pulmonary venous connection. **A,** The coronary sinus *(C)* received all pulmonary blood and contrast media with subsequent opacification of the right atrium *(RA).* **B,** The large azygos vein *(arrow)* connected to all pulmonary veins.

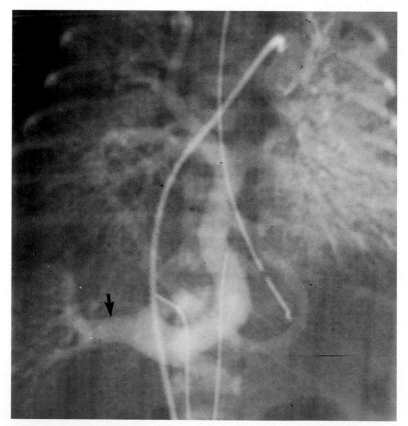

Fig. 9-44   Total anomalous pulmonary venous connection below the diaphragm. In the levophase of a pulmonary angiogram, all pulmonary veins join and pass through the esophageal hiatus of the diaphragm to connect to the portal vein *(arrow).* The intense blush of the lungs indicates slow blood flow.

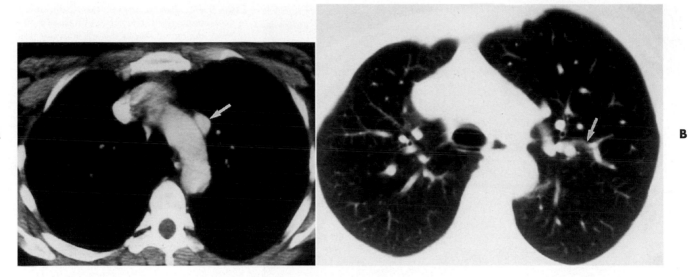

Fig. 9-45 Anomalous pulmonary vein draining the left upper lobe. **A,** The oval density adjacent to the aorta *(arrow)* is an anomalous vein which connects to the left innominate vein. **B,** Lung windows show the tortuous peripheral course to the left side of the mediastinum.

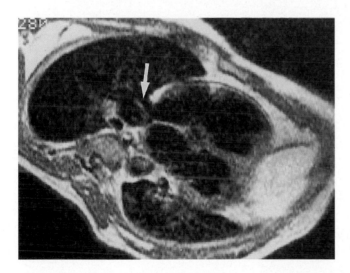

Fig. 9-46 Partial anomalous pulmonary venous connection to the right atrium. A long-axis image perpendicular to the interventricular septum shows a right pulmonary vein *(arrow)* entering the right atrium. The interatrial septum is intact. (From Miller SW, Brady TJ, Dinsmore RE et al: Cardiac magnetic resonance imaging: the Massachusetts General Hospital experience, *Radiol Clin North Am* 23:745-764, 1985.)

connects to the right superior vena cava or azygos vein. The right inferior vein may connect with either the inferior or superior vena cava, a hepatic vein, or occasionally the azygos vein. The left lung veins connect to an anomalous vertical vein draining into the left innominate vein, the coronary sinus, or the hemiazygos vein (Fig. 9-47). Although these examples are typical, there are many variations in number, size, and connections of the pulmonary veins. The atrial septum is usually intact. Conversely, if an

atrial septal defect is present, about 10% of these patients will have a pulmonary venous anomaly.

The chest radiograph is usually normal because the pulmonary-to-systemic flow ratio is generally less than 2:1. When an entire lung is drained by an anomalous connection, the main pulmonary arteries and peripheral branches are enlarged similar to a left-to-right shunt. In this case, the right ventricle is enlarged while the other cardiac chambers and the vena cava are equivocally dilated. The isolated lower lobe veins that connect to the inferior vena cava present the most striking radiographic abnormalities. The anomalous vein is almost always seen on the right side but may be a left-sided structure. In curving medially and inferiorly through the lung, the vein has been likened to a scimitar because, unlike a normal pulmonary artery, it increases in diameter as it goes to the base of the lung (Fig. 9-48). The hypogenetic lung syndrome is a rare congenital anomaly that consists of an anomalous pulmonary venous connection of the right lung to the inferior vena cava; it is associated with hypoplasia of the right lung and its bronchus and pulmonary artery. The heart is secondarily rotated toward the right hemithorax because of the small right lung. The right lung may have abnormal lobation, frequently having two rather than three lobes. This condition is also called the pulmonary venolobar syndrome.

You can detect the anomalous pulmonary veins angiographically in several ways. The catheter from the femoral vein can explore the right atrium and adjacent systemic veins and document the anomaly either by the position of the catheter or by a small hand injection of contrast material. Anomalous veins connecting to the right atrium are impossible to distinguish angiographically from an atrial

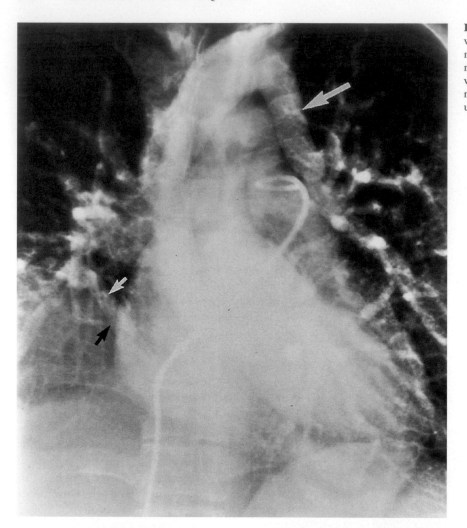

Fig. 9-47 Partial anomalous pulmonary venous connections. The venous phase of a pulmonary angiogram shows the left superior pulmonary vein connecting to the left innominate vein *(large arrow)*. The right inferior pulmonary vein *(small arrows)* joins the right atrium at the inferior vena caval junction.

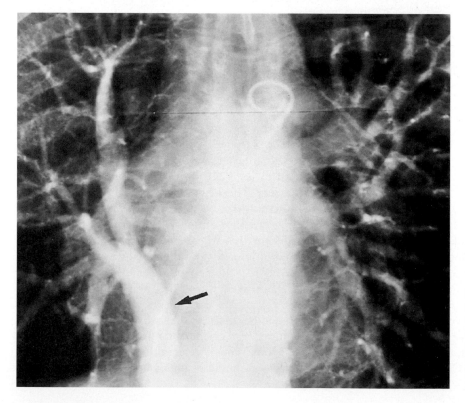

Fig. 9-48 Scimitar sign. The venous phase of a pulmonary arteriogram shows all of the right pulmonary veins *(arrow)* connecting to the inferior vena cava. As it courses inferiorly, the size of the vein becomes larger in contradistinction to the pulmonary arteries which become smaller as they pass toward the lung base.

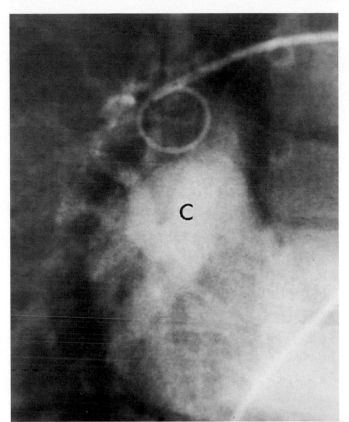

A

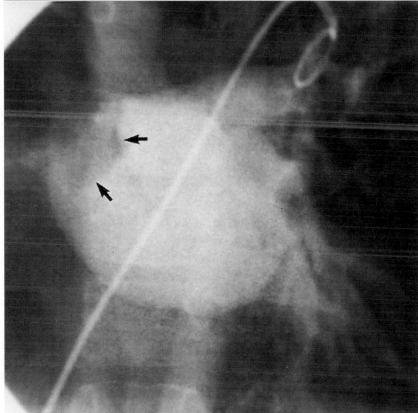

B

Fig. 9-49 Atrial septal defect and anomalous pulmonary vein. **A,** After selective right pulmonary artery injection, the confluence *(C)* of the right pulmonary veins projects behind the superior vena cava–right atrium junction. The right atrium is opacified before the left atrium. **B,** The venous phase of a selective left pulmonary angiogram reveals normal drainage of the left pulmonary veins into the left atrium. The filling defect in the left atrium *(arrows)* is caused by unopacified blood crossing a sinus venosus atrial septal defect in a right-to-left direction.

septal defect without contrast injection. Because the atrial septum runs obliquely from right to left in a posterior to anterior direction, the course of a catheter passing through an atrial septal defect into the right pulmonary veins is nearly identical to that of one passing from the inferior vena cava through the right atrium into the anomalous vein. If contrast material demarcates the superior and right lateral border of the left atrium before it passes through the atrial septal defect, then you have identified the right pulmonary veins that connect normally to the left atrium. Similarly, injection into an anomalous right superior pulmonary vein will outline the lateral border of the superior vena cava and right atrium without visualization of the oval left atrium. You can elicit the opposite effect by performing a superior vena cavogram and noting the filling defect of the unopacified blood entering that portion of the superior vena cava or right atrium where the anomalous pulmonary vein connects.

Pulmonary angiography is a common examination for locating all of the pulmonary veins. If the right atrium is visible during the levophase, an anomalous pulmonary vein or an atrial septal defect or both must be present (Fig. 9-49). When a partial anomalous pulmonary venous connection to the superior vena cava or right atrium exists, an atrial septal defect occurs in 90% of patients, whereas when the anomalous vein connects to the inferior vena cava, only 15% have an atrial septal defect. A technique of localizing the anomalous pulmonary vein with respect to the atrial septal defect involves placing a catheter into the right pulmonary vein from an inferior vena caval approach. Using cranial angulation with the hepatoclavicular or "four-chamber" view, the atrial septum is projected in profile so that the connection of the vein to the atrium is seen during a 10-ml injection.

Box 9-4   Cardiotypes

Determine atrial situs by analyzing abdomen and tracheobronchial tree

- S   solitus
- I   inversus
- A   ambiguous

Determine ventricular situs

- D   d-loop or solitus
- L   l-loop or inverted
- X   X-loop or undiagnosed

Determine aortic situs in relation to pulmonary valve

- D   Normally related great arteries with aorta to the right of the pulmonary artery
- L   Inverted great arteries with aorta to left of pulmonary arteries
- A   Aortic valve is directly anterior to pulmonary valve

Notation (atria, ventricles, great arteries)

Examples

Normal	(S,D,D)
D-TGA	(S,D,D)
L-TGA	(S,L,L)
Situs inversus	(I,L,L)
Asplenia, dextrocardia, TGA	(A,L,L)

(From Van Praagh R, Weinberg PM, Smith SD, et al: Malpositions of the heart. In Emmanouilides GC, Riemenschneider TA, Allen HD, et al (editors): Moss and Adams heart disease in infants, children, and adolescents including the fetus and young adults, ed 5, Baltimore, 1995, Williams & Wilkins.)

Cardiotyping

At this point in the segmental analysis of the heart, the atrial and ventricular situs, the atrioventricular connections, the ventriculoarterial connections, and the position of the aorta are known. This data can be expressed in a notation developed by Van Praagh to categorize all possible types of hearts (Box 9-4). The situs of the atria, as indicated by the position of the abdominal viscera and the trachea and lungs, are designated as solitus (S), inversus (I), or ambiguous (A). The ventricular situs is characterized as a d-loop (D), l-loop (L), or an undiagnosed loop (X). The position of the aorta in relation to the pulmonary valve is to the right (D), to the left (L), or directly anterior (A). These three letters are written in sequence (atrial situs, ventricular situs, aortic situs). Examples are a normal heart (S,D,D), a dextrotransposition of the great arteries (S,D,D), and a congenitally corrected transposition of the great arteries or levotransposition (S, L, L) where the d- and l- indicate the aortic position.

SEPTAL DEFECTS, HYPOPLASIAS, AND ATRESIAS

Atrial Septal Defects

Defects in the atrial septum are a common congenital malformation that allows an abnormal passage of blood between the two atria. These defects occur at several sites in the atrial septum. Atrial septal defects are also an integral part of many congenital malformations, a few of which are total anomalous pulmonary venous connection, transposition of the great arteries, and tricuspid atresia, and occasionally of acquired defects such as mitral stenosis. In the Lutembacher syndrome, the enlarging left atrium from rheumatic mitral stenosis stretches the rim of a patent but functionally closed foramen ovale so that a left-to-right shunt develops.

Most patients with atrial septal defects are diagnosed after 6 months of age, in contrast to patients with ventricular septal defects and atrioventricular caval defects, which are clinically evident earlier. Atrial septal defects may be undetected until pregnancy when normal pulmonary blood flow is increased.

Patent foramen ovale

A patent foramen ovale is a normal structure that has a flap of tissue permitting passage of blood in utero from the right atrium to the left atrium. After birth, when left atrial pressure exceeds that in the right atrium, this flap is held closed and, in most people, gradually fuses with the rest of the atrial septum after the first year of life. However, in about one fourth of adults, the foramen ovale remains patent, placing these patients at risk for paradoxical emboli.

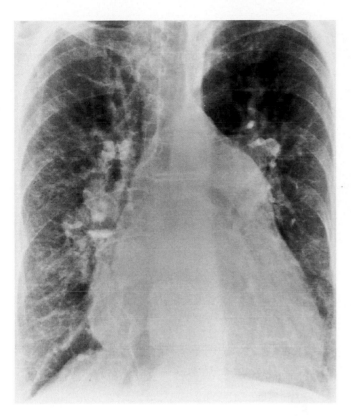

Fig. 9-50   Atrial septal defect. The increased transverse diameter of the heart reflects the large right atrium on the right side and the large right ventricle on the left side. The pulmonary artery pressures were normal, illustrating that the size of the pulmonary arteries can reflect either a large shunt or pulmonary hypertension.

Ostium secundum and primum defects

An *ostium secundum atrial septal defect* is an absence or deficiency of tissue in the region of the fossa ovalis. An *ostium primum atrial septal defect* is medial and adjacent to the crus and both atrioventricular valves. This abnormality is associated with developmental defects in the endocardial cushions that contribute to the inferior atrial septum. If all endocardial cushions are deficient, associated defects occur in the superior ventricular septum as well as in the leaflets and chordal attachments of both the mitral and tricuspid valves.

Sinus venosus defects

A *sinus venosus atrial septal defect* occurs in the superior and lateral portion of the atrial septum adjacent to the connection with the right pulmonary veins. Because of this location, anomalies of pulmonary venous connection are commonly found in the triangle defined by the superior vena cava, the interatrial septum, and the right superior pulmonary vein.

Less common defects

Less common atrial defects are those between the fossa ovalis and the inferior vena cava and in the region of the coronary sinus. An absent coronary sinus, connection of the left superior vena cava to the left atrium, and a large atrial septal defect make up this unusual developmental complex.

Chest film features

The classic chest film features of an atrial septal defect (Fig. 9-50) are enlargement of the right atrium, the right ventricle, and all segments of the pulmonary arteries ("shunt vascularity"). Because the chest film does not accurately reflect the size of the right atrium and ventricle, the heart size may appear normal. These signs of enlargement are apparent when the flow through the pulmonary artery is at least two times that through the aorta. The large size of the main pulmonary artery is usually striking when compared with the normal size of the aortic arch. There is no enlargement of the left heart in a simple atrial septal defect unless there are other complications. For example, when the right ventricle is enlarged due to increased volume, there is a distortion of the geometry of the left ventricle so that mitral prolapse and occasionally mitral regurgitation ensue. Similarly, in an atrioventricular canal defect, the left atrium and ventricle are enlarged when either a ventricular septal defect or mitral regurgitation causes volume overload in these chambers.

When cyanosis results from pulmonary arterial hypertension (Eisenmenger syndrome), the pulmonary arteries become quite large. However, evaluating the size of the hilar pulmonary vessels is not a reliable way of differentiating pulmonary arterial hypertension with a small left-to-right shunt from normal pulmonary artery pressures with a torrential shunt. When an Eisenmenger syndrome causes blood to flow in a reverse direction (from the right to the left atrium), the heart becomes smaller. Radiographic signs of pulmonary arterial hypertension at this stage include calcification of the pulmonary arteries (Fig. 9-51), aneurysmal dilatation of the hilar branches, and a serpentine course of the lower lobe pulmonary arteries.

Imaging techniques and features

Imaging of atrial septal defects involves aligning the plane of the atrial septum or observing the abnormal passage of the catheter through the defect. Alternatively, the right atrium may be opacified during a pulmonary arteriogram. The angiography of atrial septal defects starts with passing a catheter from the femoral vein through the atrial defect into the right upper pulmonary vein. Secundum defects are best seen in the long-axis oblique projection (70-degree left anterior oblique and 20-degree cranial). Primum defects are imaged in the four-chamber view (40-degree left anterior oblique and 40-degree cranial). In the four-chamber view (Fig. 9-52), you can see the entire atrial septum: superiorly from the entrance of the right upper pulmonary vein and infcri-

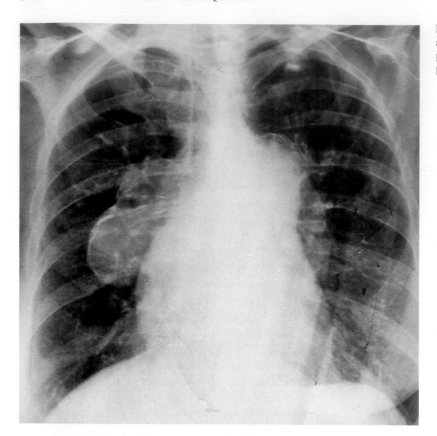

Fig. 9-51   Eisenmenger syndrome resulting from an atrial septal defect. The heart size is small. The hilar pulmonary arteries are aneurysmal and calcified. The peripheral pulmonary arteries are nearly invisible.

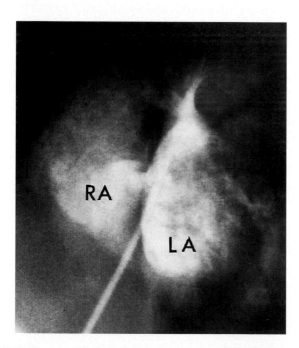

Fig. 9-52   Angiography of atrial septal defect. In the left anterior oblique cranial view, a catheter was passed from the inferior vena cava through the secundum atrial septal defect into the right upper pulmonary vein. Contrast passes across the defect from the left atrium *(LA)* to the right atrium *(RA)*. In this view, the secundum atrial septal defect is in the central part of the atrial septum. A sinus venosus defect would be present in the upper one third of the septum, while an atrioventricular canal defect would be in the lower one third of the septum.

orly to the tricuspid valve. With a catheter in the right upper pulmonary vein, contrast material streams along the left atrial side of the septum and then through the defect to opacify the right atrium. Injections into the body of the left atrium or its appendage do not outline the atrial septum as well since much of the contrast material goes directly through the mitral valve. In these projections, if the interatrial septum is divided into thirds, a sinus venosus defect will occur in the upper third, a secundum defect will occur in the middle third, and a primum defect will occur in the lower third.

In the same manner, MRI shows these three types of atrial septal defects in the plane aligned perpendicular to the septum. From an axial multislice series of images, a first set of oblique images is obtained oriented to the interventricular septum—these are images parallel to the septum. A second set of oblique images is then acquired from the first set along the axis of the mitral valve to the left ventricular apex—these images are the "four-chamber view," or perpendicular to the septum. As with echocardiography, the four-chamber view in MRIs has venosus, secundum, and primum defects in the upper, middle, and lower third of the interatrial septum, respectively. A pitfall in MRI of secundum defects is that an intact septum may have signal dropout in the fossa ovale because the septum is less than a pixel thick and has too few protons to generate a signal. If a secundum defect is suspected, a flow-sensitive sequence should also be obtained to confirm blood passing through the signal void.

Atrioventricular Septal Defects

Atrioventricular septal defects, also called endocardial cushion defects and atrioventricular canal defects, consist of atrial and ventricular septal defects together with clefts in the anterior mitral and septal tricuspid leaflets.

Complete atrioventricular canal defects

In the complete form of atrioventricular septal defect, the mitral and tricuspid valves may be formed into a single large common valve, or they may have separate annuli. The mitral valve has a deficiency or cleft in the anterior leaflet, while the tricuspid valve has a cleft in its septal leaflet. This division results in five leaflets, two of which bridge from the left to the right ventricle. A posterior leaflet extends from the posterior papillary muscle of the left ventricle to the right posterior papillary muscle of the right ventricle. The anterior leaflet extends from the medial papillary muscle of the right ventricle to the anterolateral papillary muscle of the left ventricle. The anterior leaflet may be divided with chordae tendineae going to the septum and to the papillary muscles, or it may be undivided with no attachments to the septum. The combination of defects makes the size of the mitral orifice appear two or three times as large as that of the aortic valve.

The complete form includes unequal inlet and outlet lengths of the ventricular septum, a malorientation of the aortic valve relative to the atrioventricular valves, atrial and ventricular septal defects, and a deficiency and malattachment of part of the right and left atrioventricular valves. The complete form of an atrioventricular canal defect, which constitutes about 20% of all types of canal defects, has an atrial septal defect which communicates with a ventricular septal defect. The atrioventricular valve may be common or be partitioned by the tricuspid and mitral annuli. Among patients with a complete atrioventricular canal defect, 50% to 80% have Down syndrome. Of patients with Down syndrome, 40% have an atrioventricular septal defect. (See Fig. 9-53.)

Partial or incomplete atrioventricular canal defects

A partial or incomplete atrioventricular canal defect has separate mitral and tricuspid orifices, and may have atrial or ventricular septal defects, or both, and clefts in the mitral and tricuspid valve leaflets. About two thirds of all patients with an atrioventricular canal defect have the partial form. The most common partial form is an ostium primum atrial septal defect and a cleft in the anterior (septal) leaflet of the mitral valve.

Segmental analysis

The atrial septal defect is of the ostium primum variety, involving the central portion of the atria adjacent to the atrioventricular valves. This type of atrial defect, inferior to that of the ostium secundum type, is found below the fossa ovalis. The central part of the defect extends to the annuli of the atrioventricular valves so that no intervening tissue is present between the hinge point of the

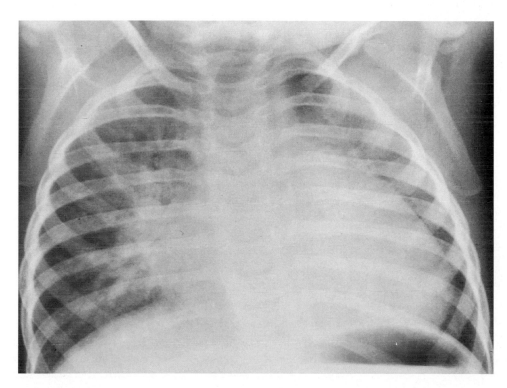

Fig. 9-53 Chest film in atrioventricular canal defect. The hilar vessels at 3 years of age are large and indistinct because of pulmonary edema surrounding them. The heart is globally enlarged.

valve leaflets and the atrial septal defect. At times the defect may also include the fossa ovalis and other more superior portions of the atrial septum. A common atrium exists when the entire atrial septum is absent. This entity is associated with a cleft in the anterior leaflet of the mitral valve and frequently with a persistent left superior vena cava.

The ventricular septal defect extends from the annuli of the atrioventricular valves inferiorly to involve not only the posteromedial portion of the septum but also the inferior free wall, and posterolaterally to the lateral portion of the mitral annulus. The membranous part of the septum may be either normal or deficient and is anterior and superior to the canal type of ventricular septal defect.

The mitral valve is displaced toward the apex of the left ventricle, as compared with the aortic valve. The papillary muscles are in front of one another rather than in the anterolateral and posteromedial locations. In the normal heart, the distance from the aortic valve to the apex is the same as that from the mitral valve to the apex. The ratio of the length of the left ventricular inflow tract to the outflow tract may vary from 0.5 to almost 1.0 (in the normal heart, this ratio is 1.0). In the complete form of atrioventricular septal defect, the ratio tends to be between 0.5 and 0.7, and in the partial form is

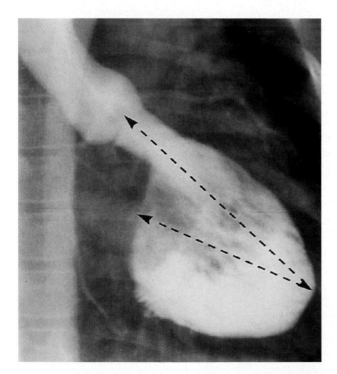

Fig. 9-54 Distinctive displacement of the mitral valve toward the apex in atrioventricular canal defect. The length from the mitral valve to the apex is 80% of that from the aortic valve to the apex. In the normal heart, these lengths are equal. In this diastolic frame, the aortic valve is closed and the mitral valve is opened. The elongated subaortic region is the gooseneck deformity.

between 0.7 and 0.9 (Fig. 9-54). The mitral leaflets are quite redundant and scalloped. Rarely, this extra valve tissue can appear as a tumor mass and obstruct the outflow tract. Because of the cleft, the mitral regurgitation may go directly into the right atrium through the atrial septal defect rather than into the left atrium.

The outflow tract of the left ventricle is usually deviated anteriorly and to the right side. Compared with the normal heart in which the direction of blood through the aortic valve is toward the right shoulder, the direction in a canal defect is more horizontal and toward the right pectoral region.

Chest film abnormalities

The appearance of the heart and lungs on the chest film reflects the abnormal blood flow (see Fig. 9-53). Since there is a left-to-right shunt across an atrial or ventricular septal defect, or across both, all segments of the pulmonary arteries are enlarged. All four chambers of the heart are large, reflecting not only the flow through the septal defect but also mitral and tricuspid regurgitation. When a combination of high cardiac output and mitral regurgitation coexist, interstitial and alveolar pulmonary edema may be visible, particularly in the hilar regions, even though the left atrial pressure is normal.

On chest film it is often impossible to distinguish a secundum atrial septal defect or an isolated membranous ventricular septal defect from either the complete or partial form of atrioventricular canal defect. There are, however, several clues on the chest film that may suggest the latter (Table 9-4). First, the age of the patient is helpful in that it is unusual in a person less than a few months old for a secundum atrial septal defect to produce visible large pulmonary vessels and signs of congestive heart failure, whereas canal defects may be associated with signs of heart failure within the first few weeks of life. Second, the left atrium is not visibly enlarged in a secundum atrial septal defect; this feature, however, is typical of an atrioventricular septal defect

Table 9-4	Distinguishing features of acyanotic shunt lesions	
Lesion	Chamber Enlargement	Dilated Aorta
Atrial septal defect	Right atrium Right ventricle	No
Ventricular septal defect	Left atrium Left ventricle Right ventricle	No
Patent ductus arteriosus	Left atrium Left ventricle	Yes

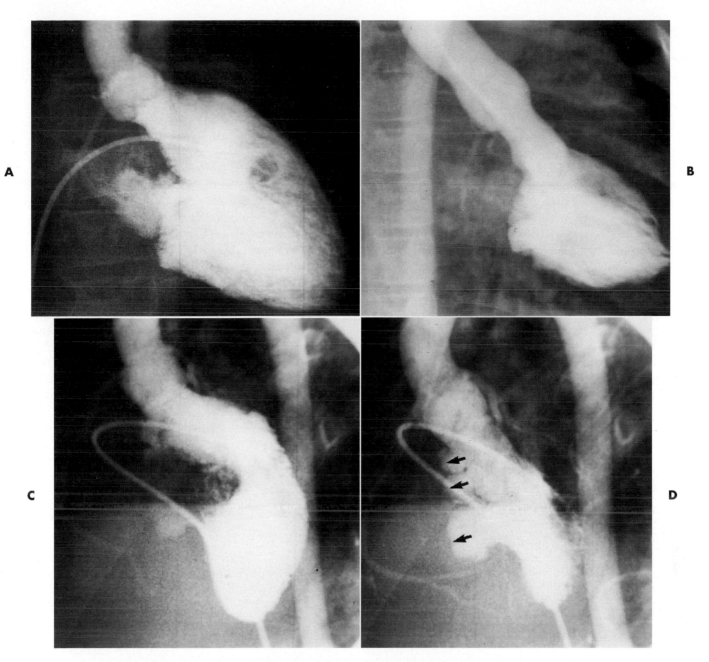

Fig. 9-55 Partial atrioventricular canal defect. Diastolic (**A** and **C**) and systolic (**B** and **D**) frames in the right anterior oblique projection (**A** and **B**) and the four-chamber left oblique projection (**C** and **D**) show the septal, inferior, and posterior deficiency of the left ventricle that constitutes the gooseneck deformity. An ostium primum atrial septal defect and a cleft anterior leaflet of the mitral valve are present with mild mitral regurgitation. The diameter of the mitral valve is about three times the aortic valve diameter. Note the redundant scalloped mitral valve *(arrows)*.

with mitral regurgitation. Third, an enlarged right atrium is not a feature of a simple ventricular septal defect but is present in an atrioventricular septal defect when there is either an atrial septal defect or a left ventricular–right atrial defect. These findings, coupled with left axis deviation of the QRS complex on the electrocardiogram, are very likely to represent some type of atrioventricular septal defect.

Angiographic features

The angiographic features of atrioventricular canal defects were first recognized in a classic paper by Baron et al. in 1964. They described the diagnostic pattern in the left ventriculogram as a "gooseneck" deformity and explained how this resulted from a deficiency in the inferior interventricular septum. The characteristic deformity in the left ventricle is visible in the right anterior oblique projection and is accentuated in diastole. The left ventricular inflow is concave and not straight as it is in the normal heart. This concave edge represents in part the apically displaced mitral valve; it has a serrated edge, which is the redundant leaflet of tissue pulled by the chordae tendineae. A radiolucent horizontal line in the mitral valve represents the cleft of the anterior leaflet. These features are present with or without a ventricular septal defect and also persist after surgical closure of the atrial and ventricular septal defects (Fig. 9-55).

By adding cranially angled projections, you can design the angiographic evaluation to determine the definite existence of an atrioventricular septal defect, the extent of the deficiency of the atrial and ventricular septa, the amount of mitral regurgitation, the presence of separate or common annuli of the atrioventricular valves, and whether their leaflets are divided or attached to the remaining septum. Angiography consists of left ventricular injections in the standard right anterior oblique and the cranially angled left anterior oblique projections (the four-chamber view). Additional injections into the right superior pulmonary vein in the angled left anterior oblique view may show the full extent of the atrial septal defect. Right ventriculography is usually not necessary but will show the free wall attachment of the tri-

cuspid valve and the right side of the common atrioventricular valve.

The right anterior oblique left ventriculogram, performed with the venous catheter passing across the atrial septal defect, demonstrates the relation between the atrioventricular valve and the left ventricular inflow and outflow tracts. The anterior leaflet of the mitral valve is denoted by the cleft and its septal attachments. In contrast, the posterior part of the mitral valve lies beside the left circumflex artery. Both of these leaflets appear concave and contribute to the gooseneck deformity. Therefore, the characteristic shape of the base of the left ventricle results from a deficiency of the diaphragmatic and posterior wall as well as from the defect of the septum.

In the cranially angled left anterior oblique projection, the mitral valve is en face to the septum, in contrast to the normal heart in which it is on the posterior heart border and away from the septum.

The presence of a ventricular septal defect is determined by locating the most apical portion of the mitral valve and analyzing its connection with the septum. If contrast material passes below this attachment into the right ventricle, a ventricular septal defect is present. In the infant, this observation is difficult because torrential regurgitation into the left atrium and then into the

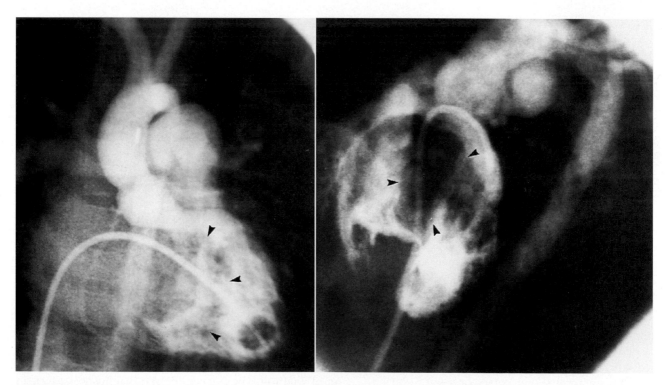

Fig. 9-56   Complete atrioventricular canal. Left ventricular angiography was performed by passing the catheter across the atrial septal defect into the left ventricle. Diastolic frames in the frontal **(A)** and left anterior oblique **(B)** projections show the gooseneck deformity of the outflow region. In systole there was simultaneous opacification of the pulmonary arteries and aorta. The open common atrioventricular valve *(arrowheads)* straddles the ventricular septum.

right heart may obscure the site of a small ventricular septal defect.

The morphology of the atrioventricular valves is best demonstrated in the hepatoclavicular view. When separate mitral and tricuspid valves exist, the septal leaflet forms the right border of the left ventricular outflow tract. When there is a common atrioventricular valve, contrast material passes from the left ventricle into the right ventricle beneath the leaflets of the common valve (Fig. 9-56). The leaflets may be attached to the septum or may form a continuous bridge from the superior rim of the common valve. The chordal attachments of the common leaflet may extend to their adjacent ventricular papillary muscles, the lip of the ventricular septal defect, or may cross into the opposite ventricle. The partial form of this malformation, in which the chordae attach on opposite sides of the septum, is the straddling atrioventricular valve.

MRI features

In the four-chamber view perpendicular to the interventricular septum, spin echo sequences will show defects at the junction of the interatrial and interventricular septum (Fig. 9-57). White blood sequences, which are sensitive to movement, are needed to assess valve regurgitation and shunt flow.

Ventricular Septal Defects

In 1879 Henri Roger described the clinical signs of a small ventricular septal defect. Shortly thereafter,

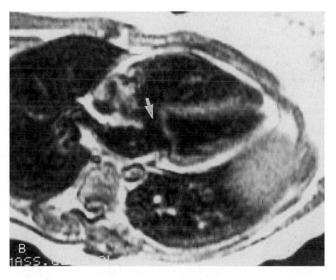

Fig. 9-57 MRI of atrial septal defect. A cardiac-gated image in a plane perpendicular to the long axis of the septum shows a primum defect *(arrow)* adjacent to the mitral and tricuspid valves. The mitral valve is closed, indicating a diastolic frame. (From Miller SW, Brady TJ, Dinsmore RE et al: Cardiac magnetic resonance imaging: the Massachusetts General Hospital experience, *Radiol Clin North Am* 23:745-764, 1985.)

Eisenmenger reported a patient with a large ventricular septal defect and cyanosis. Today their names are used as eponyms to describe the entities at the opposite ends of the clinical spectrum that result from defects in the ventricular septum. Although bicuspid aortic valve is more prevalent, ventricular septal defect is the most common congenital heart defect with symptoms in the neonate.

Classifications

Several surgical and pathologic classifications have divided these defects into supracristal and infracristal varieties. However, the crista supraventricularis is not always identified in its entirety by imaging. In addition, the ventricular septum is curvilinear so that other landmarks, such as the mitral and aortic valves, are more readily recognizable. To overcome these problems, Soto in 1980 devised a classification that divides the left ventricle into the inlet part near the mitral valve, the muscular portion, and the outflow tract portion below the aortic valve. Using this way of dividing the ventricle, defects in the posterior ventricular septum are those associated with atrioventricular septal defects. Muscular defects have slight overlap with defects in the other categories but are mainly holes of varying sizes between the trabeculations of the two ventricles. Ventricular septal defects in the left ventricular outflow region mainly occur in the membranous part of the septum. In complex defects, such as tetralogy of Fallot, the defect extends into the crista and occasionally into the muscular septum. Isolated membranous defects, viewed from the right ventricular side, are infracristal in location. The least common defect is in the supracristal location below the pulmonary valve. Also called conoventricular defects, these malformations are frequently associated with malalignment between the ventricular septum and the conal septum that separates the aortic from the pulmonary valves.

Chest film findings

In all types of ventricular septal defects, the appearance of the heart and lungs on the chest radiograph depends on the flow and pressure in the pulmonary artery. In small shunts that represent less than a 2:1 shunt to the pulmonary artery, the chest film is usually normal. In larger shunts, cardiac size increases roughly in proportion to the amount of the shunt. The left ventricular apex projects to the left and inferiorly and posteriorly. The left atrium is enlarged and can be seen as a double density behind the right atrium. The main pulmonary artery and all pulmonary vessels increase in size depending on the degree of the blood flow (Fig. 9-58). If pulmonary vascular obstruction increases so that blood flow reverses and becomes a right-to-left shunt (Eisenmenger physiology), the heart size becomes smaller. At this point, the central pulmonary arteries appear as

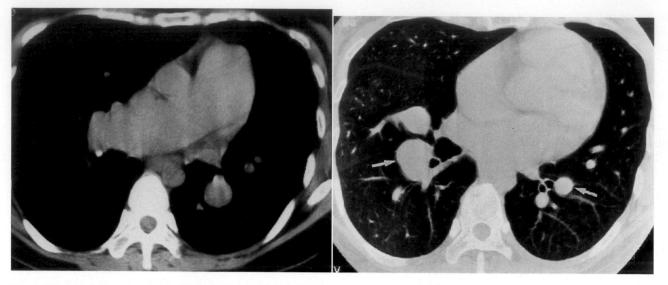

Fig. 9-58   Central pulmonary arteries in Eisenmenger syndrome. **A,** The main and right pulmonary arteries are more than twice as large as the ascending aorta and clearly exceed the 3 cm upper limits of normal. **B,** The hilar pulmonary arteries *(arrows)* are two to four times as large as their corresponding bronchus.

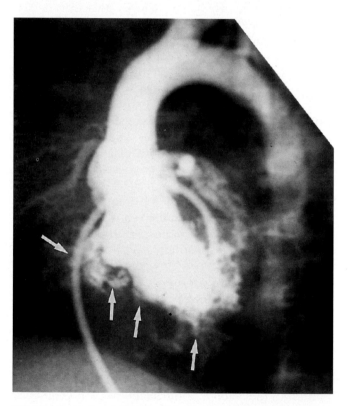

Fig. 9-59   Multiple ventricular septal defects. The *lower three arrows* point to defects in the muscular septum, while the *upper arrow* outlines a membranous defect.

aneurysms and, rarely, may be calcified. The basilar pulmonary arteries tend to elongate when pulmonary artery hypertension occurs, resulting in a serpentine course. The right ventricle, seen mainly on the lateral chest film, also enlarges as the size of the shunt increas-es. Both ventricles have a corresponding increase in diastolic volume and a similar ejection fraction.

Imaging features

The angiographic evaluation shows the size and location of these ventricular defects. The optimal projection to show the septum is with cranial angulation in the left anterior oblique view, the four-chamber view, or long-axis oblique view. The four-chamber view demonstrates the posterior portion of the septum, while the long-axis oblique view places the anterior septum in profile.

Muscular ventricular septal defects typically appear on angiography as thin small jets of contrast material that pass directly into the right ventricle. These defects are usually located in the apical half of the ventricular septum, but may exist adjacent to the membranous septum at its trabeculated edge (Fig. 9-59). Although these defects usually range from a few millimeters to a centimeter in size, most of the muscular septum may be absent, making a common ventricle. Small muscular defects, which are seen as thin streams into the right ventricle, are visible throughout most of systole. If the defects are tiny, the contracting trabeculations may close these holes so that they are visible on ventriculography only during the early part of systole.

Defects in the membranous septum are seen in the outflow tract inferior to the aortic valve and medial to the mitral valve. From the right ventricular side, the septum is deficient below the crista and behind and adjacent to the sepal leaflet of the tricuspid valve. During a left ventriculogram the path of contrast material is seen going through the septum, then apically down the right ventricular side of the septum (Fig. 9-60). This "waterfall"

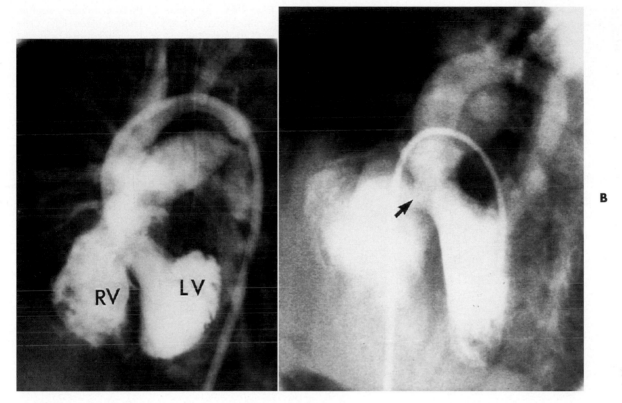

Fig. 9-60 Angiographic approaches to membranous ventricular septal defect. **A,** The catheter is passed retrograde through the hypoplastic aortic arch into the left ventricle *(LV)*. The injection opacifies the right ventricle *(RV)* and the large pulmonary arteries. **B,** Left ventriculography was performed by passing the catheter from the inferior vena cava through a patent foramen ovale. By filming in the left anterior oblique projection with steep cranial angulation, the ventricular septum is elongated and shows the subaortic membranous defect *(arrow)*.

motion is typical of a membranous defect and opacifies the entire right ventricle when the size of the defect is moderate. When the pulmonary artery pressures are normal, left-to-right shunting is visible during the left ventriculogram in both systole and diastole, although the major portion of contrast media crosses the ventricular septal defect in systole. If the peak right ventricular pressure is within 30 mm Hg of that in the left ventricle, transient right-to-left shunting occurs during isovolumetric relaxation. When pulmonary vascular obstruction ensues with systemic pulmonary artery pressures and cyanosis (Eisenmenger syndrome), most of the blood flow is from the right ventricle into the left ventricle; the degree of opacification depends less on the size of the defect than on the pressure gradient between the ventricles.

Supracristal or subpulmonary ventricular septal defects have a high incidence of associated anomalies. These include aortic regurgitation, aneurysm of the aortic sinus of Valsalva, prolapse of the right aortic cusp, and the Taussig-Bing anomaly, which is a double-outlet right ventricle with the pulmonary artery adjacent to the ventricular septal defect. In contrast to the other types of ventricular septal defects, the right oblique view best

shows the supracristal defect below the pulmonary valve. The ventricular septum is malaligned with the plane of the crista which causes the semilunar valves to obscure one another during angiography in the long-axis oblique projection. The orthogonal right oblique projection is necessary to show the relation of the ventricular septal defect to the semilunar valves.

Aneurysms of the membranous septum look like a windsock (Fig. 9-61) and project into the ventricle adjacent to the septal leaflet of the tricuspid valve. These aneurysms, which appear to represent closing membranous defects, are frequently round and smooth-walled but may have a scalloped and irregular margin. The aneurysm may connect to the right ventricle through its center, or it may be completely closed allowing no communication between the ventricles. Rarely, the aneurysms extend into the right atrium. Common lesions associated with a membranous septal aneurysm are aortic insufficiency with prolapse of a cusp into a portion of this aneurysm, bacterial endocarditis, and (rare) right ventricular outflow obstruction and tricuspid regurgitation. In views other than the left anterior oblique projection, the aneurysms may appear as masses adjacent to either the aortic or

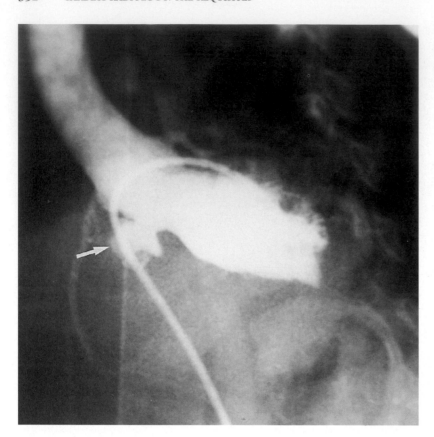

Fig. 9-61 Aneurysm of the membranous septum resulting from a closed ventricular septal defect. The left anterior oblique view shows a subaortic saccular aneurysm *(arrow)* projecting into the right ventricle.

mitral valve. Masses in the right atrium and right ventricle represent the other side of the sac.

Left ventricular–right atrial shunting is an unusual type that is the result of tricuspid valve abnormalities, including clefts or perforations in the septal leaflet adjacent to a perimembranous ventricular septal defect and aneurysms in the membranous septum. The long-axis oblique view demonstrates the ventricular septal defect and its aneurysms, while the reciprocal right anterior oblique projection shows the jet of contrast medium from the left ventricle to the right atrium. Left ventricular–right atrial shunting associated with a perimembranous ventricular septal defect is different from that with atrioventricular canal defects. Only in the latter does left ventriculography show a cleft in the anterior leaflet of the mitral valve and a deficiency in the basilar part of the interventricular septum.

Patent Ductus Arteriosus

The ductus arteriosus is a portion of the sixth aortic arch in the fetus that connects the left pulmonary artery to the descending aorta. In fetal life, about 84% of the blood entering the pulmonary artery passes across the ductus into the descending aorta. About 12 to 24 hours after birth, the ductus is functionally closed through contraction of its muscular wall. Anatomic closure follows 1 to 2 weeks later. For unknown reasons the ductus arte-

riosus may remain patent, particularly in infants of low birth weight because of prematurity, in infants with the respiratory distress syndrome, and in maternal exposure to rubella.

Characteristics

The altered hemodynamics that arise from a persistent ductus arteriosus depend on the size of the ductus and the ratio of the pulmonary-to-systemic vascular resistance. In fetal life, the shunt created by the ductus is from right to left because of the high pulmonary vascular resistance. Shortly after birth, the complex changes that happen in the first few minutes in the lungs result in a lowered pulmonary arterial pressure of one fourth to one sixth of the aortic pressure. A left-to-right shunt is thereby created through the patent ductus. This results in varying degrees of overcirculation to the lungs, left atrium, left ventricle, and the ascending and arch portions of the aorta. If the ductus does not close and an Eisenmenger reaction to the increased pulmonary flow results, the pulmonary vascular resistance again exceeds the systemic resistance and causes a right-to-left shunt across the ductus arteriosus.

The diameter and length of the ductus arteriosus varies considerably depending on whether partial closure has occurred. In the newborn infant, the ductus is nearly the size of the descending aorta and may be mistaken for the aortic arch because of the size similarity.

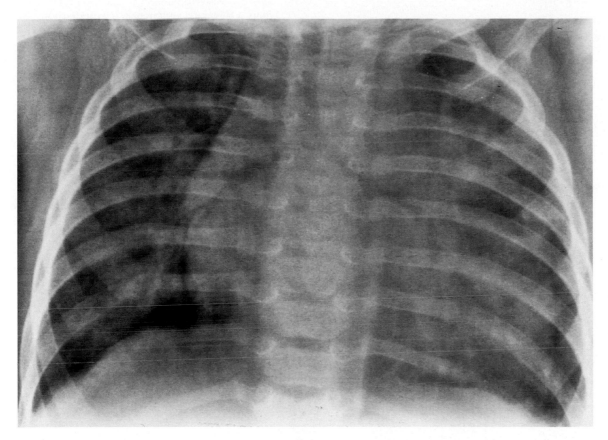

Fig. 9-62   Patent ductus arteriosus in children. The typical chest film shows a large heart with the apex to the left and inferior. The enlarged pulmonary vessels are hazy, reflecting a mild degree of pulmonary edema. The aortic contour is obscured by the thymus.

The length of the ductus is also quite variable and ranges from several centimeters to an aortic-pulmonary fistula without any intervening neck.

Complications

The major complication related to an isolated patent ductus arteriosus is the development of pulmonary arterial hypertension with resultant right-to-left flow reversal with cyanosis. Rare complications include aneurysm with thrombosis or rupture of the ductus, bacterial aortitis, and aortic dissection beginning at the ductus. Distal thromboembolism can originate from an aneurysm of the ductus arteriosus, and left phrenic nerve compression may be caused by an adjacent aneurysm.

Infant chest film abnormalities

The radiographic signs of a persistent patent ductus have a rough correlation with the degree of pulmonary circulation. In the infant and young child, the hilar and segmental pulmonary arteries are enlarged, when not obscured by the thymus (Fig. 9-62). When the shunt is greater than 2:1, perihilar pulmonary edema may begin to develop from the high cardiac output in the infant and may progress to generalized alveolar edema. Con-

comitant cardiac changes include an enlarged cardiac silhouette with cardiothoracic ratios greater than 0.55. In the infant, the differentiation of individual enlarged chambers is frequently difficult; however, on the lateral view left atrial enlargement can be detected by the posterior displacement of the left mainstem bronchus. Other noninvasive tests, such as the echocardiogram, show more accurately that the left atrium is enlarged and has an anteroposterior diameter exceeding that of the aorta. In the normal newborn infant, the anteroposterior left atrial dimension is less than that of the adjacent ascending aorta.

Adult chest film abnormalities

Because the mediastinum is not obscured by the thymus in the adult, other radiologic signs may point to the existence of a patent ductus arteriosus. The "ductus bump" is a localized dilatation adjacent to the descending aorta next to its arch at the entrance of the ductus. Embryologically, this dilatation is thought to be distinct from the involuted end of the right aortic arch. The large ascending aorta and arch may elongate so that the ascending aorta and innominate artery are visible on the right side of the mediastinum, while the left subclavian

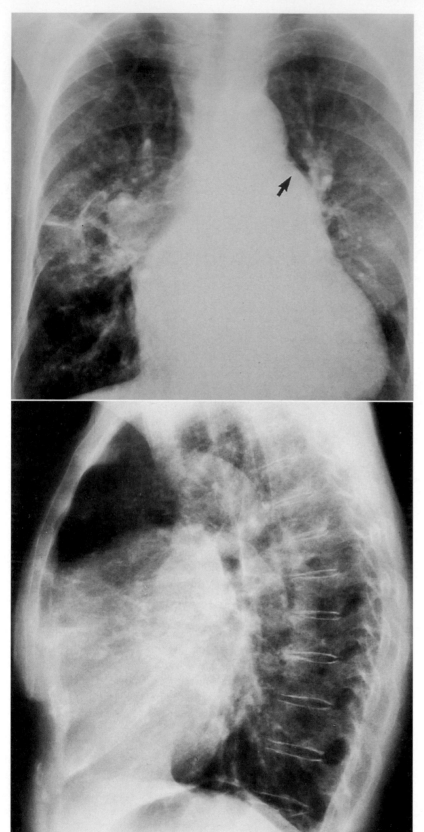

Fig. 9-63 Calcified patent ductus arteriosus *(arrow).* Posteroanterior **(A)** and lateral **(B)** chest films. Moderate pulmonary hypertension has enlarged the hilar arteries and the right ventricle. The large aortic arch indicates the site of the shunt is extracardiac.

artery projects into the left lung apex. Assuming an isolated left-to-right shunt is present, the large aortic arch indicates that the shunt is extracardiac; for example, a patent ductus arteriosus is present rather than an atrial or ventricular septal defect. An aortopulmonary septal defect (a connection between the ascending aorta and the main pulmonary artery) produces similar findings, but the amount of the shunt usually is larger. Rarely, a linear or circular calcification exists in the region of a ductus arteriosus (Fig. 9-63). The significance of this deposi-

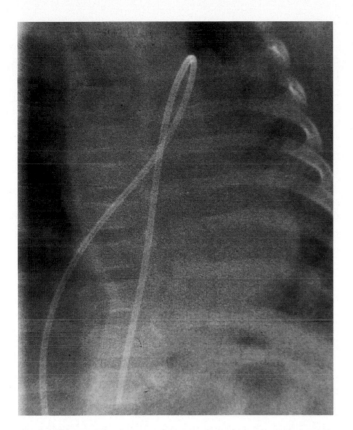

Fig. 9-64 Catheter position in patent ductus arteriosus. The catheter enters from the inferior vena cava, passes through the right heart and ductus, and ends in the distal aorta. Note that the catheter does not pass through the aortic arch.

tion of calcium usually is unclear; it may be a result of either an episode of aortitis or atherosclerosis at the aortic end of the duct. A calcified ligamentum arteriosus implies a closed ductus.

Angiographic examination

In the cardiac catheterization laboratory, a patent ductus arteriosus can be evaluated by cineangiography in several ways. A catheter advanced up the inferior vena cava can usually be manipulated out the pulmonary artery, through the duct, and into the descending aorta. In the frontal projection, the shape of the catheter looks like a musical G-clef (Fig. 9-64).

When the flow through the ductus arteriosus is left to right, if the duct is not seen with ultrasound, aortography provides the best visualization of the ductus (Fig. 9-65) and of associated juxtaductal abnormalities, such as aortic coarctation. Similarly, when the flow is reversed, a pulmonary artery injection defines the ductal anatomy, but the proximal aortic arch is usually not visualized. The flow through the ductus recorded by angiography depends on the force of the injection as well as the natural direction of shunting. In addition, most shunts have some degree of bidirectional flow so that contrast material occasionally seems to oscillate from aorta to pulmonary artery and back.

A patent ductus arteriosus may exist with other more complex cardiac defects. When a ventricular septal defect exists, a left ventriculogram is inadequate for identifying a

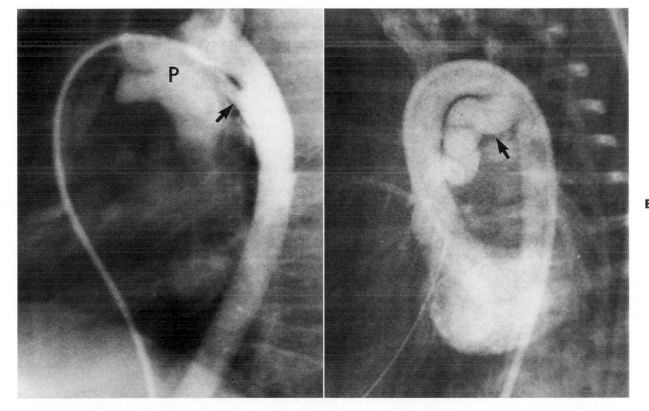

Fig. 9-65 Angiography of patent ductus arteriosus. **A,** A catheter was passed through the pulmonary artery *(P)* into a small short ductus *(arrow)*. **B,** Following a left ventricular injection, a long, redundant ductus *(arrow)* is seen below the aortic arch.

patent ductus arteriosus. In this case, the mixing through the ventricular septal defect will opacify the arch of the aorta and the main right and left pulmonary arteries nearly simultaneously, thereby obscuring the ductus. In this situation and in other connections between the aorta and pulmonary artery, such as truncus arteriosus, aortic-pulmonary window, or other aortic-pulmonary fistulas, an injection must be made in the descending aorta at the mouth of the suspected ductus. In a similar fashion, the rare anomaly of a bilateral ductus arteriosus, which forms a vascular ring around the trachea and esophagus, necessitates an injection in the proximal descending aorta with 30 to 40 degrees of cranial angulation to project both ductus from their respective aortic arches in the right and left anterior oblique projection.

Single Ventricle

Definition

It is not surprising that the definition of single ventricle or a univentricular heart is controversial given its extreme complexity. Van Praagh and colleagues believe that each cardiac chamber can be recognized by its gross morphologic characteristics; the ventricles are named by their trabecular pattern and not by their vessels or valves of entry or exit. Shinebourne et al. (1980) and Soto et al. (1979) argue that univentricular hearts possess only one ventricular chamber, which is connected to the atrial chambers. The latter group considers a normal ventricle to have an inlet segment, a trabecular portion, and an outlet segment. By their definition, a chamber is a ventricle if it contains an inlet segment and a trabecular portion, and the inlet arbitrarily must have at least one half of an atrioventricular valve entering this segment. Depending on the ventricular morphology, this malformation is also called double-inlet left ventricle and double-inlet right ventricle, or when such a distinction cannot be made, a primitive ventricle.

A *single ventricle* is a heart with two atria but only one ventricular chamber. Both mitral and tricuspid valves, or a common atrioventricular valve, connect the atria with the ventricle. Excluded from this definition of single ventricle are mitral atresia and tricuspid atresia. In the univentricular heart, the ventricle may be of a left ventricular, right ventricular, or indeterminate type, depending on its trabecular type.

A rudimentary chamber may be adjacent to the ventricle but not connected to the atrioventricular valves. If this chamber is attached to the aorta or pulmonary artery, it is called an *outlet chamber*. If it is connected to neither the atrioventricular valves nor the semilunar valves, the chamber is called a *trabecular pouch*.

Because of the primitive nature of single ventricular hearts, it is not always possible to identify the morphologic features of the ventricle by imaging. Generally, the right ventricular type has more trabeculations, but because the other ventricle is absent, there is no comparison within the same heart to be certain which ventricle remains.

The univentricular heart of the left ventricular type is the most frequent and occurs in both noninverted and inverted forms. In noninverted ventricles, the right ventricular infundibulum, although quite variable in size, is adjacent to the tricuspid valve in a posterolateral position. An inverted ventricle has a blind pouch in the ventricle that projects anteriorly and is distinctly separate from the atrioventricular valve, similar to the inverted ventricles in congenitally corrected transposition of the great arteries.

In univentricular hearts of the right ventricular type, the rudimentary chamber is posterior and either to the right or left of the main chamber. This trabecular pouch tends to be quite small and can easily be missed by confusing its vestigial septum with a papillary muscle.

A *common ventricle* is not a single ventricle because the atrioventricular valves enter separately on each side of the rudimentary interventricular septum. The interventricular septum has either single or multiple large defects with the remaining ventricular muscle having recognizable elements of right ventricular morphology on one side and of left ventricular morphology on the other.

Associated anomalies are quite common in single ventricle. About two thirds have either valvular or subvalvular pulmonary stenosis, while a small number have pulmonary atresia. In univentricular hearts of the left ventricular type, there is usually aortic obstruction when the aorta arises from an outlet chamber. Anomalous pulmonary venous connections, patent ductus arteriosus, and levomalposition of the aorta are frequent enough that additional selective injections are worthwhile to make the identifications.

Chest film features

The signs of single ventricle on the frontal chest film are indirect, reflecting the amount of intracardiac shunting and the degree of pulmonary stenosis or pulmonary arterial hypertension from vascular obstruction. In situs solitus and noninversion of the ventricles, there is an enlarged cardiomediastinal silhouette. The ventricular apex may point inferiorly in a "left ventricular pattern," or it may point to the left and superiorly with a notch between the lateral heart and diaphragm in a typical "right ventricular pattern." The left atrium is usually enlarged with signs of a double density on the right side of the cardiac silhouette and posterior displacement of the left mainstem bronchus. If transposition of the great arteries is also present, the superior mediastinum is frequently quite narrow; in infancy this pattern has been ascribed to a relative diminution in the amount of thymus. When the aorta is levotransposed, the left side of the mediastinum still retains its distinctive convex shape.

An inverted ventricle is the only distinctive sign of single ventricle that separates it from all other types of congenital heart disease on a chest film with a large heart and shunt vascularity. The trabecular pouch or rudimentary outflow chamber is anterior, superior, and to the left. In this position, the outflow chamber has a convexity separate from the other cardiac chambers, projecting where the left atrial appendage normally would be (Fig. 9-66). This bulge extends along the lateral border of the cardiac silhouette for a distance equal to and frequently greater than does the usual enlarged left atrial appendage. The pulmonary vasculature has a shunt pattern unless there is severe pulmonary stenosis. The hilar arteries are quite large, particularly those on the right side, which are not hidden behind other mediastinal structures.

Angiographic examination

The cineangiographic evaluation starts with a biplane ventriculogram in the frontal and lateral projections (Fig. 9-67). However, the cranially angled views in the left anterior oblique projection better delineate the straddling atrioventricular valves and the trabecular pouch (Fig. 9-68). Selective injections in the subaortic and subpulmonary regions or in the trabeculated pouch help to determine whether the great arteries originate from an outlet chamber.

The atrioventricular valves are best identified by seeing the leaflets open and close. Secondary signs of the location of an atrioventricular valve are the appearance of nonopacified blood entering the ventricle, particularly if the catheter passed through the valve for the ventricular injection. Since both atrioventricular valves enter a common chamber, the two valves are identified by having the catheter pass through one of them and seeing the pulmonary venous return with its washout of contrast material pass through the other. A common atrioventricular valve is suspected if only one large annulus is identified and if both systemic and pulmonary venous blood passed through this common orifice. Atrial injections are useful in excluding mitral or tricuspid atresia if they are not identified on echocardiography.

Tricuspid Atresia

Characteristics

Tricuspid atresia is characterized by congenital absence of the morphologic tricuspid valve. This anomaly, which results in cyanosis, is always associated with a group of other malformations. There is an interatrial communication and enlargement of the left ventricle and mitral valve. The right ventricle is always hypoplastic. Variable features include a ventricular septal defect, malposition of the great arteries, abnormalities in the ventriculoarterial connections, and obstruction to pulmonary blood flow.

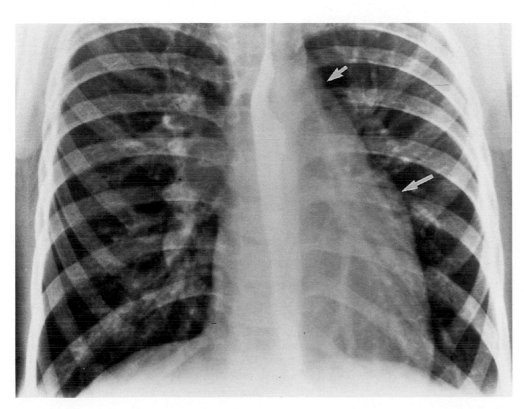

Fig. 9-66 Single ventricle. Seven-year-old child with a rudimentary outflow chamber *(long arrow)* connected to an anterior and leftward transposed aorta *(short arrow)*. The large pulmonary arteries reflect the intracardiac shunting and the moderate pulmonary hypertension.

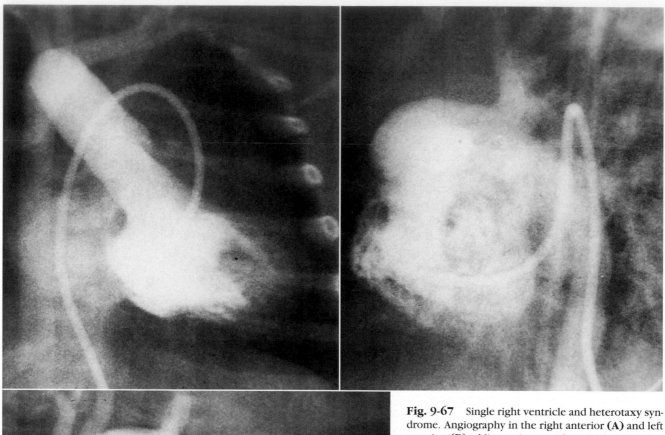

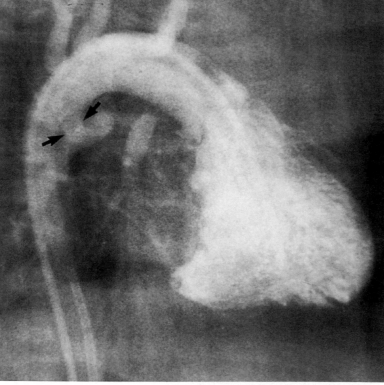

Fig. 9-67   Single right ventricle and heterotaxy syndrome. Angiography in the right anterior (**A**) and left anterior (**B**) oblique views with cranial angulation was performed with a venous catheter which passed through a left-sided inferior vena cava and hemiazygos continuation. The trabeculated ventricle has a subaortic conus with discontinuity between the common atrioventricular valve and the semilunar valve. **C,** Retrograde catheterization through the right aortic arch revealed that both pulmonary arteries came from a patent ductus arteriosus *(arrows).*

Anatomy

The anatomy of specific defects in tricuspid atresia varies depending on the presence of other associated anomalies. The right atrium is separated from the right ventricle by a membrane or area of fibrosis. Occasionally,

a dimple exists on the right atrial side with a slight invagination in the region where the tricuspid valve should be. A patent foramen ovale is the interatrial communication in two thirds of those with tricuspid atresia, while the remainder have secundum or primum atrial

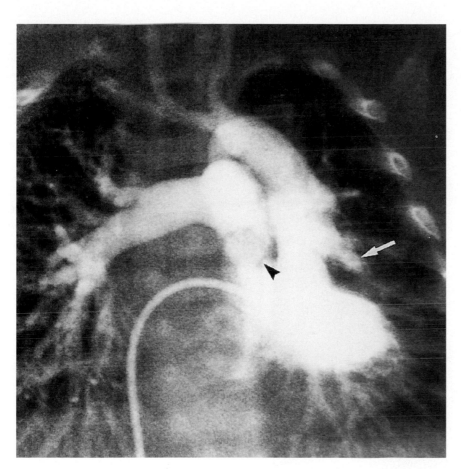

Fig. 9-68   Single ventricle with outlet chamber. The levotransposed aorta originates from a small outlet chamber *(arrow)*. The diameter of the atrioventricular valve is more than twice that of the semilunar valves, indicating a single common inlet valve. Infundibular *(arrowhead)* and valvular pulmonary stenosis is present.

septal defects. These atrial defects are frequently restrictive, and since systemic blood must pass through this defect to reach the lungs, the atrial defect serves as one source of obstruction to pulmonary blood flow. Both the left ventricle and the mitral valve are relatively large compared with the remainder of the heart. The left ventricle is both dilated and hypertrophied and occupies the diaphragmatic and anterolateral positions in the mediastinum that are usually taken by the right ventricle. In addition, the remainder of the left ventricle lies in its usual lateral and posterior location. The right ventricle is always hypoplastic, ranging from a moderate-sized chamber in some hearts to a thin sinus only a few millimeters long in the most extreme cases. A ventricular septal defect may be present, and when it exists, frequently serves as another location to obstruct pulmonary blood flow. In the absence of a ventricular septal defect, the lungs are supplied by a patent ductus arteriosus and other bronchial collaterals.

Transposition of the great arteries occurs in 20% to 30% of cases of tricuspid atresia. In dextrotransposition, the aorta connects to the right ventricular side of the ventricular septal defect and is anterior to the main pulmonary artery.

Common malformations that occur with tricuspid atresia are:

- Patent ductus arteriosus
- Transposition of the great arteries
- Left superior vena cava
- Coarctation of the aorta
- Juxtaposition of the atrial appendages

In summary, tricuspid atresia without transposition is a complex of anomalies in which the blood entering the right atrium passes across an interatrial defect into the left atrium, left ventricle, and then into the lungs either through a ventricular septal defect into the right ventricle or through the aorta and into a patent ductus arteriosus. With transposition of the great arteries, the returning blood in the cavae goes from the right atrium through the atrial septal defect to the left atrium, to the left ventricle, and into the pulmonary artery.

Chest film abnormalities

The chest film in tricuspid atresia illustrates that phrases such as "left (or right) ventricular enlargement," which are appropriate for acquired diseases, are inappropriate in discussing certain types of congenital heart disease. The position, size, and relation of the

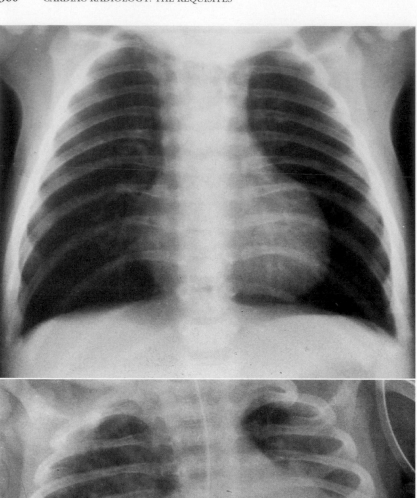

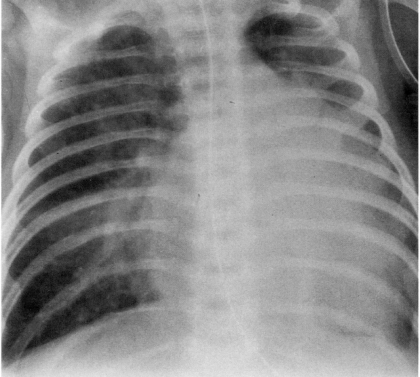

Fig. 9-69 Tricuspid atresia with and without pulmonary stenosis. **A,** The size and shape of the heart and pulmonary vessels appear normal on the posteroanterior chest film even though moderate pulmonary stenosis was identified by angiography. **B,** The large heart and central pulmonary arteries indicate increased pulmonary blood flow from the intracardiac shunt. There is no other lesion in this patient, but tricuspid atresia with transposition of the great arteries has the same appearance.

chambers in tricuspid atresia are not those of a normal adult heart. Yet the cardiac silhouette sometimes has an apex that points inferiorly and to the left, which in acquired heart disease resembles left ventricular enlargement. Other cases of tricuspid atresia have a cardiac silhouette that resembles the *coeur en sabot* appearance of right ventricular enlargement in tetralo-

gy of Fallot. Obviously, since the right ventricle is never enlarged in tricuspid atresia, this latter interpretation is fallacious. Similarly, when the ventricles are inverted or transposition of the great arteries is present, the usual position of the heart and mediastinal structures is altered so that their position in the cardiomediastinal silhouette may be unknown. In these instances, reference to a particular chamber of the heart on the chest film may be incorrect.

The size of the heart on the frontal radiograph is typically normal to slightly enlarged in tricuspid atresia (Fig. 9-69). The right atrial segment has slight rounding at the superior vena caval border, indicating atrial enlargement. The inferior half of the right atrial segment has a straight or sometimes concave appearance, the latter suggesting juxtaposition of the atrial appendages. When there is decreased pulmonary flow, the pulmonary artery segment is flat or concave. In this situation, the heart size tends to be normal, and the cardiac silhouette may appear to have an uplifted apex. This *coeur en sabot* shape is identical to that seen in tetralogy of Fallot. When pulmonary artery flow is increased, indicating no obstruction to pulmonary flow, the overall heart size may become quite large, and transposition of the great arteries is quite likely.

The pulmonary vascular markings in tricuspid atresia reflect the amount of pulmonary blood flow. In 60% to 70% of all cases of tricuspid atresia, there is diminished pulmonary vasculature. This sign indicates that there is obstruction to pulmonary blood flow at the interatrial or interventricular septal defects or at the level of the patent ductus arteriosus and other bronchial collaterals. Increase in size of the peripheral pulmonary vessels in comparison with those in the hila, along with accessory signs such as rib notching, suggest collateral flow.

Angiographic findings

The angiographic evaluation in tricuspid atresia involves a right atrial injection to establish the diagnosis. It requires a left ventricular injection to identify the size and location of a ventricular septal defect, the relation of the great arteries, and pulmonary stenosis or atresia. Typically, a catheter from the femoral vein is passed into the right atrium, but the right ventricle cannot be entered. Care should be taken that the catheter is in the right atrium and not in an azygos continuation of the inferior vena cava. Advancing the catheter allows it to pass through the interatrial communication and into the left ventricle. An aortogram is used to demonstrate a patent ductus arteriosus or bronchial collateral vessels.

Right atrial angiography in the frontal projection delineates most of the features of tricuspid atresia (Fig. 9-70). The flow of contrast material is from right atrium to left atrium to left ventricle; the right ventricle opacifies later than the left ventricle. A triangular lucency representing the right ventricle exists inferiorly between the medial border of the right atrium and the opacified left ventricle. This defect is typical of tricuspid atresia but may rarely be seen in congenital tricuspid stenosis (Fig. 9-71).

In tricuspid atresia, the left ventriculogram shows a large chamber and mitral valve. The ventricular septal defect, if present, usually is between the membranous septum and the lower muscular septum (Fig. 9-72). In the lateral view, origin of the aorta anterior to the pulmonary artery indicates transposition. The pulmonary valve and subpulmonary region may be more clear on a cranially angled left anterior oblique projection.

Blood flow from right atrium to left atrium may be seen in conditions other than tricuspid atresia. The morphology of the tricuspid region and not the flow pattern should determine the diagnosis. When mean right ventricular pressures are higher than those in the right atrium, a right atrial injection will not flow directly into the right ventricle, even though the tricuspid valve is fully patent. Such conditions exist when the pulmonary arterial or right ventricular pressures are quite high, as in pulmonary atresia, Ebstein anomaly, pulmonary arterial hypertension (Eisenmenger syndrome), and right ventricular infarct.

Pulmonary Atresia with Intact Ventricular Septum

Congenital pulmonary atresia with an intact ventricular septum is an uncommon malformation that results in complete obstruction to right ventricular outflow. Blood from the superior and inferior vena cava must pass through an interatrial communication to reach the left atrium and ventricle. The total cardiac output for both the lungs and systemic circulation is pumped by the left ventricle. The pulmonary circulation, and therefore oxygenation of the blood, is largely dependent on a patent ductus arteriosus and, to a minor extent, the bronchial arteries that anastomose to secondary pulmonary arteries. The sizes of the ductus arteriosus, the central pulmonary arteries, and the interatrial communication determine the amount of blood that reaches the lungs.

Although the malformation is called atresia of the pulmonary valve, both the associated anomalies and the resultant hemodynamic burden cause abnormalities in all cardiac chambers, the pulmonary arteries, and the aorta. The radiologic presentation, particularly on the chest film, is quite variable, and the kinds of abnormalities depend largely on the size of the right ventricle.

Classification

A useful division is to classify into one group those patients who have a small right ventricle and into another group those who have a large right ventricle. The tricuspid valve associated with a tiny right ventricle is small in proportion to the right ventricular chamber and is usually competent. In contrast, when the right ventricle is large, so are the components of the tricuspid apparatus. In this latter case, tricuspid regurgitation is invariably present. Because the pressure in a right ventricle with pulmonary atresia and intact septum is usually suprasystemic, estimating the amount of tricuspid regurgitation

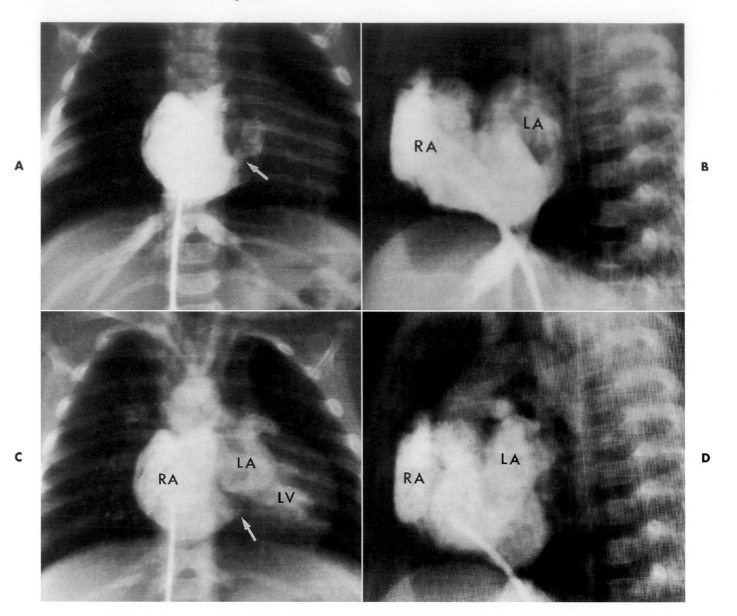

Fig. 9-70   Right atrial angiography in tricuspid atresia. **A,** Frontal view superimposes the right atrium on the left atrium. No flow enters the right ventricle. The coronary sinus is seen faintly *(arrow).* **B,** Lateral view projects the right atrium *(RA)* in front of the left atrium *(LA).* **C** and **D,** Later simultaneous frames show left ventricular and aortic opacification. Note the notch *(arrow)* between the right atrium and left ventricle *(LV).*

from an injection into a hypertensive ventricle may be fraught with inaccuracies.

Another way of classifying this malformation is to divide the right ventricle into an inlet portion, a trabecular part, and a conus. In pulmonary atresia with an intact ventricular septum, the trabecular portion or conus, or both, can be absent. The pulmonary valve is always absent. The remaining part—the tricuspid apparatus—is always present and can be sized. The diameter of the tricuspid annulus often correlates well with the size of the right ventricle and with the presence or absence of the trabecular and conal portions of the right ventricle.

Anatomic features

The right atrium is always large. When the right ventricular cavity is small and the tricuspid valve competent, the right atrium tends to be only mildly enlarged, while tricuspid regurgitation with a large right ventricle tends to produce extreme enlargement of the right atrium. The attachment of the tricuspid valve may resemble an Ebstein anomaly with the posterior leaflet attaching apically at a distance from the tricuspid annulus. Usually the interatrial communication is a patent foramen ovale, although true atrial septal defects are occasionally present. The left side of the heart and the ascending aorta

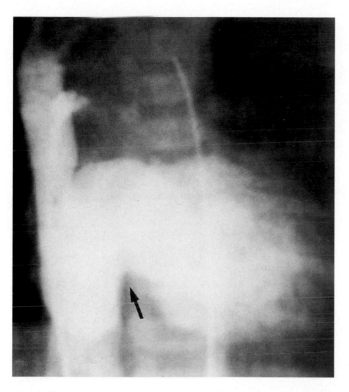

Fig. 9-71   Congenital tricuspid stenosis. Hypoplasia of the tricuspid valve may also create a notch *(arrow)* between the right atrium and right ventricle.

and arch are larger than normal, reflecting the increased cardiac output to both the systemic and pulmonary circulations. As a general rule, when either aortic or pulmonary hypoplasia or atresia is present, the uninvolved great artery is always compensatorily large and, in fact, serves as a marker for hypoplasia of the other vessel.

The size of the ascending aorta, which is normally slightly smaller than the main pulmonary artery, may have up to six times the diameter of the main pulmonary artery. Hypoplasia of the main pulmonary artery frequently extends into the right and left pulmonary arteries. The size of the arteries within the lung parenchyma reflects the blood flow through them. However, in general, patients with pulmonary atresia with an intact ventricular septum tend to have a pulmonary trunk of normal diameter, in contrast to those patients with pulmonary atresia with a ventricular septal defect who have a very small pulmonary trunk.

Chest film abnormalities

The typical features of pulmonary atresia on the chest film are a large cardiac silhouette, a concave pulmonary artery segment, and diminished pulmonary vasculature (Fig. 9-73). The severity of each of these abnormalities depends on the degree of obstruction in the pulmonary circuit and the competence of the tricuspid valve. The

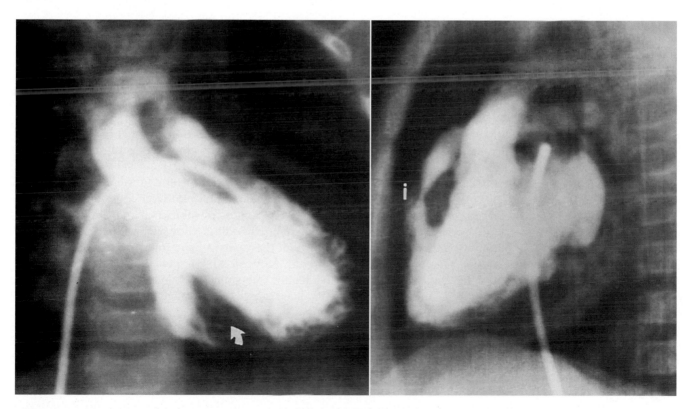

Fig. 9-72   Left ventriculography in tricuspid atresia. Simultaneous frames show the aortic and pulmonic connections. The ventricular septal defect is low in the muscular septum. The right ventricle is hypoplastic. Severe infundibular *(i)* and annular pulmonary stenosis and small pulmonary arteries are present. Note the distinctive interventricular notch *(arrow)*.

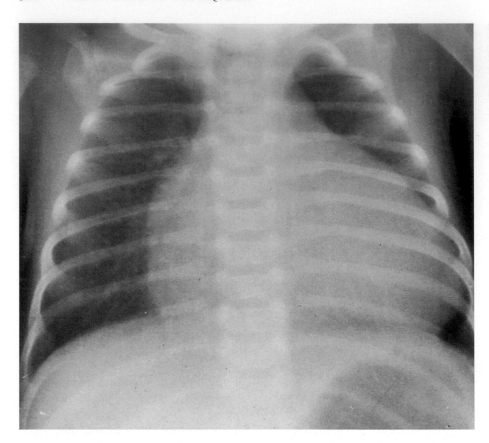

Fig. 9-73 Pulmonary atresia with intact ventricular septum. The large heart separates this lesion from isolated pulmonary stenosis, which has a normal-sized cardiac silhouette. The pulmonary vessels, partially obscured by the heart, are small.

pulmonary vessels at birth are visibly small, and in extreme cases, the pulmonary vessels beyond the hila are invisible. The pulmonary artery segment in older children appears concave, reflecting the hypoplasia of the main and left pulmonary arteries. In newborns, the thymus may obscure the entire superior mediastinum so that the true pulmonary artery segment and the hila are not visible. When atresia of the pulmonary valve is associated with a normal-sized main pulmonary artery, the pulmonary artery segment is straight.

The left ventricular apex in pulmonary atresia is projected inferiorly and to the left, reflecting mild to severe left ventricular enlargement. The right ventricle, whether small or of normal size, is not part of the cardiac silhouette on the frontal film. The right atrial segment has an exaggerated convexity and reflects the degree of right atrial enlargement. In those 80% who have a small right ventricle, the right atrium is only mildly to moderately enlarged. In the remaining 20% with an enlarged right ventricular cavity, the right atrium may be so large as to touch the lateral thoracic wall. This latter pattern of a giant cardiac silhouette with striking enlargement of the right atrium and decreased pulmonary vascularity is pathognomonic of tricuspid regurgitation from right ventricular outflow obstruction. The only malformations in which this occurs to this degree are pulmonary atresia with intact ventricular septum, tricuspid atresia, severe forms of Ebstein anomaly, congenital dysplasia of

the right ventricular wall (Uhl anomaly), and intrapericardial teratoma.

Angiographic examination

Angiographic evaluation is needed to establish the diagnosis and to size the right ventricular cavity and main pulmonary arteries in preparation for surgical correction. Right atrial injections are generally inadequate to fully define all of the constituents of pulmonary atresia. Since the pressure in the right ventricle is elevated, its cavity usually does not fill and therefore can not be sized. The angiographic catheter extending from the inferior vena cava is positioned within the right ventricle, thereby excluding tricuspid atresia. Depending on the size of the cavity, a hand injection or pressure injection with reduced volume generally shows an irregular and highly trabeculated chamber and documents the pulmonary atresia and intact septum (Fig. 9-74). The amount of contrast material opacifying the right atrium reflects the degree of tricuspid regurgitation. A severely dilated right atrium and reflux into the superior or inferior vena cava are signs of severe tricuspid insufficiency.

A striking appearance on the right ventriculogram are sinusoids leading to the coronary arteries (Fig. 9-74). These connections between the right ventricle and the coronary arteries alter the coronary flow and produce ischemia. Left coronary artery flow in the normal heart is mainly diastolic. In pulmonary atresia, the coronary flow

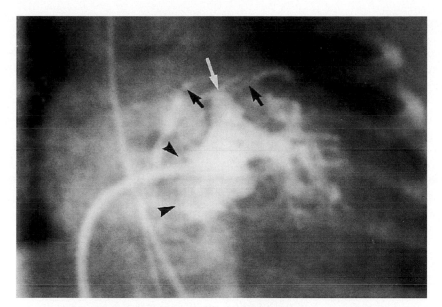

Fig. 9-74 Right ventriculogram in pulmonary atresia with an intact ventricular septum. The right ventricle with its tricuspid annulus *(arrowheads)* is small and heavily trabeculated. Mild tricuspid regurgitation outlines a large right atrium. Several characteristic sinusoids *(black arrows)* are traversing the myocardium. The *white arrow* points to the atretic pulmonary valve.

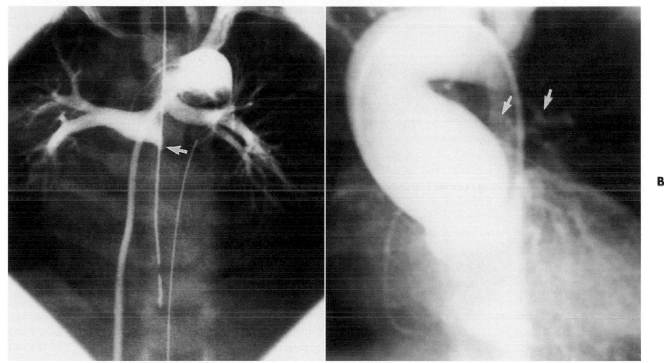

Fig. 9-75 Pulmonary valve atresia. **A,** In a left anterior oblique projection, a catheter from the aorta has been passed across a patent ductus arteriosus into the main pulmonary artery. No washout of contrast media through the pulmonary valve *(arrow)* is visible during systole. The pulmonary arteries have midline continuity. The passage of a catheter across a ductus should probably be deferred and an aortogram done instead before 1 month of age so that the ductus does not suddenly close from spasm. **B,** The large aorta is a hallmark of this malformation. The small pulmonary arteries *(arrows)* fill from bronchial collaterals.

from the hypertensive right ventricular sinusoids partially reverses the normal antegrade direction in the coronary arteries, leading to inadequate oxygenation of the myocardium and myocardial infarction.

The central pulmonary arteries have a characteristic "seagull" shape when the pulmonary valve is atretic. The right and left pulmonary arteries are the wings of the bird, the main pulmonary artery is the head, and the atretic valve is the beak (Fig. 9-75). Selective left ventricular angiography usually shows the size of the pulmonary arteries as they fill through the patent ductus. If the pulmonary arteries are not seen, an aortogram done near the ductus in the frontal projection should delineate both right and left pulmonary arteries. If you perform serial filming, photographic subtraction may be useful to recognize nonconfluence of the right and left pulmonary arteries. If you cannot see the pulmonary arteries with ventriculography or aortography, then pulmonary vein wedge angiography should be performed. The pulmonary veins are entered through an atrial septal defect or across an intact atrial septum with a transseptal technique, or by a retrograde aortic approach. After wedging an end-hole catheter into a pulmonary vein, inject contrast medium 0.4 ml/kg body weight at a rate of 2 to 4 ml/sec. This technique demonstrates whether the right and left pulmonary arteries are confluent across the midline and therefore influences the type of corrective surgery. If the pulmonary arteries are confluent, a conduit between the right ventricle and the confluence might be constructed, whereas if the arteries are not confluent, a systemic-pulmonary artery anastomosis might be attempted.

Tetralogy of Fallot

The most common cyanotic heart lesion that is recognized in the month after birth, the tetralogy of Fallot, represents roughly 10% of all congenital heart defects. Étienne-Louis Fallot in 1888 described the combination of defects that bears his name: pulmonary stenosis, a ventricular septal defect, an aorta displaced to the right, and a thick-walled right ventricle. Earlier, in 1671, Stenson reported this malformation, and in 1777 Sandfort described its clinical features in an infant who was normal at birth but became cyanotic after the first year of life. The subsequent history of this lesion and the fascinating surgical attempts to correct it were related by Helen Taussig, who with Alfred Blalock devised the subclavian artery-to-pulmonary artery anastomosis. From a different viewpoint, Van Praagh and associates in 1970 proposed that this condition is actually a "monology" with hypoplasia of the crista supraventricularis (distal conal septum) accounting for the infundibular pulmonary stenosis and the subjacent ventricular septal defect. The aorta then develops more to the right in the position normally occupied by the fully developed crista.

Characteristics

The location and severity of pulmonary stenosis, along with an associated ventricular septal defect, allow a spectrum of abnormalities to be grouped as tetralogy of Fallot. The common hemodynamic abnormality is right-to-left shunt through the ventricular septal defect, which is caused by right ventricular outflow obstruction. The variety of conditions seen with pulmonary stenosis and a ventricular septal defect may lead to diagnostic confusion when there are extremes of pulmonary stenosis. With

mild pulmonary stenosis, a left-to-right shunt occurs through the ventricular septal defect. Although this combination of lesions has been called acyanotic tetralogy of Fallot, its embryology and morphology are different. A similar condition, at least hemodynamically, results from acquired infundibular stenosis secondary to a ventricular septal defect with a hyperdynamic right ventricle (the Gasul phenomenon). At the other extreme of pulmonary stenosis, the pulmonary valve and the central pulmonary arteries may be atretic, a defect previously called a type 4 truncus arteriosus or pseudotruncus.

Anatomy

The pulmonary stenosis in a tetralogy of Fallot is infundibular and usually also is valvular; in most cases they coexist. When predominantly infundibular stenosis exists, the type of stenosis may be loosely grouped into three patterns. First, there may be a discrete narrowing or muscle bar between the body of the right ventricle and the infundibulum, creating an infundibular chamber. The second pattern is a diffusely narrowed infundibulum which appears elongated and is usually associated with a hypoplastic pulmonary valve and annulus. The third type of infundibulum is short and narrow with the ventricular septal defects subjacent to the pulmonary valve. Stenosis at the valve level is nearly always present but its severity may range from mild to complete atresia. There is a high frequency of bicuspid or unicuspid pulmonary valves, which occur in about 70% of those with tetralogy. While the pulmonary annulus is usually hypoplastic, the leaflet size ranges from complete atresia to normal. Congenital absence of the pulmonary valve leaflets in tetralogy consists of a stenosis at the annular level and aneurysmal dilatation of the central and hilar pulmonary arteries.

The pulmonary arteries are typically diffusely small but may have focal stenoses in the main or hilar branches. The left pulmonary artery may be completely absent. When pulmonary atresia occurs, the blood supply to the lungs comes through the ductus arteriosus, collateral channels, the bronchial arteries, or aortopulmonary arteries from the descending thoracic aorta. In this situation, the most frequent site of pulmonary artery stenosis is in the hilar region at the point of branching into upper and lower lobes.

The ventricular septal defect in tetralogy of Fallot is below the aortic valve on the left ventricular side and adjacent to the hypoplastic parietal band on the right ventricular side. The defect extends anteriorly as a misalignment of the crista, although it encompasses the membranous part of the septum. The defect relates to the septal leaflet of the tricuspid valve and to the right coronary cusp of the aortic valve. This relationship offers an explanation for the occasional aortic regurgitation in which the aortic cusps, usually the right, become fused into the upper part of the ventricular septal defect.

The overriding of the aorta results from an aortic root that is rotated more anterior and to the right than normal. The abnormal aortic position is more severe as hypoplasia of the infundibulum becomes more marked. Aortic dextrorotation may so severe that as much as 75% of the aorta is projected over the right ventricle. It is important to differentiate hearts with extreme overriding of the aorta from those with double-outlet right ventricle, but this may be quite difficult. In tetralogy of Fallot there is aortic-mitral continuity, while double-outlet right ventricle has a bilateral conus which is identified by contractile muscle interposed between the aortic and mitral valves. Of some help in distinguishing these entities angiographically is the fact that in extreme overriding the anterior aspect of the aortic valve plane tilts superiorly because the posterior aspect is anchored to the mitral annulus; in contrast, the plane of the aortic valve in double-outlet right ventricle is typically perpendicular to the axis of the body.

Right ventricular hypertrophy in tetralogy of Fallot is not seen at birth. Variable degrees of hypertrophy then become gradually apparent with an increase in the size of the trabeculation and of the thickness in the free wall and ventricular septum. The inflow tract adjacent to the tricuspid valve usually has normal size, while the body of the right ventricle may be quite small because of the encroachment of numerous trabeculations.

Anomalies associated with tetralogy of Fallot are:

- Left superior vena cava
- Atrial septal defect
- Patent foramen ovale
- Aberrant left anterior descending coronary artery coming across the infundibulum from the right coronary artery
- Right aortic arch

Right aortic arch, when identified on the chest radiograph of a cyanotic person, provides suggestive evidence of tetralogy. Of all the congenital heart defects that produce cyanosis, tetralogy of Fallot and truncus arteriosus are each associated with a 25% incidence of right aortic arch.

Chest film abnormalities

Distinctive features in the chest film can provide substantial evidence for the precatheterization diagnosis of tetralogy of Fallot. Important signs relate to the status of the pulmonary vasculature, the shape of the main pulmonary artery segment, the size of the heart, the appearance of the cardiac apex, and which side the aortic arch is on (Fig. 9-76). The size of the hilar and parenchymal pulmonary arteries roughly corresponds to the amount of blood reaching the lungs. Extremely small pulmonary arteries on either the posteroanterior or lateral film indicate a difficult surgical repair and imply that blood flow

may be coming from a ductus arteriosus or aortopulmonary collaterals. Normal-sized pulmonary arteries generally indicate that the pulmonary stenosis is infundibular. In older persons who have not undergone operation, rib notching is virtually diagnostic of aortopulmonary collaterals via the intercostal arteries.

When the pulmonary valve, annulus, and main pulmonary artery are small, the pulmonary artery segment is always concave (in the normal person, it is straight to slightly convex). The degree of concavity relates directly to the size of the main pulmonary artery segment. In pulmonary atresia the chest film has a deep concave notch between the aortic arch and the left atrial appendage segment.

The size of the cardiac silhouette is normal in the classic tetralogy with moderate pulmonary stenosis and a large ventricular septal defect. A large heart size is seen at both ends of the spectrum of pulmonary stenosis in the child. In minimal pulmonary stenosis with a torrential ventricular septal defect, both ventricles enlarge from the high cardiac output; this variety tends to be acyanotic. In pulmonary atresia or severe stenosis, the size of the ventricular septal defect determines the overall heart size. With a small restrictive septal defect, tricuspid regurgitation and an atrial shunt will increase the size of the other chambers. In the adult who has not undergone surgery, an increasing heart size frequently heralds the onset of right ventricular dysfunction.

The classic *coeur en sabot* shape of the heart in tetralogy consists of an uplifted apex with interposed lung between the inferior surface of the heart and the hemidiaphragm. This appearance of the apex is not constant, particularly in adults or those with extreme pulmonary stenosis or atresia. In these last two groups, the left ventricle also tends to enlarge from a poorly compliant myocardium and from increased flow (Fig. 9-77). The uplifted apex of the heart may also be seen in a normal person: a lordotic view will project the apex away from the diaphragm, and hyperaerated lungs may interpose between the heart and diaphragm.

You can usually ascertain the side of the aortic arch on the frontal chest film when you cannot see the tracheal air column. In neonates, the trachea buckles away from the side of the arch on expiration. In children and adults, the side of the arch is determined in the usual fashion by the asymmetry of tissue at the level of the aortic arch. When a right aortic arch is suspected, a barium esophagogram can be helpful. An isolated right aortic arch with a normal heart has a retroesophageal left subclavian artery; the barium-filled esophagus is deviated anteriorly by the anomalous left subclavian artery. In over 96% of instances of right aortic arch associated with tetralogy of Fallot, there is no retroesophageal anomalous artery. The branching pattern of the aortic arch then is a mirror image of the normal left aortic arch, that is, the

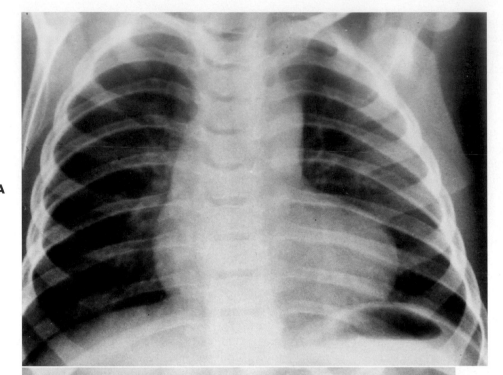

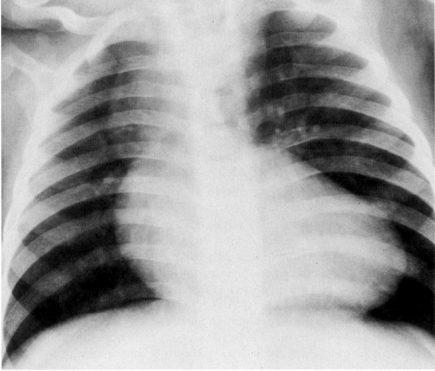

Fig. 9-76   Tetralogy of Fallot in the infant. **A,** Typical chest film shows an uplifted cardiac apex *(coeur en sabot)*, cardiothoracic ratio less than 0.5, concave main pulmonary artery segment, and small pulmonary arteries. The aortic arch is on the left side. **B,** Pulmonary atresia with ventricular septal defect has a cardiothoracic ratio greater than 0.5 with a large right atrium.

order of vessels is the left innominate artery, the right carotid artery, and the right subclavian artery.

Angiographic examination

The ventricular septal defect is best seen on the left anterior oblique projection with cranial angulation (long-axis oblique view) so as not to foreshorten the ven-tricular septum. With either a right or left ventricular injection, the ventricular septal defect can be seen extending from the aortic valve inferiorly to the muscular ventricular septum (Fig. 9-78). The malalignment of the infundibular septum with the aorta and pulmonary trunk projects the parietal band anteriorly and differentiates this type of ventricular septal defect from a mem-

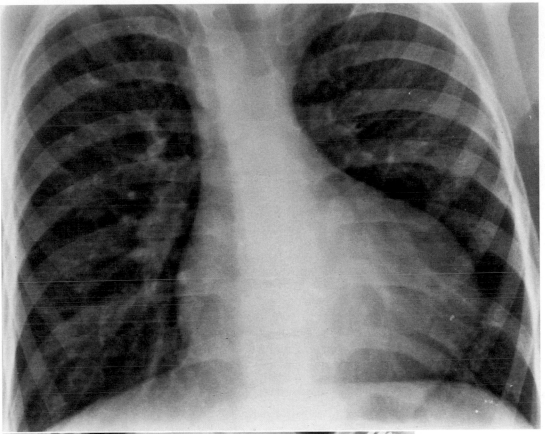

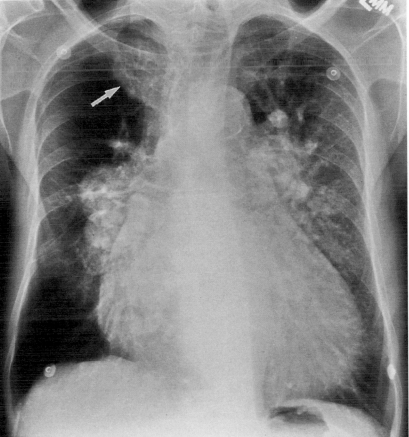

Fig. 9-77   Tetralogy of Fallot in the adult. **A,** The heart is mildly enlarged with an uplifted apex. The main pulmonary artery segment is straight and the hilar arteries are slightly small. The aortic arch is right-sided. **B,** Moderate pulmonary stenosis, moderate pulmonary hypertension, and a bidirectional ventricular shunt are atypical features of tetralogy in this cyanotic 67-year-old man. Note the differential size of the peripheral right and left pulmonary arteries. Large internal mammary artery collaterals *(arrow)* connect to the hila.

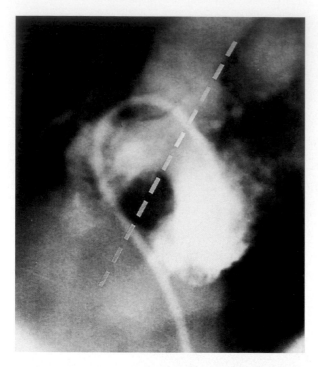

Fig. 9-78 Overriding aorta in tetralogy of Fallot. A left ventriculogram in the cranial left anterior oblique projection was performed with the catheter going through a patent foramen ovale. A line drawn through the interventricular septum locates most of the aortic valve over the right ventricle. In the normal heart, there is less than 25% aortic overriding.

branous septal defect. In the left anterior oblique projection, the aortic valve straddles or overrides the ventricular septum to quite a variable degree. Follow the plane of the interventricular septum as it intersects the aortic valve to measure the amount of overriding. The following associated defects that are important to evaluate are best visualized in the cranial left anterior oblique view:

- Position and size of ventricular septal defects
- Morphology of infundibular and valvular pulmonary stenosis
- Hypoplasia or atresia of the pulmonary arteries
- Confluence of the pulmonary arteries across the midline
- Aortic mitral separation to distinguish from double-outlet right ventricle
- Aberrant left coronary artery from the right coronary artery
- Right- or left-sided aortic arch
- Atrioventricular canal defect

Visualization of the bifurcation of the main pulmonary artery is best accomplished by right ventriculography with 40 degrees of cranial angulation in the posteroanterior projection or in the hepatoclavicular view (40 degrees cranial and 40 degrees left anterior). These views place the pulmonary valve, main pulmonary

artery, and both central branches in the same plane perpendicular to the x-ray beam (Fig. 9-79). When pulmonary atresia is present, selective catheterization of the bronchial and intercostal arteries that supply the lungs may show the location of all the pulmonary blood supply. The right and left pulmonary arteries may not connect across the mediastinum. In the older child and adult, MRI is an excellent modality to search for small mediastinal arteries. Although spin echo images usually are diagnostic, the imaging of small pulmonary arteries and aortopulmonary collaterals may require flow-sensitive techniques.

Approximately 5% of patients with tetralogy of Fallot have surgically important coronary anomalies. The most common major anomaly is the origin of the left anterior descending artery from the right coronary artery. In this anomaly, the aberrant artery courses over the usual site of infundibulotomy. The surgeon attempts to avoid transecting the anterior descending artery in this location because a major left ventricular infarction would usually result. In infants, the coronary arteries are visualized by aortography, by passing the transvenous catheter into the aortic root from the right ventricle and ventricular septal defect. With about 1.5 ml/kg of contrast material delivered over 1 second, both coronary arteries are routinely visualized in the left anterior oblique or lateral projection. You should not use the right anterior oblique projection because it casts both coronary arteries on each other and makes the left anterior descending artery fallaciously appear as though it originated from the right coronary artery. In older children and adults, selective catheterization of the coronary arteries is easily performed in the usual manner from a femoral artery approach.

Severe pulmonary lesions

Obstruction to pulmonary outflow can occur at many locations: (1) muscle bands in the body of the right ventricle, (2) in the infundibulum (Fig. 9-80), (3) at the pulmonary valve and annulus, (4) as diffuse pulmonary artery hypoplasia, and (5) as segmental stenoses or atresias in the main and hilar arteries. The extreme form of tetralogy of Fallot—pulmonary atresia with ventricular septal defect—has erroneously been called truncus arteriosus type 4 or pseudotruncus (Fig. 9-81). The spectrum of pulmonary lesions includes atresia of the right ventricular outflow tract and pulmonary valve, atresia of the main pulmonary arteries so that the right and left pulmonary arteries are continuous across the midline, and atresia of the main and proximal pulmonary arteries so that the right and left pulmonary arteries are not connected centrally (Fig. 9-82).

After demonstrating the status of the right ventricular outflow tract and ventricular septal defect with right ventriculography, the major problem is to then define the collaterals originating from the aorta which supply all of

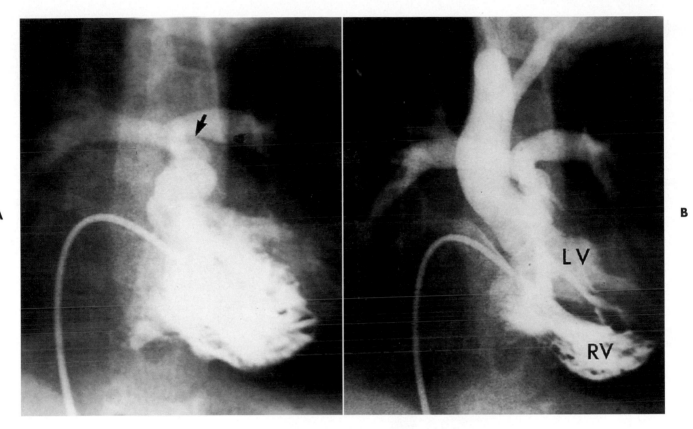

A   **B**

Fig. 9-79 Tetralogy of Fallot on right ventriculography. **A,** Early frame shows a hypoplastic infundibulum and a stenosis *(arrow)* in the main pulmonary artery. **B,** Later, the right aortic arch with mirror-image branching fills through the ventricular septal defect. *RV* = right ventricle; *LV* = left ventricle.

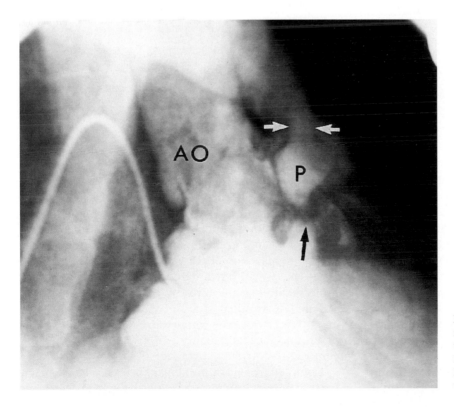

Fig. 9-80 Tetralogy of Fallot with severe pulmonary obstruction. In the right oblique projection there is systolic occlusion of the infundibulum *(black arrow).* The pulmonary annulus *(P)* is hypoplastic and has a jet *(white arrows)* through the stenotic pulmonary valve. *AO* = aorta.

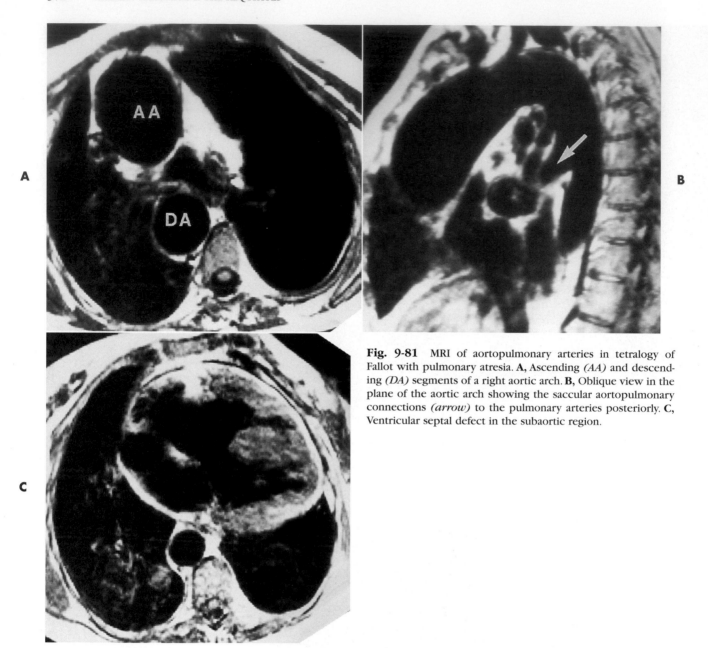

Fig. 9-81 MRI of aortopulmonary arteries in tetralogy of Fallot with pulmonary atresia. **A,** Ascending *(AA)* and descending *(DA)* segments of a right aortic arch. **B,** Oblique view in the plane of the aortic arch showing the saccular aortopulmonary connections *(arrow)* to the pulmonary arteries posteriorly. **C,** Ventricular septal defect in the subaortic region.

the pulmonary arteries. Serial large-film angiography (or MRI) in this situation is superior to cineangiography because it offers a large field size and the ability to use photographic subtraction. If the central arteries are not visualized with this technique, or if the proximal central pulmonary artery was occluded by previous shunt surgery, pulmonary vein wedge angiography may be required. Each pulmonary vein is injected in turn until you can visualize the central pulmonary arteries adequately enough to estimate their size and distribution.

Postoperative evaluation

Total repair of tetralogy of Fallot includes closing the ventricular septal defect and enlarging the right ventricular infundibulum and pulmonary valve annulus, usually with a patch. Evaluation of residual ventricular septal defects is similar to that for any other ventricular communication, namely, with a left ventriculogram in a cranially angled left anterior oblique view. A dehiscence of the septal patch usually is visualized as a small jet directed into the right ventricle. Abnormalities in the outflow tract of the right ventricle include residual stenosis, aneurysm of the patch graft (Fig. 9-83), false aneurysm at the border of the patch, and localized akinesis of a segment of the adjacent right ventricle.

Complete repair of pulmonary atresia with ventricular septal defect involves closing the septal defect and

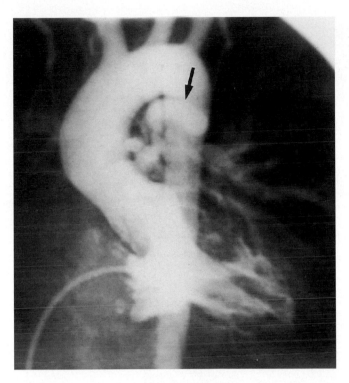

Fig. 9-82 Tetralogy of Fallot with pulmonary atresia. The right ventriculogram opacifies the aorta through the ventricular septal defect. Aortic collaterals *(arrow)* and possibly a patent ductus supply the tiny pulmonary arteries.

placing a valve conduit between the body of the right ventricle and the main pulmonary artery. Postoperative complications of this operation include false aneurysms at the suture lines and kinking or stenosis of the conduit. These complications involving the conduit are visible with right ventriculography in the frontal and lateral projections. Left ventricular function may be diminished after tetralogy repair. If an anomalous left anterior descending artery was transected, a left ventricular infarct of variable size usually ensues involving the septum, apex, or anterolateral wall. Left ventricular function may be abnormal after operation, even with normal coronary arteries and in the absence of electrocardiographic evidence of infarction.

Surgical systemic shunts to the pulmonary arteries are evaluated with selective angiography. By placing the catheter into the subclavian artery with a transfemoral retroaortic approach, you can inject a subclavian-pulmonary artery (Blalock-Taussig) shunt (Fig. 9-84). Pertinent angiographic observations include the patency of the subclavian-pulmonary arterial anastomosis, stenoses at the anastomotic site, and the distribution and size of the pulmonary arteries. With the aortic catheter passed through the anastomosis into the right pulmonary artery, a forceful injection usually causes reflux back across the anastomosis into the aorta.

Hypoplastic Left Heart Syndrome

A variety of obstructive lesions in the left side of the heart have been grouped under terms such as *hypoplasia of the aortic tract complex, hypoplastic left heart syndrome,* and *hypoplastic left ventricle syndrome.* These names describe a group of lesions that are characterized by one or more of the following: (1) mitral atresia or stenosis, (2) a small left ventricle, (3) aortic atresia or stenosis, and (4) hypoplastic aortic arch, including preductal coarctation and aortic arch interruption. Important clinical factors are the size of the left ventricle, a patent ductus arteriosus, and an atrial septal defect to decompress the pulmonary veins. There are also many associated anomalies. The clinical expression of this group of lesions is congestive heart failure in the first week of life, occasionally accompanied by mild cyanosis.

Characteristics

These lesions generally have an intra atrial communication and a patent ductus arteriosus. A small patent foramen ovale usually provides a path for passage of blood from the left atrium to the right atrium, although other types of atrial septal defects are occasionally present. The ductus arteriosus tends to be large and supplies the path for right-to-left passage of blood from the pulmonary artery to the systemic circulation. Given the increased flow through the right heart, the right atrium and right ventricle are always enlarged.

In aortic atresia with an intact ventricular septum, the left ventricle and ascending aorta are quite hypoplastic. The mitral valve may be either atretic or hypoplastic. The size of the left ventricular chamber varies from a slitlike sinus if mitral atresia is present, to a small chamber, which is frequently seen as myocardial sinusoids when the mitral valve is patent. An unusual variant occuring in about 4% of hearts with aortic atresia is that they also have a ventricular septal defect. This additional lesion allows the left ventricle to develop to nearly normal size. There may be either atresia of the mitral valve or a normally developed mitral valve in patients with aortic valve atresia and ventricular septal defects. The ventricular septal defects may include a membranous defect, complete atrioventricular canal defect, and conoventricular malalignment defect. While the ascending aorta is usually quite small when aortic valve atresia exists, it rarely may be normal-sized.

The mitral valve is atretic in about one fourth of those patients with aortic valve atresia. However, the aortic valve may be normal when the mitral valve is absent. The region of the mitral valve is represented as a membrane or fused leaflets, occasionally with a central dimple. As with aortic atresia, the left atrium is usually quite small and the right atrium, right ventricle, and pulmonary

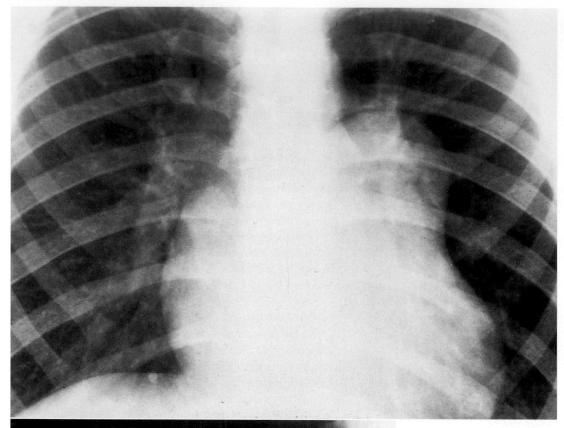

A

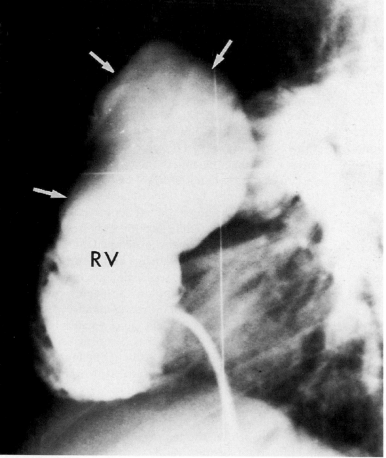

B

RV

Fig. 9-83 Aneurysm of the right ventricular outflow region after tetralogy repair. **A,** The pulmonary annulus was widened with a pericardial patch which subsequently stretched. **B,** The large patch aneurysm *(arrows)* was akinetic and extended superiorly from the body of the right ventricle *(RV)*. (Courtesy of Kenneth E. Fellows, M.D.)

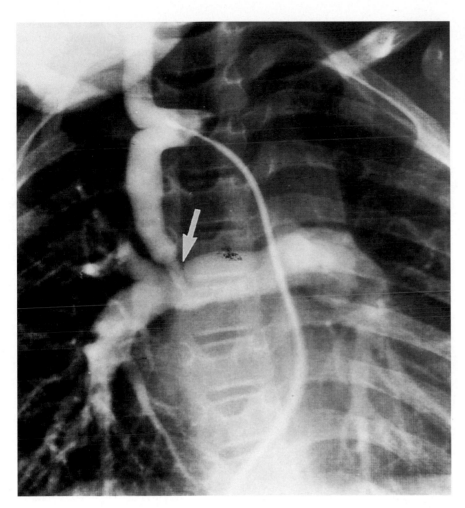

Fig. 9-84 Blalock-Taussig shunt in tetralogy of Fallot. An inferior vena cava catheter enters the right subclavian artery after going across the ventricular septal defect into the aorta. The pulmonary artery anastomosis is stenotic *(arrow).*

artery are large. In mitral atresia, transposition of the great arteries and pulmonary stenosis are frequently present. Persistent left superior vena cava and other forms of anomalous pulmonary venous connection are common. If the interatrial communication is not restrictive, the hemodynamic picture resembles that of single ventricle.

Chest film abnormalities

The typical chest film in this heterogeneous group of lesions shows a large cardiac silhouette with signs of pulmonary edema (Fig. 9-85). The right ventricle is large and may produce a configuration of a *coeur en sabot* with an uplifted apex and a lung partially interposed between the heart and the diaphragm. This appearance is also quite variable so that even with a hypoplastic left ventricle, the apex may enlarge directly to the left. In newborn infants, the size of the thoracic aorta, particularly when it is small, is impossible to determine on the chest film because the thymus obscures this region. Additionally, malpositions of a normal-sized aorta, as in transposition of the great arteries, may also have a narrow superior mediastinal silhouette. The lungs usually show signs of pulmonary edema, particularly in the perihilar regions.

The hilar vessels are usually enlarged and indistinct. For this reason, it may be difficult to distinguish venous from arterial hypertension based on vessel size.

Angiographic examination

The best initial approach is with cross-sectional echocardiography because catheterization and angiography in babies with the hypoplastic left heart syndrome are potentially hazardous. These infants usually have mild to moderate pulmonary edema. The entire systemic output passes through the patent ductus arteriosus if any part of the left heart is atretic. Passage of a catheter across the ductus may partially occlude it and can potentially cause spasm.

The standard procedure for catheterization uses either the umbilical artery line or a percutaneous transfemoral arterial line to place a catheter in the thorax for aortography. The left atrium can be entered through the atrial septal defect. The type of intracardiac angiography depends on the particular lesions present and the ability of the catheter to be manipulated into the left atrium and right ventricle. In general, a left atrial injection is useful to document mitral atresia (Fig. 9-86). When the left ventri-

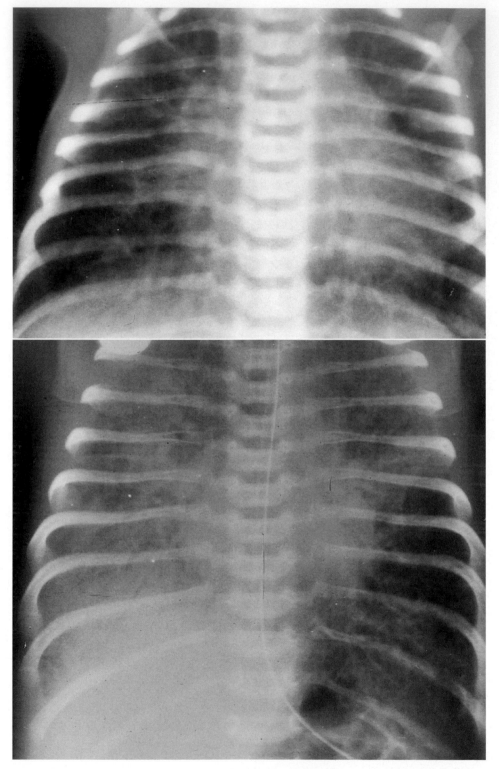

Fig. 9-85 Hypoplastic left heart syndrome with mitral atresia. **A,** The heart is enlarged and the pulmonary vessels are slightly hazy, suggesting minimal pulmonary edema. **B,** The heart is of normal size but severe pulmonary edema exists. The difference between these two patients is that the patient in **B** has a restrictive atrial septal defect which prevents decompression of the left atrial hypertension.

cle can be entered with a venous catheter placed across the interatrial communication, a left ventriculogram with a hand injection will show the size of this chamber. If, after these injections, the baby appears to be a candidate for surgery, right ventriculography may be helpful in identifying pulmonary stenosis and transposition complexes.

Aortography typically shows a hypoplastic aortic arch and ascending aorta which opacify in a retrograde direction when the catheter tip is placed in the aortic isthmus (Fig. 9-87). The contrast material in the aortic root and ascending aorta has slow washout because of the reduced, nearly absent forward flow. The absence of

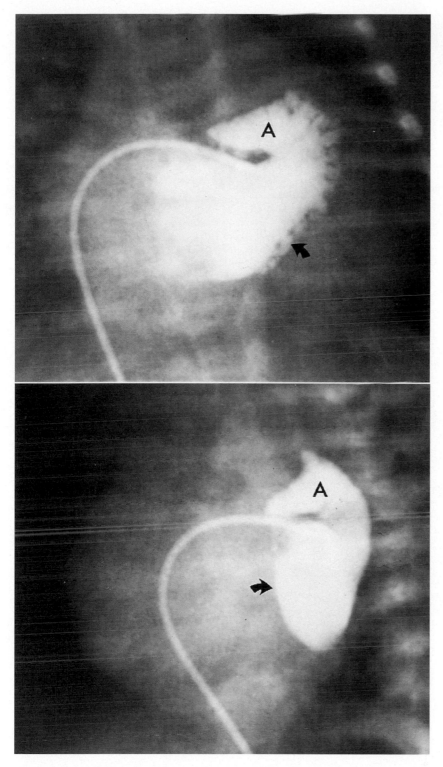

Fig. 9-86 Mitral atresia in hypoplastic left heart syndrome. Left atrial injection in the **(A)** posteroanterior and **(B)** lateral projections with the catheter passing through the atrial septal defect delineates the borders of the atretic mitral valve *(arrows)*. No contrast media passed into the left ventricle. Note the triangular left atrial appendage *(A)*.

a negative filling defect above the hypoplastic aortic valve is diagnostic of aortic atresia. If there is any forward flow through the aortic valve, a small washout of unopacified blood will occur above the aortic annulus. Usually the ductus arteriosus also fills on this retrograde injection. Failure to see the subclavian and carotid arteries may suggest an aortic arch interruption. Passing a

venous line up to the inferior vena cava and into the left atrium through the interatrial communication will document mitral atresia. The left atrium with its appendage will characteristically appear oval with no connection to the left ventricle. An occasional dimple or irregularity is seen at the atretic mitral valve. On later frames, contrast material passes across the interatrial septum to opacify

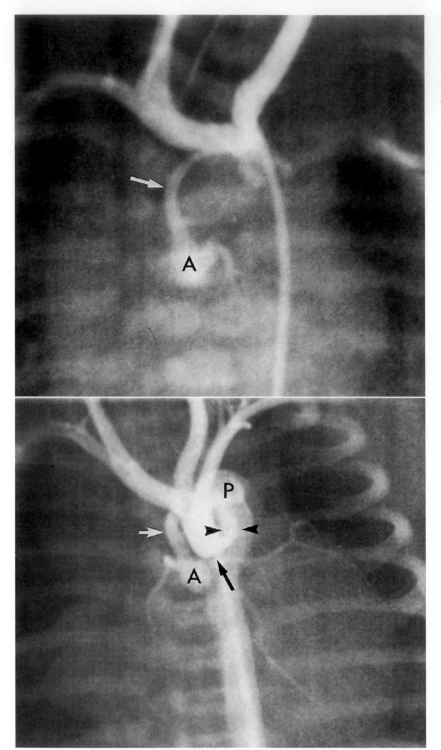

Fig. 9-87 Aortic atresia demonstrated with retrograde aortography. **A,** The aortic valve is atretic and the ascending aorta *(white arrow)* is severely hypoplastic. **B,** The main pulmonary artery *(P)* fills through a patent ductus arteriosus *(arrowheads)*. A coarctation *(black arrow)* is distal to the ductus. *A* = aortic annulus, *white arrow* = ascending aorta.

the right atrium. If a normal-sized left ventricle is encountered with aortic atresia, a ventricular septal defect probably is present, indicating the need for angled left anterior oblique projections to define the location of the defect.

MRI, in addition to ultrasound, is useful to delineate noninvasively the aorta and intracardiac defects in the hypoplastic left heart syndrome (Fig. 9-88). After light sedation, cardiac-gated images are obtained in the plane of the aorta. Additional images may be needed in the four-chamber view to image the interatrial and interventricular septa. Gradient-recalled pulse sequences with magnitude and phase reconstruction can identify small septal shunts and patency of hypoplastic valves.

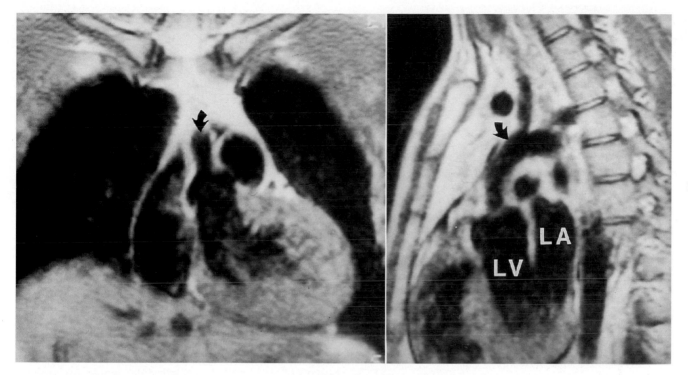

Fig. 9-88   Hypoplastic aorta. Cardiac-gated spin echo MRI in the **(A)** coronal and **(B)** lateral planes show the hypoplastic ascending aorta and arch *(arrows)*, which are 10 mm in diameter in this adult. The aortic root has normal dimensions. Severe hypertrophy of the left ventricle is seen in midsystole. *LV* = left ventricle; *LA* = left atrium.

DIFFERENTIAL DIAGNOSIS IN CONGENITAL HEART DISEASE

Pattern Recognition and Triangulation Approach

Benjamin Felson, one of the fathers of chest radiology, had his "Aunt Minnie" approach. With me, my Aunt Mary serves the same purpose. When I see her walking toward me, I do not need to analyze her hairstyle, the dress she wears, or her comfortable shoes. There is no differential diagnosis. I know in a millisecond that it is my Aunt Mary and nobody else. In cardiac radiology, some lesions are just as distinctive (Box 9-5). Of course, the more expert you are, the longer is your list of "Aunt Marys." One can debate whether a scimitar sign is present, but if it is, it is an anomalous pulmonary vein and nothing else. The more nonspecific an abnormality is on an image, the wider net that must be cast for possible diagnoses.

At least for the chest film, most patterns of cardiac disease are not uniquely diagnostic. Many image patterns are specific, for example, pulmonary edema, so a list of possible diagnoses can be made. Some images have features of more than one pattern. For example, the chest film of a patient with pulmonary artery hypertension may have features that are similar to shunt vascularity. Finally, some images do not have classifiable patterns. In spite of these

difficulties, the first step in differential diagnosis is to classify the heart shape, lung vessels, and other information on the film into one of the standard patterns.

How do you construct a differential diagnosis if the chest film shows pulmonary venous hypertension and a large left atrium? (An even harder question: How do you remember the gamut of the many abnormal patterns that are seen in heart disease?) One way is to look at the many parts of the disease and thereby construct the whole. Here is one way: First, analyze the image so that the findings can be placed into a pattern. In the foregoing example, the pattern is pulmonary venous hypertension and a large left atrium. Second, construct a list of possible diagnoses. Third, use other imaging tests or clinical information to narrow the list. In the case of pulmonary venous hypertension and a large left atrium, the major abnormality should be an obstruction at the mitral valve. Adding clinical information—the patient is an adult—puts rheumatic mitral stenosis or atrial fibrillation at the top of the list while the less common left atrial myxoma has a lower probability. But if the chest film is of an infant, then coarctation with or without the hypoplastic left heart syndrome, anomalous coronary artery from the pulmonary artery, or possibly a partial atrioventricular canal defect might constitute a short list.

Diagnosis from angiography or cross-sectional imaging is largely recognizing the cardiac and vascular structures, their connections with one another, and the abnormal physiology that results. In cardiac diagnosis, leaving aside nuclear scans, physiologic function is expressed in pulmonary vascular patterns, cardiac contraction, and valvular stenosis and regurgitation.

The five types of pulmonary patterns are:

- High output (shunt vascularity)
- Pulmonary arterial hypertension
- Pulmonary venous hypertension
- Normal
- Decreased pulmonary flow

Box 9-5   Some Common "Aunt Marys" in Cardiac Imaging

CHEST FILM

Scimitar sign of total anomalous pulmonary venous connection (TAPVC)
Anomalous origin of the left pulmonary artery from the right pulmonary artery (pulmonary sling) on the lateral view as a mass between the trachea and esophagus
Pneumopericardium
Coarctation of the aorta
Snowman sign of TAPVC to the left innominate vein

ANGIOGRAPHY

Coronary artery stenosis
Left ventricular aneurysm
Gooseneck sign of atrioventricular canal defect
TAPVC to the portal vein
Mitral valve prolapse
Domed bicuspid valves of aortic stenosis and pulmonic stenosis
Apically displaced tricuspid valve in Ebstein anomaly
Left atrial myxoma on the atrial septum
Coarctation of the aorta

ECHOCARDIOGRAPHY

Hypertrophic cardiomyopathy
Mitral valve prolapse
Left ventricular aneurysm on the four-chamber view
Domed bicuspid valves of aortic stenosis and pulmonic stenosis
Left atrial myxoma on the atrial septum
Pericardial effusion

MAGNETIC RESONANCE IMAGING

Truncus arteriosus
Aortic dissection
Coarctation of the aorta
Lipomatous hypertrophy of the interatrial septum (LHIS)
Hypertrophic cardiomyopathy in the four-chamber view
Left atrial myxoma on the atrial septum

Occasionally more than one pattern exists. For example, both shunt vascularity and pulmonary venous hypertension can be present in infants with endocardial cushion defect. The combination of the shunt vascularity and pulmonary arterial hypertension patterns constitutes the Eisenmenger reaction.

Analysis of cardiac contractility is typically expressed as an ejection fraction. To measure this quantity, end diastole and end systole must be located. The signs of diastole and systole are:

Systole	Diastole
Open aortic valve	Closed aortic valve
Closed mitral valve	Open mitral valve

End-diastolic volume is the largest ventricular volume and occurs at the peak of the atrial contraction. On a cineangiogram, the left ventricle has its largest volume at the "atrial kick" in late diastole after atrial contraction has added the last 20% of ventricular inflow. On cardiac-gated MRI, any image taken less than 100 ms from the R wave is considered an end-diastolic image. An end-systolic image is taken about 300 to 350 ms after the R wave. Do not try to judge systole or diastole by the volume of the ventricles as a middiastolic frame will record the same volume as a midsystolic one.

A jet through the valve with doming of the leaflets makes the diagnosis of a stenotic valve on magnitude-reconstructed MRI or angiographic image. However, the quantitation of the amount of stenosis is usually not accurate by these methods but can be estimated with Doppler ultrasound or phase magnetic resonance analysis.

Valve regurgitation is subjectively graded by the amount of contrast that flows backward on the angiogram or by the amount of disturbance of the backward jet as seen on color flow Doppler echocardiography or gradient echo MRI:

Grade	Severity	
1	Mild	Slight regurgitation with partial opacification of the chamber adjacent to the valve
2	Moderate	Faint opacification of the entire chamber with clearing on the next couple of beats
3	Moderately severe	Dense opacification of the chamber for several beats before clearing begins
4	Severe	Regurgitation occurs as if no valve is present. The contrast in the regurgitant chamber is more dense than the forward flow. For mitral regurgitation, left ventricular contrast flows into pulmonary veins.

Segmental Analysis

Begin the differential diagnosis by extracting all pertinent information from the image and then classify the type of pulmonary vasculature and the shape of the heart. A typical schema for chest film analysis follows:

1. Categorize the pulmonary vascular pattern
   A. Increased pulmonary flow
   B. Pulmonary artery hypertension
   C. Pulmonary venous hypertension
   D. Normal
   E. Decreased pulmonary flow
2. Mediastinal contours
   A. Pulmonary artery segment—convex, straight, or concave
   B. Cardiac apex—left- or right-sided
   C. Aorta—left- or right-sided
3. Abdomen
   A. Abdominal situs—solitus, inversus, or ambiguous

By Pulmonary Pattern

The five types of pulmonary patterns then form the beginning of a diagnostic list:

A-1. Increased pulmonary blood flow (shunt vascularity) without cyanosis
1. Atrial septal defect
   a. Secundum (at the location of a patent foramen ovale)
   b. Primum (part of atrioventricular canal defect)
   c. Sinus venosus (at junction of superior vena cava, interatrial septum, and right upper lobe pulmonary vein)
2. Ventricular septal defect
   a. Membranous, perimembranous
   b. Atrioventricular canal defect
   c. Muscular
   d. Malalignment (tetralogy of Fallot)
   e. Supracristal
3. Atrioventricular canal defect (endocardial cushion defect)
   a. Primum atrial septal defect
   b. Ventricular septal defect of the canal type
   c. Cleft anterior leaflet of mitral valve
   d. Cleft septal leaflet of tricuspid valve
4. Patent ductus arteriosus
5. Aortopulmonary septation
6. Ruptured sinus of Valsalva aneurysm with regurgitation into right atrium or right ventricle
7. Pulmonary shunts
   a. Partial anomalous pulmonary venous connection (PAPVC)

   b. Pulmonary arteriovenous fistula, small
8. Systemic shunts
   a. Iatrogenic femoral artery—vein fistula
   b. Large arteriovenous malformations
9. Noncardiac high-output states
   a. Pregnancy
   b. Anemia
   c. Thyrotoxicosis
   d. Beriberi
   e. Pheochromocytoma
   f. Paget's disease

The gamut for cyanotic heart disease classically starts with the five T's:

1. Tetralogy of Fallot
2. Transposition of the great arteries
3. Truncus arteriosus
4. Total anomalous pulmonary venous connection
5. Tricuspid atresia

Of these five, in their classic form, only tetralogy of Fallot has decreased pulmonary flow. The others have normal to increased pulmonary blood flow. Exceptions abound in congenital heart disease, so that pulmonic stenosis in any of these lesions can change the pulmonary pattern to that of decreased flow. Tetralogy of Fallot can have a shunt vascularity pattern if the pulmonary valve is absent.

A-2. Increased pulmonary blood flow (shunt vascularity) with cyanosis
1. Dextrotransposition of the great arteries
2. Total anomalous pulmonary venous connection (TAPVC) above diaphragm
3. Truncus arteriosus
4. Tricuspid atresia with transposition
5. Double-outlet right ventricle
6. Single ventricle

The pattern of pulmonary artery hypertension is enlargement of the central pulmonary arteries and normal size of the parenchymal branches. With cross-sectional imaging, the upper limit of normal of the main pulmonary artery within 2 SD is 3 cm.

B. Pulmonary Artery Hypertension
1. Eisenmenger syndrome
2. Secondary to pulmonary venous hypertension
3. Chronic pulmonary parenchymal disease
4. Pulmonary emboli from thrombi, tumor, or foreign substances
5. Primary

Pulmonary edema from congenital heart disease is caused by obstruction in or distal to the pulmonary veins. A list can be made in order of blood flow: at the pulmonary veins, left atrium, left ventricle, aortic valve, or aorta. The list can be reordered by time of presentation. Pulmonary edema within a day of birth from cardiac causes is frequently the hypoplastic left heart syndrome, TAPVC below the diaphragm, or a cardiomyopathy. At 1 week, the onset of edema is more likely a large shunt such as a patent ductus arteriosus, coarctation, or severe aortic stenosis. At 6 months, the anomalous coronary artery from the pulmonary artery causing left ventricular failure should be considered.

C. Pulmonary Venous Hypertension
  1. Hypoplastic left heart syndrome
     a. Pulmonary vein stenosis or atresia
     b. Cor triatriatum
     c. Supramitral ring
     d. Congenital mitral stenosis or atresia
     e. Hypoplastic left ventricle
     f. Aortic stenosis or atresia
     g. Hypoplastic aorta
     h. Coarctation
  2. Obstructed TAPVC (below the diaphragm)
  3. Myocarditis
  4. Left coronary artery originating from pulmonary artery leading to left ventricular infarct and failure (Bland-White-Garland syndrome)
  5. Cardiomyopathies causing increased filling pressure
     a. Dilated cardiomyopathy from myocarditis
     b. Restrictive cardiomyopathy from glycogen storage disease
     c. Hypertrophic cardiomyopathies
        1. Idiopathic hypertrophic subaortic stenosis
        2. Muscular dystrophies
  6. High-output failure
     a. Thyrotoxicosis and other metabolic diseases
     b. Peripheral arteriovenous fistulas
  7. Mediastinal tumor compressing pulmonary veins

Many cardiac lesions, if they have a trivial expression, have a normal vascular pattern. Minor valvular stenosis and regurgitations and small left-to-right shunts are common examples. Some lesions depend on age at presentation. Coarctation recognized in the newborn typically has a chest film with pulmonary edema, whereas an adult presentation will have normal lung appearance.

D. Normal Pulmonary Vascularity
  1. Left-to-right shunt with aortic-pulmonary flow less than 2:1
  2. Aortic stenosis in adults
  3. Coarctation
  4. Pulmonary stenosis
  5. Corrected transposition of the great arteries
  6. Cardiac and pericardial tumors

Decreased pulmonary flow is identified by small pulmonary arteries. The main pulmonary artery segment is concave, the hilar vessels are hypoplastic, and the parenchymal arteries and veins are difficult to see. To cause cyanosis from heart disease, the patient must have both obstruction to pulmonary blood flow and a shunt pathway causing blood to flow from the right side of the heart to the left side.

E. Decreased Pulmonary Blood Flow
  1. Tetralogy of Fallot
  2. Tricuspid atresia
  3. Ebstein anomaly and patent foramen ovale
  4. Pulmonary atresia
  5. Hypoplastic right heart syndrome
  6. Eisenmenger syndrome
  7. Any complex malformation with both obstruction to flow through the right side of the heart or pulmonary arteries *and* shunt lesion
     Examples: truncus arteriosus with pulmonary stenosis, Uhl anomaly with patent foramen ovale

By Age

After the chest film has been analyzed segmentally and the pulmonary pattern identified, the list of differential diagnoses should be ordered by the probability of the disease being present. The age at presentation and the prevalence of the disease help to complete the triangle of diagnosis: image analysis, a list of differential diagnoses, and correlation with the clinical circumstances:

In the first week
  Cardiomyopathies and myocarditis
     Intrapartum asphyxia
     Diabetes
  Hypoplastic left heart syndrome
  Interrupted aortic arch
  Myocarditis
  Obstructed TAPVC
  Transposition of the great arteries
  Tricuspid atresia
  Ebstein anomaly
  Pulmonary atresia and intact ventricular septum (duct-dependent)

In the first month
  Large patent ductus arteriosus
  Coarctation
  Atrioventricular canal defects
  Large ventricular septal defects
  Tetralogy of Fallot
  Unobstructed TAPVC
  Pulmonic stenosis, severe
  Double-outlet right ventricle
  Single ventricle

At several months
Atrial septal defects
Left coronary artery from the pulmonary artery
Truncus arteriosus
Pulmonic stenosis, moderate

At several years
Atrial septal defect
PAPVC
Coarctation
Aortic stenosis from bicuspid aortic valve

In adults
Aortic stenosis from bicuspid aortic valve
Ebstein anomaly
Pulmonic stenosis
Atrial septal defect
Aortic regurgitation from Marfan syndrome
Coarctation
Pulmonic stenosis

By Prevalence

The prevalence of acyanotic congenital heart disease is as follows:

Disease	Rate per 10,000 live births
Ventricular septal defect	14.18
Pulmonic stenosis	5.17
Endocardial cushion defect	4.03
Atrial septal defect	3.78
Aortic stenosis and bicuspid aortic valve	2.78
Coarctation of aorta	2.09
Patent ductus arteriosus	0.94

The prevalence of cyanotic congenital heart disease is as follows:

Disease	Rate per 10,000 live births
Tetralogy of Fallot	3.53
Dextrotransposition of the great arteries	2.73
Hypoplastic left heart	1.54
Tricuspid and pulmonary atresia	1.33
Truncus arteriosus	0.69
TAPVC	0.59
Double-outlet right ventricle	0.49

The overall distribution of heart malformations is as follows:

Malformation	Percent
Ventricular septal defect	28
Atrial septal defect	10
Pulmonary valve stenosis	10

The overall distribution of heart malformations—cont'd

Malformation	Percent
Patent ductus arteriosus	10
Tetralogy of Fallot	10
Aortic stenosis	7
Coarctation of the aorta	5
Transposition of the great arteries	5
Other	15
Total	100

Data from Ferencz C, Neill CA: Cardiovascular malformations: prevalence at live birth. In Freedom RM, Benson LN, Smallhorn J (eds): Neonatal heart disease, London, 1992, Springer-Verlag, and Ferencz C, Rubin JD, McCarter RJ et al: Congenital heart disease: prevalence at live birth, *Am J Epidemiol* 121:31-36, 1985.

SUGGESTED READINGS

Books

Amplatz K, Moller JH, Castaneda-Zuniga WR: *Radiology of congenital heart disease,* vol 1, New York, 1986, Thieme Medical Publishers.

Elliott LP: *Cardiac imaging in infants, children, and adults,* Philadelphia, 1991, JB Lippincott.

Emmanouilides GC, Riemenschneider TA, Allen HD et al: *Moss and Adams heart disease in infants, children, and adolescents including the fetus and young adults,* ed 5, Baltimore, 1995, Williams & Wilkins.

Farre JR: *Pathological researches. Essay I. On malformations of the heart,* London, 1814, Longman, Hurst, Rees, Orme & Brown, p 28.

Freedom RM, Benson LN, Smallhorn JF: *Neonatal heart disease,* London, 1990, Springer-Verlag.

Freedom RM, Culham JAG, Moes CAF: *Angiocardiography of congenital heart disease,* New York, 1984, Macmillan.

Higgins CB, Silverman NH, Kersting-Sommerhoff BA et al: *Congenital heart disease. Echocardiography and magnetic resonance imaging,* New York, 1990, Raven Press.

Perloff JK, Child JS: *Congenital heart disease in adults,* Philadelphia, 1991, WB Saunders.

Soto B, Pacifico AD: *Angiocardiography in congenital heart malformations,* Mount Kisco, NY, 1990, Futura.

Spindola-Franco H, Fish BG: *Radiology of the heart: cardiac imaging in infants, children, and adults,* New York, 1985, Springer-Verlag.

Swischuk LE: *Differential diagnosis in pediatric radiology,* Baltimore, 1994, Williams & Wilkins.

Swischuk LE, Sapire DW: *Basic imaging in congenital heart disease,* ed 3, Baltimore, 1986, Williams & Wilkins.

Tonkin ID: *Pediatric cardiovascular imaging,* Philadelphia, 1992, WB Saunders.

Journals

Arciniegas JG, Soto B, Coghlan HC et al: Congenital heart malformations: sequential angiographic analysis, *AJR Am J Roentgenol* 137:673, 1981.

Attie F, Soni J, Ovseyevitz J et al: Angiographic studies of atrioventricular discordance, *Circulation* 62:407, 1980.

Ayres SM, Steinberg I: Dextrorotation of the heart. An angiographic study of forty-one cases, *Circulation* 27:268, 1963.

Babbitt DP, Cassidy GE, Godard JE: Rib notching in aortic coarctation during infancy and early childhood, *Radiology* 110:169, 1974.

Baron MG, Wolf BS, Steinfeld L et al: Endocardial cushion defects: specific diagnosis by angiocardiography, *Am J Cardiol* 13:162, 1964.

Beerman LB, Park SC, Fischer DR et al: Ventricular septal defect associated with aneurysm of the membranous septum, *J Am Coll Cardiol* 5:118-123, 1985.

Blieden LC, Randall PA, Castaneda AR et al: The "gooseneck" of the endocardial cushion defect: anatomic basis, *Chest* 65:13, 1974.

Brandt PWT, Calder AL, Barratt-Boyes BG et al: Double outlet left ventricle. Morphology, cineangiographic diagnosis and surgical treatment, *Am J Cardiol* 38:897, 1976.

Bull C, DeLeval MR, Mercanti C et al: Pulmonary atresia and intact ventricular septum: a revised classification, *Circulation* 66:266, 1982.

Calcaterra G, Anderson RH, Lau KC et al: Dextrocardia—Value of segmental analysis in its categorisation, *Br Heart J* 42:497, 1979.

Calder LS, Van Praagh R, Van Praafh S et al: Truncus arteriosus communis. Clinical, angiocardiographic and pathologic findings in 100 patients, *Am Heart J* 92:23, 1976.

Carey LS, Elliot LP: Complete transposition of the great vessels. Roentgenographic findings, *AJR Am J Roentgenol* 91:529, 1974.

Collett RW, Edwards JE: Persistent truncus arteriosus: A classification according to anatomic types, *Surg Clin North Am* 29:1245, 1949.

Crupi G, Macartney FJ, Anderson RH: Persistent truncus arteriosus. A study of 66 autopsy cases with special reference to definition and morphogenesis, *Am J Cardiol* 40:569, 1977.

De la Cruz MV, Berrazueta MR, Arteaga M et al: Rules for diagnosis of atrioventricular discordances and spatial identification of ventricles. Crossed great arteries and transposition of the great arteries, *Br Heart J* 38:341, 1976.

Didier D, Higgins CB, Fisher MR et al: Congenital heart disease: Gated MR imaging in 72 patients, *Radiology* 158:227, 1986.

Dinsmore RE, Wismer GL, Guyer D et al: Magnetic resonance imaging of the interatrial septum and atrial septal defects, *AJR Am J Roentgenol* 145:697, 1985.

Dotter CT, Steinberg I: Angiocardiography in congenital heart disease, *Am J Med* 12:219, 1952.

Elliott LP, Bargeron LM Jr, Soto B et al: Axial cineangiography in congenital heart disease, *Radiol Clin North Am* 18:515, 1980.

Elliott LP, Neufeld HN, Anderson RC et al: Complete transposition of the great vessels. I. An anatomic study of sixty cases, *Circulation* 27:1105, 1963.

Fellows JE, Freed MD, Keane JF et al: Results of routine preoperative coronary angiography in tetralogy of Fallot, *Circulation* 51:561, 1975.

Figley MM: Accessory roentgen signs of coarctation of the aorta, *Radiology* 62:671, 1954.

Fisher MR, Hricak H, Higgins CB: Magnetic resonance imaging of developmental venous anomalies, *AJR Am J Roentgenol* 145:705, 1985.

Freedom RM, Culham G, Rowe RD: The criss-cross and superoinferior ventricular heart: an angiographic study, *Am J Cardiol* 42:620, 1978.

Glancy DL, Morrow AG, Simon AL et al: Juxtaductal aortic coarctation. Analysis of 84 patients studied hemodynamically angiographically and morphologically after 1 year, *Am J Cardiol* 51:537, 1983.

Gross GW, Steiner RM: Radiographic manifestations of congenital heart disease in the adult patient, *Radiol Clin North Am* 29:103, 1991.

Guit Gl, Kroon HM, van Voorthuisen AE, Steiner RM et al: Congenitally corrected transposition in adults with left atrioventricular valve incompetence, *Radiology* 155:567-570, 1985.

Ivemark BI: Implications of agenesis of the spleen on the pathogenesis of contruncus anomalies in childhood: an analysis of the heart; malformations in the splenic agenesis syndrome, with fourteen new cases, *Acta Paediatr Scand* Suppl 104:1, 1966.

Jaffe RB: Complete interruption of the aortic arch: 1. Characteristic of radiographic findings in 21 patients, *Circulation* 52:714, 1975.

Jaffe RB: Complete interruption of the aortic arch: 2. Characteristic angiographic features with emphasis on collateral circulation to the descending aorta, *Circulation* 53:161, 1976.

Jaffe RB: Systemic atrioventricular valve regurgitation in corrected transposition of the great vessels, *Am J Cardiol* 37:395, 1976.

Jaffe RB, Scherer JL: Supracristal ventricular septal defects: spectrum of associated lesions and complications, *AJR Am J Roentgenol* 128:629, 1977.

Kersting-Sommerhoff BA, Seelos KC, Hardy C et al: Evaluation of surgical procedures for cyanotic congenital heart disease by using MR imaging, *AJR Am J Roentgenol* 155:259, 1990.

Kiely B, Filler J, Stone S et al: Syndrome of anomalous venous drainage of the right lung to the inferior vena cava. A review of 67 reported cases and three new cases in children, *Am J Cardiol* 20:102, 1967.

Kirks DR, Currarino G, Chen JTT: Mediastinal collateral arteries: important vessels in coarctation of the aorta, *AJR Am J Roentgenol* 146:757, 1986.

Landing BH, Lawrence TK, Payne VC Jr et al: Bronchial anatomy in syndromes with abnormal visceral situs, abnormal spleen and congenital heart disease, *Am J Cardiol* 28:456, 1971.

Lavin N, Mehta S, Liberson M et al: Pseudocoarctation of the aorta: an unusual variant with coarctation, *Am J Cardiol* 24:584, 1969.

Leung MP, Baker EJ, Anderson RH et al: Cineangiographic spectrum of Ebstein's malformation: its relevance to clinical presentation and outcome, *J Am Coll Cardiol* 11:154-161, 1988.

Liao PK, Edwards WD, Julsrud PR et al: Pulmonary blood supply in patients with pulmonary atresia and ventricular septal defect, *J Am Coll Cardiol* 6:1343-1350, 1985.

Liberthson RR, Pennington DG, Jacobs M et al: Coarctation of the aorta: review of 234 patients and clarification of management problems, *Am J Cardiol* 43:835, 1979.

Link KM, Herrera MA, D'Souza VJ et al: MR imaging of Ebstein anomaly: results in four cases, *AJR Am J Roentgenol* 150:363, 1988.

McCartney JF, Shinebourne EA, Anderson RH: Connexions, relations, discordance, and distorsions, *Br Heart J* 38:323, 1976.

Neye-Bock S, Fellows KE: Aortic arch interruption in infancy: radio- and angiographic features, *AJR Am J Roentgenol* 135:1005, 1980.

Partridge JB, Scott O, Deverall PB et al: Visualization and measurement of the main bronchi by tomography as an objective indicator of thoracic situs in congenital heart disease, *Circulation* 51:188, 1975.

Patterson W, Baxley WA, Karp RB et al: Tricuspid atresia in adults, *Am J Cardiol* 49:141, 1982.

Piccoli GP, Gerlis LM, Wilkinson JL et al: Morphology and classification of atrioventricular defects, *Br Heart J* 42:621, 1979.

Randall PA, Moller JH, Amplatz K: The spleen and congenital heart disease, *AJR Am J Roentgenol* 119:551, 1973.

Rao PS: A unified classification for tricuspid atresia, *Am Heart J* 99:799, 1980.

Rao PS: Dextrocardia: systematic approach to differential diagnosis, *Am Heart J* 102:389, 1981.

Rose V, Izukawa T, Moes CAF: Syndromes of asplenia and polysplenia. A review of cardiac and non-cardiac malformations in 60 cases with special reference to diagnosis and prognosis, *Br Heart J* 37:840, 1975.

Rothko K, Moore GW, Hutchins GM: Truncus arteriosus malformation: a spectrum including fourth and sixth aortic arch interruptions, *Am Heart J* 99:17, 1980.

Sanders C, Bittner V, Nath PH et al: Atrial septal defect in older adults: atypical radiographic appearance, *Radiology* 167:123-127, 1988.

Sato K, Ohara S, Tsukaguchi I et al: A criss-cross heart with concordant atrioventricular-arterial connections, *Circulation* 57:396, 1978.

Shea PM, Lutz JF, Vieweg WVR et al: Selective coronary arteriography in congenitally corrected transposition of the great arteries, *Am J Cardiol* 44:1201, 1979.

Shinebourne EA, Lau KC, Calcaterra G et al: Univentricular heart or right ventricular type: clinical, angiographic and electrocardiographic features, *Am J Cardiol* 46:439, 1980.

Shinebourne EA, Macartney FJ, Anderson RH: Sequential chamber localization—Logical approach to diagnosis in congenital heart disease, *Br Heart J* 38:327, 1976.

Simpson IA, Chung KJ, Glass RF et al: Cine magnetic resonance imaging for evaluation of anatomy and flow relations in infants and children with coarctation of the aorta, *Circulation* 78:142, 1988.

Sloan RD, Cooley RN: Coarctation of the aorta. The roentgenologic aspects of one hundred and twenty-five surgically confirmed cases, *Radiology* 61:701, 1953.

Smyth PT, Edwards JE: Pseudocoarctation, kinking or buckling of the aorta, *Circulation* 46:1027, 1972.

Soto B, Bargeron LM Jr, Paacifico AD et al: Angiography of atrioventricular canal defects, *Am J Cardiol* 48:492, 1981.

Soto B, Becker AE, Moulaert AJ et al: Classification of ventricular septal defects, *Br Heart J* 43:332, 1980.

Soto B, Bertranou EG, Bream PR et al: Angiographic study of univentricular heart of right ventricular type, *Circulation* 60:1325, 1979.

Soto B, Pacifico AS, Souza AD et al: Identification of thoracic isomerism from the plain chest radiograph, *AJR Am J Roentgenol* 131:995, 1978.

Squarcia U, Ritter DG, Kincaid OW: Dextrocardia: angiographic study and classification, *Am J Cardiol* 32:965, 1973.

Stanger P, Rudolph AM, Edwards JE: Cardiac malpositions. An overview based on study of sixty-five necropsy specimens, *Circulation* 56:159, 1977.

Taussig HB: Tetralogy of Fallot: early history and late results, *AJR Am J Roentgenol* 133:423, 1979.

Thiene G, Gallucci V, Macartney FJ et al: Anatomy of aortic atresia. Cases presenting with a ventricular septal defect, *Circulation* 59:173, 1979.

Tonkin IL, Kelley MJ, Bream PR et al: The frontal chest film as a method of suspecting transposition complexes, *Circulation* 53:1015, 1976.

Tynan MJ, Becker AB, Macartney FJ et al: Nomenclature and classification of congenital heart disease, *Br Heart J* 41:544, 1979.

Van Mierop LHS, Eisen S, Schiebler GL: The radiographic appearance of the tracheobronchial tree as an indicator of visceral situs, *Am J Cardiol* 25:432, 1970.

Van Praagh R: What is the Taussig-Bing malformation? (editorial), *Circulation* 38:445, 1968.

Van Praagh R: Terminology of congenital heart disease. Glossary and commentary (editorial), *Circulation* 56:139, 1977.

Van Praagh R, Durnin RE, Jockin H et al: Anatomically corrected malposition of the great arteries (S,D,L), *Circulation* 51:20, 1975.

Van Praagh R, Van Praagh S: Isolated ventricular inversion. A consideration of the morphogenesis, definition and diagnosis of nontransposed and transposed great arteries, *Am J Cardiol* 17:395, 1966.

Van Praagh R, Van Praagh S, Nebesar RA et al: Tetralogy of Fallot: underdevelopment of the pulmonary infundibulum and its sequelae, *Am J Cardiol* 26:25, 1970.

Van Praagh R, Van Praagh S, Vlad P et al: Anatomic types of congenital dextrocardia. Diagnostic and embryologic implications, *Am J Cardiol* 13:510, 1964.

Van Praagh R, Van Praagh S, Vlad P et al: Diagnosis of the anatomic types of single or common ventricle, *Am J Cardiol* 15:345, 1965.

Wilkinson JL, Acerete F: Terminological pitfalls in congenital heart disease. Reappraisal of some confusing terms, with an account of a simplified system of basic nomenclature, *Br Heart J* 35:1166, 1973.

Winer-Muram HT, Tonkin ILD: The spectrum of heterotaxic syndromes, *Radiol Clin North Am* 27:1147, 1989.

Woodring JH, Howard TA, Kanga JF: Congenital pulmonary venolobar syndrome, *Radiographics* 14:349, 1994.

CHAPTER 10

Thoracic Aortic Diseases

Aortic Anatomy and Size

Aortic Aneurysms

Shape

Size and types

Chest film findings

Acquired Diseases

Aortic dissection

Classifications

Complications

Pathologic causes and contributing factors

Plain film findings

Tomographic imaging

Magnetic resonance imaging

Angiography

Catheter approach

Signs of dissection

Surgical treatment

Annuloaortic ectasia and Marfan syndrome

Root enlargement

Marfan syndrome presentation

Radiologic techniques

Sinus of Valsalva aneurysms

Etiology

Calcification

Complications

Aortitis

Takayasu's Aortitis

Classifications

Imaging assessment

Other types of aortitis

Ankylosing spondylitis

Behçet disease

Cardiovascular syphilis

Infected aortic aneurysms

Thoracic cardiovascular trauma

Penetrating wounds

Blunt trauma

Aortic tears

Cardiac injury

Thoracic atherosclerotic aneurysms

Appearance

Location

Imaging

Penetrating aortic ulcer

Congenital Anomalies

Left aortic arch

Right aortic arch

Double aortic arch

Pulmonary artery sling

Hemitruncus

Coarctation of the aorta

Imaging Diagnosis

Classifications

Characteristics

Chest film abnormalities

Imaging examination

Pseudocoarctation

Aortic arch interruption

Characteristics

Classifications

Chest film abnormalities

Imaging examination

Suggested Readings

Just as a primary cardiac problem can affect other organ systems, systemic disease or an abnormality in another organ system can secondarily cause cardiac dysfunction. Deciding which is the primary abnormality can pose a diagnostic dilemma. For example, in a patient with aortic regurgitation, is the cause intrinsic aortic valve disease with secondary aortic dilatation, or is it an aortic aneurysm with dilatation of the aortic annulus that prevents coaption of the aortic leaflets? It is generally better to do noninvasive tests first (such as chest radiography, computed tomography [CT], echocardiography, and magnetic resonance imaging [MRI]) before angio-

Table 10-1   Size of the normal adult thoracic aorta (cm)*

	Mean	Upper limit of normal†
Aortic root	3.7	4.0
Ascending aorta	3.2	3.7
Descending aorta	2.5	2.8

From Aronberg DJ, Glazer HS, Madsen K, et al: Normal thoracic aortic diameters by computed tomography, *J Comput Assist Tomogr* 8:247, 1984; and Drexler M, Erbel R, Muller U, et al: Measurement of intracardiac dimensions and structures in normal young adult subjects by transesophageal echocardiography, *Am J Cardiol* 65:1491, 1990.
†Two standard deviations above the mean.

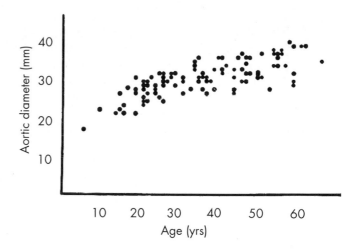

Fig. 10-1   Size of the normal ascending aorta. The diameter of the middle of the ascending aorta was measured from 100 normal angiocardiograms performed in the left anterior oblique projection. Note the wide range and increasing caliber with advancing age. (From Dotter CT, Steinberg I: The angiocardiographic measurement of the normal great vessels, *Radiology* 52:353-358, 1949.)

graphy, to examine the aorta and the aortic root. These diseases require imaging of the thoracic aorta to size the aortic annulus and to detect stenoses or enlargement of the aorta (in addition to aortic valvular stenosis), fistulas to the cardiac chambers or systemic vessels, and intrinsic aortic wall abnormalities.

AORTIC ANATOMY AND SIZE

The *sinus* part of the aorta includes the three sinuses of Valsalva above the aortic leaflets. The *aortic annulus* is that part of the fibrous skeleton of the heart to which the aortic leaflets attach. The *ascending aorta* extends from the sinuses of Valsalva to the brachiocephalic artery. The *sinotubular ridge* is the junction between the sinuses of Valsalva and the tubular ascending aorta. Most aortic diseases do not cross the sinotubular ridge but involve either the sinuses below or the ascending aorta above. The major exception is the annuloaortic ectasia seen in Marfan syndrome. The *aortic arch* is the transverse segment from which the brachiocephalic, left carotid, and left subclavian arteries originate. The *aortic isthmus* is the segment between the left subclavian artery and the ductus arteriosus or ligamentum arteriosus. The *descending aorta* begins after the ductus and ends at the aortic hiatus of the diaphragm. Most of the ascending aorta is within the pericardium.

The size of the aorta is often critical for diagnosing aortic disease. Several measurements are useful in identifying the upper range of normal. On the frontal chest film the distance between the left border of the trachea and the lateral border of the aortic arch is always less than 4 cm in adults and usually less than 3 cm in those less than 30 years of age. On an aortogram or tomographic scan of the ascending aorta, the normal diameter should be less than 4 cm (Table 10-1). Longitudinal

enlargement is more difficult to quantitate but is manifest by tortuosity, occasional kinking or buckling, and displacement into the adjacent lung or mediastinum.

The diameter of the normal adult aorta has a wide range that gradually increases with age (Fig. 10-1).

In children less than 2 months old, the aortic isthmus—that portion from the left subclavian artery to the ligamentum arteriosum—is normally smaller than the adjacent descending aorta. This appearance looks like a preductal coarctation, but actually is the normal development of the fetal aorta as it remolds following ductal closure. The increased blood flow in the fetus presumably enlarges the descending aorta adjacent to the ductus arteriosus. A normal isthmus may have a diameter equal to 40% of the ascending aorta, although most normal neonatal aortic arches are slightly larger than this.

AORTIC ANEURYSMS

Shape

Geometrically shaped like a cylinder, the aorta can dilate in two directions: radially and longitudinally. Symmetric radial dilatation is a *fusiform aneurysm*. Longitudinal enlargement causes a tortuous aorta. The term *ectatic aorta* is appropriate when the diameter of the aorta is greater than the mean but less than 2 standard deviations (SD) above the mean diameter. Ectatic aortas have both transverse and longitudinal enlargement and are seen in the elderly when the elastic media and other components of the wall are either lax or starting to degenerate.

Size and Types

There are a number of definitions of aneurysm, but most are keyed on the size at which there is potential for rupture (Fig. 10-2). An aortic diameter greater than 1.5 times normal is a commonly accepted definition of aneurysm. For practical purposes, aneurysms in the ascending aorta are greater than 5 cm and those in the descending aorta are greater than 4 cm. A *saccular aneurysm* is an eccentric dilatation that involves one side of the aorta (Fig. 10-3). For example, most infected aneurysms are saccular. The most common is a *fusiform aneurysm* that involves the entire circumference of the aorta. It can occur in a short segment or can involve the entire aorta. *True aneurysms* have all elements of the aorta incorporated into the wall of the aneurysm. *False aneurysms* have a perforation into the intima and media. An example is an aortic transection from trauma. A radiologic description of the aneurysm includes the location and extent, the type, and, in conjunction with the clinical history, the cause. Box 10-1 lists the common associations, but many aneurysms fall into several categories. Atherosclerotic aneurysms are usually fusiform and occur in the inferior parts of the aorta, but may be saccular. Infected aneurysms may be either true or false. Syphilitic aneurysms can be either saccular or fusiform.

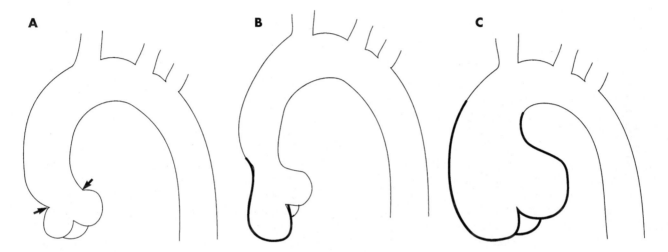

Fig. 10-2   Aortic root aneurysms. **A,** Drawing of the normal thoracic aorta, sinotubular ridge *(arrows),* and the aortic root with the sinuses of Valsalva. **B,** Aortic root aneurysm involving the right sinus of Valsalva. The aneurysm ends at the sinotubular ridge. **C,** Annuloaortic ectasia dilates uniformly all three sinuses of Valsalva and extends into the ascending aorta. The sinotubular ridge is no longer identified as a distinct notch.

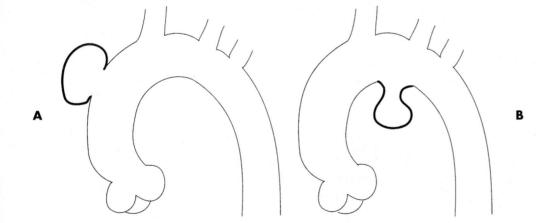

Fig. 10-3   Saccular aneurysms. **A,** The saccular aneurysm on the greater curvature of the ascending aorta has a discrete neck and involves only a small segment of the aortic circumference. **B,** The saccular aneurysm on the lesser curvature of the arch of the aorta can extend into or compress the adjacent trachea and esophagus, pulmonary arteries, pericardium, and recurrent laryngeal nerve.

Box 10-1   Aneurysms of the Thoracic Aorta

BY LOCATION

Sinuses of Valsalva

Infected
Congenital
Trauma
Annuloaortic ectasia

Ascending aorta

Aortitis
Takayasu's disease
Syphilis
Trauma
Annuloaortic ectasia
    Marfan syndrome
    Ehlers-Danlos syndrome

Aortic Arch

Trauma
Infection
Syphilis
Of patent ductus arteriosus
Coarctation
Takayasu's disease
Duct of Kommerell from aberrant right subclavian
    artery

Descending aorta

Atherosclerosis
Infected
Inflammatory
    Syphilis
    Takayasu's disease

BY SHAPE

Saccular

Trauma
Infected
Of ductus arteriosus
Syphilis
Penetrating ulcer

Fusiform

Cystic medial necrosis
Atherosclerosis

BY INTEGRITY OF THE AORTIC WALL

True

Cystic medial necrosis
Atherosclerosis
Collagen-vascular disease
    Rheumatoid arthritis
    Ankylosing spondylitis
Aortitis

False

Trauma
Infected
Penetrating ulcer
Rupture
After aortotomy

The list is not inclusive but serves as a starting point for diagnosis and management.

Chest Film Findings

The chest film is one of the first examinations obtained when thoracic aortic aneurysm, dissection, or transection is suspected, even though its sensitivity and specificity for these diagnoses are widely variable. The purpose of the chest film is to assess the size of the aorta and to identify a rupture. A valuable use of the chest film is to follow the mediastinal contours over a time interval to detect an increasing mediastinal width (Box 10-2). Tracheal or bronchial compression can be suspected when these structures are extrinsically deviated (Fig. 10-4). Compression of a pulmonary artery is recognized by unilateral pulmonary oligemia. For most of its thoracic course, the lesser curvature of the aorta is not visible on the chest film so the only signs of aortic enlargement are

Box 10-2   Chest Film Signs of Thoracic Aortic Aneurysm

Saccular mass contiguous with the aorta
Wide superior mediastinum
Rightward displacement of the ascending aorta into the
    right lung
Aortic arch diameter greater than 4 cm
Wide or tortuous left para-aortic stripe
Tracheal or bronchial deviation
Rightward deviation of the esophagus
Extrinsic compression of the trachea or esophagus

those of the greater curvature displacing adjacent structures. Other signs appear when the aorta has ruptured into the mediastinum. Unilateral pleural fluid or pericardial fluid usually indicates impending exsanguination or cardiac tamponade. Rupture into the mediastinum is ini-

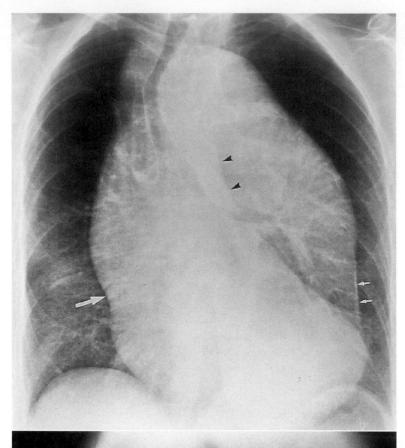

A

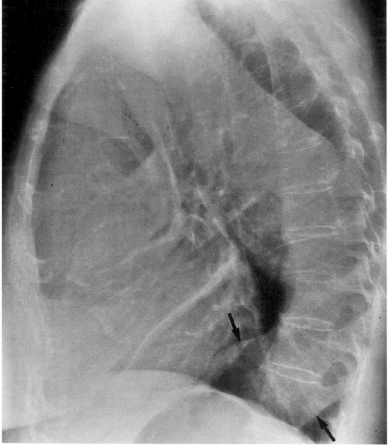

B

Fig. 10-4 Fusiform aneurysm of the entire thoracic aorta. **A,** The ascending aorta as it exits the heart *(large arrow)* extends into the right lung. The trachea is displaced to the right side and is moderately narrowed by the aortic arch. The left paravertebral stripe *(arrowheads)* represents the posterior lung as it extends into the vertebral sulcus behind the aneurysm. A streak of calcium *(small arrows)* in the intima at the interface of the lung and aorta denotes a thin aortic wall. **B,** On the lateral view the anterior mediastinum is completely filled to the retrosternal border by the ascending portion of the aneurysm. Because the descending aorta at the diaphragm still has a fusiform aneurysm *(arrows),* it is highly probable that the entire abdominal aorta also is aneurysmal.

Box 10-3   Chest Film Signs of Aortic Rupture or Transection

Left pleural cap
Wide mediastinum with obliteration of soft tissue lines
    and stripes
Wide paratracheal stripe
Unilateral pleural fluid
Large cardiac silhouette
Depression of left main stem bronchus
Deviation of nasogastric tube

---

tially constrained by the tissue in the mediastinum and pleural compartments. The chest film signs of aortic rupture are those of mediastinal hemorrhage (Box 10-3).

ACQUIRED DISEASES

Aortic Dissection

Though Morgagni recognized aortic dissection at necropsy over 200 years ago, even today it may be difficult to diagnose and it certainly remains a therapeutic enigma. Most aortic dissections, or dissecting hematomas, at least in their early stages are not aneurysms because they are not a localized enlargement of the aorta. You should reserve the term *dissecting aneurysm* for those cases in which the aorta (usually the false channel) is actually dilated. The clinical picture of a person with abrupt, severe chest pain associated with a loss of one or more peripheral pulses strongly suggests dissection; however, atypical onset of myocardial infarction, pulmonary or systemic emboli, musculoskeletal syndromes, and other chest pain syndromes may mimic the presence of aortic dissection, and therefore aortic imaging is mandatory for a definitive diagnosis. Similarly, a small percentage of dissections are "silent," occurring without pain, and are discovered only from an abnormal chest film. In these cases, other types of thoracic aneurysm, penetrating aortic ulcer, or nonvascular mediastinal disease must be distinguished from aortic dissection.

Morphologically, separation of the media from the adventitia for a variable length along the aorta characterizes dissections. Most dissections have a tear in the intima which allows a column of blood to advance and fill the false channel. A few dissections, however, have no tear in the true lumen and presumably have arisen from a hemorrhage in the vasa vasorum.

Almost all dissections arise in either the ascending aorta about a centimeter above the sinotubular ridge, or in the descending aorta at or just beyond the aortic isthmus. Spontaneous dissections that originate elsewhere in the abdominal aorta, coronary, renal, carotid, and other arterial beds are uncommon.

The intimal tear into the false channel usually is single but variations abound so that multiple entry and distal reentry tears are frequently observed by aortic imaging and at necropsy. Although most tears go distally, the aorta can dissect in a retrograde direction. If the dissection reaches the aortic root, it may rupture into the aortic root causing cardiac tamponade, occlude the right coronary artery, or create aortic regurgitation. Dissections in the ascending aorta usually follow the greater curvature of the aortic arch; the false channel forms anteriorly on the right side in the ascending aorta and then follows a spiral course to the posterior and left lateral portion of the descending thoracic aorta. Although its distal extent is quite variable, the false channel frequently proceeds on the left side to compromise the left renal artery and left iliac artery.

Classifications

The DeBakey classification is based on the extent of the dissection. Type I dissections involve the ascending aorta and extend around the arch distally. Type II dissections are limited to the ascending aorta. Type III begin beyond the arch vessels. The Stanford classification divides dissections by their proximal extent. Stanford type A are those involving the ascending aorta, regardless of whether the primary entry tear exists distally and extends in a retrograde direction into the ascending aorta. Stanford type B begin after the arch vessels and is the same as DeBakey type III. With this schema, proximal dissections are seen more frequently in necropsy series and distal dissections are reported in greater number in clinical series, probably because these patients survive longer. The distinction of proximal from distal dissection is important because patients with distal dissection have a better outcome with medical treatment, while those with proximal dissection live longer after surgical treatment.

Complications

Aortic rupture into the pericardium, pleural space, or mediastinum can be suggested on the plain chest film by a large heart diameter, pleural fluid, and a wide mediastinum. This heralds the need for immediate pericardiocentesis and other cardiopulmonary supportive measures. A dissection can partially or completely occlude a branch of the aorta by compression of the true channel by the false channel or by adjacent compression from an intimal flap. Any artery arising from the aorta can be occluded, but the right coronary artery and the three arch vessels are commonly affected. Surgical treatment aims at preventing retrograde tear into the heart and pericardium by resecting the segment that contains the entry tear. An interposition graft is then inserted, collapsing the false channel distally. Dissections in the aortic root are treated with a composite graft with the prosthetic aortic valve sewn to the graft and the coronary arteries replanted into the sides of the graft.

When there is dissection of the ascending aorta, over half the patients have aortic regurgitation which contributes to hemodynamic instability. Aortic regurgitation can be caused by an asymmetric tear that misaligns one leaflet below the other, by a tear that results in a flail leaflet, or by disruption of the annulus with subsequent lack of coaptation of the leaflets. Subsequent proximal dissection may extend into the walls of the heart, producing a fistula between the aorta and the atria or the right ventricle.

Pathologic causes and contributing factors

The cause of aortic dissection is frequently ascribed to cystic medial necrosis, although a more accurate histologic description is a degeneration of the media with loss of elastic tissue and muscle cells. Cystic medial degeneration may occur as an isolated disease or it may be part of a generalized connective tissue disease as in Marfan syndrome or Ehlers-Danlos syndrome. Cystic medial lesions are associated with Marfan syndrome, the leading cause of dissection in persons under age 40 years. The major abnormality associated with aortic dissection is systemic hypertension, which is present in about 70% of patients. Other associated abnormalities include congenital bicuspid aortic valves, coarctation of the aorta, Turner syndrome, pregnancy, and aortic surgery.

Plain film findings

The plain film findings of dissection are indirect but can suggest the need for further evaluation (Fig. 10-5). An abnormally wide mediastinum, separation of calcium from the wall of the aortic arch, a left apical pleural cap, pleural fluid, and displacement of the trachea and esophagus from the midline are important characteristics of a thoracic aortic abnormality. However, the chest film findings are insensitive for the detection of aortic dissection; nearly one fifth of patients with dissection have normal chest films.

Tomographic imaging

Computed tomography with intravenous contrast, MRI, and echocardiography all have excellent sensitivity and specificity for detecting aortic dissection, but each has limitations specific to its technology. Optimal CT imaging is with intravenous contrast on a spiral scanner (Fig. 10-6). Spiral CT requires a correctly timed bolus of contrast media and has streak artifacts from the pulsating aortic wall that can mimic the intimal flap.

Magnetic resonance imaging

MRI does not require intravenous contrast and has more options to characterize the extent of the dissection. The imaging plane can be placed parallel to that of the aorta in addition to the coronal and axial slices.

"White blood" gradient echo sequences and phase reconstruction techniques can help identify slowly flowing blood in the false channel. Its major limitation is the resolution of the arch vessels so that the distal extent of the dissection into small arteries is frequently not shown.

Because of slow blood flow, clotted false channels, and occasionally the twisted shape of the intimal flap, aortic dissection can be difficult to distinguish from other types of aneurysm and aortitis (Fig. 10-7). MRI is particularly useful in these situations because different pulse sequences and reconstruction techniques can be exploited to produce a distinction between flowing blood and static tissue. Spin echo sequences producing "black blood" images easily show the intimal flap when there is moderate flow in both channels. But in regions of slowly flowing blood, the signal in that region may be similar to tissue in the aortic wall and adjacent mediastinum. A number of techniques exist that can image very slow velocity differences and separate nonmoving and clotted blood in the false channel from slow-moving blood. Even echo rephasing, the fortuitous occurrence of velocity compensation in the second echo, is recognized as a higher signal intensity in the second echo in regions of slowly flowing blood (Fig. 10-8). A caveat is that failure of the signal intensity on the second echo to be greater than the first echo image is often observed in regions of complex velocity changes such as those that occur in vortices and eddies around bends in the aorta.

One of the most sensitive ways to make the distinction between thrombus and slowly flowing blood is to reconstruct the original data as a phase image. All MRIs are generated as complex numbers, which are typically reconstructed as magnitude images. However, the same data can be displayed as a phase image, which then becomes a picture of velocity of the tissue within each pixel. The phase image needs to be interpreted with the magnitude image in order to identify the area of concern where a thrombosed channel may be present. Changes in signal intensity, including alternating white to black phase breaks in the phase image, indicate flowing blood (Fig. 10-9).

Another strategy that can be quite helpful is to obtain a gradient echo cine study through the area that has questionable flow in the standard spin echo image. With velocity compensation, the gradient echo pulse sequence should be obtained at only one slice to avoid the inflow of partly saturated spins from a neighboring slice (Fig. 10-10).

Unlike the other techniques, transesophageal echocardiography can be done at the bedside. The major advantage over the other techniques is the quantitation of aortic regurgitation with color flow Doppler. Its disadvantage is that the aortic arch cannot be completely imaged with either the transthoracic or transesophageal technique.

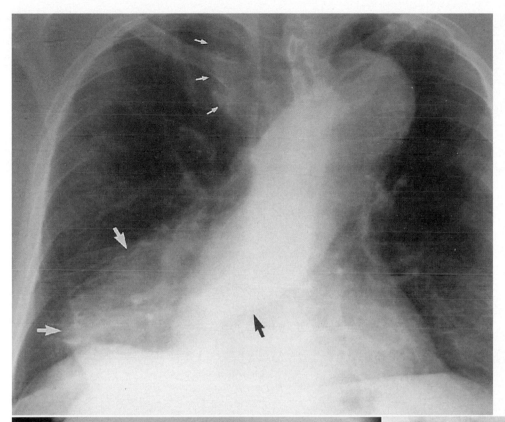

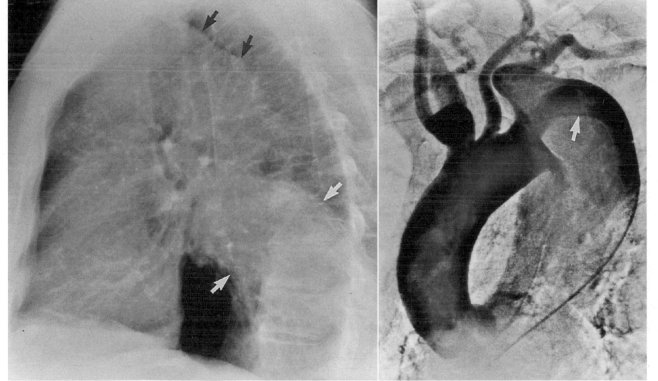

Fig. 10-5 Aortic dissection and aneurysm. **A,** The chest film shows an aortic aneurysm beginning at the aortic arch and extending distally in a tortuous aorta that crosses to the right side of the thorax *(large arrows)* before returning to the midline to enter the aortic hiatus of the diaphragm. A mass in the right paratracheal region *(small arrows)* suggests an aneurysm in the brachiocephalic artery. **B,** The lateral chest film shows a scalloped appearance to the distal aortic arch *(black arrows)*. The mass in the posterior thorax *(white arrows)* is the aorta passing in front of the spine behind the left atrium to make a bend in the right side of the chest before returning to the midline. **C,** An angiographic subtraction image shows the small brachiocephalic aneurysm. The dissection begins after the left subclavian artery with an intimal flap *(arrow)*. The superior extent of the saccular aneurysm adjacent to the left subclavian artery is also visible on the chest film in the supraclavicular region.

Angiography

When dissection is suspected, the purpose of angiography is to establish a diagnosis, visualize the proximal and distal extent, and identify serious complications. The decision whether to treat dissection medically or surgically depends on many factors. Typically, the dissection involving the proximal aorta is treated surgically and the dissection in the descending aorta is treated medically. Therefore, the thoracic image must delineate the extent of the dissection and,

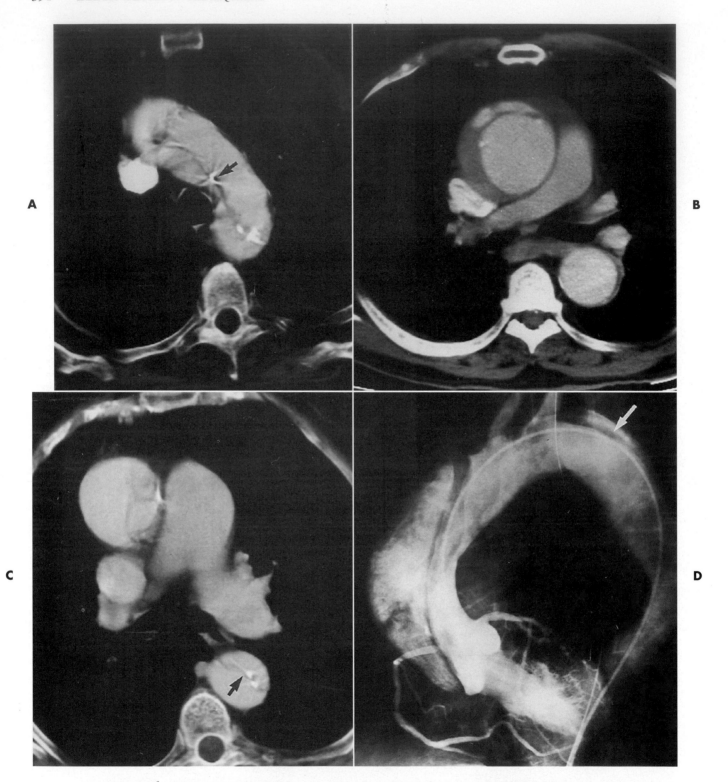

Fig. 10-6   CT signs of aortic dissection. **A,** At the aortic arch level, intravenous contrast outlines calcium *(arrow)* in the intimal flap between the two channels. **B,** A nonopacified hematoma is posterior to two components of the false channel in the ascending aorta. **C,** At the level of the main pulmonary artery, a separate dissection has a displaced, calcified intima *(arrow)*. **D,** An angiogram confirmed a type A dissection beginning in the aortic root and causing severe aortic regurgitation. Both coronary arteries fill from the true channel. A separate entry *(arrow)* after the left subclavian artery partly occludes it. (Courtesy of John A. Kaufman, M.D.)

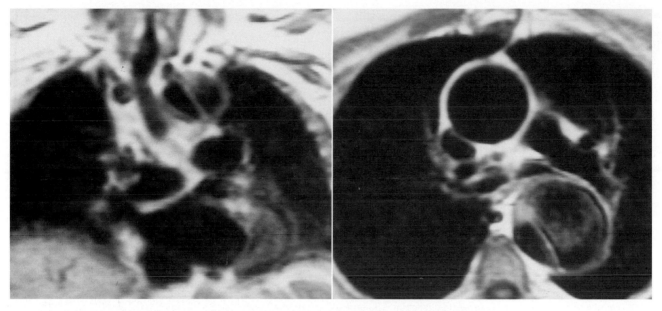

Fig. 10-7 Double-channeled aortic dissection. **A,** Spin echo images show the intimal flap in the aortic arch, which is delineated by a "black blood" signal void from flowing blood in both the true and false channel. **B,** An axial view shows the dissection limited to the descending aorta, a Stanford type B. The false channel is larger than the true channel and has some signal intensity because of slower blood velocities.

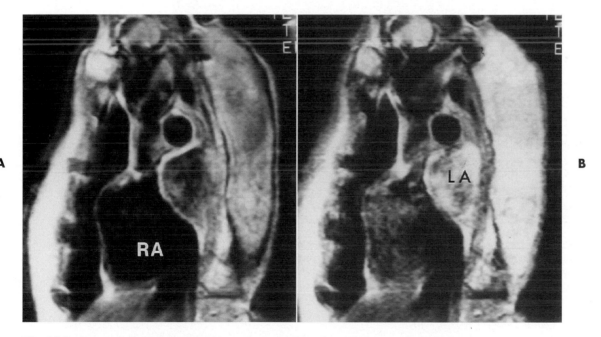

Fig. 10-8 Even-echo rephasing. Signal intensity in the false channel of an aortic dissection increases from the first echo image **(A)** to the second echo image **(B)** indicating slowly flowing blood. This effect is also seen in the left atrium *(LA)* and right atrium *(RA)*. (From Miller SW, Holmvang G: Differentiation of slow flow from thrombus in thoracic magnetic resonance imaging, emphasizing phase images, *J Thorac Imaging* 8:98-107, 1993.)

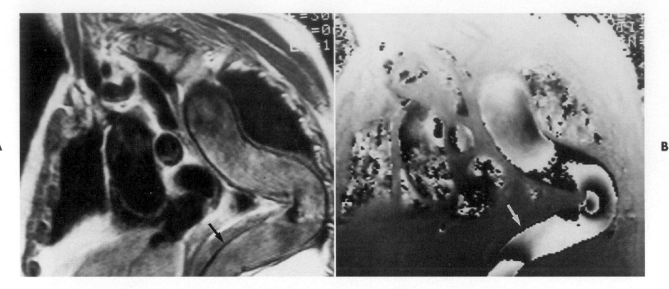

Fig. 10-9 Magnitude and phase images. **A,** Increased signal intensity from the blood is seen in a spin echo image of a tortuous aorta with an aortic dissection. The intimal flap *(arrow)* begins at the acute bend in the aorta near the diaphragm. Note the signal void in the eddy flow at the inner wall of this bend. **B,** Concentric circular phase breaks at the bend in the aorta are generated by nonuniform blood velocity. The false channel of the dissection after the bend in the aorta *(arrow)* has the same signal intensity as the adjacent mediastinum, indicating thrombosis of this channel. (From Miller SW, Holmvang G: Differentiation of slow flow from thrombus in thoracic magnetic resonance imaging, emphasizing phase images, *J Thorac Imaging* 8:98-107, 1993.)

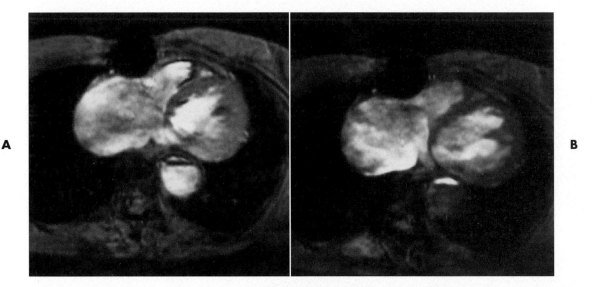

Fig. 10-10 Gradient echo cine study of aortic dissection. **A,** In midsystole there is a "white blood" signal indicating flow in the descending aorta in both the small anterior true channel and the larger posterior false channel. **B,** In diastole, the signal intensity in the false channel is almost absent, indicating much slower flow than in the anterior true channel. The variation in signal intensity in the false channel through the cardiac cycle establishes that it is not thrombosed. (From Miller SW, Holmvang G: Differentiation of slow flow from thrombus in thoracic magnetic resonance imaging, emphasizing phase images, *J Thorac Imaging* 8:98-107, 1993.)

in particular, determine if it involves the ascending aorta.

Catheter approach The site of catheterization will depend on which pulses are present. If no extremity pulses are felt, a pulmonary angiogram with delayed fol-low-through may show the dissection. However, a general principle is that angiography should be performed with an injection as close to the abnormality as possible, and therefore a femoral, axillary, or brachial arterial approach is preferred. Since the left iliac artery is most frequently involved with a dissection, the preferred route is a percutaneous transfemoral approach from the right side.

The ultimate goal is to place the catheter in the true lumen of the aorta about 2 cm above the sinotubular ridge of the aortic root. The identification of the true channel cannot always be ascertained from catheter location, the size of the channel, or the speed of blood flow alone because the false channel may compress the true channel in unusual ways. Separation of a catheter from the greater curvature of the aortic arch by a centimeter or more confirms the presence of an abnormality. The false channel generally has less flow velocity than the true channel and therefore fills later. Another sign that the false channel is opacified is that there are no arteries originating from it.

Although there has been much concern about the potential consequences of injecting into the false channel (such as possible extension of the dissection or aor-

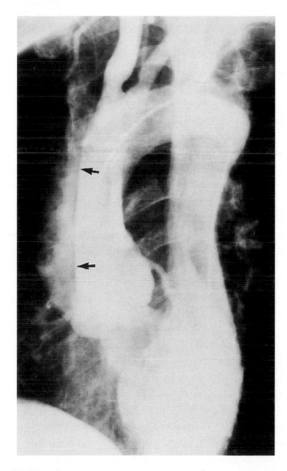

Fig. 10-11 Aortic dissection. The lucency representing the intimal flap *(arrows)* extends from the aortic root around the arch. The false channel is less dense than the true lumen and occupies the greater curvature of the aortic arch. Aortic regurgitation has opacified the left ventricle. (Courtesy of Christos A. Athanasoulis, M.D.)

tic rupture), a more important criterion for a safe angiographic injection is the rapid washout of contrast material during the test injection. This assures a large-capacity reservoir for the contrast agent, allowing a safe injection. At times, even on the final angiogram, it is not possible to determine which is the true or which is the false channel; however, you can still perform an adequate and safe angiogram as long as a high-pressure injection is not made into a cul-de-sac. Either the true or false channel may be the main conduit, and therefore filming should extend about 20 seconds to see late filling. If only one channel appears to fill, either the false channel is clotted or it is a retrograde dissection with a distal entry point. Another injection, distal to the first, in the descending aorta with filming over the thorax should opacify the false channel if it is patent. Based on clinical presentation, an abdominal aortogram may be appropriate to search for complications involving the arteries to the gut, kidneys, and legs.

Signs of dissection   The intimal flap, a lucency several millimeters thick outlined by contrast on both sides, is the hallmark of dissection. You can often identify the actual entry from one channel into another or into multiple channels, and the subsequent flow of blood in either an antegrade or retrograde direction. This intimal tear may extend only a few centimeters (Fig. 10-11) or may extend the entire length of the aorta, even into peripheral vessels (Fig. 10-12). The leaflets of the aortic valve, particularly with annuloaortic ectasia or Marfan syndrome, may be effaced and appear as a lucency; the large aortic leaflets can be difficult to distinguish from a true intimal tear in the aortic root, particularly if large-film technique is used. Cineangiography usually resolves this problem. True tears may be further differentiated by their origin above the sinotubular ridge and extension backward into the valve.

An ulcerlike projection from the aorta may represent an early sign of dissection, although other types of aneurysms, including those caused by infection and penetrating atherosclerotic ulcer, may be associated with this finding. The base of the ulcer represents the defect in the intima leading to a thrombosed false channel (Fig. 10-13). In the descending aorta where side branches originate, the ulcer may be an occlusion or detachment of the intima from an intercostal artery.

The false channel may not opacify during angiography and, therefore, may present as a thick wall (usually >1 cm) along the greater curvature of the aorta (Fig. 10-13). An eccentric wall thickness greater than 1 cm is unusual in a clotted atherosclerotic or syphilitic aneurysm or aortitis. You may occasionally see an unopacified channel if the injection was made proximal to the entry tear and the distal dissection has extended in a retrograde direction. Before the diagnosis of a thrombosed false channel is made, an injection should

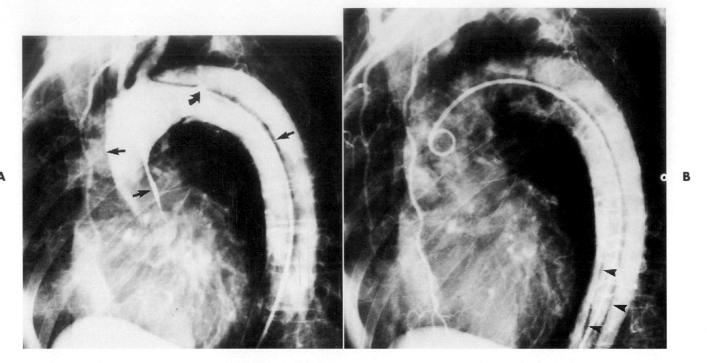

Fig. 10-12 Aortic dissection. Early **(A)** and late **(B)** films show the intimal flap *(arrows)* extending from the aortic root distally into the abdomen. The *curved arrow* points to one of several communications between the false channel on the greater curvature and the true channel medially. Note the multiple intimal tears *(arrowheads)* in the descending aorta.

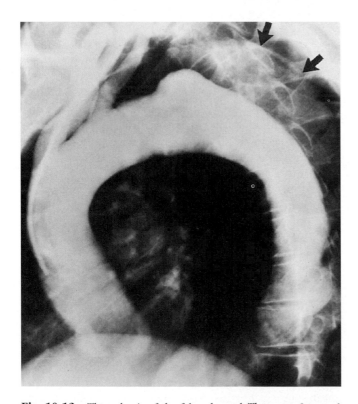

Fig. 10-13 Thrombosis of the false channel. The mass *(arrows)* on the greater curvature never opacified on delayed films. The diameter of the false channel is greater than that of the aorta. The small, saccular aneurysm in the aortic arch may represent a site of rupture into the false channel.

be made with the catheter at the level of the diaphragm to search for retrograde flow from a distant entry site. The thrombosed false channel has been called a "healed" dissection and is less liable to rupture late. Initially, the true channel is frequently smaller than the false channel, although either may enlarge to greater than the normal aortic width, then justifying the term *dissecting aneurysm.*

Aortic regurgitation may result from three mechanisms (Fig. 10-14): (1) the circumferential tear may widen the aortic root so that the leaflets cannot coapt in diastole (Fig. 10-15); (2) if the dissection is asymmetric, one leaflet may be depressed below the plane of the valve, thus producing an asymmetric regurgitation (Fig. 10-16); and (3) the leaflet may be disrupted by the false channel, producing a flail leaflet (Fig. 10-17).

In addition to occluding or transecting any vessels from the aorta, a dissection may compromise other mediastinal vessels. The expanding hematoma of the false channel may compress the right pulmonary artery. Similarly, it may both displace and compress the superior vena cava. On the left side of the mediastinum, because the false channel extends posterolaterally, the pulmonary veins are occasionally compressed. If this abnormality leads to reduced flow through the left lung, then a dissection may be confused with pulmonary embolism on a ventilation-perfusion lung scan.

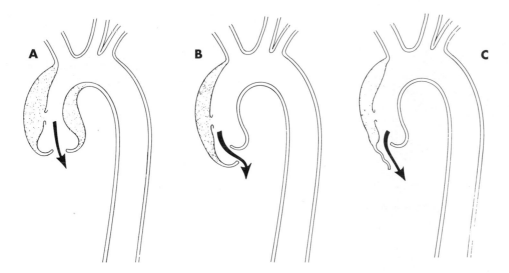

Fig. 10-14 Mechanisms of aortic regurgitation in aortic dissection. **A,** Circumferential tear with widening of the aortic root and separation of the aortic cusps. **B,** Displacement of one aortic cusp substantially below the level of the others by the pressure of the dissecting hematoma. **C,** Actual disruption of the aortic annulus leading to a flail cusp. (From Slater EE, DeSanctis RW: The clinical recognition of dissecting aortic aneurysm, *Am J Med* 60:625-633, 1976.)

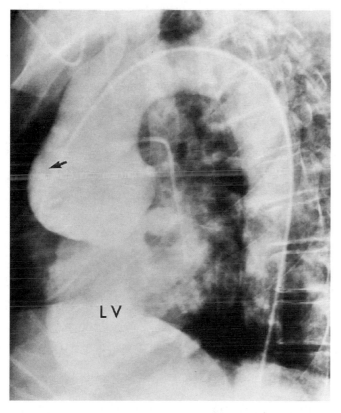

Fig. 10-15 An intimal flap *(arrow)* of a dissection in association with annuloaortic ectasia has resulted in severe regurgitation into the left ventricle *(LV)*.

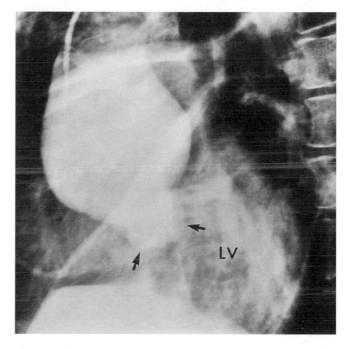

Fig. 10-16 Annuloaortic ectasia and aortic dissection, with the intimal flap seen on other films, caused prolapse of one of the aortic cusps *(arrows)*. The left ventricle *(LV)* is opacified by mild aortic regurgitation.

Surgical treatment

The primary goals of surgical treatment of dissection are to prevent extension back to the heart and pericardium and prevent aortic rupture. The usual surgical procedure in the ascending aorta is to replace it with a prosthetic graft. If there is also aortic regurgitation, a composite graft is used, consisting of an aortic valve prosthesis sewn into the proximal end of the graft; the proximal coronary arteries are then transected and replanted into the graft (Bentall procedure). Angiography after surgery may show the distal intimal flap with normal or reduced flow in the false channel, or a thrombosed false channel. Also, extension of the dissec-

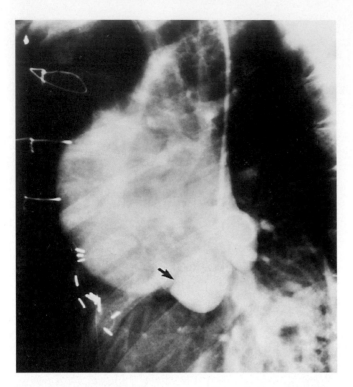

Fig. 10-17 Aortic dissection *(arrow)* occurred along with a false aneurysm from an aortotomy for an aortocoronary bypass graft. The distortion of the annulus resulted in severe aortic regurgitation.

tion, enlargement of the aneurysm, or reduction in blood flow from an aortic branch may occur in spite of the proximal graft replacement. After surgery, over 80% of dissections will retain the opacification of both the true and false lumina, suggesting the presence of additional distal fenestrations.

Annuloaortic Ectasia and Marfan Syndrome

Root enlargement

In Marfan syndrome, the sentinel vascular abnormalities in the aorta are aortic regurgitation, fusiform dilatation of the aorta, and dissection. These are represented pathologically by cystic medial necrosis. Degeneration of the aortic media leads to dilatation of the annulus. The aortic leaflets are spread apart and aortic regurgitation ensues. However, patients who do not have other features of Marfan syndrome may have annuloaortic ectasia. The term *annuloaortic ectasia* describes pear-shaped dilatation of the sinuses of Valsalva and the proximal aorta. Persons without the Marfan syndrome but with annuloaortic ectasia are usually male (by a 2:1 ratio) and are typically first seen after age 40. Those with Marfan syndrome have clinical symptoms at a much younger age. The aorta in homocystinuria may have an identical appearance.

Marfan syndrome presentation

In contrast to isolated annuloaortic ectasia, Marfan syndrome is a generalized disorder of connective tissue demonstrating autosomal dominant inheritance and manifested by cardiovascular, ocular, and skeletal abnormalities. Involvement of the cardiovascular system occurs in more than half of affected adults. Dilatation of the aortic annulus and ascending aorta are usually the first abnormal signs. Later, aortic regurgitation appears, which may ultimately cause left ventricular failure. Aortic dissection is a common complication and is frequently the cause of death. Mitral regurgitation is the most common cardiac abnormality in children and is due to redundant, elongated chordae tendineae and overly large leaflets that produce prolapse of the leaflets into the left atrium. You may occasionally see calcification of the mitral annulus in children.

Radiologic techniques

Many of the clues to the diagnosis of Marfan syndrome are frequently visible on the chest film (Fig. 10-18). On the frontal film, the thoracic cage appears large and elongated with large-volume lungs. The heart may be shifted to the left from a narrow anteroposterior thoracic diameter. In normal young adults less than 20 years of age, the aorta should be inapparent. In contrast, aortic elongation and ectasia in this age group are common signs of Marfan syndrome. Cardiomegaly is usually nonspecific and may reflect only the pectus excavatum, but aortic regurgitation from annuloaortic ectasia and mitral regurgitation from prolapsing mitral leaflets are common conditions that pathologically enlarge the heart. On the lateral film, a pectus excavatum is frequently identified as well as a narrow thoracic diameter.

Marfan patients without symptoms are easily observed with serial MRI every 6 to 12 months. Surgical referral is usually undertaken if a previously stable aortic aneurysm begins to enlarge or if the aortic arch and descending aorta exceed a diameter of 5 cm. MRI allows detection of the onset of annuloaortic ectasia (Fig. 10-19) with dilatation of the aortic root and ascending aorta, as well as visualization of a dissection. Aortic regurgitation can be observed and quantitated with velocity-encoded pulse sequences. Observations on the aortic root and quantitation of aortic regurgitation can also be made by echocardiography.

Aortography is usually reserved for urgent clinical situations where noninvasive imaging was inconclusive. Some surgeons request coronary angiography to evaluate whether a dissection extended near or into the coronary arteries. Occasionally, aortography can identify an entry site of a dissection that was not apparent on other methods (Fig. 10-20).

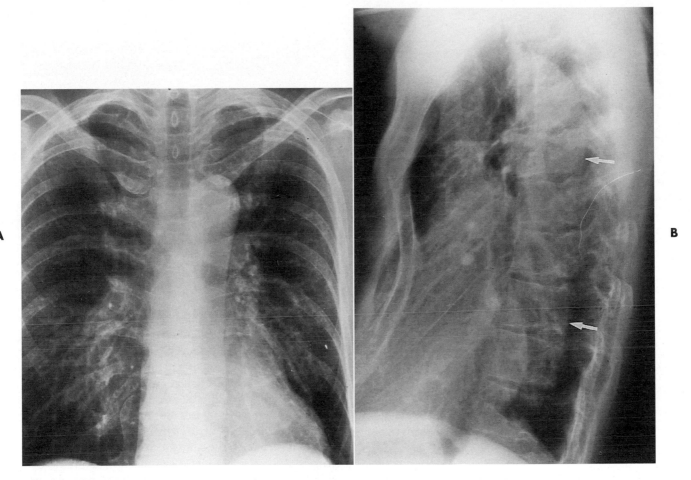

Fig. 10-18 Marfan syndrome. **A,** The elongated thorax and the apparent large lungs are nonspecific and somewhat insensitive skeletal signs. The heart has slight levocardia. The aortic arch is slightly dilated. **B,** The pectus excavatum and narrow anteroposterior diameter of the thorax have displaced the heart into the left side of the thorax. The posterior rounding of the left ventricle does not necessarily indicate enlargement but may be caused by the posterior displacement of the heart. Note the dilated aorta *(arrows)* from the arch to the diaphragm.

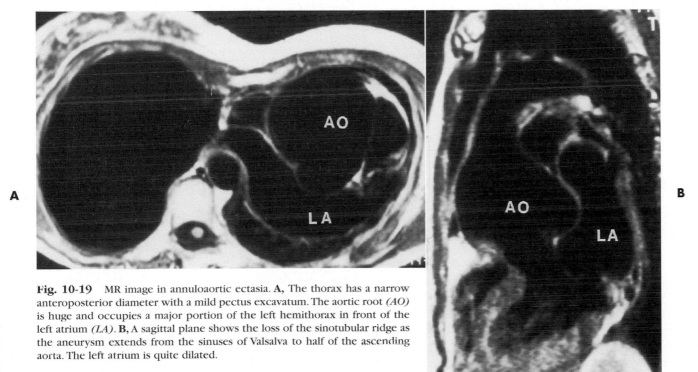

Fig. 10-19 MR image in annuloaortic ectasia. **A,** The thorax has a narrow anteroposterior diameter with a mild pectus excavatum. The aortic root *(AO)* is huge and occupies a major portion of the left hemithorax in front of the left atrium *(LA)*. **B,** A sagittal plane shows the loss of the sinotubular ridge as the aneurysm extends from the sinuses of Valsalva to half of the ascending aorta. The left atrium is quite dilated.

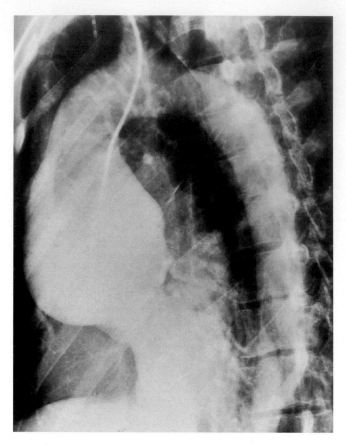

Fig. 10-20 Annuloaortic ectasia. The aneurysm involves both the sinuses of Valsalva and the proximal half of the ascending aorta. The dilatation of the annulus has secondarily caused aortic regurgitation. The left ventricle is enlarged and is densely opacified, indicating a severe degree of insufficiency.

<table>
<tr><td>

Box 10-4   Sinus of Valsalva Aneurysms

Congenital—single cusp involved with normal aorta
  Localized deficiency of the tissue in the aortic
    annulus
  Retraction of a cusp into a closing ventricular septal
    defect
Inherited—all cusps involved with annuloaortic ectasia
  Marfan syndrome
  Ehlers-Danlos syndrome
Acquired—saccular false aneurysms
  Aortic root abscess with endocarditis
  Luetic aortitis
  Aortic dissection

</td></tr>
</table>

Sinus of Valsalva Aneurysms

Etiology

Dilatation of one or all of the sinuses of Valsalva may be associated with abnormalities in the aortic valve or the aorta. These aneurysms may be classified radiologically as *discrete* (localized to the sinuses) or *annuloaortic* (involving both the aortic root and the ascending aorta). The classic type is annuloaortic ectasia with a pear-shaped configuration of the aortic root and equal dilatation of all sinuses.

An outline of sinus of valsava aneurysms is presented in Box 10-4. Discrete aneurysms that involve a single sinus are usually congenital (Fig. 10-21), although rarely dilatation of two or all three sinuses may also be congenital. These are generally less than 4 cm in diameter and involve mainly the right sinus. The tissue in the aortic annulus adjacent to the leaflet histologically has sparse fibroelastic elements and grossly may have fenestrations through the cusp. A sinus of Valsalva aneurysm can develop as a consequence of a ventricular septal defect. One of the ways a ventricular septal defect can

close spontaneously is to form fibrous tissue around its edges. As the membranous ventricular septal defect becomes smaller, the adjacent leaflet of the aortic valve is pulled inferiorly into the defect. The clinical consequence of the developing leaflet prolapse is that the left-to-right shunt through the ventricular septal defect is transformed to that of aortic regurgitation.

Acquired discrete aneurysms usually involve all three sinuses if they are a consequence of a generalized inflammatory process; for example, syphilis or an immune complex aortitis. Aortic root abscesses are actually false aneurysms since they erode through the aorta into cardiac or mediastinal tissue.

Since the sinuses of Valsalva lie completely within the cardiac silhouette, the discrete type of aneurysm is not visible on the plain chest film. If the ascending aorta is also dilated, the right side of the mediastinum will have the characteristic convexity of the aorta as it extends into the adjacent lung.

Calcification

Calcification of the sinuses of Valsalva above the aortic leaflets is rare. If there is also extensive aortic calcification, this indicates syphilitic aortitis. Mild calcification of the nondilated sinuses and flecks in the ascending aorta suggest the presence of type II hyperlipoproteinemia. Rarely, congenital or nonsyphilitic aneurysms in the aortic root may calcify.

Complications

Aortic regurgitation is the main complication of progressive dilatation of the aortic annulus and the resultant lack of coaptation of the leaflets. Any type of sinus of Valsalva aneurysm can rupture into an adjacent structure. The onset is abrupt with severe aortic regurgitation or a torrential left-to-right shunt. Most sinus aneurysms rupture into the right sinus; they perforate anteriorly into the right ventricular outflow

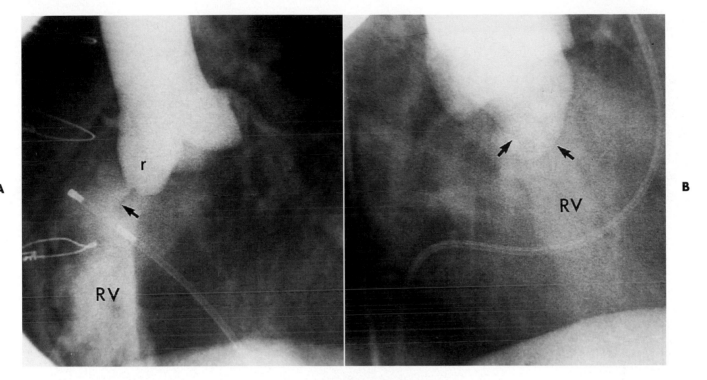

Fig. 10-21   Two examples of rupture of a congenital sinus of Valsalva aneurysm into the right ventricle *(RV)*. **A,** A supravalvular aortogram in the left oblique projection opacifies the right ventricle. The right sinus *(r)* of Valsalva is large, indicating a congenital origin. A jet *(arrow)* of contrast densely opacifies the right ventricle. No aortic regurgitation occurred. **B,** Large right sinus *(arrows)* has a "windsock" shape and extends into the right ventricle. A ventricular septal defect was present in infancy but closed spontaneously. The size of the fistulous connection is small as judged by the degree of right ventricular opacification.

tract, dissect into the ventricular septum, or perforate posteriorly in the right atrium. Aneurysms of the non-coronary sinus rupture into the right atrium. Rupture of the left sinus into the left atrial appendage is extremely rare. When an aneurysm ruptures, aortography shows contrast medium entering the cardiac chamber and opacifying downstream structures on subsequent films (Fig. 10-22). Both a left ventriculogram and an aortogram may be necessary to distinguish a ventricular septal defect with aortic regurgitation from a ruptured sinus of Valsalva aneurysm. The contrast in the right ventricle from an aortogram could have passed into the left ventricle from aortic regurgitation and then across a ventricular septal defect, or it could have flowed directly from the aorta through the rupture into the right ventricle.

Since an aneurysm of the right sinus of Valsalva can compress and distort adjacent structures, significant hemodynamic complications can occur as the aneurysm dilates. Right coronary artery compression, superior vena cava obstruction, right ventricular outflow obstruction, and endocarditis can produce dramatic clinical events.

Aortitis

A number of clinical syndromes have vasculitis that involves the aorta. Most of these diseases are either associated with or caused by immune complexes deposited in the vessel wall. Intimal proliferation and fibrosis, degeneration of the elastic fibers, round cell infiltration, and occasionally giant cells usually allow a specific histologic diagnosis. The gross changes, except in Takayasu's disease, are far less specific, regrettably so because these are the features seen on angiography and cross-sectional imaging. Aortitis produces aneurysms in many portions of the aorta and its related branches. They are usually fusiform but occasionally saccular. Takayasu's disease is the only aortitis that produces stenoses in the thoracic aorta. Significant stenoses in the aortic arch are well known in the acquired disease: aortic dissection, false aneurysms from laceration of the aortic arch after a motor vehicle accident, infected aortic aneurysms with abscess formation, Behçet's disease, and rarely atherosclerotic and syphilitic disease.

Dilatation of the ascending aorta is one of the earliest signs of aortitis, but it is not specific for aortitis because

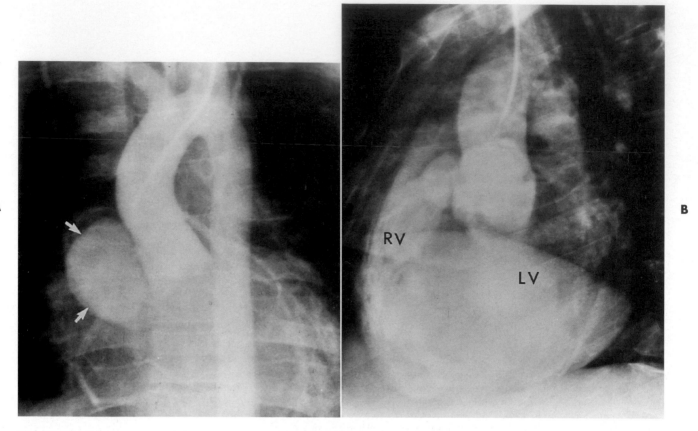

Fig. 10-22   False aneurysm of the sinus of Valsalva from aortic root infection. **A,** An unruptured abscess cavity *(arrows)* fills from the aorta and compresses the right atrium and ventricle. **B,** In a different patient, the aortic root abscess has ruptured into the right ventricle *(RV).* Aortic regurgitation is moderate. In both examples, all three sinuses of Valsalva have similar size, making a congenital etiology unlikely. The point of rupture was through the aortic annulus above the leaflet.

systemic hypertension and aortic valve disease also widen the aorta.

Takayasu's aortitis

Takayasu was a Japanese ophthalmologist who in 1908 described a woman with an unusual arteriovenous network in the retina. Similar findings and with absence of peripheral pulses have given this disease the names pulseless disease, aortic arch syndrome, middle aortic syndrome, occlusive thromboaortopathy, and atypical coarctation.

Classifications   There are four types of Takayasu's aortitis (Fig. 10-23). The Shimizu-Sano or type 1, is characterized by stenoses throughout the aortic arch and the innominate, carotid, and subclavian arteries. Type 2, or Kimoto type, shows segmental stenoses in the descending thoracic and abdominal aortas, including in the renal arteries. The Inada, or type 3, includes stenoses of both the aortic arch and the distal thoracic and abdominal aorta. Pulmonary artery stenoses with any aortic involvement define the disease as type 4. The most prevalent

type of Takayasu's disease is type 3 (55%), followed by type 2 (11%) and type 1 (8%). About half of these patients have pulmonary stenoses. Aortic regurgitation is usually mild, although it may occasionally be severe.

Imaging assessment   Because of its diffuse and widespread nature, you may need both MRI and angiography to assess its extent and severity. Biplane thoracic aortograms or gradient echo MRI will detect aortic regurgitation and aortic arch stenosis (Figs. 10-24 and 10-25). Abdominal aortography or magnetic resonance angiography will outline renal artery involvement and evaluate the arteries to the legs and gastrointestinal tract (Fig. 10-26). Occasionally, you will need angiography and ventilation-perfusion scans to assess pulmonary involvement.

The earliest change seen on the angiogram is an irregularity or narrowing of the aortic lumen even though there is no pressure gradient. MRI frequently shows a thickened aortic wall. More severe stenoses have collateral circulation with reconstitution of distal vessels. Associated aneurysms may be either saccular or fusiform and show an irregular dilatation of a long segment of the

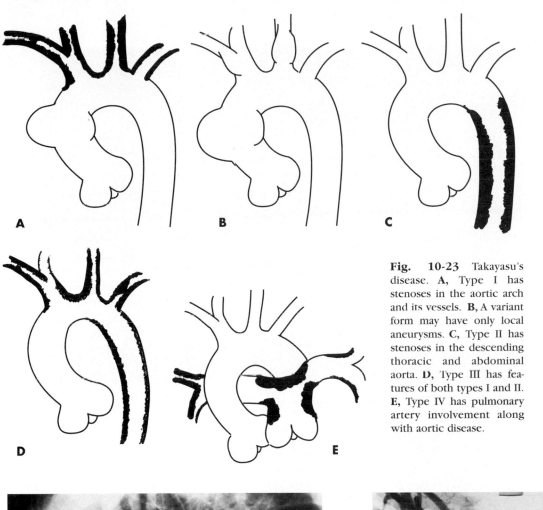

Fig. 10-23 Takayasu's disease. **A,** Type I has stenoses in the aortic arch and its vessels. **B,** A variant form may have only local aneurysms. **C,** Type II has stenoses in the descending thoracic and abdominal aorta. **D,** Type III has features of both types I and II. **E,** Type IV has pulmonary artery involvement along with aortic disease.

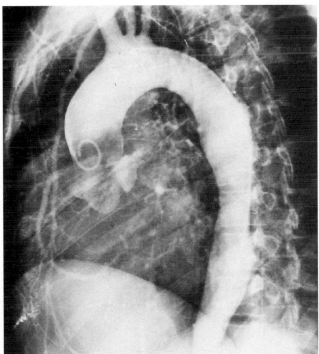

Fig. 10-24 Takayasu's aortitis. The lumen of the descending aorta is irregular and narrow from the isthmus to near the diaphragmatic hiatus.

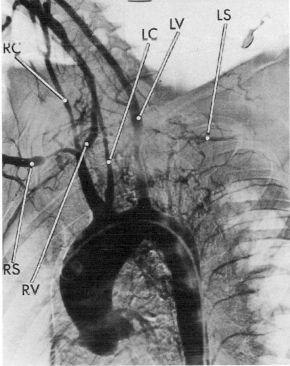

Fig. 10-25 Takayasu's arteritis. Photographic subtraction of multiple irregular and fusiform stenoses present in the subclavian, carotid, and vertebral arteries. The left subclavian artery is occluded and fills from collaterals. Note the several small mediastinal collateral vessels above the aortic arch. *RS* = right subclavian artery; *LS* = left subclavian artery; *RC* = right carotid artery; *LC* = left carotid artery; *RV* = right vertebral artery; *LV* = left vertebral artery.

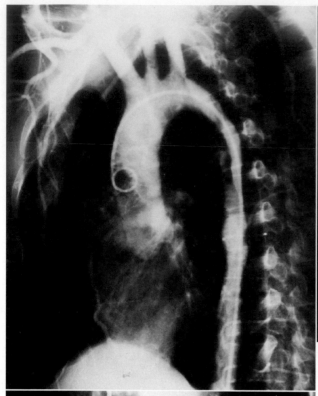

A

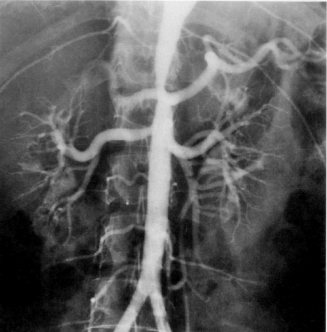

B

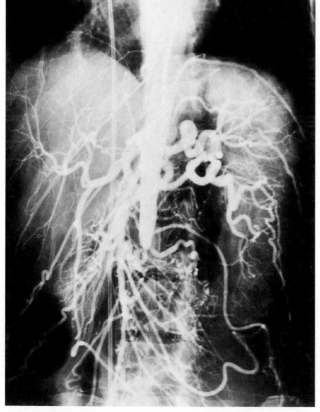

C

Fig. 10-26 Thoracoabdominal aortitis. Thoracic **(A)** and abdominal **(B)** aortograms show a stenosis in a long segment of the aorta extending across the aortic hiatus of the diaphragm. **C,** Another patient had complete occlusion of the aorta below the renal arteries. Abundant mesenteric and retroperitoneal collateral channels opacified the iliac arteries on later films.

aorta. A distal stenosis in the aorta may secondarily produce proximal aortic dilatation, so it may be difficult to distinguish a concomitant aortitis of the proximal aorta from secondary dilatation of a normal aortic wall as a result of a more distal stenosis.

Other types of aortitis

Inflammation of the media and adventitia is common in the acute phase in all types of aortitis. As healing progresses, the damaged tissue is replaced by collagen. The collagen forms part of the scar, retracts, crinkling the inti-

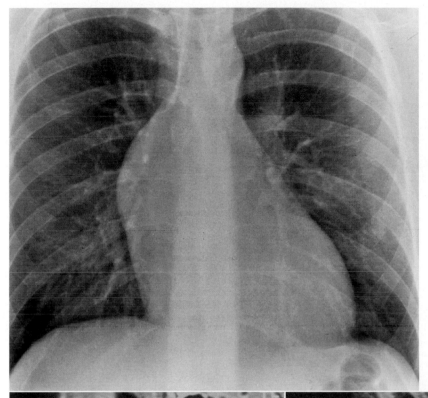

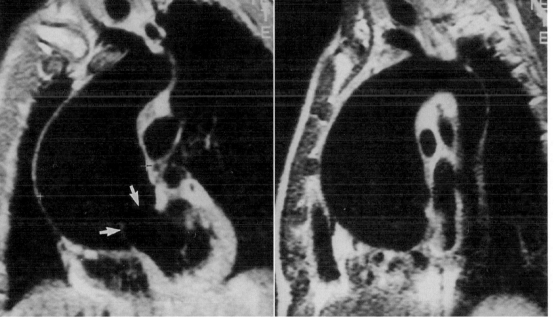

Fig. 10-27 Reiter syndrome. **A,** The aneurysmal ascending aorta projects anteriorly and obscures the right hilum. **B,** MRI with spin echo sequence in an oblique plane parallel to the aorta shows the aneurysmal ascending aorta with its thin anterior wall. The stenotic bicuspid aortic valve *(arrows)* is domed in this systolic frame. **C,** An adjacent image shows mild ectasia in the aortic arch and a normal descending aorta.

ma, and creates the "tree bark" appearance of the luminal surface of the aorta seen in all types of aortitis. Much later, superimposed atherosclerosis and degenerative calcification represent the endstage of the inflammatory process. From an imaging perspective, the aorta dilates in response to the weakened structural support of its wall (Fig. 10-27). As a rule, the ascending aorta dilates more than the arch, and the abdominal aorta is little involved (the opposite of atherosclerosis). As healing progresses, the aortic wall may become quite thick (Fig.

10-28). Aortic rupture can occur as a consequence of any type of aortic dilatation from aortitis. Aortic regurgitation mainly is from dilatation of the aortic annulus, but there may be inflammatory valvutitis and bacterial endocarditis. As listed in Box 10-5, giant cell arteritis, ankylosing spondylitis, rheumatoid arthritis, the aortitis associated with rheumatic fever, relapsing polychondritis, Reiter syndrome, and syphilis all may produce aortic regurgitation and dilatation of the ascending aorta and arch. The aorta may be involved in the collagen diseases of sys-

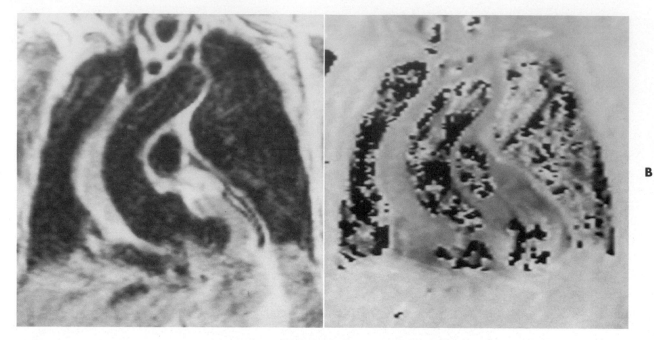

Fig. 10-28   Giant cell aortitis. **A,** A magnitude image of a spin echo image shows a high signal intensity in the thick wall of the ascending aorta. In order to distinguish slowly flowing blood from solid tissue, a phase image **(B)** was constructed that has the same gray intensity in the aortic wall as in the nonmoving chest wall, indicating no flow. The salt-and-pepper appearance of the lungs and blood in the aorta reflect a statistical noise from tissue with very low signal. A thrombosed false channel of a dissection could have a similar appearance.

Box 10-5   Diseases That May Produce Aortitis with Dilatation of the Ascending Aorta and Aortic Regurgitation

Takayasu's aortitis
Giant cell aortitis
Ankylosing spondylitis
Rheumatoid arthritis
Rheumatic fever
Relapsing polychondritis
Reiter syndrome
Syphilis
Behçet disease

---

temic lupus erythematosus, scleroderma, and rarely in ulcerative colitis or psoriasis. Although these entities pathologically and clinically are rather specific, the major angiographic finding is fusiform and symmetric dilatation of the aorta.

Ankylosing spondylitis   Ankylosing spondylitis affects that portion of the aorta behind the sinuses of Valsalva (Fig. 10-29). The process extends downward to the aortic cusps, which becomes thickened, and upward a few centimeters in the ascending aorta. Ankylosing spondylitis is one kind of severe aortitis that crosses the distinct junction of the sinotubular ridge as it dilates the aortic root and ascending aorta. In contrast to syphilis, the scarring process in ankylosing spondylitis involves the sinuses of Valsalva, both the free edge and the base of the aortic leaflets, and extends below the aortic valve to the mitral annulus. In syphilis, the scarring begins above the sinuses of Valsalva and only the free edge of the aortic valve is thickened and curled.

Behçet disease   Behçet disease is a rare vasculitis with oral, skin, and genital ulcers, eye lesions, aneurysms of the aorta and pulmonary arteries, and occlusion of the vena cava. Although any of the medium-sized and large arteries may be involved by this disease, the aorta and pulmonary arteries are the most common site (Fig. 10-30). The ostium of arteries originating from the aorta may be stenosed or occluded. The Hughes-Stovin syndrome with pulmonary aneurysms and venous thrombosis may be the same disease as Behçet's disease without the oral and genital ulcers. Other similar entities are the aortic aneurysms and brachiocephalic stenoses in Takayasu's disease.

Cardiovascular syphilis   The hallmark of cardiovascular syphilis is aortitis, which is the consequence of spirochete infection of the aortic media with subsequent inflammation and scarring. Later, focal medial necrosis ensues, along with intimal fibrous proliferation. In this late phase, there are no spirochetes, but scarring of the aortic wall and loss of elastic tissue produce a weakness in the wall, which is (paradoxically) quite thick. Superimposed on the intima is severe atherosclerosis with plaques and calcification. Both the incidence and

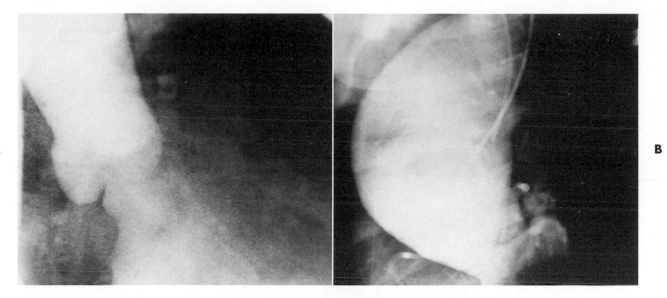

Fig. 10-29   Aortitis mainly involving the ascending aorta. **A,** Dilatation of the aortic annulus by ankylosing spondylitis has resulted in severe aortic regurgitation. **B,** Giant cell aortitis has produced a 10-cm-diameter aneurysm extending from the aortic root to the innominate artery. Moderate aortic regurgitation was present on other films.

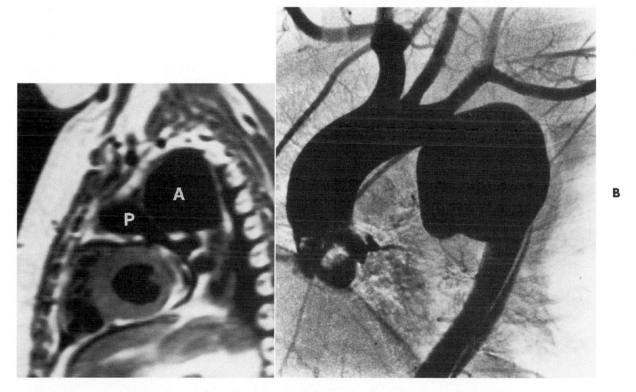

Fig. 10-30   Behçet disease. **A,** MR image shows a large aneurysm in the aortic arch *(A)* which partially compresses the left pulmonary artery *(P)* inferiorly. **B,** A photographic subtraction of the thoracic aortogram identifies the neck of the aneurysm beginning after the left subclavian artery and extending 10 cm into the descending aorta.

severity of aortitis are greatest in the ascending aorta, followed by the arch, descending aorta, and rarely, the upper abdominal aorta. This distribution differs from pure atherosclerosis, in which the lower abdominal aorta is most likely to be severely affected.

The aortitis of syphilis characteristically involves the ascending aorta and begins above the sinotubular ridge. The sinotubular ridge is preserved and does not dilate. The diagnosis of aortitis rests on two signs: calcification and dilatation. Calcification, which occurs in about 25%

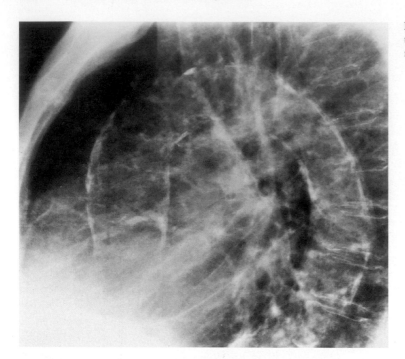

Fig. 10-31 Luetic aortitis. Extensive "eggshell" calcification extends from the aortic annulus through the entire thoracic aorta.

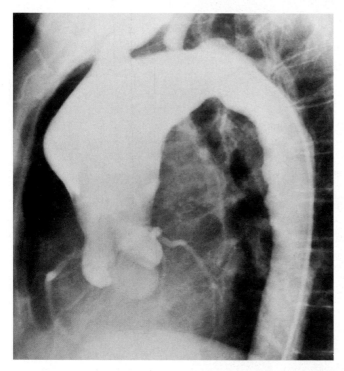

Fig. 10-32 Luetic aneurysm. The fusiform aneurysm in the ascending aorta does not involve the aortic root. The thoracic aorta was densely calcified on preliminary films. The descending aorta is unusually jagged and rough from severe superimposed atherosclerosis. The aortic leaflets are thick and have a slight jet through them. On later films, mild regurgitation opacified the left ventricle. (Courtesy of Arthur C. Waltman, M.D.)

of those with luetic aortitis, is initially thin with sharp margins. Later, when severe atherosclerosis has developed, there are larger, irregular chunks of calcium. The calcification tends to occur along the anterolateral wall

of the aorta, but in later stages involves the entire circumference (Fig. 10-31). Calcification of the ascending aorta is also seen in pure atherosclerosis and, rarely, in Takayasu's arteritis so that neither its presence nor absence is diagnostic. However, a densely calcified ascending aorta from the sinuses of Valsalva to the arch vessels is typical of the severe, superimposed atherosclerosis of cardiovascular syphilis.

Aortic aneurysm occurs in about half of patients with cardiovascular syphilis and is mainly found in the thoracic aorta (Fig. 10-32). Counting multiple aneurysms, approximately 50% occur in the ascending aorta, 30% in the arch, 15% in the descending aorta, and less than 5% in the abdominal aorta. These aneurysms may rupture into or compress the adjacent superior vena cava, bronchi, esophagus, pulmonary artery, and pleural and pericardial cavities. The sinuses of Valsalva may be the site of syphilitic aneurysms either with primary involvement or with extension of the dilated ascending aorta. In contrast to sinus dilatation from cystic medial necrosis, luetic involvement of the sinuses may be eccentric. Although the shape of the aneurysms is unpredictable, they tend to be eccentric and saccular. In the series of Steinberg and colleagues, of 60 luetic aneurysms, 43 (72%) were saccular and 17 (28%) had fusiform dilatation.

Aortic regurgitation is the most frequent complication of syphilitic aortitis, occurring in 60% of those with cardiovascular syphilis. The edges of the leaflets are also thickened and do not coapt, but calcification of the leaflets usually does not occur unless there is concomitant rheumatic or atherosclerotic disease. Regurgitation can also result from dilatation of the aortic annulus with separation of the valve commissures. Although the aortic regurgitation may be mild to severe, aortic stenosis is not a feature of aortic valve disease.

Coronary artery ostial stenosis from syphilis does not extend into the coronary artery itself, but rather results from abundant intimal thickening in the sinuses of Valsalva. Twenty-six percent of patients in Heggtveit's series had luetic coronary ostial stenosis. These stenoses may produce myocardial ischemia, but necropsy study shows little evidence that this occurs. Occasionally, the coronary arteries may be aneurysmal, a finding that may reflect the primary disease or the secondary aortic regurgitation.

Infected aortic aneurysms

In 1885, William Osler used the term *mycotic aneurysm* to describe an infectious process involving an arterial wall. This designation has been replaced by the term *infected aneurysm* to include organisms of both bacterial and fungal origin. Infected aneurysms occur in persons of all ages, although they are usually seen in adults. Aneurysms caused by bacterial infection in children are usually associated with an underlying congenital abnormality, such as coarctation of the aorta, Marfan syndrome, or sinus of Valsalva aneurysm. Such aneurysms can also arise in an aorta damaged by trauma, as from previous aortotomy or at the tip of an indwelling catheter. In adults, a predisposing condition is almost always present since aortic involvement is extremely rare in overwhelming septicemia. Bacterial endocarditis, occurring on a substrate of either congenital or rheumatic heart disease or intravenous drug addiction is a predisposing factor. Vascular

infection may also arise by contiguous spread from adjacent empyema or infected lymph nodes; this is the usual pathophysiology of a tuberculous aneurysm.

Since the shape, size, and location of an aneurysm are not specific for infection, any aneurysm is a candidate for the site of the infection in a patient with the clinical manifestations of a systemic infection. The causative organism usually is *Staphylococcus aureus, Escherichia coli,* or a *Salmonella* species and less frequently *Pseudomonas, Staphylococcus epidermidis, Streptococcus vividans,* and tuberculosis. Fungal infections with *Candida* or *Aspergillus* may occur in an immunodeficient patient.

The most prevalent site of infected aneurysm is the femoral arteries, although infections are commonly located in the thoracic and abdominal aorta. The most frequent location in the thorax is the lesser curvature of the aortic arch in the region of the ligamentum arteriosum. This type of aneurysm occurs at the junction of the aorta with a patent ductus arteriosus and at the site of a coarctation. In the latter case, the aneurysm is frequently located just distal to the coarctation since aneurysms occurring as part of the coarctation are proximal, and an aneurysm occurring in the poststenotic segment in the jet stream is prone to be infected. The aortic root is a common location for infection in patients with aortic valve disease. These aneurysms are located in the sinuses of Valsalva and extend outward into the adjacent mediastinum.

Abscesses in the valve ring within the myocardium are difficult to image (Fig. 10-33). These patients have active infective endocarditis on one or more valves, usually the aortic valve, and there is always valvular regurgi-

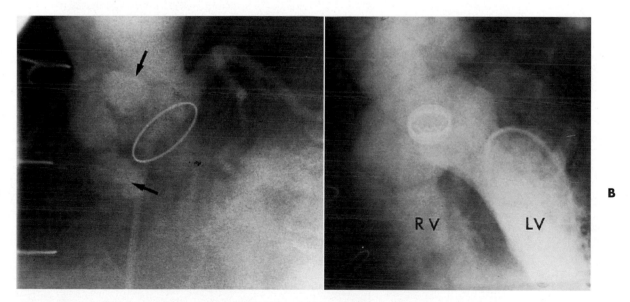

Fig. 10-33 Aortic root abscess from prosthetic endocarditis. **A,** Two saccular abscesses *(arrows)* are adjacent to a Hancock porcine aortic valve. The inferior abscess is within the interventricular septum. Moderate aortic regurgitation is present. **B,** The entire aortic root around the prosthetic aortic valve is an abscess cavity. Severe aortic regurgitation fills the left ventricle *(LV)*. A wide fistula connects the aortic root with the right ventricle *(RV)*.

tation. The angiographic detection depends on seeing the deformity of the valve ring or its displacement by the abscess cavity. In the aortic region, the valve ring abscess usually lies behind the aortic valve adjacent to the left atrium and mitral annulus (Fig. 10-34).

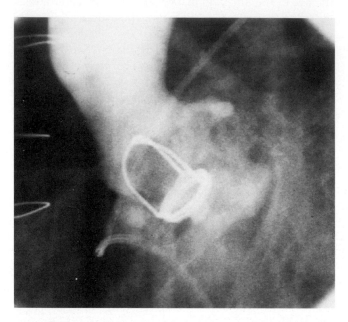

Fig. 10-34   Aortic valve ring abscess. The irregular filling of contrast medium around the Starr-Edwards aortic valve is a large necrotic cavity from endocarditis on the prosthetic valve.

An infected aneurysm is usually saccular, although it may be any shape, including fusiform (Fig. 10-35). It may not be possible to distinguish between a saccular true aneurysm and a false aneurysm that has perforated into the mediastinum. In the thorax, two thirds of these aneurysms are apparent on plain chest films that show mediastinal enlargement. Accessory findings include tracheal deviation and adjacent gas density. Infected aneurysms in the aortic root may be difficult to distinguish from the normal curvature of the sinuses of Valsalva. In these patients, you should perform biplane aortography to search for the eccentric outpouching. Because of the adjacent inflammatory response, aortic root abscesses have a thick wall which can be imaged with CT or MRI.

The natural history of infected aneurysms is expansion and subsequent rupture. Infections originating primarily in the mediastinum may rupture into adjacent structures, causing arteriovenous fistula or exsanguination into a bronchus. Rupture into the left pleural space occurs because of the left-sided descent of the descending aorta. A para-aortic mediastinal or pleural abscess may secondarily rupture into the aorta. One of the complications of a tuberculous lymph node is erosion into the aorta. Bone erosion of the anterior portion of the vertebral bodies and lateral displacement of the mediastinal lines are accessory signs of a chronic and slow-growing tuberculous aneurysm.

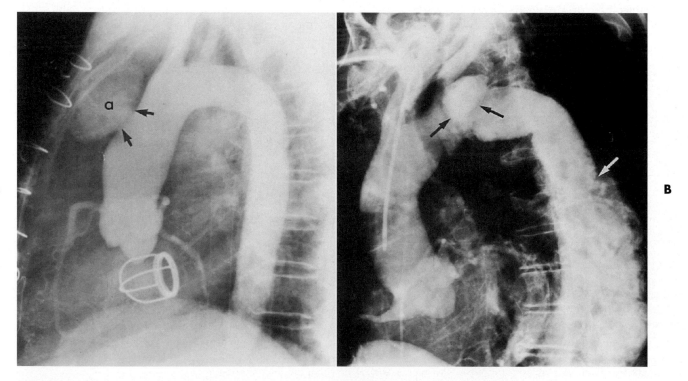

Fig. 10-35   False aneurysms. **A,** The ascending aorta is concave and displaced posteriorly by an 8-cm hematoma or abscess in the anterior mediastinum near the aortotomy site. The cavity *(a)* filled through a 1-cm defect in the aortic wall *(arrows)*. **B,** A saccular cavity *(black arrows)* developed at the proximal anastomosis of an aortic graft placed because of a dissection. The *white arrow* marks the distal anastomosis.

Thoracic cardiovascular trauma

Penetrating wounds   Since ancient times, physicians have recognized penetrating wounds of the heart and great vessels. In his *Natural History,* Pliny* wrote of Aristomenes who lived about 300 B.C.:

> It is related that certain men are born with hairy hearts, and that no others are of greater energy, for example, Aristomenes, The Messenian, who killed 300 Lacaedaemonians. Wounded and captured once, he escaped through a cave in a quarry, following the narrow passage used by foxes. Captured a second time, when his guards were overcome by sleep, he rolled to the fire and burned off his thongs together with some of his body. When he was captured a third time, the Lacaedaemonians cut out his heart while he still lived, and a hairy heart was found.

With early diagnosis and treatment, modern medical and surgical techniques have enabled some victims to survive injuries to the heart and aorta. The sequelae of penetrating wounds to the heart include cardiac tamponade, left-to-right shunts usually between the ventricles, valve injuries, true and false ventricular aneurysms, coronary artery lacerations and occlusions, and retained foreign bodies. When there is emergent surgery for stab wounds to the heart, postoperative angiography may be necessary to check for unsuspected communications between chambers or to the great vessels. When the injury penetrates the anterior chest wall, it commonly punctures the right ventricle or left anterior descending coronary artery; the left ventricle, right atrium, and left atrium are less frequently harmed.

Penetrating trauma due to medical procedures or devices is becoming increasingly common with widespread use of indwelling intravenous and interarterial catheters, including the intraaortic balloon pump. Cardiac tamponade from perforation of the right ventricle by a pacing electrode is a recognized complication of cardiac pacing. Catheter fragments may migrate to a distal vascular bed and perforate the vessel wall to form a false aneurysm or cause an arterial dissection.

The purpose of imaging in evaluating penetrating cardiovascular trauma is several fold: (1) to identify the type and extent of arterial or venous injury; (2) to identify and quantitate damage to the cardiac valves; (3) to visualize lacerations of the heart, coronary arteries, or great vessels; (4) to identify and quantitate the existence of cardiac tamponade; (5) to locate the entry and exit of arteriovenous fistulas or fistulas into other organs or nonvascular parts of the body; (6) to retrieve intravascular foreign objects; and (7) to attempt to control bleeding elsewhere (e.g., interventional angiography with catheter-controlled bleeding in pelvic fractures).

The type of imaging performed in a trauma situation obviously depends on the clinical setting. In certain kinds of trauma, multiple vascular injuries are likely to be present, for example, with gunshot wounds and severe automobile accidents. In these situations, it is wise to consider the possibility of multiple cardiac and arterial injuries and to perform adequate imaging to delineate their extent.

Blunt trauma   Blunt trauma to the heart and great vessels is frequent in severe automobile accidents in which there is high-speed deceleration on impact, in falls from a great height, and in blast and percussive injuries. If cardiac injury is absent, about 20% of these victims will survive a traumatic aortic rupture for a variable amount of time. Of those who survive, the rupture is usually at the site of the aortic isthmus, whereas in those who died it is more often in the ascending aorta.

Aortic tears   Although the aorta may be torn in any location, in over 90% of nonpenetrating trauma cases that survive the point of the laceration is the isthmus. It is here that the relatively mobile ascending aorta and arch join the rigid descending aorta which is fixed by the pleura, resulting in a plane of shear. The tears at the isthmus are usually transverse but are occasionally ragged or spiral. When the aorta is completely ruptured, the distal end may retract several centimeters so that the intervening vascular channel is composed entirely of periadventitial and pleural tissue (Fig. 10-36). Lesser injuries that may be imaged include intimal hemorrhage with laceration and, occasionally, intravascular thrombus attached to the isthmus. A partial rupture will produce a false aneurysm that is eccentric and saccular. When the laceration is complete, a traumatic aortic rupture will appear as a fusiform aneurysm, in which case the bulge represents not the vessel wall but the retropleural and mediastinal containment of the false aneurysm. As with all false aneurysms, there is the potential to expand and rupture, a process that can happen quickly or extend over many years. In the 10% of patients with traumatic rupture of the aorta from blunt trauma, the origins of the innominate, left carotid, or left subclavian arteries are injured, occasionally with other injury to the ascending aorta. The innominate artery injury may be a pseudoaneurysm at its origin or in its proximal segment. This artery may also be occluded, in which case collateral circulation comes from the circle of Willis and flows retrograde into the ipsilateral vertebral artery.

The imaging evaluation in the diagnosis of suspected aortic transection remains controversial even after hundreds of articles analyzing the role of the chest film, CT, transesophageal ultrasound, and angiography. The imaging of each patient needs to be individualized according to the amount of trauma, the cardiovascular stability of the patient, and the medical resources available. Several guidelines appear to have reasonable reliability in the triage of patients with blunt chest injury. The chest film is a useful first step in mild trauma, in addition to identifying lung and musculoskeletal injuries, because if it is

---

*Quoted in Spodick DH: Medical history of the pericardium: the hairy hearts of hoary heroes, *Am J Cardiol* 26: 447, 1970.

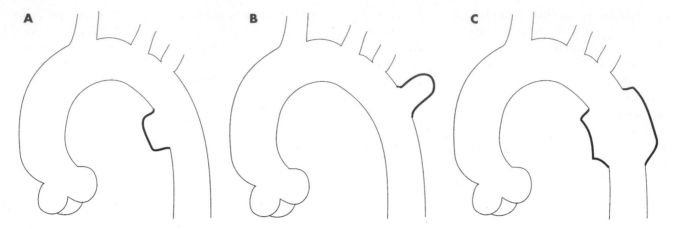

Fig. 10-36   Traumatic aortic laceration. **A,** An incomplete tear in the aortic isthmus involves only the inferior curve of the aorta. **B,** An incomplete tear may occur in the greater curve of the aorta opposite the ligamentum arteriosum. **C,** A complete transection of the aorta has a circumferential false aneurysm in the aortic isthmus.

normal with no signs of mediastinal hemorrhage, then it is quite unlikely that an aortic tear is present. If, however, in spite of the negative chest film, the amount of trauma or its mechanism was potentially sufficient to tear the aorta, then CT or angiography is required for definitive diagnosis. In like manner, normal findings on chest CT with intravenous contrast virtually exclude aortic injury. If the CT shows mediastinal widening or hemorrhage, the diagnostic possibilities are arterial injury, which requires surgery, or rupture of small mediastinal veins, which does not. In these instances, aortography, although not fool-proof, is the accepted practice (Fig. 10-37).

Cardiac injury   Blunt trauma to the heart and peri-cardium is seen indirectly on chest films with signs of cardiac tamponade and ventricular dysfunction (Box 10-6). An enlarging cardiac silhouette or pulmonary edema implies cardiac injury. In general, echocardiography and angiography are needed to analyze the site and physio-logic extent of the trauma.

Damage to the cardiac valves occurs much less fre-quently with nonpenetrating chest trauma. The aortic valve may be disrupted along the base of the leaflets or by laceration of the middle or edge of a cusp (Fig. 10-38). Damage to the mitral and tricuspid valves is rare and is associated with varying degrees of leaflet stability, culmi-nating in a flail leaflet when a papillary muscle is ruptured.

Myocardial ischemia after blunt trauma is a sign of coronary artery injury. The task of cardiac imaging is to distinguish among cardiac contusion, myocardial infarc-tion from preexisting coronary artery disease, and direct traumatic injury to the coronary artery. Coronary arteri-ography may demonstrate normal coronary arteries, indi-cating that there is a contusion of the heart. There may be coronary tears, dissections, or extrinsic stenoses from an adjacent hematoma. When an artery is transected, the distal ends constrict in a natural attempt to reduce blood

---

Box 10-6   Blunt Cardiac Trauma

PERICARDIUM

Laceration laterally with communication with the
   pleural space
Laceration of the diaphragmatic pericardium with
   herniation of the abdominal contents into the
   pericardium
Tamponade

MYOCARDIUM

Rupture
   Cardiac chamber into the pericardium
   Interventricular septum
   Papillary muscle
   Cardiac valve
Laceration or contusion
Ventricular aneurysm
   True aneurysm from coronary occlusion or from
      contusion
   False aneurysm from penetrating trauma

CORONARY ARTERIES

Laceration
Occlusion
Fistula

---

flow so that arteriographic visualization may be subtle. After injury to the coronary arteries ventriculography may show abnormalities such as ventricular aneurysm, pseudoaneurysm, or papillary muscle dysfunction. After a penetrating injury, there may be arteriovenous fistulas, either to the adjacent coronary vein or into the coronary sinus, right atrium, or right ventricle.

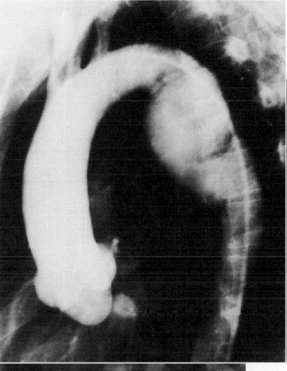

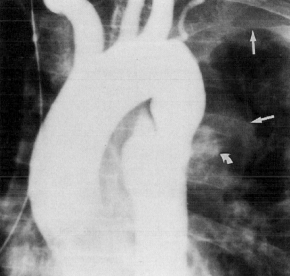

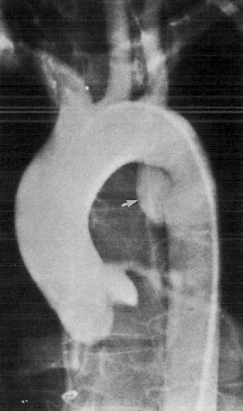

Fig. 10-37   Aortic transection from a motor vehicle accident. **A,** The complete transection is in the aortic isthmus after the left subclavian artery. The large false aneurysm represents the parietal pleura, which is the only constraining tissue preventing rupture into the pleural space. **B,** The transection occurred obliquely and produced retropleural elevation by the extending hematoma, manifested by mediastinal and apical capping *(straight arrows).* A jet of contrast media *(curved arrow)* is coming through the tear. **C,** An incomplete traumatic laceration *(arrow)* can look similar to an aortic diverticulum. Clinical history and cross-sectional imaging are needed to make this distinction.

Thoracic atherosclerotic aneurysms

Appearance   Atherosclerotic thoracic aneurysms can be either saccular or fusiform. The saccular variety involves expansion of only a portion of the wall and looks like an eccentric blister when viewed in tangent (Fig. 10-

39). The most common type is the fusiform aneurysm in which the entire aortic segment is cylindrically dilated (Fig. 10-40). The thin wall of the aortic aneurysm may appear thick because of a laminated thrombus within the sac. The aortic lumen may not be dilated if the aneurysm

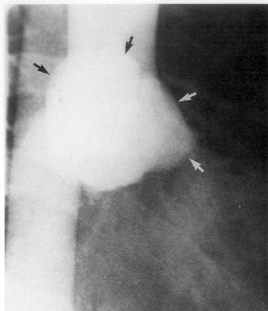

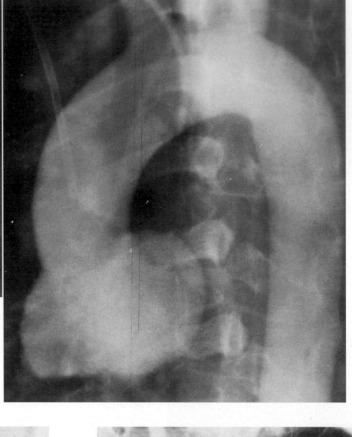

A

B

Fig. 10-38 Traumatic laceration of the aortic root. **A,** Two false aneurysms (*white* and *black arrows*) are separated by a thin membrane. The distortion of the cuspal attachments has created mild aortic regurgitation. **B,** In the left anterior oblique projection, the disrupted aortic root is expanded in both anterior and posterior directions.

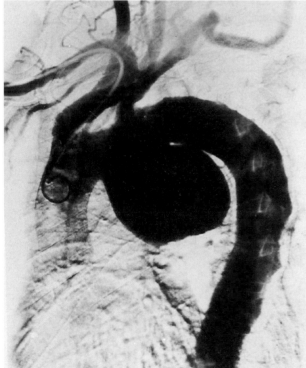

Fig. 10-39 Saccular atherosclerotic aneurysm. A photographic subtraction of an aortogram shows a 7-cm-diameter saccular aneurysm on the lesser curvature of the aortic arch. The aneurysm originates opposite the left subclavian artery and compresses and distorts adjacent mediastinal structures.

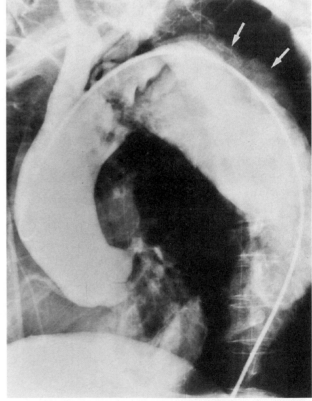

Fig. 10-40 Fusiform atherosclerotic aneurysm. The ascending aorta is mildly dilated and slight aortic regurgitation fills the left ventricle. The fusiform aneurysm extends from the left subclavian artery distally and was followed below the diaphragm on other injections. The irregular lucency in the arch is caused by poor mixing of blood and contrast media around a large plaque. Note the thick wall (*arrows*) representing intraluminal thrombus.

contains an intra-aneurysmal thrombus. In such cases, the correct diagnosis of thrombus in an aneurysm may hinge on locating intimal calcifications in the wall of the aorta, which is widely separated by thrombus from the apparent lumen, or on finding an adjacent soft tissue mass that is concentric to the aneurysm.

Location   Atherosclerosis of the thoracic aorta is usually confined to the transverse arch and descending aorta. If the entire aorta is evaluated, the greatest amount of atherosclerosis, aneurysms, and occlusions is in the infrarenal section with decreasing frequency of atherosclerotic disease in the suprarenal segment, the descending aorta, and the arch. Atherosclerotic plaques, seen angiographically as intimal irregularity and luminal narrowing, are regularly seen in persons from all countries where malnourishment is not a major problem. Fine linear calcifications in both the ascending and descending aorta are more commonly seen with uncomplicated atherosclerosis. The diseases that are associated with the greatest extent of atherosclerotic change in the ascending aorta are type II hyperlipoproteinemia, syphilis, and diabetes mellitus. In type II hyperlipoproteinemia, the calcific deposits involve the sinuses of Valsalva and aortic cusps, but rarely produce aortic stenosis. Diabetes mellitus and syphilis also may result in extensive plaques in the ascending aorta. Severe calcification confined to the ascending aorta as seen on a chest radiograph represents dystrophic calcification from any inflammatory process, including atherosclerosis. An aortitis such as Takayasu's disease may calcify after many years.

Imaging   Imaging in the diagnosis of atherosclerotic thoracic aortic aneurysms is performed with spiral CT, MRI (Fig. 10-41), or biplane angiography. With MRI, the oblique image plane can be rotated to show the entire aorta. The images should show:

- The relation of the aneurysm to adjacent mediastinal structures
- Involvement of the head and neck arteries
- The presence of associated lesions such as coarctation
- The location of other unsuspected aortic aneurysms.

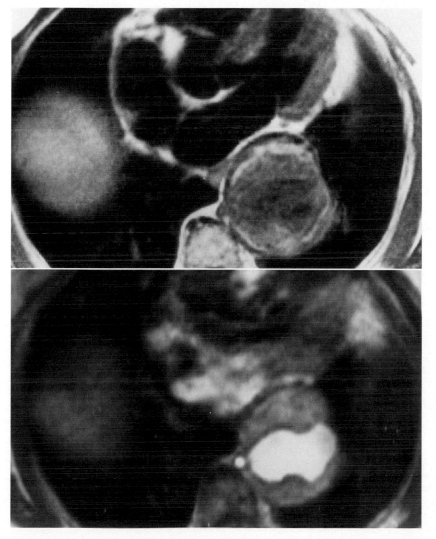

Fig. 10-41   Thoracic aortic aneurysm with thrombus. **A,** Spin echo pulse sequence poorly differentiates the lumen of the aorta from thrombus because of slowly flowing blood. **B,** With flow-related enhancement, the moving blood appears bright and is clearly distinguishable from adjacent thrombus. (From Miller SW, Holmvang G: Differentiation of slow flow from thrombus in thoracic magnetic resonance imaging, emphasizing phase images, *J Thorac Imaging* 8:98-107, 1993.)

Roughly half of those patients with thoracic aneurysms also have abdominal aneurysms. Therefore, when there is possible thoracic surgery you should perform abdominal imaging to screen for multiple aneurysms.

Penetrating aortic ulcer

One of the complications of atherosclerosis is a penetrating atherosclerotic ulcer that results when a choles-

terol plaque ruptures into the lumen of the aorta and dissects into the aortic media, disrupting the internal elastic lamina. The hematoma in the media extends for a variable distance and may penetrate the aortic wall but be contained by the adventitia. At this stage, the ulcer is a contained rupture or a pseudoaneurysm. Uncommonly, the aortic ulcer may perforate through the adventitia and rupture into the pleural space. Most penetrating aortic

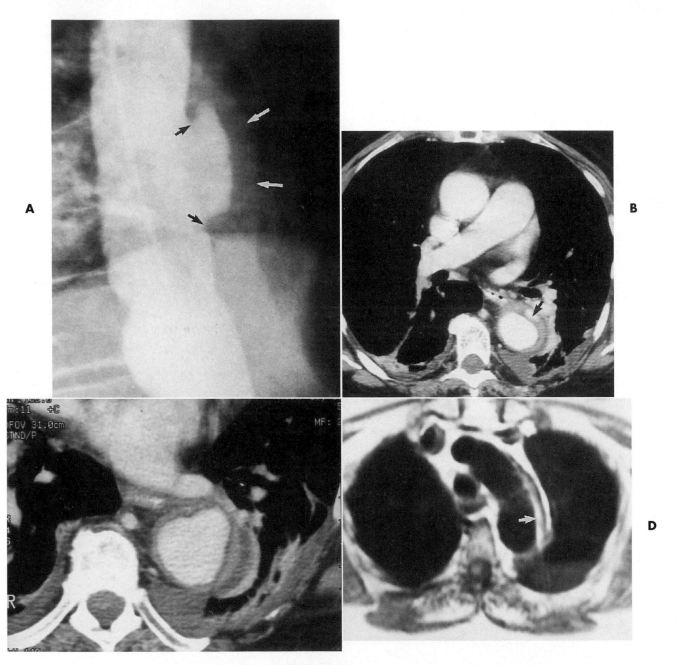

Fig. 10-42   Penetrating atherosclerotic ulcer. **A,** A lateral thoracic aortogram shows an ulcerated plaque with a broad neck *(black arrows)* near the diaphragm. A thick anterior wall *(white arrows)* displaces the para-aortic pleura anterior to the ulcer. **B,** The thick wall in the descending aorta on the CT scan has a focal region of high signal *(arrow)* and a crescentic band of lesser intensity in the dissecting hematoma. **C,** The alternating bands of signal intensity indicate hemorrhage into the aortic media. **D,** A band of high signal intensity *(arrow)* in the aortic arch on spin echo MR image is part of the extension of the penetrating ulcer. The high signal intensity reflects the subacute hemorrhage. (Courtesy of S. Mitchell Rivitz, M.D.)

ulcers occur in the descending thoracic aorta in an area of severe atherosclerosis, although rarely they are present in the ascending aorta and in the abdominal aorta.

The clinical presentation is frequently the sudden onset of severe chest pain that is similar to myocardial infarction or aortic dissection. Characteristically, these patients are elderly and have diffuse arteriosclerosis and hypertension. Coronary artery disease, cerebral vascular disease, and peripheral vascular occlusions are common features.

The chest film frequently shows diffuse or focal enlargement of the descending thoracic aorta with a widened mediastinum. If the aortic ulcer is leaking, there may be pleural effusions. On CT, penetrating ulcers appear as focal excavation within an area of mural thickening. The aortic wall is frequently thickened and displaced inward. Extensive adjacent calcification and ragged edges help to distinguish this entity from aortic dissection. Intravenous contrast may flow into a crescentic intramural hematoma which can extend into the mediastinum. Since multiple ulcers may be present, the entire aorta should be imaged.

A subacute hematoma in the wall of the aorta can be characterized with MRI by high signal intensity on both T1- and T2-weighted images. As the methemoglobin is further degraded and absorbed, the signal intensities will return to those of adjacent tissues (Fig. 10-42).

CONGENITAL ANOMALIES

The thoracic aorta and the branches from the aortic arch have many common variants. Most of these anomalies, including a mirror-image right aortic arch, produce no clinical symptoms. Aortic arch vascular malformations produce two types of symptoms: (1) dyspnea and dysphagia associated with compression of the trachea and esophagus, and (2) arterial obstruction or stenosis with signs of ischemia to the arms or head. A vascular ring is formed if the trachea and esophagus are encircled by the aortic arch and its ductus arteriosus and branches. All of these anomalies are rare, but a few of the more common variations will be illustrated.

The imaging evaluation of a suspected vascular ring begins with a chest film and a barium esophagogram. The right aortic arch is easily identified on adult chest films. A posterior indentation of the barium-filled esopohagus at the level of the aortic arch suggests a retroesophageal vascular structure. A small imprint implies a retroesophageal subclavian artery and a larger impression is the aorta between the esophagus and spine. Double aortic arch usually has a higher and larger impression on the right side of the esophagus compared with the smaller and inferior left-sided convexity. Most complex arch anomalies require cross-sectional imaging or angiography to

map the entire anomaly prior to surgery. These anomalies can be difficult to analyze and frequently require multiple projections. With angiography, cranially angled oblique views will project the ductus below the aortic arch. With MRI, coronal, axial, and oblique views in the plane of the aorta arc needed to trace each vascular structure through the mediastinum in relation to the trachea.

Left Aortic Arch

There are many normal variations of the origins of the aortic arch arteries. The right and left carotid arteries, the right and left subclavian arteries, and the left vertebral artery can all originate separately from the aortic arch or be joined or originate with their nearest neighbor. An aberrant right subclavian artery is seen in about 1% of persons and usually goes behind the esophagus but may pass between the esophagus and trachea or may go anterior to the trachea (Fig. 10-43). The origin of the right subclavian artery, if it is dilated, is called a diverticulum of Kommerell (Fig. 10-44).

The *aortic diverticulum* is on the inferior curvature of the aortic arch in the isthmus (Fig. 10-45). In the embryo the right side of the double aortic arch rejoined the left arch to form the descending aorta. The aortic diverticulum is the obliterated end of the right arch. A *ductus diverticulum* is the obliterated aortic end of the ductus arteriosus. These diverticula may enlarge and be confused with an aortic aneurysm or a traumatic laceration.

Right Aortic Arch

The right aortic arch passes to the right side of the trachea and esophagus and usually recrosses to the left side posteriorly in the middle of the thorax behind the right

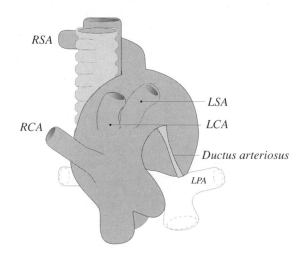

Fig. 10-43 Left aortic arch with aberrant right subclavian artery going behind the esophagus. *RSA* = right subclavian artery; *RCA* = right carotid artery; *LSA* = left subclavian artery; *LCA* = left carotid artery; *LPA* = left pulmonary artery.

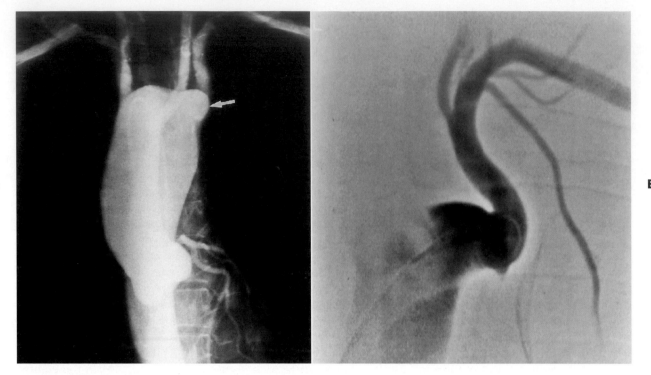

Fig. 10-44   Diverticulum of Kommerell. **A,** An anteroposterior angiogram shows a round convexity *(arrow)* at the origin of the left subclavian artery. **B,** An oblique angiogram with the catheter at the origin of the left subclavian artery shows its large conical origin. A diverticulum of Kommerell can also exist at the origin of an aberrant right subclavian artery with a left arch and an aberrant left subclavian artery with a right arch.

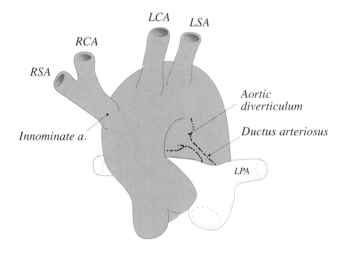

Fig. 10-45   Left aortic arch with aortic diverticulum connected to a left ductus arteriosus. *RSA* = right subclavian artery; *RCA* = right carotid artery; *LCA* = left carotid artery; *LSA* = left subclavian artery; *LPA* = left pulmonary artery.

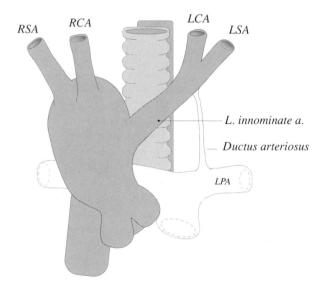

Fig. 10-46   Right aortic arch with mirror-image branching.

pulmonary artery to descend into the abdomen on the left side. If the heterotaxia syndrome is present, the aortic arch may continue on the right side into the abdomen.

Mirror-image branching from a right aortic arch is almost always associated with congenital heart disease. The order of origin of the branches is typically a left bra-

chiocephalic artery, right carotid artery, and right subclavian artery (Fig. 10-46). The ductus arteriosus goes from the left subclavian artery to the left pulmonary artery in front of the trachea and does not cause a vascular ring. About 25% to 50% of patients with truncus arteriosus will have a right aortic arch with mirror-image branching, and about 25% with tetralogy of Fallot will have this type of right aortic arch. A rare variation of mirror-image branching with right aortic arch has an aortic diverticulum behind the esophagus, which connects with the left ductus arteriosus, completing the vascular ring.

The most common type of right aortic arch has an aberrant retroesophageal left subclavian artery (Fig. 10-47). If a left ductus connects this left subclavian artery to the left pulmonary artery, a vascular ring is formed. Although there is a potential for compression of the trachea and esophagus if a left ductus persists, most patients are asymptomatic. The incidence of congenital heart disease with this type of right arch is less than 2%.

An unusual right aortic arch anomaly has a stenosis in the left subclavian artery. The left subclavian artery may arise from the left pulmonary artery (isolation of the left subclavian artery) or may have a stenosis near the aortic diverticulum (Fig. 10-48).

A right aortic arch is identified on the chest film as a right paratracheal mass which displaces both the trachea and esophagus leftward (Fig. 10-49). The barium-filled esophagus is displaced anteriorly on the lateral film if there is an aberrant left subclavian artery. The para-aortic stripe in the upper middle mediastinum is present on the right side and absent on the left. In the lower thorax above the diaphragm the aorta crosses to the left side and the left para-aortic stripe again becomes visible. On CT and MRI the aortic arch arteries can be traced from their origins to map their position in relation to the trachea and esophagus (Fig. 10-50).

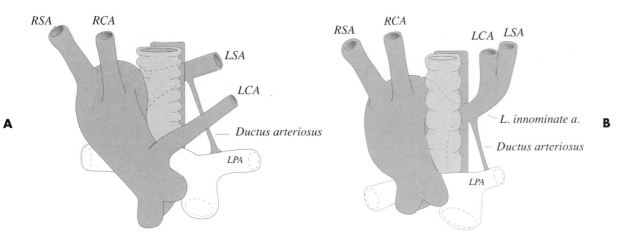

Fig. 10-47 Right aortic arch with an aberrant retroesophageal left subclavian artery (**A**), and a retroesophageal aortic isthmus and aberrant left innominate artery (**B**).

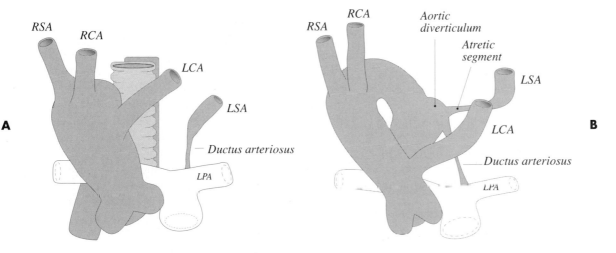

Fig. 10-48 Left subclavian artery stenosis associated with right aortic arch. **A,** The left subclavian artery originates from a left ductus arteriosus (isolation of the left subclavian artery). If the left ductus is closed, the left subclavian artery blood comes from a subclavian steal from retrograde flow down the left vertebral artery from the circle of Willis. **B,** A stenotic or atretic proximal segment of the left subclavian artery originates from an aortic diverticulum.

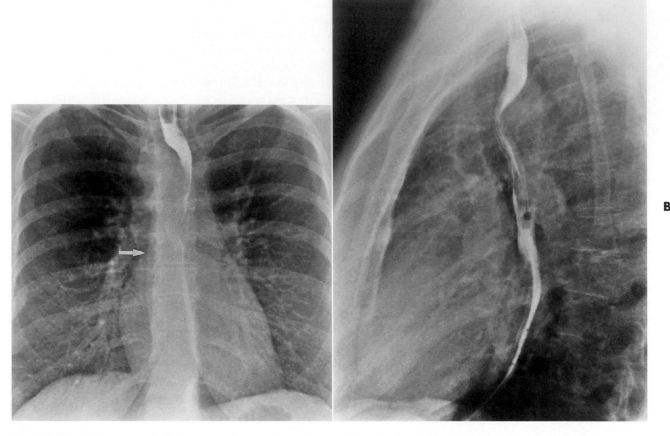

Fig. 10-49   Right aortic arch. **A,** Barium in the esophagus deviates leftward around the right aortic arch. The right arch also displaces the trachea to the left. The right para-aortic stripe *(arrow)* is on the right side of the spine until it crosses to the midline above the diaphragm. **B,** The lateral chest film shows anterior deviation by the aortic arch of both the trachea and the esophagus by the aortic isthmus.

Double Aortic Arch

The ascending aorta may split into right and left aortic arches, which pass on both sides of the trachea to join posteriorly behind the esophagus (Fig. 10-51). In most cases, the right arch is larger and higher than the left arch. Although double aortic arch is rarely associated with congenital heart disease, there is frequently compression and malacia of the trachea. The plain chest film may show bilateral paratracheal masses with compression of the intervening trachea. A barium esophagogram shows bilateral indentations by the two aortic arches along the lateral sides of the esophagus with the right side superior and larger than the left side.

The angiographic picture of a double aortic arch is an "Aunt Mary." The characteristic double-looped aorta is visualized with either a left ventriculogram or aortogram (Fig. 10-52). MRI is more complex but also shows the heart and mediastinal structures (Fig. 10-53).

Pulmonary Artery Sling

Aberrant origin of the left pulmonary artery from the right pulmonary artery is part of an unusual anomaly in which the left pulmonary artery passes between the trachea and the esophagus (Fig. 10-54). The diagnosis can occasionally be made on a lateral chest film taken during a barium swallow so that the aberrant left pulmonary artery is a mass between the trachea and the esophagus. Most patients have cardiovascular and tracheoesophageal anomalies. The major respiratory abnormality usually is a significant stenosis in the right mainstem bronchus and the tracheal bifurcation. In the compressed trachea and bronchus the cartilage may be formed abnormally because that segment of the bronchus usually remains stenotic even after surgical relocation of the aberrant pulmonary artery. The radiologic features of air trapping from the stenotic bronchus include an opaque right upper lobe caused by poor clearing of fetal fluid and lobar emphysema with a hyperlucent right or left lung.

Hemitruncus

Hemitruncus is the anomalous origin of one pulmonary artery from the ascending aorta. If the right pulmonary artery comes from the aorta, the chest film shows huge right pulmonary arteries and normal left pulmonary arteries. Anomalous origin of the left pul-

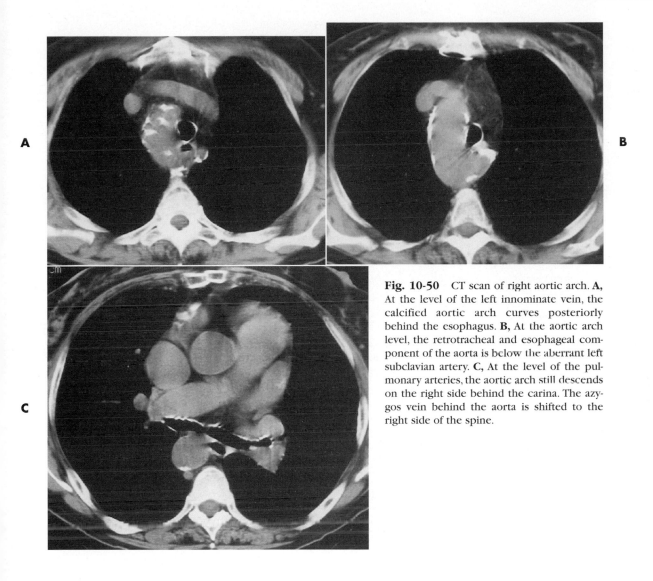

Fig. 10-50 CT scan of right aortic arch. **A,** At the level of the left innominate vein, the calcified aortic arch curves posteriorly behind the esophagus. **B,** At the aortic arch level, the retrotracheal and esophageal component of the aorta is below the aberrant left subclavian artery. **C,** At the level of the pulmonary arteries, the aortic arch still descends on the right side behind the carina. The azygos vein behind the aorta is shifted to the right side of the spine.

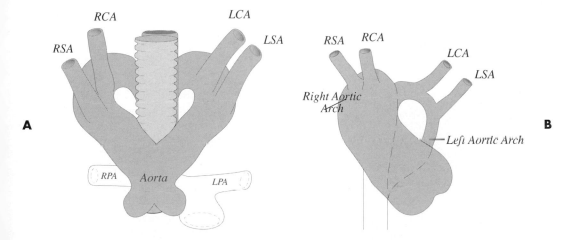

Fig. 10-51 Double aortic arch. **A,** Each aortic arch has the same size with the carotid arteries originating before the subclavian arteries. **B,** The more common type of double aortic arch has a larger and higher right arch with hypoplasia of the left aortic arch.

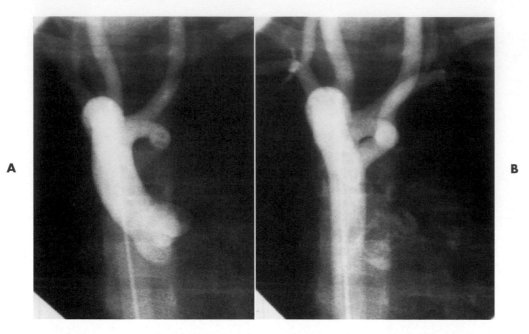

Fig. 10-52 Angiogram of double aortic arch. **A,** An injection into the ascending aorta with filling of the aortic root shows a larger right arch which is higher than the smaller left arch. **B,** The descending phase of the angiogram shows the posterior bifurcation as both aortic arches join to form the descending aorta.

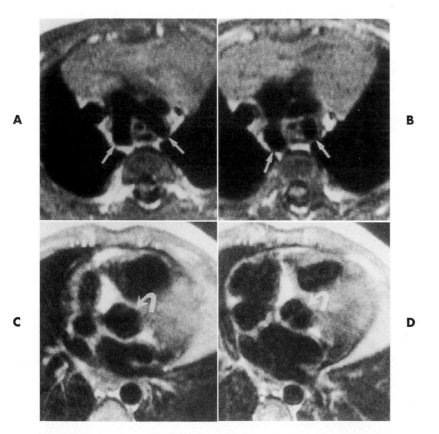

Fig. 10-53 MR image of double aortic arch. Transverse spin echo MRI scans show a double aortic arch (*straight arrows,* **A** and **B**) and bicuspid aortic valve *(curved arrows)* in systole **(C)** and diastole **(D)**. (From Fellows KE, Weinberg PM, Baffa JM, et al: Evaluation of congenital heart disease with MR imaging: current and coming attractions, *AJR Am J Roentgenol* 159:925-931, 1992.)

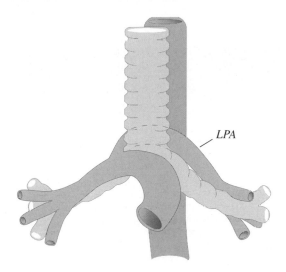

Fig. 10-54 Pulmonary artery sling. The left pulmonary artery originates from the right pulmonary artery and passes between the trachea and esophagus. This location of the aberrant pulmonary artery frequently creates a stenosis in the trachea and right mainstem bronchus.

monary artery from the aorta occurs in tetralogy of Fallot with right aortic arch.

Coarctation of the Aorta

In 1791 Paris delivered a paper on the pathology of coarctation. Although the clinical and pathologic signs of collateral flow in coarctation were known in the nineteenth century, the radiologic recognition of rib notching and the abnormal mediastinal silhouette were not firmly established until nearly 30 years after the first chest films were taken. In 1928, Abbott described the rib notching from enlarged intercostal vessels and the size discrepancy between the aortic arch and the descending aorta at the level of the left subclavian artery. Some of the first angiographic examinations were performed for coarctation in 1941.

Imaging diagnosis

In current medical practice, the diagnosis of coarctation that is suggested on physical examination is confirmed by imaging. The chest film in the adult frequently shows the notched aortic isthmus, but this sign is usually not seen in the infant. In infants, the evaluation of coarctation is typically made by echocardiography. In children and adults, MRI and occasionally angiography provide additional important information and may modify the medical and surgical management. These additional observations include associated aortic arch anomalies, aberrant subclavian vessels, atypical or long-segment aortic stenoses, and patent ductus arteriosus. At times, abundant collaterals that are evident on angiography were undetected by the physical examination or from the chest film. When minimal collaterals are present, the surgical approach may change from a primary

repair to a bypass graft around the coarctation in order to protect the blood supply to the spinal canal.

Classifications

There are numerous classifications of coarctation based on the age of the patient, the position of a patent ductus arteriosus in relation to the coarctation, and the length of the coarctation. Most of these schemata, including the classification into infantile or adult types, have limited usefulness in patient management because there is great variability within the categories, and the adult type of coarctation is frequently present in infants. Preductal and postductal coarctation are meaningful if the ductus is patent. Box 10-7 is a useful list of imaging observations that includes ductal patency, extent of collaterals, aortic arch anomalies, and coarctation in unusual locations.

Characteristics

The typical coarctation occurs in the aortic isthmus. This segment of the aorta between the origin of the left subclavian artery and the ductus is normally slightly small in the fetus and newborn. The fetal configuration of the isthmus produces a diameter that is roughly three fourths of the diameter of the descending thoracic aorta. Three months after birth, the fetal configuration of the isthmus is gone and the aortic arch has the same diameter throughout. The coarctation consists of an obstructing membrane on the greater curvature of the aorta opposite the ductus or ligamentum arteriosum. Typically, the lesser curvature of the aorta, which includes the site of the ductus, is retracted medially toward the left pulmonary artery. Beyond the obstruction there is usually a short segment that is dilated and may rarely be aneurysmal. The aorta proximal to the coarctation may be enlarged either congenitally or from hypertension. The dilatation may include the innominate, carotid, and subclavian vessels. More than half have tubular hypoplasia of the transverse portion of the aortic arch, beginning after the innominate artery and ending at the coarctation. In this configuration, the innominate, carotid, and subclavian arteries are dilated and may be as large as the transverse aortic arch.

The position of a patent ductus arteriosus with respect to the coarctation affects both the clinical presentation and the imaging interpretation. A ductus arteriosus may originate proximal, distal, or adjacent to a coarctation. If the coarctation is distal to the ductus arteriosus, blood flow is initially from the aorta to the pulmonary arteries in a left-to-right direction. If later the pulmonary vascular resistance increases because of an Eisenmenger reaction, the shunt may become bidirectional or reversed. If the coarctation is proximal to the ductus arteriosus, flow through the ductus will depend on the size of the ductus and the difference between the pulmonary and systemic vascular resistances. In this situation, the blood flow is frequently from the pulmonary artery to the descending aorta, a state that produces cyanosis in the lower half of the body. Oxygenated blood from the left ventricle goes to the aortic arch arteries, while deoxygenated blood from the right ventricle goes through the ductus to the lower body. A juxtaductal coarctation produces a complex pattern of blood flow which may vary dynamically as the pulmonary and systemic vascular resistances change with daily activity.

Stenosis or the anomalous origin of a subclavian artery distal to the coarctation results in an inequality in pulses and blood pressures in the two arms. A rare condition that produces equal blood pressures in both arms is the anomalous origin of both subclavian arteries below the coarctation. Coarctation at multiple sites or in the distal tho-

---

Box 10-8   Anomalies Associated with Aortic Coarctation

COMMON

Bicuspid aortic valve with stenosis and regurgitation
Patent ductus arteriosus
Ventricular septal defects
Turner syndrome

RARE

Transposition of the great arteries
Double outlet right ventricle
Shone syndrome (parachute mitral valve, supramitral ring, aortic valve stenosis, and aortic coarctation)

---

racic and abdominal aorta probably represents an embryologically different malformation such as neurofibromatosis, or an acquired disease such as Takayasu's aortoarteritis. Mucopolysaccharidosis (Hurler and Scheie syndromes) may have long tubular segmental stenoses in the aorta resembling those seen in Takayasu's disease.

Congenital bicuspid aortic valve is frequently associated with coarctation. One fourth to one half of those patients with aortic coarctation will also have a bicuspid aortic valve. Anomalies associated with aortic coarctation are listed in Box 10-8.

Fatal complications of aortic coarctation include bacterial aortitis at the site of the coarctation, aortic dissection, aneurysm of the ductus with rupture, and distal thromboembolism. Fatal left ventricular failure may occur from hypertensive heart disease or from stenosis and regurgitation of a bicuspid aortic valve. Since the carotid arteries are hypertensive, aneurysms in the circle of Willis may develop and rupture.

Chest film abnormalities

Plain film findings have their angiographic counterpart and are particularly useful in searching for the extent of collateral supply. The thoracic aorta shows an abnormal contour on the chest film in roughly 60% of patients with coarctation. The "figure 3 sign" is the undulation in the distal aortic arch at the site of the coarctation (Fig. 10-55). The distal convexity in this region represents the poststenotic dilatation. There is considerable variability in the size of the ascending aorta and in the upper half of the figure 3 sign. The ascending aorta may be large, normal, or invisible on the chest film, reflecting the wide morphologic variety of aortic coarctation. Because the left subclavian artery dilates in response to the hypertension on the proximal side of the coarctation, this vessel is frequently visible as it swings from the mediastinum toward the apex of the left lung.

Rib notching is the result of enlarged and tortuous intercostal arteries that serve as collateral channels. The notches are an exaggeration of the neurovascular groove

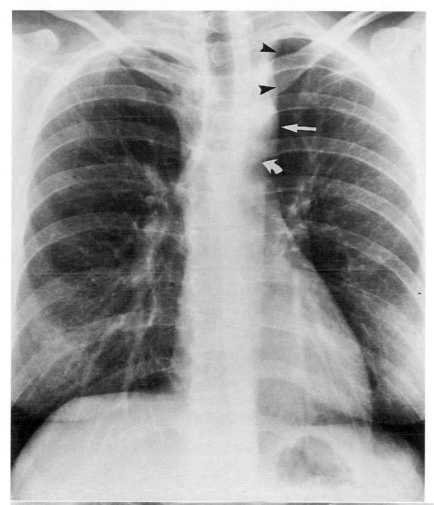

A

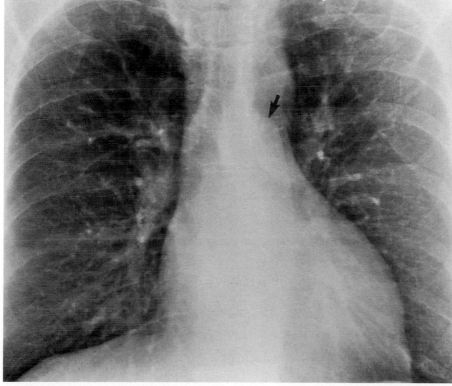

B

Fig. 10-55 Coarctation of the aorta. **A,** Minimal rib notching is present. The arch of the aorta *(straight arrow)* is unusually large and the left subclavian artery *(arrowheads)* has elongated into the left apex. The site of the coarctation *(curved arrow)* is the deep concavity in the descending aorta. **B,** The para-aortic stripe has a deep indentation *(arrow)* posteriorly behind the pulmonary artery segment.

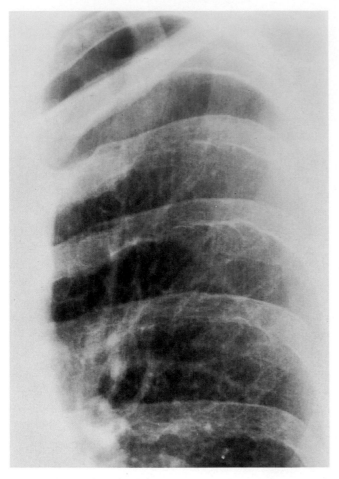

Fig. 10-56   Rib notching from coarctation occurs in the middle and lateral parts of the posterior ribs. Notching only in the medial rib adjacent to the costovertebral junction may be a normal variant.

in the inferior aspect of the rib (Fig. 10-56). The degree of notching ranges from minimal undulations, which are variations of normal findings without coarctation, to deep ridges in the inferior rib margin. A small notch near the costovertebral joint is normal, so that the more lateral the notching, the more likely it is pathologic. Rarely, the intercostal artery is so tortuous that it notches the superior aspect of the adjacent inferior rib. Rib notching is uncommon before the age of 6 years and its frequency increases with age, so most adults have this sign. The notching may occur at scattered sites and is usually not present on all ribs. After surgical repair of the coarctation, rib notching regresses as the bone is remodeled and the collateral vessels become smaller.

The intercostal arteries that serve as collateral channels originate from the descending aorta. For this reason, the first and second ribs do not have notches because their intercostal arteries come from the superior intercostal artery, which originates from the subclavian artery, above the coarctated site. Unilateral rib notching implies the presence of an anomalous subclavian artery. Notching of the left ribs only occurs when an aberrant right subclavian artery originates below the coarctated segment. Unilateral notching of the right ribs exists when the coarctation originates between the left carotid and left subclavian arteries. The size and extent of the notching reflects the amount of collateral blood flow through the intercostal arteries. When the coarctation is mild, no notching may be present; conversely, severe stenosis in the adult almost always has some element of rib notching.

In infancy, the abnormal mediastinal contours are invisible because of the overlying thymus. The typical

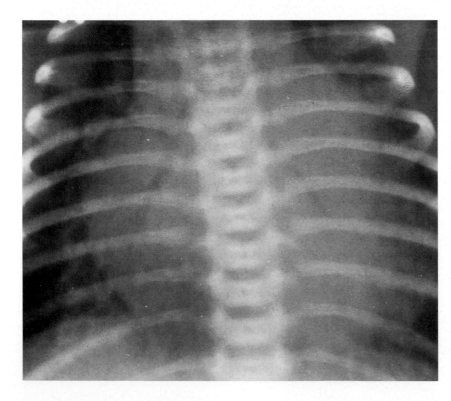

Fig. 10-57   Coarctation in a 2-month-old infant. The large cardiac silhouette and the indistinct pulmonary vessels reflect congestive heart failure. The wide mediastinum, particularly on the right side, is the thymus. The site of the coarctation (the "figure 3 sign") is typically not visible at this age. (From Miller SW: Aortic arch stenoses: coarctation, aortitis, and variants, *Appl Radiol* 24:15-19, 1995.)

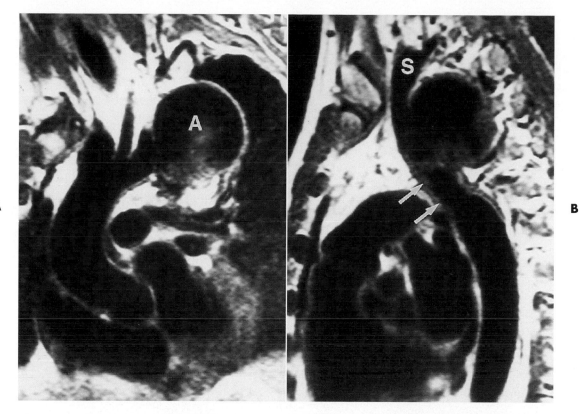

Fig. 10-58 Pseudoaneurysm after surgery for repair of a coarctation. **A,** A spin echo sequence in the plane of the ascending aorta shows a large saccular aneurysm *(A)* in the aortic isthmus. **B,** A parallel slice, which includes the descending aorta, shows the origin of the left subclavian artery *(S)* at the neck of the aneurysm. The grafted segment *(arrows)* is intact above a poststenotic dilatation of the aorta.

chest film displays signs of congestive heart failure with a large cardiac silhouette and perihilar pulmonary edema (Fig. 10-57). The extent of both of these findings depends on the severity of the coarctation and the patency of the ductus arteriosus. A barium esophagogram may be useful to outline the medial side of the aorta. The barium in the esophagus, when fully distended, has a reversal of the figure 3 sign. The sharp lateral outpouching represents the site of the coarctation and the inferior area of constriction represents the poststenotic dilatation of the aorta.

Imaging Examination

In the infant, most coarctations are easily seen with ultrasound. In the suprasternal plane, echodense tissue narrows the aortic isthmus from its posterior aspect. Continuous wave Doppler beam interrogation allows calculation of the pressure gradient across the stenosis.

MRI is the preferred vascular study in older children and adults as it has no ionizing radiation and can image long segments of the aorta (Fig. 10-58). Because the stenosis typically is severe and the aorta tortuous at the poststenotic segment, the technique must be tailored to the pathologic findings. Slice thickness should be about 5 mm. The coronal plane images are useful to show the extent and size of collaterals. A multislice series then is designed from the axial stack to obtain a series of oblique images parallel to the long axis of the aorta centered on the coarctated segment. Gradient echo sequences (Fig. 10-59) in the

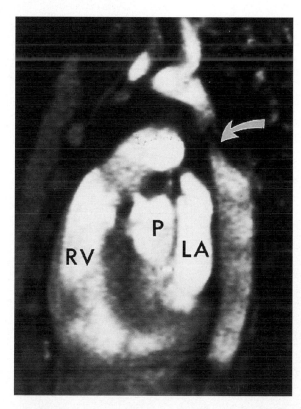

Fig. 10-59 Gradient echo image of an aortic coarctation. In the sagittal plane, which contains the right ventricle *(RV)*, left pulmonary artery *(P)*, and the left atrium *(LA)*, the aortic isthmus has a long stenosis *(arrow)* beginning distal to the left subclavian artery.

aortic plane can produce images similar to those of aortography. Visualization of a jet indicates a significant stenosis and pressure gradient across the coarctation.

Aortography gives the highest resolution of the coarctated segment, the aortic arch vessels, and the flow through the collateral channels (Fig. 10-60). The catheter from the femoral artery can almost always be advanced through the coarctated segment with a guidewire and positioned in the ascending aorta. Retrograde flow of contrast material then outlines the aortic root and identifies any bicuspid aortic valve. The left anterior oblique projection with cranial angulation projects a ductus inferior to the aortic arch (Fig. 10-61). In small patients, cineangiography is quicker and offers ready review of

the videotape. In adults, either cineangiography or large-size serial filming can be used to image the entire thorax. In the latter instance a delayed sequence of up to 10 to 12 seconds is desirable to include late collateral opacification. At the conclusion of a retrograde aortogram, you should record a measurement of the pressure gradient across the stenotic segment. Box 10-9 lists the elements demonstrated in an aortogram.

The collateral circulation influences the extent of upper extremity hypertension and the amount of circulation to the lower half of the body. The major routes of collateral flow are through the subclavian arteries and through bridging collaterals in the mediastinum around the coarctated site. These routes vary considerably from patient to

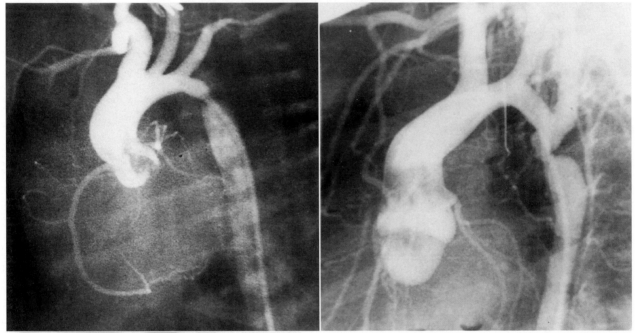

Fig. 10-60 Aortography of three variations of aortic coarctation filmed in the left anterior oblique projection. **A,** Aortic valve stenosis is indicated by the domed leaflets of the bicuspid valve and the poststenotic dilatation of the ascending aorta. The transverse arch is frequently hypoplastic before the coarctation. **B,** The bicuspid aortic valve is oriented in an anteroposterior direction. There is pronounced poststenotic dilatation after the coarctation. Large internal mammary arteries and bridging mediastinal vessels are visible. **C,** The transverse arch has normal size. A small diverticulum *(arrow)* represents the obliterated ductus arteriosus.

patient even when the degree of coarctation is similar. Numerous bridging mediastinal vessels are frequent when other considerably longer pathways are poorly visualized.

A common collateral channel is for blood to flow from the subclavian arteries to the internal mammary

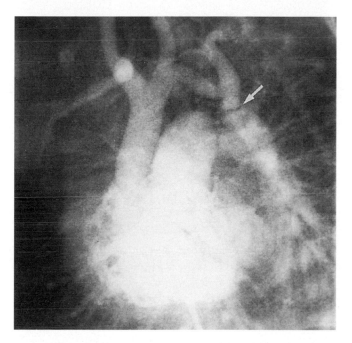

Fig. 10-61 Cranial angulation for demonstrating coarctation of the aorta. In this double outlet right ventricle filmed in the long axial oblique projection, the coarctation *(arrow)* is projected above the left pulmonary artery. The transverse aortic arch is hypoplastic.

arteries, then in a retrograde direction in the intercostal arteries to the descending aorta (Fig. 10-62). This pathway is responsible for the radiologic signs of large, undulating soft tissue in the retrosternal region on the lateral chest film and for the presence of rib notching. Obviously, if a subclavian artery originates anomalously in the low-pressure region below the coarctation, there will be no collateral flow in that side of the thorax. Another collateral pathway involves the thyrocervical and costocervical arteries, which originate from the subclavian artery. These vessels course through the scapular region to join intercostal arteries in the inferior thoracic region. Collateral pathways that are rarely seen on angiography include the superior and inferior epigastric arteries, which form a bridge from the intercostal arteries to the lumbar and iliac arteries, and the anterior spinal artery and other communicating arteries adjacent to the spinal cord.

The extent and size of the collateral channels that are angiographically visible roughly correspond to the age of

Box 10-9 Aortic Coarctation Evaluation
Site and length of the coarctation
Extent of tubular narrowing of transverse aortic arch
Location of anomalous arch vessels
Location of ductus
Extent of collateralization about the coarctation

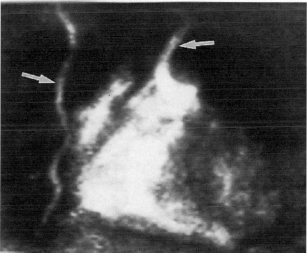

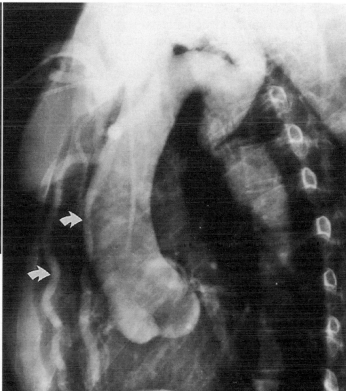

A

B

Fig. 10-62 Collateral vessels in coarctation. **A,** A gradient echo image shows large bilateral internal mammary arteries *(arrows)* in a coronal plane that also includes the right ventricle. **B,** Thoracic aortography opacifies large internal mammary arteries *(arrows)*.

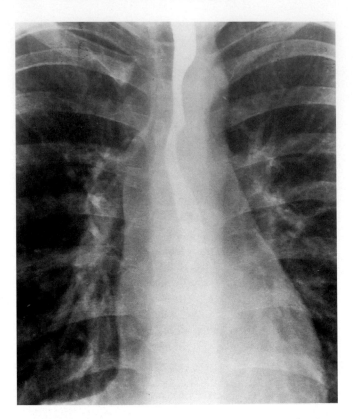

Fig. 10-63   Pseudocoarctation. Barium in the esophagus exhibits the "reverse 3 sign" outlining the medial site of the aortic indentation in the descending aorta. The para-aortic stripe is slightly widened laterally. No rib notching is present and no pressure gradient exists across the aortic isthmus.

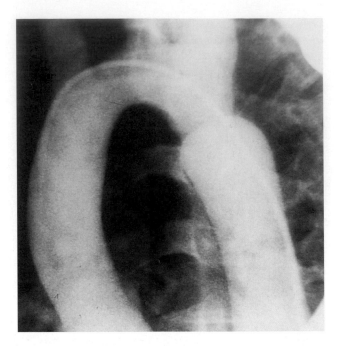

Fig. 10-64   Aortogram of pseudocoarctation. The local indentation after the left subclavian artery narrows the lumen by 25% and has a 5 mm Hg gradient

the patient and the severity of the stenosis. Large and tortuous intercostal vessels are common in the adult but are rarely seen in infants. When the coarctation is distal to the ductus, collateral circulation forms during fetal life. Collateral circulation may be absent when the coarctation is proximal to the ductus.

Pseudocoarctation

Pseudocoarctation is a term used by Dotter and Steinberg to denote a lesion that has the same morphology as the classic coarctation but does not produce obstruction. This anomaly has a buckling of the aorta at the isthmus with little or no pressure gradient across it. All features of a true coarctation, including the figure 3 sign, may be seen in pseudocoarctation except that there is no rib notching or sign of collateral flow (Fig. 10-63). Coarctations that have a focal constriction of less than 50% have no pressure gradient across them and have no evidence of collateral flow (such as rib notching). The chest film has a mediastinal mass that is an elongated and high aortic arch. A gradient of less than 30 mm Hg is acceptable for the diagnosis of pseudocoarctation.

Pseudocoarctation may be two separate aortic anomalies. One type may be a true coarctation without a pressure gradient. The embryologic abnormality that causes coarctation presumably had only a minor expression that produced the intimal infolding and distal dilatation (Fig. 10-64). The second type may be an abnormal elongation of the thoracic aorta which is kinked at the ligamentum attachment (Fig. 10-65).

Aortic Arch Interruption

Characteristics
Complete interruption of the aortic arch is a rare congenital anomaly characterized by discontinuity of the arch between the proximal ascending aorta and the distal descending aorta. The ductus arteriosus is frequently patent and is the connection to the distal arch and descending aorta. This anomaly usually has three defects: (1) ventricular septal defect, (2) patent ductus arteriosus, and (3) arch interruption. The DiGeorge syndrome of thymic hypoplasia, bicuspid aortic valve, hypoplastic left ventricle, and truncus arteriosus is frequently associated with aortic arch interruption. Unlike severe coarctation, there is no residual connection between the ascending and descending aorta.

Classifications
The site of the arch interruption determines classification into one of three types (Fig. 10-66). Type A has the interruption distal to the left subclavian artery. In a vari-

ation of this type, the right subclavian artery arises from the descending aorta or the pulmonary artery. In type B, the interruption is after the left common carotid artery. The left subclavian artery arises from the descending aorta. This variety is the most common form of interrupted arch; its variations include forms in which the right subclavian artery comes from the right pulmonary artery via a right ductus, and another variation where the right subclavian artery connects to the descending aorta.

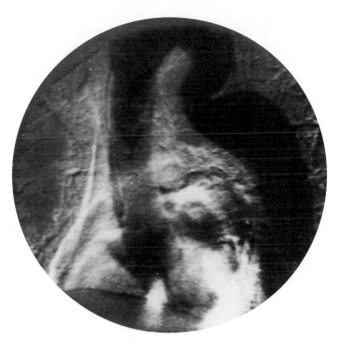

Fig. 10-65   Pseudocoarctation and cervical aortic arch. In the left anterior oblique projection, the elongated cervical aortic arch extends above the clavicle, then is kinked in the aortic isthmus, and has moderate ectasia in the descending segment. (From Miller SW: Aortic arch stenoses: coarctation, aortitis, and variants, *Appl Radiol* 24:15-19, 1995.)

Type C interruption is a discontinuity of the aortic arch distal to the innominate artery. The left carotid and left subclavian arteries connect to the descending aorta.

Chest film abnormalities

The plain chest film is characterized by nonspecific features that include cardiomegaly, increased pulmonary blood flow, and pulmonary edema. Details of the aortic arch are usually invisible even when no obvious thymus is present. In older patients, the trachea is frequently midline, reflecting a hypoplastic ascending aorta. The pulmonary artery is quite large and the aortic arch invisible, creating a deep notch in the aortic-pulmonary recess. On a well-penetrated film, the descending aorta may appear to end at the level of the main pulmonary artery. In older patients, rib notching, either bilateral or unilateral, depends on the site of the arch interruption and the origin of the subclavian arteries.

Imaging examination

Since this is mostly a disease of neonates, echocardiography is the modality that ordinarily makes the diagnosis. The aortic arch assessed from the suprasternal area is scanned for continuity and for a large ductus arch.

The characteristic angiographic features depend on the anatomic type of interruption and the collateral flow to arteries not attached to the proximal aorta. In type A interruption with all brachiocephalic vessels arising from the ascending aorta, the angiographic appearance of these vessels resembles the letter V or W. There is a deep notch filled by the left lung between the large main pulmonary artery and the left subclavian artery. In type B interruption, the V configuration is formed by the two carotid arteries (Fig. 10-67).

Collateral circulation is identified by delayed filming and resembles that seen in aortic coarctation. With type

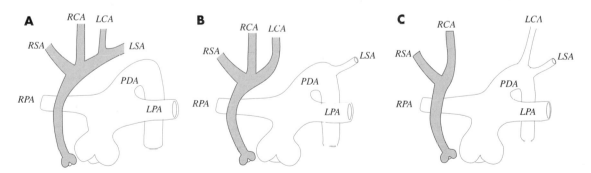

Fig. 10-66   Complete interruption of the aortic arch. **A,** Type A: Interruption of the aortic arch distal to the origin of the left subclavian artery with the descending aorta connecting to the ductus arteriosus. **B,** Type B: Interruption distal to the left common carotid artery with the left subclavian artery arising from the descending aorta. **C,** Type C: Interruption distal to the right innominate artery with the left common carotid and left subclavian arteries arising from the descending aorta. *LPA* = left pulmonary artery; *RPA* = right pulmonary artery; *PDA* = patent ductus arteriosus; *RSA* = right subclavian artery; *RCA* = right carotid artery; *LCA* = left carotid artery; *LSA* = left subclavian artery.

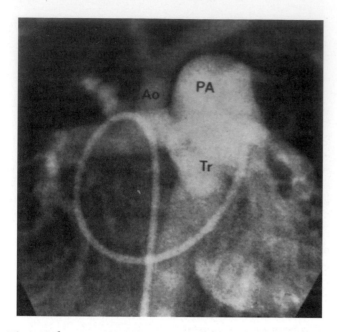

Fig. 10-67 Type B aortic arch interruption. The catheter is above the truncal valve *(Tr)* in an infant with a Van Praagh type 4 truncus arteriosus. The aorta *(Ao)* is small and is interrupted distal to the left common carotid artery. Both subclavian arteries arose from the descending aorta. The brachiocephalic arteries form the V sign. A large patent ductus arteriosus functions as the aortic arch. *PA* = pulmonary artery. (From Neye-Bock S, Fellows KE: Aortic arch interruption in infancy: radio- and angiographic features, *AJR Am J Roentgenol* 135:1005-1010, 1980.)

A interruption and normal origin of the subclavian arteries, the collateral pathways are identical to aortic coarctation, particularly when the ductus is partly or completely closed. In older children, there may be bilateral rib notching. With type B interruption with the left subclavian artery connected to the descending aorta, collateral flow should promote rib notching only on the right side. A subclavian steal phenomenon may be visible with retrograde flow down the left vertebral artery to opacify the left subclavian artery. In a similar fashion, retrograde flow in any brachiocephalic artery may theoretically be visible if it attaches to the low-pressure side of the aortic interruption.

SUGGESTED READINGS

Books

Doroghazi RM, Slater EE (eds): *Aortic dissection,* New York, 1983, McGraw-Hill.

Lande A, Berkmen YM, McAllister HA Jr: *Aortitis: clinical, pathologic, and radiographic aspects,* New York, 1986, Raven Press.

Lindsey J Jr: *Diseases of the aorta,* Philadelphia, 1994, Lea & Febiger.

Lindsay J Jr, Hurst JW: *The aorta,* New York, 1979, Grune & Stratton.

Shuford WH, Sybers RG: *The aortic arch and its malformations: with emphasis on the angiographic features,* Springfield, Ill, 1974, Charles C Thomas.

Steward JR, Kincaid OW, Edwards JE: *An atlas of vascular rings and related malformations of the aortic arch,* Springfield, Ill, 1964, Charles C Thomas.

Yao JST, Pearce WH: *Aneurysms: new findings and treatments,* Norwalk, Conn, 1994, Appleton & Lange.

Journals

Berdon WE, Baker DH: Vascular anomalies and the infant lung: rings, slings, and other things, *Semin Roentgenol* 7: 39-64, 1972.

Bissett GS, III, Strife JL, Kirks DR, et al: Vascular rings: MR imaging, *AJR Am J Roentgenol* 149: 251-256, 1987.

Cigarroa JE, Isselbacher EM, DeSanctis RW, et al: Medical progress. Diagnostic imaging in the evaluation of suspected aortic dissection: old standards and new directions, *AJR Am J Roentgenol* 161:485-493, 1993.

DeSanctis RW, Doroghazi RM, Austen WG, et al: Aortic dissection, *N Engl J Med* 317:1060-1067, 1987.

Dinsmore RE, Liberthson RR, Wismer GL, et al: Magnetic resonance imaging of thoracic aortic aneurysms: comparison with other imaging methods, *AJR Am J Roentgenol* 146:309, 1986.

Dotter CT, Steinberg I: Angiocardiography in congenital heart disease, *Am J Med* 12:219, 1952.

Dotter CT, Steinberg I: The angiographic measurement of the normal great vessels, *Radiology* 52:353, 1949.

Fisher RG, Bladlock F, Ben-Menachem Y: Laceration of the thoracic aorta and brachiocephalic arteries by blunt trauma: report of 54 cases and review of the literature, *Radiol Clin North Am* 19:91, 1981.

Fisher RG, Chasen MH, Lamki N: Diagnosis of injuries of the aorta and brachiocephalic arteries caused by blunt chest trauma: CT vs aortography, *AJR Am J Roentgenol* 162:1047-1052, 1994.

Godwin JD, Turley K, Herfkens RJ, et al: Computed tomography for follow-up of chronic aortic dissections, *Radiology* 139:655, 1986.

Gomes AS, Lopis JF, George B, et al: Congenital abnormalities of the aortic arch: MR imaging, *Radiology* 165:691-695, 1987.

Groskin S, Maresca M, Heitzman ER: Thoracic trauma, in McCort JJ, Mindelzun RE (eds): *Trauma radiology,* New York, 1990, Churchill Livingstone.

Heggtveit HA: Syphilitic aortitis: a clinicopathologic autopsy study of 100 cases, *Circulation* 29: 346-355, 1964.

Hilgenberg AD: Trauma to the heart and great vessels, in Burke JF, Boyd RJ, McCabe CJ (eds): *Trauma management: early management of visceral, nervous system, and musculoskeletal injuries,* St Louis, 1988, Mosby–Year Book, pp 153-175.

Ishikawa K: Diagnostic approach and proposed criteria for the clinical diagnosis of Takayasu's arteriopathy, *J Am Coll Cardiol* 12:964-972, 1988.

Jaffee RB: Complete interruption of the aortic arch: 1. Characteristic radiographic findings in 21 patients, *Circulation* 52:714, 1975.

Jaffee RB: Complete interruption of the aortic arch: 2. Characteristic angiographic features with emphasis on collateral circulation of the descending aorta, *Circulation* 53:161, 1976.

Kampmeier RH: Saccular aneurysm of the thoracic aorta. A clinical study of 633 cases, *Ann Intern Med* 12:624, 1938.

Kazerooni EA, Bree RL, Williams DM: Penetrating atherosclerotic ulcers of the descending thoracic aorta: evaluation with CT and distinction from aortic dissection, *Radiology* 183:759-765, 1992.

Kersteing-Sommerhoff BA, Higgins CB, White RD, et al: Aortic dissection: sensitivity and specificity of MR imaging, *Radiology* 166:651-655, 1988.

Kirks DR, Currarino G, Chen JTT: Mediastinal collateral arteries: important vessels in coarctation of the aorta, *AJR Am J Roentgenol* 146:757-762, 1986.

Lande A: Takayasu's arteritis and coarctation of the descending thoracic and abdominal aorta: a critical review, *AJR Am J Roentgenol* 127:227, 1976.

Liberthson RR, Pennington DG, Jacobs M, et al: Coarctation of the aorta: review of 234 patients and clarification of management problems, *Am J Cardiol* 43:835, 1979.

Liu YQ: Radiology of aortoarteritis, *Radiol Clin North Am* 23:671-688, 1985.

Lupi-Herrera E, Sanchez-Torres G, Marcushamer J, et al: Takayasu's arteritis. Clinical study of 107 cases, *Am Heart J* 93:103, 1977.

Miller SW, Holmvang G: Differentiation of slow flow from thrombus in thoracic magnetic resonance imaging, emphasizing phase images, *J Thorac Imaging* 8:98-107, 1993.

Movsowitz HD, Lampert C, Jacobs LE, et al: Penetrating atherosclerotic aortic ulcers, *Am Heart J* 128:1210-1217, 1994.

Neye-Bock S, Fellows KE: Aortic arch interruption in infancy: radio- and angiographic features, *AJR Am J Roentgenol* 135:1005, 1980.

Park JH, Chung JW, Im JG, et al: Takayasu arteritis: evaluation of mural changes in the aorta and pulmonary artery with CT angiography, *Radiology* 196:89-93, 1995.

Park JH, Han MC, Bettmann MA: Arterial manifestations of Behçet disease, *AJR Am J Roentgenol* 143:821-825, 1984.

Parmley LR, Thomas WM, Manion WC, et al: Nonpenetrating traumatic injury of the aorta, *Circulation* 15:405-410, 1958.

Petasnick JP: Radiologic evaluation of aortic dissection, *Radiology* 180:297-305, 1991.

Raptopoulos V: Chest CT for aortic injury: may be not for everyone, *AJR Am J Roentgenol* 162:1053-1055, 1994.

Roberts WC: Aortic dissection: anatomy, consequences, and causes, *Am Heart J* 101:195, 1981.

Simoneaux SE, Bank ER, Webber JB, et al: MR imaging of the pediatric airway, *Radiographics* 15:287-298, 1995.

Slater EE, DeSanctis RW: The clinical recognition of dissecting aortic aneurysm, *Am J Med* 60:625-633, 1976.

Smyth PT, Edwards JE: Pseudocoarctation, kinking or buckling of the aorta, *Circulation* 46:1027, 1972.

Soulen RL, Fishman EK, Pyeritz RE, et al: Marfan syndrome: evaluation with MR imaging versus CT, *Radiology* 165:697-701, 1987.

Steinberg I, Dotter CT, Peabody G, et al: The angiographic diagnosis of syphilic aortitis, *AJR Am J Roentgenol* 62:655, 1949.

Taylor DB, Blaser SI, Burrows PE, et al: Arteriopathy and coarctation of the abdominal aorta in children with mucopolysaccharidosis: imaging findings, *AJR Am J Roentgenol* 157:819-823, 1991.

Tunaci A, Berkman YM, Gökmen E: Thoracic involvement in Behçet's disease: pathologic, clinical, and imaging features, *AJR Am J Roentgenol* 164:51-56, 1995.

Vasile N, Matheier D, Keita K, et al: Computed tomography of thoracic aortic dissection: accuracy and pitfalls, *J Comput Assist Tomogr* 10:211, 1986.

Walker TG, Geller SC: Aberrant right subclavian artery with a large diverticulum of Kommerell: a potential for misdiagnosis, *AJR Am J Roentgenol* 149:477-478, 1987.

White RD, Ullyot DJ, Higgins CB: MR imaging of the aorta after surgery for aortic dissection, *AJR Am J Roentgenol* 150:87-92, 1988.

Yamada I, Numano F, Suzuki S: Takayasu arteritis: evaluation with MR imaging, *Radiology* 188:89-94, 1993.

Yamada T, Tada S, Harada J: Aortic dissection without intimal rupture: diagnosis with MR imaging and CT, *Radiology* 168:347-352, 1988.

Yamato M, Lecky JW, Hiramatsu K, et al: Takayasu arteritis: radiographic and angiographic findings in 59 patients, *Radiology* 161:329-334, 1986.

Yucel EK, Steinberg FL, Egglin TK, et al: Penetrating aortic ulcers: diagnosis with MR imaging, *Radiology* 177:779-781, 1990.

Index

A

Abdominal aorta, echocardiography, 80-81
Abscesses
  aortic, 286, 411-412
  pericardial, 276, 278
Acquired immunodeficiency syndrome, cardiac lesions in, 286-287
Africans, aneurysms in, 238
Age, diagnosis and, 382-383
Aging, cardiac effects of, 4-6
AIDS, cardiac lesions in, 286-287
Akinesis, 203, 240
Alveolar edema, 31, 35
Amplatz catheter, 124
Anatomically corrected malposition of great arteries, 334
Anatomy
  for angiography, 129-144
  aorta, 387
  for magnetic resonance imaging, 103-122
  pericardial, 264-265
  in pulmonary atresia with intact ventricular septum, 362-363
  in tetralogy of Fallot, 366-367
  in tricuspid atresia, 358-359
Aneurysms
  aortic
    atherosclerotic, 388, 415-418
    chest film findings, 389-391
    infected, 388, 411-412
    shape, 387
    sinus of Valsalva, 402-403
    size and types, 388-389
    syphilitic, 410
  coronary, 217
  dissecting, 391, 398
  echocardiography, 73, 80
  left ventricular, 200
    definition and pathologic correlation, 235
    false aneurysm, 238
    imaging signs, 235
    in septal rupture, 241, 243
    thrombi and, 233
  membranous septal, 351-352
  resection, ventriculography after, 238
Angina pectoris, 213, 215
Angiography, 123-146; see also
  Aortography; Ventriculography
  aortic regurgitation, 162-163
  aortic stenosis
    congenital valvular, 153

    subvalvular, 158-160
  bypass grafts, 230-231
  cardiac chambers
    characteristics, 138
    left atrium, 138, 140
    left ventricle, 138, 140-141
    right atrium, 137-138
    right ventricle, 138-140
  cardiac valves
    aortic valve, 144
    mitral valve, 141-143
    pulmonary valve, 143
    tricuspid valve, 141
  catheterization techniques, 124
  cineangiography, 124, 126
  congenital heart disease
    atrial septal defects, 343-344
    atrioventricular septal defects, 347-349
    complete dextrotransposition of great arteries, 320, 323-325
    congenitally corrected transposition of great vessels, 313-317
    differential diagnosis, 379-380
    double-outlet right ventricle, 326-327
    hypoplastic left heart syndrome, 375-378
    patent ductus arteriosus, 355-356
    pulmonary atresia with intact ventricular septum, 364-366
    pulmonary veins, abnormal connections, 336-337, 339-342
    single ventricle, 357
    tetralogy of Fallot, 143, 368, 370
    tricuspid atresia, 361
    truncus arteriosus, 330
    ventricular septal defects, 350-352
  contraindications, 124
  coronary
    atherosclerosis, 202-203, 206
    collateral vessels, 213
    interpretation of arterial stenoses, 208, 210
    spasm, 215-216
    uses and analysis, 201-202
  coronary anatomy
    cardiac veins, 136-137
    left coronary artery, 133-135
    right coronary artery, 129-133
  Ebstein anomaly, 196
  indications, 123-124
  mitral regurgitation, 175
  mitral stenosis, 168

  projection positions, 126-127
  radiation exposure and protection, 127-129
  technical factors, 128
  thoracic aortic disease
    aortic arch interruption, 433-434
    aortic dissection, 393, 396-398
    coarctation of aorta, 430-432
Angioplasty; see Percutaneous transluminal coronary angioplasty
Angiosarcomas, 79, 284
Ankylosing spondylitis, 40, 408
Annuloaortic ectasia, 396, 400, 402
Anticoagulation, with stent placement, 257-258
Aorta
  anatomy and size, 387
  atresia, in hypoplastic left heart syndrome, 373
  coarctation; see Coarctation of aorta
  congenital anomalies, 419-434
  diseases; see also Thoracic aortic diseases
    echocardiography, 80-81
  levotransposed, 334
  pulmonary artery and, 304, 307
  rupture or transection, chest film signs, 391
  tears, 413-414
  in tetralogy of Fallot, 367
Aortic aneurysms
  atherosclerotic, 388, 415-418
  chest film findings, 389-391
  infected, 388, 411-412
  shape, 387
  sinus of Valsalva, 402-403
  size and types, 388-389
  syphilitic, 410
Aortic arch, 387
  double, 422
  interruption, 433-434
  left, 419
  magnetic resonance imaging, 103-104
  right, 367-368, 419-421
  in truncus arteriosus, 330
Aortic arch syndrome, 404
Aortic dissection, 391
  angiography, 393, 396-398
  classifications, 391
  complications, 391-392
  magnetic resonance imaging, 392
  pathologic causes and contributing factors, 392
  plain film findings, 392

Aortic dissection—cont'd
   surgical treatment, 399-400
   tomographic imaging, 392
Aortic diverticulum, 419
Aortic isthmus, 387
Aortic regurgitation, 162
   angiographic technique, 162-163
   aortic dissection and, 392, 398
   causes, 163-165
   chest film findings, 162
   color Doppler detection, 35
   echocardiography, 67-69
   imaging findings, 163
   magnetic resonance imaging tech-
      nique, 163
   with prosthetic aortic valves, 165-167
   pulmonary vasculature and, 25
   in sinus of Valsalva aneurysm, 402-403
   in syphilitic aortitis, 410-411
Aortic root abscess, 286
Aortic stenosis
   echocardiography, 65-67
   in hypertrophic cardiomyopathy, 291
   subvalvular
      angiographic findings, 158-159
      causes, 151
      in double-outlet right ventricle,
         325, 327
      pathologic abnormalities, 158
      unusual subaortic obstruction, 159-
         160
   supravalvular, 160
      associated lesions, 160-162
      classifications, 160
   valvular, 149-151
      acquired, 156-157
      causes, 151
      chest film findings, 151
      congenital, 153-154
      imaging features, 153
Aortic valve
   angiography, 144
   bicuspid, 16-17, 153, 165, 426
   magnetic resonance imaging, 107-108
Aortic valve disease
   calcifications, 15-17, 65, 153, 156-157
   degenerative, 163-164
   echocardiography, 65-69
   infective endocarditis, 164
Aortic valvuloplasty, percutaneous, 261-
   262
Aortitis, 403-404
   Takayasu's, 403, 404-406
   types, 406-411
Aortography
   annuloaortic ectasia and Marfan syn-
      drome, 400
   coarctation of aorta, 430-432
   complete dextrotransposition of great
      arteries, 324

hypoplastic left heart syndrome, 376-
   378
truncus arteriosus, 330
Aortopulmonary septation, 333
   anatomically corrected malposition of
      great arteries, 334
   hemitruncus arteriosus, 330, 333
   truncus arteriosus, 329-330
Apical imaging planes for echocardiography, 49
   Doppler examination, 53-54
Arrhythmogenic right ventricular dysplasia, 287, 288
Arterial switch operation, 324
Ascending aorta, 387
ASH, 291, 292
Asplenia, 299, 307, 309-311
Asymmetric septal hypertrophy, 291, 292
Atherectomy, directional coronary, 252
Atherosclerosis, coronary
   aneurysms and, 217
   angiography, 201-203, 206, 210
   extent and location, 203-206
   morphology, 206-208
Atherosclerotic thoracic aneurysms
   appearance, 415-417
   imaging, 417-418
   location, 417
Atria; see also Left atrium; Right atrium
   morphology and position, 302, 307
   myxomas, 79, 280
   thrombi, echocardiography, 80
Atrial septal defects, 342; see also
   Atrioventricular septal defects
   chest film features, 343
   echocardiography, 81-84
   imaging techniques and features, 343-
      345
   less common defects, 343
   magnetic resonance imaging, 108, 111
   ostium secundum and primum
      defects, 343
   patent foramen ovale, 342
   sinus venosus defects, 343
Atrioventricular connections, morphology, 304
Atrioventricular discordance, 311-319
Atrioventricular septal defects, 84
   angiographic features, 347-349
   chest film abnormalities, 346-347
   complete atrioventricular canal
      defects, 345
   magnetic resonance imaging features,
      349
   partial or incomplete atrioventricular
      canal defects, 345
   segmental analysis, 345-346
Atypical coarctation, 404
Axial projections, in congenital heart
   disease, 127

Azygos vein
   cardiac tamponade and, 271
   magnetic resonance imaging, 104

B

Balloon angioplasty; see Percutaneous
   transluminal coronary angioplasty
Balloon valvuloplasty; see Percutaneous
   aortic valvuloplasty; Percutaneous
   mitral balloon valvuloplasty
Behçet disease, 408
Bentall procedure, 399
Beriberi, 25
Bernoulli theorem and simplified
   Bernoulli equation, 59
Bicuspid aortic valve, 16-17, 153, 165, 426
Bicuspid pulmonary valve, 183
Blalock-Hanlon procedure, 324
Blalock-Taussig shunt, 36, 373
Bland-White-Garland syndrome, 222, 225
Blood flow
   coronary, 210-213
   pulmonary; see Pulmonary vasculature
Blunt cardiovascular trauma, 413, 414
Boot-shaped heart (coeur en sabot), 10,
   360, 361, 367, 375
Bradycardia, 212
Bypass grafting, coronary, 226
   complications, 228, 230
   imaging techniques, 230-231
   internal mammary artery grafts, 226-
      227
   saphenous vein grafts, 227-228

C

Calcifications, 15
   aortic valve, 15-17, 65, 153, 156-157
   in aortitis, 409-410
   ascending aorta, 417
   coronary, 21-23
   in ductus arteriosus region, 354-355
   left atrial, 18
   left ventricular thrombi, 233
   mitral annulus, 17, 62
   mitral valve, 17, 62, 168
   myocardial, 17-18
   pericardial, 18-21, 272, 274
   sinus of Valsalva, 402
   tricuspid, 191
Candida, 194
Cardiac and pericardial calcifications,
   15-23
Cardiac chambers
   angiography evaluation
      characteristics, 138
      left atrium, 138, 140
      left ventricle, 138, 140-141
      right atrium, 137-138

right ventricle, 138-140
echocardiography evaluation
  left atrium, 56-57
  left ventricular systolic function, 56
  left ventricular volume, 54-56
  normal linear dimensions, 54
  right atrium, 58
  right ventricle, 57-58
enlargement, 6-8
  in interventricular septum rupture, 240
  left atrium, 10-11
  left ventricle, 11-15
  right atrium, 8
  right ventricle, 10
morphology, 302-304
thrombus in, 286
Cardiac connections and positions, 307-311
Cardiac contractility, analysis, 380
Cardiac injury, 414
Cardiac malpositions, 299
Cardiac masses, 278-286
Cardiac output, Doppler echocardiography and, 56
Cardiac shape and size, 4-15, 200
Cardiac surgery, 36
Cardiac tamponade, 266, 270-271
Cardiac valves, angiography
  aortic valve, 144
  mitral valve, 141-143
  pulmonary valve, 143
  tricuspid valve, 141
Cardiac veins, anatomy on angiography, 136-137
Cardiomyopathies, 278, 287
  classifications, 287
  dilated, 74, 235, 288, 290, 296
  distinguishing features, 296
  echocardiography, 74-76
  hypertrophic, 74-75, 290-292, 296
  imaging abnormalities, 292-296
  left ventricular abnormalities in, 296
  restrictive, 75-76, 274-276, 288-290, 291, 296
Cardiothoracic ratio, 6
Cardiotyping, 342
Cardiovascular syphilis, 408-411
Catheter-induced spasm, 216-217
Catheterization, for angiography, 124
  in aortic dissection, 396-397
Catheters
  balloon dilatation, 248-249
  coronary sinus and, 41
  left superior vena cava and, 43
Central pulmonary arteries, 23-24
Chambers; *see* Cardiac chambers
Chest films, 3-4
  aortic regurgitation, 162
  congenital heart disease

atrial septal defects, 343
atrioventricular septal defects, 346-347
complete dextrotransposition of great arteries, 320
differential diagnosis, 379
hypoplastic left heart syndrome, 375
patent ductus arteriosus, 353-355
pulmonary atresia with intact ventricular septum, 363-364
pulmonary vasculature and heart shape analysis, 381
pulmonary veins, abnormal connections, 335-337, 339
single ventricle, 356-357
tetralogy of Fallot, 367-368
tricuspid atresia, 359-361
truncus arteriosus, 330
ventricular septal defects, 349-350
Ebstein anomaly, 196
interventricular septum rupture, 240
ischemic heart disease, 200-201
mitral regurgitation, 174-175
mitral stenosis, 167-168
pericardium, normal, 265-266
pulmonary stenosis, 180-182
thoracic aortic disease
  annuloaortic ectasia and Marfan syndrome, 400
  aortic aneurysms, 389-391
  aortic arch interruption, 433
  aortic dissection, 392
  coarctation of aorta, 426-429
tricuspid stenosis, 191
valvular aortic stenosis, 151
Children; *see also* Congenital *entries*
  angiography, 123, 128
  cardiopulmonary appearance, 4-5
  Kawasaki disease, 217
  magnetic resonance imaging, 97
  primary tumors, 279
Chordae tendinae, 142-143
  in mitral regurgitation, 174, 176
Cineangiography, 124, 126
Circle of Vieussens, 131
Coarctation of aorta, 425
  anomalies associated with, 426
  characteristics, 426
  chest film abnormalities, 426-429
  classifications, 425
  diagnosis, 425
  imaging evaluation, 425, 429-432
Coeur en sabot, 10, 360, 361, 367, 375
Coils, for coronary artery fistulas, 262
Collateral vessels, coronary, 213
Common ventricle, 356
Complete transposition of great arteries (dextrotransposition), 320
  angiographic anatomy, 320, 323-325
  echocardiography, 88-89

surgical procedures, 325
Computed tomography
  aortic dissection, 392
  calcifications
    coronary, 23
    pericardial, 19, 21
  pericardium
    effusion, 266
    normal, 265
Congenital anomalies
  coronary arteries, 221
    of origin, 221-225
    of origin and course, 225-226
    of termination, 226
  thoracic aorta, 419
    aortic arch interruption, 433-434
    coarctation of aorta, 425-432
    double aortic arch, 422
    hemitruncus, 422
    left aortic arch, 419
    pseudocoarctation, 432
    pulmonary artery sling, 422
    right aortic arch, 419-421
Congenital heart disease, 298-385
  axial projections in, 127
  cyanotic defects with increased pulmonary arterial flow, 27
  differential diagnosis
    by age, 382-383
    pattern recognition and triangulation approach, 379-380
    by prevalence, 383
    by pulmonary pattern, 381-382
    segmental analysis, 380-381
  echocardiography
    atrial septal defects, 81-84
    complete transposition of great arteries, 88-89
    double outlet right ventricle, 90-91
    patent ductus arteriosus, 86-87
    tetralogy of Fallot, 87-88
    truncus arteriosus, 89-90
    univentricular heart, 91-92
    ventricular septal defects, 84-86
  left ventricular inflow obstruction, 172-174
  malpositions and abnormal connections
    aortopulmonary septation anomalies, 329-334
    atrioventricular discordance, 311-319
    cardiac connections and positions, 307-311
    cardiotyping, 342
    partial transposition of great arteries, 324-329
    pulmonary veins, abnormal connections, 334-342
    ventriculoarterial discordance, 319-324

Congenital heart disease—cont'd
  pericardial absence, 276
  segmental analysis of malformations, 299
    associated malformations, 307
    atrial morphology, 302
    atrioventricular connections, 304
    cardiac axis and visceral situs, 299-302
    diagnostic approach, 299
    relations of great arteries, 304, 307
    ventricular morphology, 302-304
    ventriculoarterial connections, 307
  septal defects, hypoplasias, and atresias
    atrial septal defects, 342-345
    atrioventricular septal defects, 345-349
    hypoplastic left heart syndrome, 373-378
    patent ductus arteriosus, 352-356
    pulmonary atresia with intact ventricular septum, 361-366
    single ventricle, 356-357
    tetralogy of Fallot, 366-373
    tricuspid atresia, 357-361
    ventricular septal defects, 349-352
  tricuspid valve in, 192, 194-197
  valvular aortic stenosis, 153-154
Congenitally corrected transposition of great vessels, 313
  angiographic anatomy and technique, 313-317
  coronary artery patterns, 317-318
  isolated ventricular inversion, 318
  straddling atrioventricular valves, 318-319
Congenital mitral stenosis, 172, 174
Congenital skeletal abnormalities, 36, 40
Congestive heart failure, 243, 266
Conoventricular defects, 349
Constrictive pericarditis, 271-272
  calcifications in, 272, 274
  restrictive cardiomyopathy vs., 274-276, 289-290
Continuity equation, 67
Conus
  bilateral, 325
  types, 307
Conus artery, anatomy on angiography, 131
Coronary arteries; see also Ischemic heart disease; Left coronary artery; Right coronary artery
  anatomy, on angiography, 129-137
  angiography; see Angiography, coronary
  atherosclerosis
    aneurysms and, 217
    angiography, 201-203, 206, 210
    extent and location, 203-206

morphology, 20-2106
blood flow
  normal, 210-211
  reserve, 212-213
  stenosis effects on, 213
  transient variations, 211-212
blunt trauma, 414
bypass grafting, 226
  complications, 228, 230
  imaging techniques, 230-231
  internal mammary artery grafts, 226-227
  saphenous vein grafts, 227-228
calcifications, 21-23
collateral vessels, 213
congenital anomalies, 221
  of origin, 221-225
  of origin and course, 225-226
  of termination, 226
in congenitally corrected transposition of great vessels, 317-318
dissection, 221
  NHLBI classification, 251
fistulas, 226, 262
interventional devices, 252-258
lesions, classification for angioplasty, 248
nonatherosclerotic disease, 210
ostial stenosis, 411
in pulmonary atresia with intact ventricular septum, 364-365
spasm, 213, 215
  angiography, 215-216
  catheter-induced vs. Prinzmetal syndrome, 216-217
stenosis
  angiography, 201-203, 206, 208, 210
  blood flow and, 213
  calcification and, 23
  extent and location, 203-206
  morphology, 206-208
  in septal rupture, 243
in tetralogy of Fallot, 370
in truncus arteriosus, 330
ventricular position and, 307-308
wall motion abnormalities and, 233
Coronary sinus, 41
  magnetic resonance imaging, 115
Coronary stents, 254, 256-258
Cor pulmonale, 41
Cor triatriatum, 172
Crista terminalis, magnetic resonance imaging, 114
CT; see Computed tomography
Cyanotic heart disease, 381
Cycled multislice multiphase spin-echo imaging, 99
Cystic fibrosis, 41
Cystic medial necrosis, 392
Cysts

cardiac, 278-279, 280
pericardial, 78, 276

D

DCA, 252, 253
DeBakey classification of aortic dissection, 391
Descending aorta, 387
Dextrocardia, 299, 302, 308
Dextrotransposition, 320
  angiographic anatomy, 320, 323-325
  echocardiography, 88-89
  surgical procedures, 325
Diabetes mellitus, 207, 417
Diastolic pseudogating, 102-103
Diazepam, 97
Dicloxacillin, 259
DiGeorge syndrome, 41, 433
Dilated cardiomyopathy, 288
  causes, 290
  echocardiography, 74
  left ventricular abnormalities in, 296
  thrombi and, 235
Dinsmore's principle, 8
Directional coronary atherectomy, 252
Dissecting aneurysm, 391, 398
Distal right coronary artery, anatomy on angiography, 131-133
Diverticulum of Kommerell, 419
Doppler echocardiography
  aortic disease, 80-81
  cardiomyopathies, 75-76
  congenital heart disease, 81-90
  ischemic heart disease, 73
  left ventricular systolic function, 56
  normal examination, 52
    apical views, 53-54
    other views, 54
    parasternal long-axis view, 52
    right ventricular inflow view, 52-53
  pericardial disease, 77-78
  valvular heart disease, 58-72
Double aortic arch, 422
Double-outlet left ventricle, 327-329
Double-outlet right ventricle, 324-327
  echocardiography, 90-91
Down syndrome, 36, 41, 345
Dressler syndrome, 201, 266, 270
Ductus arteriosus, patent; see Patent ductus arteriosus
Ductus bump, 353
Dyskinesis, 233
Dysplastic pulmonary valve, 183

E

Ebstein anomaly, 8, 194-197, 313
  chest films, 191
  echocardiography, 64

tricuspid regurgitation and, 315, 317
ECG gating, in magnetic resonance
    imaging, 98
Echocardiography, 46-95
    advantages, 46-47
    aortic diseases, 80-81
    cardiomyopathies, 74-76
    congenital heart disease, 81-92
    evaluation of cardiac chamber size
        and function
        left atrium, 56 57
        left ventricular systolic function, 56
        left ventricular volume, 54-56
        normal linear dimensions, 54
        right atrium, 58
        right ventricle, 57-58
    intracardiac masses, 78-80
    ischemic heart disease, 72-74
    mitral stenosis, 168
    normal Doppler examination, 52; see
        also Doppler
        echocardiography
        apical views, 53-54
        other views, 54
        parasternal long-axis view, 52
        right ventricular inflow view, 52-53
    normal examination, 47
        apical imaging planes, 49
        left parasternal imaging planes, 47-
            49
        right parasternal views, 50
        subcostal imaging planes, 49-50
        suprasternal imaging planes, 50
        transesophageal imaging, 50 52
    pericardial disease, 76-78
    valvular heart disease, 58-72
Echo dephasing, 103
Echo rephasing, 102
Ectatic aorta, 387
Edema, pulmonary, 30
    cardiac causes, 35
    chest radiograph, 200
    from congenital heart disease, 381-
        382
    radiologic appearance, 30-36
Ehlers-Danlos syndrome, 41, 392
Eisenmenger reaction, 380
Eisenmenger syndrome, 27-29, 343, 349,
    351
Ejection fraction, estimating, 56
ELCA, 253, 254
Elderly, cardiopulmonary appearance in,
    6
Electrocardiographic gating, in magnetic
    resonance imaging, 98
Ellis-van Creveld syndrome, 41
End-diastolic volume, 380
Endocardial cushion defects; see
    Atrioventricular septal defects
Endocarditis, 286

infective
    aortic regurgitation from, 164
    echocardiography, 71-72
Enlargement of chambers, 6-8
    in interventricular septum rupture,
        240
    left atrium, 10-11
    left ventricle, 11-15, 200
    right atrium, 8
    right ventricle, 10
Epicardium, 264
Excimer laser coronary angioplasty, 253,
    254

F

Fallot's tetralogy; see Tetralogy of Fallot
False aneurysms, 238, 388
Fibromas, 279
Fibrosarcomas, echocardiography, 79
Figure 3 sign, 426
Fistulas, coronary, 226, 262
Flail mitral leaflet, 62, 176
Flow, in magnetic resonance imaging,
    102-103
Flow ratios, pulmonary, 25
Fluid and water exchange, in pulmonary
    vein hypertension, 30
Fluoroscopy, radiation exposure from,
    127, 129
Foramen ovale, patent, 342
Friedrich ataxia, 41
Fusiform aneurysm, 387, 388

G

Gasul phenomenon, 366
Gradient-reversal acquisition, in magnet-
    ic resonance imaging, 99, 100-101,
    103
Grafting
    for aortic dissection, 399
    coronary bypass, 226-231
Great arteries
    anatomically corrected malposition,
        334
    relations of, 304, 307
    transposition; see Transposition of
        great arteries

H

Heart rate, left ventricle and, 232
Heart size and shape, 4-15, 200
Hemitruncus (arteriosus), 330, 333, 422
Heterotaxy, 41, 308-311
Heterotaxy syndrome, 299, 302, 420
High-velocity signal loss, 103
Hilar structures of pulmonary arteries,
    24

Holt-Oram syndrome, 36, 41
Homocystinuria, 41
Hughes-Stovin syndrome, 408
Hurler syndrome, 426
Hyperlipoproteinemia type II, 207, 417
Hypertension, pulmonary
    arterial, 27-30
    venous, 30-36
Hypertrophic cardiomyopathy, 290-292
    echocardiography, 74-75
    left ventricular abnormalities in, 296
Hypogenetic lung syndrome, 339
Hypoplastic left heart syndrome, 174, 373
    angiographic examination, 375-378
    characteristics, 373, 375
    chest film abnormalities, 375

I

Idiopathic hypertrophic subaortic steno-
    sis, 159
Infants; see also Congenital entries
    cardiopulmonary appearance in, 4
Infected aortic aneurysms, 411-412
Infection, pericardial effusion from, 266,
    270
Infective endocarditis
    aortic regurgitation from, 164
    echocardiography, 71-72
Infundibular stenosis, 182-183, 186-187,
    366
Inlet ventricular septal defects, 84
Innominate artery injury, 413
Innominate vein, left, magnetic reso-
    nance imaging, 103
Interatrial septum, magnetic resonance
    imaging, 108, 114
Internal mammary artery grafts, 226-227
Interstitial edema, 30-31
Interventional cardiology, 247-263
    coronary artery fistulas, 262
    newer coronary interventional
        devices, 252-258
    percutaneous aortic valvuloplasty,
        261-262
    percutaneous mitral balloon valvulo-
        plasty, 258-261
    percutaneous transluminal coronary
        angioplasty, 247-252
Interventricular septum rupture, 200,
    240-243
Intracardiac thrombus, echocardiogra-
    phy, 79-80
Intracardiac tumors, echocardiography,
    78-79
Inverted ventricle, 356, 357
Ischemic heart disease, 199-246
    angiographic interpretation of arterial
        stenoses, 208, 210
    chest radiograph, 200-201

Ischemic heart disease—cont'd
  congenital anomalies of coronary
    arteries, 221-226
  coronary aneurysms, 217
  coronary angiography, 201-203
  coronary artery spasm, 213, 215-217
  coronary blood flow determinants,
    210-213
  coronary bypass grafting, 226-231
  coronary collateral vessels, 213
  coronary dissection, 221
  echocardiography, 72-74
  left ventricular abnormalities in coro-
    nary disease, 231-233
  mitral regurgitation from coronary
    artery disease, 243-244
  morphology of coronary atherosclero-
    sis, 206-208
  myocardial bridging, 221
  rupture of interventricular septum,
    240-243
  segmental wall motion abnormalities,
    233-238
  stenosis extent and location, 203-206
  ventriculography after aneurysm
    resection, 238
Isolated ventricular inversion, 318
Isomerism, 299
Ivemark syndrome, 41

J

Jatene operation, 324
Judkins catheter, 124

K

Kaposi sarcoma, 287
Kartagener syndrome, 41
Kawasaki disease, 217
Kerley A and B lines, 31
Kommerell's diverticulum, 419
Kugel's artery, 213

L

Lead placement, ECG, in magnetic resonance imaging, 98
Leaflet abnormalities
  in Ebstein anomaly, 196
  in mitral regurgitation, 174, 175-176
Left anterior descending artery, anatomy
  on angiography, 134
Left aortic arch, 419
Left atrium
  angiography, 140
  calcifications, 18
  echocardiography, 56-57
  enlargement, 10-11, 57, 112

morphology and position, 302, 307
  thrombus, 286
Left circumflex artery, anatomy on
  angiography, 134
Left coronary artery, anatomy on angiography, 133
  left anterior descending artery, 134
  left circumflex artery, 134
Left innominate vein, magnetic resonance imaging, 103
Left main equivalent disease, 205-206
Left superior vena cava, 42-43
Left ventricle
  aneurysms, 200
    definition and pathologic correla-
      tion, 235
    false aneurysm, 238
    imaging signs, 235
    resection, ventriculography after,
      238
    in septal rupture, 241, 243
  angiography, 140-141
  in cardiomyopathy, 296
  in congenitally corrected transposi-
    tion of great vessels, 314
  in coronary disease, 231-233
  double-outlet, 327-329
  echocardiography
    regional wall motion, 72-73
    systolic function, 56
    volume, 54-56
  enlargement, 11-15, 200
  inflow obstruction, congenital abnor-
    malities causing, 172-174
  in interventricular septum rupture,
    240-243
  magnetic resonance imaging, 112, 114
  morphology, 302-304
  papillary muscles and, 244
  thrombus, 233-235, 286
Leukemia, 279
Levocardia, 299, 308
Levotransposition of great arteries, 313
  angiographic anatomy and technique,
    313-317
  coronary artery patterns, 317-318
  isolated ventricular inversion, 318
  straddling atrioventricular valves, 318-
    319
Libman-Sacks endocarditis, 286
Lipomas/lipomatous hypertrophy, 282,
  284
Long-axis view, 47
d-loop, 307
l-loop, 307-308
Loop rule, 307
Lungs; see also Pulmonary entries
  fluid exchange in, 30
  hypogenetic lung syndrome, 339

Lupus erythematosus, systemic, 286
Lutembacher syndrome, 342
Lymphomas, 279, 287

M

Magnetic resonance imaging, 96-122
  advantages, 96
  annuloaortic ectasia and Marfan syn-
    drome, 400
  aortic dissection, 392
  aortic regurgitation, 163
  atrial septal defects, 344-345
  atrioventricular septal defects, 349
  coarctation of aorta, 429
  contraindications, 96-97
  electrocardiographic gating, 98
  examination, 99-100
  flow appearance, 103
  flow effects, 102-103
  gradient direction, 101
  hypoplastic left heart syndrome, 378
  normal and pathologic anatomy, 103-
    122
  parameters, 100-101
  patient preparation, 97-98
  pericardial effusion, 266
  pericardium, normal, 265-266
  sections, 101-102
  Takayasu's aortitis, 404
  truncus arteriosus, 330
Malformations; see Congenital heart disease
Malpositions, 299
Marfan syndrome, 41, 176, 387
  aortic cusps in, 164
  aortic disease in, 80
  aortic valve leaflets in, 397
  chest film, 36
  cystic medial lesions in, 392
  presentation, 400
  radiologic techniques, 400
Masses
  cardiac, 278-286
  pericardial, 276, 278
Melanoma, 279
Membranous septal defects, 84
Membranous subaortic stenosis, 158-159
Mesocardia, 308
Metabolic disorders associated with
  heart disease, 41
Metastatic tumors, 279
Mitral annular calcification, 17, 62
Mitral regurgitation, 174
  angiography, 143, 175
  causes, 175
  chest film findings, 174-175
  color Doppler detection, 35
  from coronary artery disease, 243-244

echocardiography, 60-64
mitral valve prolapse in, 175-176
in obstructive hypertrophic cardiomyopathy, 294-295
pulmonary edema and, 35
rheumatic, 175
in septal rupture, 241, 243
Mitral stenosis, 167
causes, 167
chest film findings, 167-168
congenital abnormalities causing left ventricular inflow obstruction, 172-174
echocardiography, 55, 58-60
imaging approach, 168
rheumatic, 168
time course, 167
Mitral valve
angiography, 141-143
atresia, in hypoplastic left heart syndrome, 373, 375
calcifications, 17, 62, 168
echocardiography, 17, 60-61, 62
incomplete closure, 17, 62
prolapse, 60-61, 175-176
Mitral valvuloplasty, 258-261
MRI; see Magnetic resonance imaging
Mucopolysaccharidoses, 41
Muscular ventricular septal defects, 84
Mustard procedure, 324
Myocardial bridging, 221
Myocardial diseases
in AIDS, 286-287
cardiac masses, 278-279
cardiomyopathies, 287-296
primary tumors, 279-286
thrombus, 286
vegetations, 286
Myocardial hibernation, 203
Myocardial infarction; see also Ischemic heart disease
chest radiograph, 200
in diabetes and hyperlipoproteinemia, 207
echocardiography, 72-74
pericardial effusion after, 266, 270
Myocardial stunning, 203
Myocarditis, in AIDS, 286-287
Myocardium
blunt trauma, 414
calcifications, 17-18
Myxomas, 79, 280, 282

N

National Heart, Lung, and Blood Institute (NHLBI) coronary artery dissection classification, 251
Neurofibromatosis, 36, 41

Noonan syndrome, 41, 186
No-reflow phenomenon after PTCA, 251

O

Oblique sinus of pericardium, 264
Obstruction, pulmonary edema from, 35
Obstructive hypertrophic cardiomyopathy, 291-295
Occlusive thromboaortopathy, 404
Osteogenesis imperfecta, 36, 41
Ostium primum atrial septal defect, 81, 83, 343, 345
Ostium secundum atrial septal defect, 81, 83, 343, 346
Outlet chamber, 304, 356, 357

P

Paget disease, 25
Papillary fibroelastomas, 282
Papillary muscles
angiography, 140, 143
mitral regurgitation and, 174, 177-179, 243-244
rupture, 174, 177-178, 243-244
chest radiograph, 200
echocardiography, 73
ventriculography, 244
Parasternal imaging planes for echocardiography, 47-49, 50
Doppler examination, 52
Paravalvular regurgitation, 165
Parietal pericardium, 264
Partial transposition of great arteries
double-outlet left ventricle, 327-329
double-outlet right ventricle, 90-91, 324-327
Patent ductus arteriosus, 320, 352
angiographic examination, 355-356
characteristics, 352-353
chest film abnormalities
in adults, 353-355
in infants, 353
coarctation of aorta and, 425, 426
complications, 353
echocardiography, 86-87
in hypoplastic left heart syndrome, 373
Patent foramen ovale, 342
PAV, 261-262
Pediatrics; see Children; Congenital entries
Penetrating aortic ulcers, 418-419
Penetrating cardiovascular trauma, 413
Percutaneous aortic valvuloplasty, 261-262
Percutaneous mitral balloon valvuloplasty, 258
complications, 260

long-term follow-up, 260-261
mechanism, 260
patient preparation, 259-260
patient selection, 258-259
results, 260
Percutaneous transluminal coronary angioplasty, 247
arterial wall changes after, 247
complications, 250-251
contraindications, 250
lesion classification for, 248
patient selection, 247-248
restenosis after, 251-252
results, 249-250
technique, 248-249
Perfusion catheters, 248
Pericardial diseases
anatomy, 264-265
echocardiography, 76-78
Pericardial effusion
appearance on CT and MRI, 266
causes, 270
chest radiograph, 201
echocardiography, 76-77
normal pressure-volume relations, cardiac tamponade, and congestive heart failure, 266
syndromes
cardiac tamponade, 270-271
infection, collagen diseases, metabolic diseases, and tumors, 266
myocardial infarction, 266, 270
Pericardial tamponade, 76-77
Pericarditis
constrictive, 271-272
calcifications in, 272-274
restrictive cardiomyopathy vs., 274-276
radiation, 270
Pericardium
anatomy, 264-265
blunt trauma, 414
calcifications, 18-21, 272-274
congenital absence, 276
constriction, 77-78
cysts, 78
magnetic resonance imaging, 106
masses, 276, 278
normal appearance on chest film, CT, and MRI, 265-266
Peripartum cardiomyopathy, 288
Peripheral pulse gating, in magnetic resonance imaging, 98
Pheochromocytomas, 25
Plain films; see Chest films
Plaque morphology, 206-207
Pleural effusions, 35
PMV; see Percutaneous mitral balloon valvuloplasty

Poiseuille's equation, 210
Polysplenia, 299, 307, 309, 311
Positioning, for magnetic resonance imaging, 97-98
Posterior interventricular vein, 137
Postpericardiotomy syndrome, 270
Pregnancy, magnetic resonance imaging in, 97
Prevalence of congenital heart diseases, 383
Primary tumors, 279-286
Prinzmetal syndrome, 216-217
Progeria, 41
Prolapsing mitral leaflet syndrome, 141
Prosthetic heart valves
    aortic regurgitation and, 165-167
    echocardiography, 69-71
    mitral stenosis and regurgitation and, 179
Proximal aorta, echocardiography, 80
Pseudoaneurysms, left ventricular, 238
Pseudocoarctation of aorta, 432
PTCA; see Percutaneous transluminal coronary angioplasty
Pulmonary arteries
    acquired small, 25
    aorta and, 304, 307
    atrial septal defects and, 343
    central, 23-24
    congenitally hypoplastic, 25
    convex main, 5, 27
    diffuse hypoplasia, 189
    hypertension, 381
        causes, 29
        Eisenmenger syndrome, 27-29
        pressure measurements and pulmonary vasculature patterns, 27
        secondary to pulmonary venous hypertension, 29-30
    magnetic resonance imaging, 104-106
    in pulmonary atresia with intact ventricular septum, 365-366
    in tetralogy of Fallot, 366, 367, 370
    in truncus arteriosus, 330
Pulmonary artery sling, 422
Pulmonary atresia, 8, 182
    with intact ventricular septum, 361
        anatomic features, 362-363
        angiographic examination, 364-366
        chest film abnormalities, 363-364
        classification, 361-362
    with ventricular septal defect, 370, 372-373
Pulmonary edema, 30
    cardiac causes, 35
    chest radiograph, 200
    from congenital heart disease, 381-382
    radiologic appearance, 30-36

Pulmonary regurgitation, 191
    causes, 179
    Doppler detection, 53
    echocardiography, 69
Pulmonary stenosis, 179
    causes, 179
    chest film findings, 180-182
    in complete dextrotransposition of great arteries, 320
    in double-outlet right ventricle, 325, 327
    echocardiography, 69
    subvalvular, 179, 186-187
    supravalvular, 179, 187-189
    in tetralogy of Fallot, 366, 367
    valvular, 182-186
Pulmonary valve
    angiography, 143
    bicuspid, 183
Pulmonary vasculature, 23
    angiography, 342
    diminished, 24-25
    high-output states, 25-27
    hypertension
        arterial, 27-30
        venous, 30-36
    patterns, 380, 381-382
        determining, 23-24
Pulmonary veins
    abnormal connections, 334
        partial anomaly, 337, 339-342
        total anomaly, 334-337
    hypertension, 30, 382
        fluid and water exchange, 30
        pulmonary artery hypertension secondary to, 29-30
        radiologic appearance, 30-36
    magnetic resonance imaging, 106
Pulmonary vein wedge angiography, 366
Pulmonary venolobar syndrome, 339
Pulseless disease, 404

R

Radiation exposure and protection, 127-129
Radiation pericarditis, 270
Regional wall motion, 233
Regurgitation
    aortic; see Aortic regurgitation
    mitral; see Mitral regurgitation
    pulmonary, 191
        causes, 179
        Doppler detection, 53
        echocardiography, 69
    tricuspid, 192-194
        causes, 194
        in congenitally corrected transposition of great vessels, 315, 317
        echocardiography, 52-53, 64

valvular, grades, 380
Reiter syndrome, 40
Respiratory gating, in magnetic resonance imaging, 98
Restenosis after angioplasty, 251-252
Restrictive cardiomyopathy, 288-290, 291
    constrictive pericarditis vs., 274-276, 289-290
    echocardiography, 75-76
    left ventricular abnormalities in, 296
Rhabdomyomas, 279
Rhabdomyosarcomas, echocardiography, 79
Rheumatic heart disease, 10
    aortic regurgitation in, 163
    calcifications in, 16-17, 18
        aortic stenosis, 156-157
    mitral regurgitation in, 62, 175
    mitral stenosis in, 167, 168
    tricuspid stenosis in, 191-192
Rib notching from coarctation of aorta, 426, 428
Right aortic arch, 419-421
Right atrium
    angiography, 137-138
    appendage, magnetic resonance imaging, 107
    echocardiography, 58
    enlargement, 8
    morphology and position, 302, 307
    thrombus, 286
Right coronary artery, anatomy on angiography, 129
    conus artery, 131
    distal right coronary artery, 131-133
    sinoatrial nodal artery, 129, 131
Right ventricle
    angiography, 138-140
    in congenitally corrected transposition of great vessels, 314
    double-outlet, 90-91, 324-327
    echocardiography, 57-58, 90-91
    enlargement, 10, 57-58, 367
    magnetic resonance imaging, 111-112, 114
    morphology, 302-304
    in pulmonary atresia with intact ventricular septum, 361-362
    thrombus, 286
Right ventricular inflow view, 48
    Doppler examination, 52-53
Rotablator, 252-253
Rubella, 41
Ruptures
    aortic, 413
    chest radiograph, 200
    interventricular septum, 240-243
    papillary muscles, 174, 177-178, 243-244

chest radiograph, 200
echocardiography, 73

S

Saccular aneurysm, 388
SAM, 291-292
Saphenous vein grafts, 227-228, 230
Scheie syndrome, 426
Scoliosis, 36
Sedation, for magnetic resonance imaging, 97
Segmental analysis of cardiac malformations
　associated malformations, 307
　atrial morphology, 302
　atrioventricular connections, 304
　atrioventricular septal defects, 345-346
　cardiac axis and visceral situs, 299-302
　diagnostic approach, 299
　relations of great arteries, 304, 307
　ventricular morphology, 302-304
　ventriculoarterial connections, 307
Segmental analysis of pulmonary vasculature, 23, 25, 381
Segmental wall motion abnormalities, 233
　correlation with coronary artery disease, 233
　factors influencing wall motion, 233
　left ventricular thrombus, 233-235
　left ventricular true and false aneurysm, 235-238
Senning procedure, 324
Septal arteries, 221
Shape of heart, 4-15
Shielding from radiation, 129
Shone syndrome, 174
Short-axis view at papillary muscle level, 49
Short-axis view of base of heart, 48-49
Shunts; see also Atrial septal defects; Patent ductus arteriosus; Ventricular septal defects
　atrial, size estimation, 83-84
　Blalock-Taussig, 36, 373
　pulmonary vasculature and, 25
Sickle cell disease, 36, 40, 41
Simpson's rule, 56
Single-outlet heart, 307
Single ventricle, 304
　angiographic examination, 357
　chest film features, 356-357
　definition, 356
　echocardiography, 91-92
Sinoatrial nodal artery, anatomy on angiography, 129, 131
Sinotubular ridge, 387

Sinuses of Valsalva
　aneurysms
　　calcification, 402
　　complications, 402-403
　　echocardiography, 80
　　etiology, 402
　angiography, 144
　magnetic resonance imaging, 107-108, 111
Sinus of aorta, 387
Sinus venosus atrial septal defects, 81, 83, 343
Situs ambiguus, 299, 309
Situs inversus, 299
Situs inversus totalis, 302, 304
Situs solitus, 299
Size of aorta, 387
Size of heart
　aging and, 5-6
　cardiothoracic ratio, 6
　chamber enlargement, 6-15
　chest radiograph, 200
Skeletal abnormalities
　cardiac surgery and, 36
　congenital syndromes with heart disease, 36, 40
　syndromes and metabolic disorders associated with heart disease, 41
　thoracic cage and heart disease, 36
"Snowman" configuration, 336
Sones catheter, 124
Spasm, coronary artery, 213, 215-217
Spine abnormalities, 36
Spin-echo acquisition, in magnetic resonance imaging, 99, 100
Splenic anomalies, 299, 307, 309-311
Stanford classification of aortic dissection, 391
Staphylococcus, 194
Starr-Edwards valves, 70, 96
Stenosis
　aortic; see Aortic stenosis
　coronary; see Coronary arteries, stenosis
　infundibular, 182-183, 186-187, 366
　mitral; see Mitral stenosis
　pulmonary; see Pulmonary stenosis
　tricuspid, 191-192
　　causes, 192
　　echocardiography, 65
Stents, 254, 256-258
Sternotomy, 36
Straddling atrioventricular valves, 318-319
Stroke volume, Doppler echocardiography and, 56
Subaortic stenosis; see Subvalvular aortic stenosis
Subclavian arteries
　aortic arch interruption and, 433, 434

coarctation of aorta and, 425, 426, 428
　in left aortic arch, 419
　in right aortic arch, 421
Subcostal imaging planes for echocardiography, 49-50
Subvalvular aortic stenosis
　angiographic findings, 158-159
　causes, 151
　in double-outlet right ventricle, 325, 327
　pathologic abnormalities, 158
　unusual subaortic obstruction, 159-160
Subvalvular pulmonary stenosis, 179, 186-187
Superior vena cava, 302
Supracristal ventricular septal defects, 84
Suprasternal imaging planes for echocardiography, 50
Supravalvular aortic stenosis, 160
　associated lesions, 160-162
　classifications, 160
Supravalvular pulmonary stenosis, 179, 187-189
Syndromes associated with heart disease, 41
Syphilis, 408-411, 417
Systemic lupus erythematosus, 286
Systolic anterior motion, 291-292

T

Tachycardia, 212
Takayasu's aortitis, 403, 404, 417, 426
　classifications, 404
　imaging assessment, 404, 406
Taussig-Bing heart, 325, 327, 351
TEC, 253
Tetralogy of Fallot, 366
　anatomy, 366-367
　angiography, 143, 368, 370
　boot-shaped heart in, 10
　characteristics, 366
　chest film abnormalities, 367-368
　complete transposition of great arteries in, 320
　coronary anomalies in, 225-226
　echocardiography, 87-88
　postoperative evaluation, 372-373
　with pulmonary atresia
　　hemitruncus arteriosus vs., 333
　　truncus arteriosus vs., 330
　pulmonary valve and, 183, 186, 191
　pulmonary vasculature in, 25, 381
　right aortic arch in, 420
　severe pulmonary lesions, 370-372
　ventricular septal defect in, 349
Thalassemia major, 40
Thoracic aorta

echocardiography, 80-81
magnetic resonance imaging, 104
Thoracic aortic diseases, 386-435
  acquired
    annuloaortic ectasia and Marfan
      syndrome, 400
    aortic dissection, 391-400
    aortitis, 403-411
    atherosclerotic aneurysms, 388,
      415-418
    cardiovascular trauma, 413-414
    infected aortic aneurysms, 388, 411-
      412
    penetrating aortic ulcer, 418-419
    sinus of Valsalva aneurysms, 402-
      403
  aneurysms, 387-391
  congenital, 419
    aortic arch interruption, 433-434
    coarctation of aorta, 425-432
    double aortic arch, 422
    hemitruncus, 422
    left aortic arch, 419
    pseudocoarctation, 432
    pulmonary artery sling, 422
    right aortic arch, 419-421
Thoracic cage and heart disease, 36
Thoracotomy, posterior, 36
Thrombosis, stenting and, 258
Thrombus
  cardiac, 286
  intracardiac, echocardiography, 79-80
  left ventricular, 233-235
Thymus, age and, 4-5
Thyrotoxicosis, 25
Trabecular pouch, 356, 357
Transesophageal imaging, 50-52, 80
Transluminal extraction endarterectomy
  catheter, 253
Transposition, 307
Transposition of aorta and pulmonary
  artery, 320
Transposition of great arteries
  complete dextrotransposition, 320
    angiographic anatomy, 320, 323-325
    surgical procedures, 325
  congenitally corrected (levotransposi-
    tion), 313
    angiographic anatomy and tech-
      nique, 313-317
    coronary artery patterns, 317-318
    isolated ventricular inversion, 318
    straddling atrioventricular valves,
      318-319
  echocardiography, 88-89
  partial
    double-outlet left ventricle, 327-329
    double-outlet right ventricle, 90-91,
      324-327

in tricuspid atresia, 359
Transverse relaxation time, 100
Transverse sinus of pericardium, 264
Trauma, thoracic cardiovascular, 413-414
Treacher Collins syndrome, 41
Tricuspid regurgitation, 192-194
  causes, 194
  in congenitally corrected transposi-
    tion of great vessels, 315, 317
  echocardiography, 52-53, 64
Tricuspid stenosis, 191-192
  causes, 192
  echocardiography, 65
Tricuspid valve
  angiography, 141
  atresia
    anatomy, 358-359
    angiographic findings, 361
    characteristics, 357
    chest film abnormalities, 359-361
  Ebstein anomaly, 194-197
  echocardiography, 64-65, 197
  magnetic resonance imaging, 115, 197
  prolapse, 194
Trisomy 21, 36
Truncus arteriosus, 329-330, 420
  echocardiography, 89-90
T2, 100
Tuberculosis, pericardial calcifications
  from, 18
Tuberous sclerosis, 41
Tumors, cardiac, 278-279
  benign vs. malignant, 280
  echocardiography, 78-79
  imaging signs, 286
  malignant, 284-285
  metastatic, 279
  normal variants vs., 278
  primary, 279-284
Tunnel subaortic stenosis, 159
Turner syndrome, 41

U

Uhl anomaly, 288
Ulcers, 397
  penetrating aortic, 418-419
Ultrasonography; see Echocardiography
Univentricular heart; see Single ventricle

V

Valsalva's sinuses; see Sinuses of Valsalva
Valvular heart disease, 149-198
  aortic regurgitation, 162-167
  aortic stenosis
    subvalvular, 158-160
    supravalvular, 160-162
    valvular, 149-157

echocardiography
  aortic valve disease, 65-69
  infective endocarditis, 71-72
  mitral valve disease, 58-64
  prosthetic heart valves, 69-71
  pulmonary valve disease, 69
  tricuspid valve disease, 64-65
imaging modalities, 149
mitral regurgitation, 174-179
mitral stenosis, 167-174
pulmonary stenosis and regurgitation,
  179-191
regurgitation grades, 380
stenosis, 380
tricuspid valve disease, 191-197
Valvular pulmonary stenosis, 182-186
Valvular trauma, 414
Valvuloplasty, percutaneous
  aortic, 261-262
  mitral, 258-261
Variations of heart and mediastinum
  measurements, 6
Vegetations on heart valves, 286
Vein grafts, 227-228, 230
Ventricles; see also Left ventricle; Right
  ventricle; Single ventricle
  in dilated cardiomyopathy, 288
  morphology, 302-304
  thrombi, echocardiography, 80
Ventricular looping, 307-308
Ventricular outflow tracts, types, 307
Ventricular septal defects, 349; see also
  Atrioventricular septal defects
  chest film findings, 349-350
  classifications, 349
  in complete dextrotransposition of
    great arteries, 320
  in congenitally corrected transposi-
    tion of great vessels, 313
  in double-outlet right ventricle, 324-
    325
  echocardiography, 84-86
  imaging features, 350-352
  in tetralogy of Fallot, 366, 368, 370, 372
Ventricular septal rupture, echocardiography, 73
Ventriculoarterial connections, morphology, 307
Ventriculoarterial discordance, 319-324
Ventriculography
  after aneurysm resection, 238
  atrioventricular septal defects, 348-
    349
  complete dextrotransposition of great
    arteries, 320, 323-324
  congenitally corrected transposition
    of great vessels, 314
  interventricular septum rupture, 240
  left ventricle analysis, 231-232

papillary muscle dysfunction, 244
pulmonary atresia with intact ventric-
    ular septum, 364-366
truncus arteriosus, 330
ventricular septal defects, 350-352
Vertebral abnormalities, 36
Vieussens' circle, 131

Visceral-atrial rule, 299

W

Wall motion abnormalities, 233
    correlation with coronary artery dis-
    ease, 233

factors influencing wall motion, 233
left ventricular thrombus, 233-235
left ventricular true and false
    aneurysm, 235-238
Williams syndrome, 41, 162
Wilms tumor, 279